The American Psychiatric Association Publishing

TEXTBOOK OF
FORENSIC
PSYCHIATRY

THIRD EDITION

The American Psychiatric Association Publishing

TEXTBOOK OF
FORENSIC PSYCHIATRY

THIRD EDITION

EDITED BY

Liza H. Gold, M.D.
Richard L. Frierson, M.D.

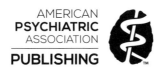

AMERICAN
PSYCHIATRIC
ASSOCIATION
PUBLISHING

Manufactured in the United States of America on acid-free paper
21   20   19   18   17   5   4   3   2   1

American Psychiatric Association Publishing
1000 Wilson Boulevard
Arlington, VA 22209-3901
www.appi.org

Library of Congress Cataloging-in-Publication Data
Names: Gold, Liza H., editor. | Frierson, Richard L., editor. | American Psychiatric
    Association Publishing, publisher.
Title: The American Psychiatric Association Publishing textbook of forensic
    psychiatry / edited by Liza H. Gold, Richard L. Frierson.
Other titles: American Psychiatric Publishing textbook of forensic psychiatry. |
    Textbook of forensic psychiatry
Description: Third edition. | Arlington, Virginia : American Psychiatric Association
    Publishing, [2018] | Preceded by American Psychiatric Publishing textbook of
    forensic psychiatry / edited by Robert I. Simon, Liza H. Gold. 2nd ed. 2010. |
    Includes bibliographical references and index.
Identifiers: LCCN 2017037789 | ISBN 9781615370672 (hardcover : alk. paper)
Subjects: | MESH: Forensic Psychiatry
Classification: LCC RA1151 | NLM W 740 | DDC 614/.15—dc23 LC record available
    at https://lccn.loc.gov/2017037789.

British Library Cataloguing in Publication Data
A CIP record is available from the British Library.

Contents

PART I
Introduction to Forensic Psychiatry

    Donald J. Meyer, M.D.
    Thomas G. Gutheil, M.D.

    Eric Y. Drogin, J.D., Ph.D.
    Carol S. Williams, LL.B. (Hons.)

    James L. Knoll IV, M.D.

    Graham D. Glancy, M.B., Ch.B., FRCPsych, FRCPC

    Madelon V. Baranoski, Ph.D.

    Barbara E. McDermott, Ph.D.

PART IV
Criminal Justice

PART V
Correctional Psychiatry and
Sex Offenders

Dedication

ROBERT I. SIMON (1934–2016)

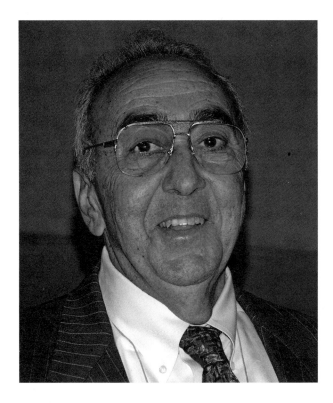

Be an opener of doors for such as come after thee.

Ralph Waldo Emerson

We dedicate this volume to Robert I. Simon, M.D., the lead editor of the first and second editions of *The American Psychiatric Publishing Textbook of Forensic Psychiatry*. Dr. Simon was awarded the American Academy of Psychiatry and the Law and the American Psychiatric Association's joint Manfred S. Guttmacher Award three times for outstanding contributions to the literature of forensic psychiatry. He was also awarded the American Psychiatric Association's Isaac Ray Award in recognition of his outstanding contributions to the fields of forensic psychiatry and the psychiatric aspects of jurisprudence.

Dr. Simon understood the need for a textbook of forensic psychiatry, particularly one accessible to general and forensic psychiatrists alike. He was the moving force behind both the first and the second editions of this text. Dr. Simon was gratified to be Editor Emeritus for this third edition and, as always, planned to make his own contribution to the text.

Contributors

Elisha R. Agee, Psy.D.
Clinical Psychologist, Institute of Law, Psychiatry, and Public Policy; University of Virginia School of Medicine, Charlottesville, Virginia

Stuart A. Anfang, M.D.
Vice Chair for Clinical Services, Department of Psychiatry, Baystate Health, Springfield, Massachusetts; Associate Professor of Psychiatry, University of Massachusetts Medical School—Baystate

Kenneth L. Appelbaum, M.D.
Director, Correctional Mental Health Policy and Research, Center for Health Policy and Research, Commonwealth Medicine; Clinical Professor of Psychiatry, University of Massachusetts Medical School

Peter Ash, M.D.
Professor and Director, Psychiatry and Law Service, Department of Psychiatry and Behavioral Sciences, Emory University, Atlanta, Georgia

Madelon V. Baranoski, Ph.D.
Professor, Law and Psychiatry Division, Department of Psychiatry, Yale University School of Medicine, New Haven, Connecticut

Arielle R. Baskin-Sommers, Ph.D.
Assistant Professor, Departments of Psychology and Psychiatry, Yale University, New Haven, Connecticut

Elissa Benedek, M.D.
Adjunct Clinical Professor of Psychiatry, University of Michigan, Ann Arbor, Michigan

Brad D. Booth, M.D., FRCPC
Assistant Professor, Division of Forensic Psychiatry, University of Ottawa, Ottawa, Ontario, Canada

John Bradford, M.D., D.P.M., FRCPC
Full Professor, Division of Forensic Psychiatry, University of Ottawa; Scientist, Royal Ottawa Institute of Mental Health Research, Ottawa, Ontario, Canada

Giovana V. de Amorim Levin, M.D., FRCPC
Assistant Professor, Division of Forensic Psychiatry, University of Western Ontario, London, Ontario, Canada

Eric Y. Drogin, J.D., Ph.D.
Department of Psychiatry, Harvard Medical School, Boston, Massachusetts

Albert M. Drukteinis, M.D., J.D.
Adjunct Associate Professor of Psychiatry, Geisel School of Medicine at Dartmouth, Director of New England Psychodiagnostics, Manchester, New Hampshire

Joel A. Dvoskin, Ph.D., ABPP
Assistant Professor (Clinical); Department of Psychiatry, University of Arizona College of Medicine, Tucson, Arizona

Judith Edersheim, J.D., M.D.
Co-Director, The Massachusetts General Hospital Center for Law, Brain and Behavior, Associate Psychiatrist, Massachusetts General Hospital; Assistant Professor of Psychiatry, Harvard Medical School, Boston, Massachusetts

Patrick Fox, M.D.
Chief Medical Officer, Colorado Department of Human Services, Denver, Colorado

Susan Hatters Friedman, M.D.
Associate Professor of Psychological Medicine, University of Auckland, Auckland, New Zealand

Richard L. Frierson, M.D.
Alexander G. Donald Professor of Psychiatry and Vice Chair for Education, Director, Forensic Psychiatry Fellowship, Department of Neuropsychiatry and Behavioral Science, University of South Carolina School of Medicine, Columbia, South Carolina

Graham D. Glancy, M.B., Ch.B., FRCPsych, FRCPC
Associate Professor, Department of Psychiatry, University of Toronto, Ontario, Canada

Liza H. Gold, M.D.
Clinical Professor of Psychiatry, Department of Psychiatry, Georgetown University School of Medicine, Washington, D.C.

Thomas G. Gutheil, M.D.
Professor of Psychiatry, Harvard Medical School, Cambridge, Massachusetts

Ryan C.W. Hall, M.D.
Assistant Professor of Medical Education University of Central Florida College of Medicine, Orlando, Florida; Affiliate Associate Professor, Department of Psychiatry, University of South Florida, Tampa, Florida; Adjunct Faculty, Barry Law School, Orlando, Florida

Annette Hanson, M.D.
Assistant Professor and Director, Forensic Psychiatry Fellowship, University of Maryland, Clifton T. Perkins Hospital, Jessup, Maryland

Kaustubh G. Joshi, M.D.
Associate Professor of Clinical Psychiatry, Department of Neuropsychiatry and Behavioral Science, University of South Carolina School of Medicine, Columbia, South Carolina

Reena Kapoor, M.D.
Associate Professor of Psychiatry, Law and Psychiatry Division, Yale School of Medicine, New Haven, Connecticut

James L. Knoll IV, M.D.
Professor of Psychiatry, Director of Forensic Psychiatry, SUNY Upstate Medical University, Syracuse, New York

Richard Martinez, M.D., M.H.
Robert D. Miller Professor of Forensic Psychiatry; Director, Forensic Psychiatry Fellowship, University of Colorado Denver Medical School, Denver, Colorado

Barbara E. McDermott, Ph.D.
Professor of Clinical Psychiatry, Department of Psychiatry and Behavioral Sciences, Division of Psychiatry and the Law, University of California, Davis, Sacramento, California

Jeffrey L. Metzner, M.D.
Clinical Professor of Psychiatry, University of Colorado School of Medicine, Denver, Colorado

Donald J. Meyer, M.D.
Associate Director of Forensic Psychiatry, Beth Israel Deaconess Medical Center, Boston, Massachusetts; Assistant Professor of Psychiatry, Harvard Medical School, Cambridge, Massachusetts

Robert D. Morgan, Ph.D.
Chair and John G. Skelton Jr. Regents Endowed Professor, Department of Psychological Sciences, Texas Tech University, Lubbock, Texas

Daniel C. Murrie, Ph.D.
Director of Psychology, Institute of Law, Psychiatry, and Public Policy; Professor of Psychiatry and Neurobehavioral Sciences, University of Virginia School of Medicine, Charlottesville, Virginia

Debra A. Pinals, M.D.
Clinical Professor of Psychiatry and Director, Program in Psychiatry, Law, and

Ethics, Department of Psychiatry, University of Michigan, Ann Arbor, Michigan

Marilyn Price, M.D.
Law and Psychiatry Service, Massachusetts General Hospital; Assistant Professor of Psychiatry, Harvard Medical School, Boston, Massachusetts

Patricia R. Recupero, J.D., M.D.
Clinical Professor of Psychiatry, Warren Alpert Medical School of Brown University; Senior Vice President Education and Training, Care New England Health System, Providence, Rhode Island

Charles L. Scott, M.D.
Chief, Division of Psychiatry and the Law, Clinical Professor of Psychiatry; Director, Forensic Psychiatry Fellowship, University of California Davis Medical Center, Sacramento, California

Michael C. Seto, Ph.D., C.Psych.
Director, Forensic Research Unit, The Royal's Institute of Mental Health Research, Director of Forensic Rehabilitation Research, Royal Ottawa Health Care Group, Ottawa, Ontario, Canada; Adjunct, University of Toronto, Ryerson University, Carleton University, University of Ottawa

Robert L. Trestman, Ph.D., M.D.
Chair of Psychiatry, Virginia Tech Carilion School of Medicine and Carilion Clinic, Roanoke, Virginia

Donna Vanderpool, M.B.A., J.D.
Vice President, Risk Management, Pro-fessional Risk Management Services, Inc., Arlington, Virginia

Stephanie A. Van Horn, Ph.D.
Doctoral Candidate, Department of Psychological Sciences, Texas Tech University, Lubbock, Texas

Barry W. Wall, M.D.
Clinical Professor of Psychiatry, Department of Psychiatry and Human Behavior, Alpert Medical School of Brown University, Providence, Rhode Island

Clarence Watson, J.D., M.D.
Clinical Associate Professor of Psychiatry, Perelman School of Medicine, University of Pennsylvania, Philadelphia, Pennsylvania

Marlynn Wei, J.D., M.D.
Private Practice, New York City; Contributing Editor, *Harvard Health*

Kenneth J. Weiss, M.D.
Robert L. Sadoff Clinical Professor of Forensic Psychiatry, Perelman School of Medicine, University of Pennsylvania, Philadelphia, Pennsylvania

Carol S. Williams, LL.B. (Hons.)
Department of Psychology, Aberystwyth University, Aberystwyth, Ceredigion, United Kingdom

Cheryl D. Wills, M.D.
Assistant Professor of Psychiatry, Case Western Reserve University, Cleveland, Ohio

Disclosures of Competing Interests

The following contributors to this book have reported no competing interests during the year preceding manuscript submission:

Stuart A. Anfang, M.D.
Kenneth L. Appelbaum, M.D.
Peter Ash, M.D.
Madelon V. Baranoski, Ph.D.
Arielle R. Baskin-Sommers, Ph.D.
Brad D. Booth, M.D., FRCPC
John Bradford, M.D., D.P.M., FRCPC
Eric Y. Drogin, J.D., Ph.D.
Albert M. Drukteinis, M.D., J.D.
Joel A. Dvoskin, Ph.D., ABPP
Judith Edersheim, J.D., M.D.
Patrick Fox, M.D.
Susan Hatters Friedman, M.D.
Richard L. Frierson, M.D.
Graham D. Glancy, M.B., Ch.B., FRCPsych, FRCPC

Liza H. Gold, M.D.
Thomas G. Gutheil, M.D.
Ryan C.W. Hall, M.D.
Annette Hanson, M.D.
Kaustubh G. Joshi, M.D.
Reena Kapoor, M.D.
James L. Knoll IV, M.D.
Richard Martinez, M.D., M.H.
Barbara E. McDermott, Ph.D.
Jeffrey L. Metzner, M.D.
Donald J. Meyer, M.D.
Robert D. Morgan, Ph.D.
Daniel C. Murrie, Ph.D.
Debra A. Pinals, M.D.
Marilyn Price, M.D.
Patricia R. Recupero, J.D., M.D.
Charles L. Scott, M.D.
Michael C. Seto, Ph.D., C.Psych.
Robert L. Trestman, Ph.D., M.D.
Donna Vanderpool, M.B.A., J.D.
Clarence Watson, J.D., M.D.
Marlynn Wei, J.D., M.D.
Kenneth J. Weiss, M.D.
Carol S. Williams, LL.B. (Hons.)
Cheryl D. Wills, M.D.

Preface

We are pleased to present the third and expanded edition of *The American Psychiatric Association Publishing Textbook of Forensic Psychiatry*. This edition is designed to be an accessible and comprehensive review of the specialty. As with the previous editions, this edition will be of value as a reference for general psychiatrists who undertake forensic work. However, the third edition can also serve as a core textbook for forensic psychiatry fellows, a reference for psychiatry residents or medical students, and a study guide for the examination to maintain board certification in forensic psychiatry for those already practicing this complicated and endlessly stimulating subspecialty.

Since the second edition was published in 2010, much has changed in the field of psychiatry; it became evident that a third and expanded edition of the textbook was needed. For example, in 2013, the American Psychiatric Association (APA) published the fifth edition of the *Diagnostic and Statistical Manual of Mental Disorders* (DSM-5; American Psychiatric Association 2013), the first major revision in 20 years of the most widely used psychiatric diagnostic classification criteria. The subspecialty of forensic psychiatry has continued to develop and mature as well, as laws evolve and new research has contributed to our understanding of human behavior.

The third edition of the *Textbook of Forensic Psychiatry* encompasses these changes and advances with updates of chapters from the second edition and 10 additional chapters of subject matter. The content of this third edition was designed to cover the major topic areas of the American Board of Psychiatry and Neurology (ABPN) certification examination in forensic psychiatry as well as the Accreditation Council for Graduate Medical Education (ACGME) program requirements for fellowships in forensic psychiatry (Accreditation Council for Graduate Medical Education 2016). Additionally, this new edition highlights the Landmark Cases in forensic psychiatry as established by the American Academy of Psychiatry and the Law (AAPL).

Although many general psychiatrists still provide forensic services, the demand for forensic specialists in many types of legal cases with psychiatric issues has increased. The emphasis on specialized fellowship training has resulted in the incorporation of the latest advances in neurosciences and brain imaging as well as legal principles and case law. Even when general psychiatrists provide forensic psychiatric services, they are increasingly being held to the same standards as forensic psychiatric specialists.

Although general and forensic psychiatry have much in common, forensic psychiatry places additional and differing demands on its practitioners. For example, the goals of clinical evaluations conducted for therapeutic purposes and those conducted for forensic purposes differ considerably. Clinical treatment relationships are established to help patients and are guided by standard medical ethics, such as nonmaleficence and confidentiality. In contrast, forensic evaluations are conducted to provide objective information to a third party, such as the courts, employers or insurers, or some other administrative or regulatory institution. Forensic evaluations are guided by a different set of ethical precepts than those guiding psychiatric treatment. Forensic psychiatric goals and precepts result in methodologies and relationships with evaluees that differ significantly from those of a purely therapeutic relationship.

Forensic Psychiatry: A Brief History

Although the recognition of the insanity defense dates back to biblical times, the practice of forensic psychiatry did not emerge in the United States and Europe until the mid–nineteenth century. The asylum movement and the emphasis on the social and psychological treatment of insanity known as "moral treatment" occurred during the first half of the nineteenth century (Porter 1997). The asylum doctors, the first psychiatrists, were referred to as "alienists" well into the twentieth century because of the public's belief that persons suffering from mental illness were "alienated" from their families and society. In addition to asylum administration and patient treatment, these physicians participated in legal proceedings by testifying in civil and criminal cases involving questions of insanity and mental disorders (Gold 2010).

Isaac Ray's seminal 1838 book, *A Treatise on the Medical Jurisprudence of Insanity* (Ray 1853/1962), was the most comprehensive and systematic presentation of the nineteenth century understanding of insanity as it related to the court system and the law (Mohr 1997). Ray was one of the original founders and an early president of the organization that became the APA. He called for an expansion in the definition of insanity to include conditions involving the emotional and volitional powers of the mind in which the power of self-government is lost or impaired. Ray's *Treatise* was widely known among the legal profession. For example, attorneys repeatedly referenced the *Treatise* in the highly publicized M'Naghten trial (Scull et al. 1996).

Ray drew no distinction between the general psychiatrist and the forensic psychiatrist. Nevertheless, Ray's *Treatise* contributed to the identification of forensic practice as one requiring a different skill set from the skills needed for general practice (Gold 2010). As Ray stated in a publication subsequent to his 1838 text, "[I]t cannot be too strongly impressed upon our minds that the duty of an expert is very different from those which ordinarily occupy our attention, and requires a kind of knowledge, and a style of reflection, not indispensable to their tolerably creditable performance" (Ray 1851, p. 55).

During the first half of the twentieth century, concerns regarding the quality of expert testimony resulted in professional action. In his 1933 presidential address to the APA, the organization's new president called for the development of a qualification board to be set up to certify specialists in psychiatry and neurology (Zonana 2012). That same year the APA and the National Committee for Mental Hygiene, at a joint meeting, voted to create an examination board. This resulted in the establishment of the American Board of Psychiatry and Neurology in 1934 (Hollender 2012).

Board Certification and Training in Forensic Psychiatry

Despite the establishment of the ABPN, the demarcation between forensic and general psychiatric practice remained undefined until more recent times. In the 1960s, the National Institutes of Health provided seed money for numerous specialty training programs, including eight in forensic psychiatry (Zonana 2012). While attending the 1968 APA meeting in Boston, Massachusetts, the directors of these forensic training programs decided that a forensic specialty professional organization should be established (Rappeport 1999). The following year, they adopted the name American Academy of Psychiatry and the Law for this new organization.

In conjunction with the development of specialty training in forensic psychiatry, the APA Committee on Psychiatry and the Law called for the establishment of a forensic psychiatry certification board in the early 1970s (Zonana 2012). In 1975, the Forensic Sciences Foundation received a grant from the U.S. Department of Justice to establish a planning process for certification in several forensic specialties, including pathology, odontology, anthropology, and psychiatry (Rappeport 1999). Members of the American Academy of Forensic Sciences and AAPL met in June 1976 and decided to establish the American Board of Forensic Psychiatry (ABFP) (Zonana 2012).

The ABFP administered written and oral certification examinations in forensic psychiatry and certified more than 260 forensic psychiatrists over the next 16 years. During this same time period, AAPL sponsored the Accreditation Council on Fellowships in Forensic Psychiatry, which accredited forensic psychiatry training programs through established standards and site visits (Zonana 2012). The American Board of Medical Specialties (ABMS) officially recognized forensic psychiatry as a subspecialty of psychiatry in 1992, allowing the ABPN to take over the forensic psychiatry certification process.

The first ABPN forensic psychiatry certification examination was administered in 1994 (Rappeport 1999; Zonana 2012). Since then, and as of this writing, ABPN has certified 2,255 psychiatrists in the subspecialty of forensic psychiatry (American Board of Psychiatry and Neurology 2015a). Official ABMS recognition of forensic psychiatry as a subspecialty also enabled ACGME to oversee the accreditation process for forensic psychiatry training fellowship programs. Currently, 44 ACGME-accredited forensic psychiatry fellowship programs are providing training in the United States. Additional fellowship programs, accredited by the Royal College of Physicians and Surgeons, provide training in Canada.

Since its establishment in 1969, AAPL has grown tremendously. As of this writing, with more than 2,000 members, AAPL is the largest forensic psychiatry professional organization. AAPL is "dedicated to excellence in practice, teaching, and research in forensic psychiatry" (American Academy of Psychiatry and the Law 2016). This organization has been on the cutting edge of many of the developments reflected in this text, such as refining concepts relevant to the insanity defense and the human rights movement's scrutiny of civil commitment and patient's rights, particularly the right to treatment (Rappeport 1999). As the legal system has increased its requests for psychiatric testimony in, for example, non-traditional matters such as divorce and custody cases, increasing numbers of general psychiatrists have turned to AAPL to provide the training needed to develop necessary forensic skills.

The Landmark Cases

In addition to covering a considerably larger number of topics, this edition of the *Textbook of Forensic Psychiatry* has been organized to incorporate the ABPN's and AAPL's Landmark Cases. The competent practice of forensic psychiatry requires a working knowledge of the main sources of law: statutes, regulations, and case law. Case law, in particular, has affected the practice of general and forensic psychiatry over the past decades. For example, case law has

- Shaped core psychiatric practices such as informed consent and confidentiality;
- Governed how mental illness is viewed and managed in criminal law;
- Protected the rights of the increasing numbers of people with mental illness in correctional settings; and
- Regulated important issues involving children, from child abuse reporting to the provision of education related services.

AAPL first established the Landmark Case list over 25 years ago to assist forensic psychiatry fellowship programs in curriculum development and in standardizing curricula among programs. The overwhelming majority of Landmark Cases involve decisions made at an appellate court level or higher; U.S. Supreme Court decisions account for two-thirds of current Landmark cases. The cases usually establish an important prec-

edent and most are applicable to general and/or forensic psychiatric practice. Most of the cases also involve important interpretations of federal laws or constitutional issues such as due process, equal protection, and cruel and unusual punishment. Fellowship programs typically teach the Landmark Cases in a didactic format with faculty that include attorneys as well as forensic psychiatrists.

The Association of Directors of Forensic Psychiatry Fellowships (ADFPF) maintains AAPL's Landmark Case list. In 1992 AAPL compiled all of these cases into a published volume. Since that time, the list of Landmark Cases has undergone three revisions (1999, 2007, and 2014). During each revision some cases were added and some were deleted, reflecting evolving legal thought regarding issues relevant to forensic practice. In 2014, several cases that had been previously deleted from the list were added back due to their historical significance. AAPL's Landmark Case list currently consists of 91 cases.

The ABPN also uses a list of Landmark Cases to guide the content outline for the subspecialty certification examination in forensic psychiatry (American Board of Psychiatry and Neurology 2015b). While the content of the exam is not solely based on Landmark Cases, the Landmark Cases relevant to the exam content are listed in the content outline that is available to prospective examinees as a study guide. The AAPL Landmark Case list and the ABPN list overlap substantially but are not identical.

This text covers all cases that appear on the AAPL Landmark Case list and the ABPN forensic psychiatry certification examination content outline. Not all the topics in this volume are associated with Landmark Cases. However, all the Landmark Cases are reviewed in the chapters discussing subjects in which particular cases are relevant. The Landmark Cases are identified in bold italic print, both at the top of each chapter in which they are discussed and throughout the text in all chapters. An index of these cases is also provided at the end of the volume for ease of reference.

Conclusion

The evolution of the fascinating subspecialty of forensic psychiatry has created multiple areas of practice that require specialized knowledge. As the practice of forensic psychiatry has become more specialized, the time has come for an expanded edition of the *Textbook of Forensic Psychiatry* directed toward teaching the precepts of forensic psychiatry in their own right. This edition is designed to be a comprehensive, accessible, and a "user-friendly" teaching tool. Chapter authors have incorporated the changes in diagnosis and diagnostic criteria found in DSM-5 and have also incorporated the Landmark Cases in a manner different than any other text.

We hope that general clinicians, especially those with some forensic interest and experience, will find much of value in these pages. Nevertheless, this third edition is also directed toward practicing forensic psychiatrists, forensic psychiatry fellows in training, general psychiatry residents, and all those interested in forensic psychiatry who wish to stay abreast of developments in this fascinating field.

Liza H. Gold, M.D.
Richard L. Frierson, M.D.

References

Accreditation Council for Graduate Medical Education: Forensic Psychiatry Programs, Academic Year 2016–2017, United States. 2016. Available at: https://apps.acgme.org/ads/Public/Reports/ReportRun?ReportId=1andCurrentYear=2016andSpecialtyId=89andIncludePreAccreditation=trueandIncludePreAccreditation=false. Accessed December 20, 2016.

American Academy of Psychiatry and the Law: Landmark cases. 2014. Available at: http://www.aapl.org/landmark_list.htm. Accessed December 20, 2016.

American Academy of Psychiatry and the Law: Welcome to AAPL. 2016. Available at: aapl.org. Accessed December 20, 2016.

American Board of Psychiatry and Neurology: Facts and statistics as of December 31, 2015. 2015a. Available at: https://www.abpn.com/about/facts-and-statistics/. Accessed December 20, 2016.

American Board of Psychiatry and Neurology: Subspecialty Examination in Forensic Psychiatry 2015 Content Blueprint. December 15, 2015b. Available at: https://www.abpn.com/wp-content/uploads/2015/01/FP2015-blueprint.pdf. Accessed December 20, 2016.

American Psychiatric Association: Diagnostic and Statistical Manual of Mental Disorders, 5th Edition. Arlington, VA, American Psychiatric Publishing, 2013

Gold LH: Rediscovering forensic psychiatry, in The American Psychiatric Publishing Textbook of Forensic Psychiatry, 2nd Edition. Edited by Simon RI, Gold LH. Washington, DC, American Psychiatric Publishing, 2010, pp 3–41

Hollender MH: The founding of the ABPN, in The American Board of Psychiatry and Neurology: Looking Back and Moving Ahead. Edited by Aminoff MJ, Faulkner LR. Washington, DC, American Psychiatric Publishing, 2012, pp 9–16

Mohr JC: The origins of forensic psychiatry in the United States and the great nineteenth-century crisis over the adjudication of wills. J Am Acad Psychiatry Law 25(3):273–284, 1997 9323654

Porter R: The Greatest Benefit to Mankind: A Medical History of Humanity. New York, WW Norton, 1997

Rappeport JR: Thirty years and still growing. J Am Acad Psychiatry Law 27(2):273–277, 1999 10400435

Ray I: Hints to the medical witness in questions of insanity. Am J Insanity 8:53–67, 1851

Ray I: A Treatise on the Medical Jurisprudence of Insanity, 3rd Edition (1853). Edited with introduction by Overholser W. Cambridge, MA, Belknap Press, 1962

Scull A, MacKenzie C, Hervey N: Masters of Bedlam: The Transformation of the Mad Doctoring Trade. Princeton, NJ, Princeton University Press, 1996

Zonana H: Forensic psychiatry, in The American Board of Psychiatry and Neurology: Looking Back and Moving Ahead. Edited by Aminoff MJ, Faulkner LR. Washington, DC, American Psychiatric Publishing, 2012, pp 151–159

Acknowledgments

Our thanks to American Psychiatric Association Publishing for the opportunity to present this revised and expanded third edition. We gratefully acknowledge our chapter authors for their outstanding contributions. It has been gratifying to collaborate again with those who have updated their original contributions and with the new authors who have contributed chapters to this edition.

I am most grateful to Richard L. Frierson, M.D., for agreeing to take on the challenge of co-editing this volume. He managed to fit painstaking chapter editing and his own writing into an incredibly busy forensic and academic schedule. The breadth and depth of his knowledge regarding forensic psychiatry was an invaluable resource. As always, I thank Ian J. Nyden and our children for their love, support, and patience.

—LHG

Thanks to Liza H. Gold, M.D., for extending me this wonderful opportunity to give back to the profession. It has been my pleasure. Thanks to Susan R. Luthren, who keeps me grounded. Thanks to my forensic trainees, past and present, who have made my work both rewarding and fun.

—RLF

PART I

Introduction to Forensic Psychiatry

CHAPTER 1

The Expert Witness

Donald J. Meyer, M.D.
Thomas G. Gutheil, M.D.

Landmark Cases

Frye v. U.S., 54 App.D.C. 46, 293 F. 1013 (1923)

Daubert v. Merrell Dow Pharmaceuticals, Inc., 509 U.S. 579, 113 S.Ct. 2786 (1993)

Kumho Tire Co. Ltd. v. Carmichael, 526 U.S. 137, 119 S.Ct. 1167 (1999)

Testimony Under Oath: The Truth and Nothing but the Truth

Psychiatrists who are called to serve as witnesses in criminal, civil, and administrative legal proceedings face complex legal rules and regulations that belie the simple oath a witness takes when being sworn in. Witnesses are often surprised to find that attorneys and judges have enormous editorial authority over the witnesses' vision of the narrative of the whole truth of the events in question. After all, the legal system calls on psychiatrists for assistance and then frequently constrains the scope and weight of their testimony.

Witnesses may be mollified by the reminder that the physician has neither the standing nor the understanding of legal procedure that a physician has of medical procedures and disease. Both law and medicine have had centuries to craft and refine their different perspectives and respective approach to ascertaining truth (Gutheil et al. 2003). "In medicine, truth is discovered. In law, truth is decided" (M. Baranoski, personal communication,

March 5, 2009). The judge in a bench trial or the jury, if empaneled, is named the trial's *finder of fact*. They, not the witnesses, are not only finders of fact but also decision makers.

Physicians are accustomed to proffering opinions to respectful listeners. In contrast, in the course of the adversarial process, physicians being cross-examined in a trial or questioned in a deposition may feel personally disrespected and hear their professional expertise and opinions questioned and dismissed. However, a thorough understanding of what the legal system expects of an individual witness, and why it expects this and not something else, will foster greater witness effectiveness and equanimity. This will assist expert psychiatrists in successfully negotiating the unfamiliar terrain of the courtroom and the law.

Types of Witnesses

Two categories of witnesses exist under the law: *fact witnesses* and *expert witnesses*. A psychiatrist may be called to testify as a fact witness or as an expert witness. Fact witnesses may testify to things they have perceived with their own five senses. For example, a treating psychiatrist might be called to testify about direct observations of the mental state of a patient in treatment who later committed a crime. This psychiatrist, serving as a fact witness, might be asked what the patient said he felt and thought, how the patient was dressed, whether the patient appeared agitated, and how the patient responded to what the psychiatrist attempted to clarify.

Treating psychiatrists typically would not be asked if an event had caused a patient's mental illness. Although treating psychiatrists might believe that they are the most informed and qualified individuals to answer that forensic question, the law has decided that fact witnesses testify only to those facts ascertained with their own five senses. If the treating psychiatrist has been called as a fact witness, the law will require that witness to adhere to those limitations.

The Federal Rules of Evidence (FRE; Federal Evidence Review 2015) were first codified in 1973 by the U.S. Supreme Court and passed by both houses of Congress in 1975 as a guide for attorneys, prosecutors, and judges about what evidence may be admitted in federal jurisdictions. The rules addressed questions of relevance, admissibility of hearsay testimony, and which party bears the burden of proof. Many states have adopted the FRE, whereas other states have chosen to develop their own evidentiary rules.

Federal Rule 702 defines the courts' expectation of testimony proffered by an expert witness in an applicable jurisdiction (Table 1–1). Before being admitted by the trial court, an expert witness will be reviewed in direct and cross-examination to clarify if the witness is qualified as defined in Rule 702.

The law has an uneasy view of experts in general and mental health experts in particular. Expert witnesses are granted testimonial latitude that fact witnesses are not. With that latitude, the legal system has concerns that an expert may gain too much authority at trial and in so doing hijack the adjudicatory decision making from the trier of fact. Experts may be chastised for invading the province of the jury. However, the legal system also profoundly needs mental health experts. Many legal determinations turn on a defendant's mental state, and most of those determinations cannot be made by the trier of fact alone. A mental health expert can assist the trier of fact in understanding facts beyond his or her everyday knowledge and experience.

TABLE 1–1.   **Federal Rule of Evidence 702: testimony by expert witness**

A witness who is qualified as an expert by knowledge, skill, experience, training, or education may testify in the form of an opinion or otherwise if

  (a)   the expert's scientific, technical, or other specialized knowledge will help the trier of fact to understand the evidence or to determine a fact in issue;

  (b)   the testimony is based on sufficient facts or data;

  (c)   the testimony is the product of reliable principles and methods; and

  (d)   the expert has reliably applied the principles and methods to the facts of the case.

Source.   Federal Evidence Review 2015, p. 30.

Expert testimony about mental states and mental illness that are beyond the knowledge and experience of the trier of fact is needed in all manner of legal issues: criminal responsibility, diminished capacity, testamentary capacity, capacity to give informed consent, commitment, and malpractice, to name a few. Mental health experts in the adjudicatory process educate the triers of fact so that they are better able to judge the facts in question. Although attorneys are zealous advocates for their clients, experts' zeal is reserved for their formation of objective, nonpartisan opinions (American Academy of Psychiatry and the Law 2005). Although experts are usually retained by one side in litigation, the intended goal and beneficiary of an expert's opinion is a better educated and informed trier of fact.

Unlike fact witnesses, expert witnesses may testify about their analysis and conclusions of facts presented at trial. They may introduce other facts relevant to the case at trial. In the case of a patient who had a manic episode secondary to an antidepressant, the expert may introduce other information about secondary mania, as, for example, in answering the question "Based on your training and experience, what could the defendant doctor have done to treat these manic symptoms and mitigate the patient's risk?" Experts also may answer hypothetical questions: "Doctor, what if the defendant had not been prescribed an an-

tidepressant?" Such questions may be far afield from the actual facts of the case and, rather than informing, can lead the jury astray. The law has been mindful that experts may be unduly confident or lack professional rigor in the methods on which they rely and in the testimony they proffer (Mossman 1999). Experts can and do sometimes introduce unreliable and prejudicial evidence to be considered by the trier of fact. Even worse, they may usurp decisions that are solely the province of the trier of fact, such as incorrectly offering opinions about a witness's credibility.

Admissibility of a Psychiatrist as an Expert and of Expert Opinions

Mindful of the risks posed by expert witnesses, American jurisprudence has developed specific procedures to help guard against these unwanted outcomes. Before a psychiatrist may testify as an expert, both the expert and the opinions to be proffered are scrutinized for admissibility. For a psychiatrist to be qualified as an expert, typically the retaining party questions the expert to document that he or she has the requisite relevant, reliable training, experience, knowledge, and skill. Merely being a psychiatrist may not be sufficient to be qualified as an expert in a given case. For example, an infectious disease expert was ruled not qualified to be an expert witness in a case that concerned treatment of *Chlamydia* (*Commonwealth of Massachusetts v. Barresi* 1999). This expert had had no direct experience with treating *Chlamydia*, and the expert's anticipated testimony relied on book learning. Book learning alone was judged an insufficient foundation on which to be qualified and admitted as an expert in this particular case. On the contrary, had the case concerned gram-negative sepsis, an illness with which the expert had direct clinical experience, the physician might have been qualified.

The trial judge is the gatekeeper who decides what evidence and testimony will be presented to or excluded from the court. Rule 702 of the FRE uses the words, "A witness who is qualified as an expert by knowledge, skill, experience, training, or education may testify." The conjunction "or" provides a degree of flexibility for the trial judge to determine whether an expert is qualified without stepping outside of the rule.

Sometimes professional codes of ethics may be used to challenge a purported expert's qualifications because these codes introduce a foundation for requiring a higher level of expertise. These codes are not binding on the trial judge, but the judge may choose to rely on them in a case in which the judge excluded an expert viewed as lacking the requisite background. For example, Ethics Guideline V: Qualifications, of the American Academy of Psychiatry and the Law (AAPL; 2005) states, "Expertise in the practice of forensic psychiatry should be claimed only in areas of actual knowledge, skills, training, and experience." AAPL used the conjunction "and," indicating that knowledge, skills, training, and experience are *all* required of a forensic expert.

The American Medical Association (AMA; 2004, p. 6), in its Council on Ethical and Judicial Affairs report on medical testimony, stated, "When physicians choose to provide expert testimony, they should have recent and substantive experience or knowledge in the area in which they testify." Even though the AMA followed the FRE's use of the conjunction "or," its ethical statement introduced a factor of time. Psychiatrists' credentials may be scrutinized for the timeliness of their experience. A psychiatrist testifying about the standard of care on a recent inpatient cannot expect to rely on experience that is many years past and not up to date.

Although these ethical codes are not binding on the judge, they may be binding on the expert. Experts who are members of professional societies that have enforceable, not merely aspirational, codes of ethics can face ethics investigations and sanctions by the respective professional society. The AMA (American Medical Association 2016) and the American Psychiatric Association (APA; 2013) both have enforceable ethical codes. AAPL's Ethics Guidelines (American Academy of Psychiatry and the Law 2005) have not been adopted by the APA and therefore are an aspirational but not an enforceable code. However, ethics complaints against AAPL members are referred to the member's District Branch of the APA for adjudication under the APA's ethics codes and procedures. Professional ethics committees have been empowered by the Health Care Quality Improvement Act (1986) as Peer Review Committees to review members' clinical work as well as members' testimony before the courts (*Austin v. American Association of Neurological Surgeons* 2001; Meyer and Price 2012).

Once the credentials of the expert have been presented to the court through direct testimony and cross-examination, the judge decides whether to admit an individual as an expert to offer testimony. Expert witness and retaining counsel typically coordinate how they will introduce the expert's credentials in a way that is coherent and meaningful to the particular case rather than simply generating a boring list of where an expert has trained and worked.

In addition to qualifications of the expert, courts scrutinize the relevance and the reliability of the opinions to be proffered by an expert. Some ordinary challenges, such as the hearsay objection (when a challenge is brought against testimony that appears to be based on something told to but not directly observed by the witness), are barred in the case of expert psychiatric testimony. Experts rely not only on what examinees tell them but also on collateral information obtained from important third parties, such as relatives, friends, coworkers, and others.

However, even when an individual has been credentialed as an expert, there is no guarantee that the expert's testimony will be admissible. In one case (*Blanchard v. Eli Lilly* 2002), a renowned psychiatric expert in suicide intended to testify that fluoxetine was the proximate cause of severe akathisia, in the midst of which the decedent patient killed her two children and then herself. The court refused to admit the expert's testimony, explaining that the expert had never treated a selective serotonin reuptake inhibitor–induced akathisia and that the expert could not identify probative information in the medical record or elsewhere that the decedent patient had symptoms of akathisia. The basis for the expert's opinion was his knowledge of case reports in the medical literature, which the court regarded as too speculative to have sufficient probative value for the facts at trial.

Frye and the General Acceptance Rule

How then does an expert meet the court's anticipated expectations of standards of admissibility? American law has long grappled with the criteria for admissibility of expert testimony, desiring the benefit of new knowledge but wary of purported knowledge that had not been adequately scrutinized. In 1923, the rule of *general acceptance by the scientific community* was written (***Frye v. U.S.*** 1923). At the time, James Frye's attorney sought to introduce the systolic blood pressure deception test, a new scientific method intended to measure witness veracity by taking sequential blood pressure measurements to ascertain whether that individual was telling the truth. Frye, a defendant in a murder trial, was subjected to this deception test and then offered the scientist who conducted the test as an expert to testify. The prosecution's objection to this testimony was sustained by the trial court judge. The appellate court affirmed the trial court ruling and in so doing established the ***Frye*** general acceptance rule:

> Just when a scientific principle or discovery crosses the line between the experimental and demonstrable stages is difficult to define. Somewhere in this twilight zone the evidential force of the principle must be recognized, and while the courts will go a long way in admitting expert testimony deduced from a well-recognized scientific principle or discovery, the thing from which the deduction is made must be sufficiently established to have gained general acceptance in the particular field in which it belongs. (***Frye v. U.S.*** 1923, 1014)

Psychiatrists wishing to testify in jurisdictions where the ***Frye*** rule is still used as a standard of admissibility should be prepared to demonstrate and defend how the opinions proffered will pass muster under the general acceptance rule.

Daubert: Relevance and Reliability

For all federal and for many state jurisdictions, admissibility criteria for expert testimony changed in 1993 when the Supreme Court decided the case of ***Daubert v. Merrell Dow Pharmaceuticals Inc.*** (1993). The plaintiff had been treated for nausea during pregnancy with Bendectin, a medication long accepted as safe during pregnancy. The plaintiff alleged that Bendectin caused serious birth defects in her children. Some of the plaintiff's scientific evidence was based on meta-analysis of other studies and had been excluded by the trial court, an exclusion affirmed by the appellate court because it did not meet the general acceptance rule.

In *Daubert*, the Supreme Court ruled that the FRE were the correct admissibility standard for determination of the reliability of expert evidence, not the *Frye* rule. Under FRE 702, quoted earlier, a trial judge pursuant to FRE 104a would assess "whether the reasoning or methodology underlying the testimony is scientifically valid and... whether that reasoning or methodology properly can be applied to the facts in issue." The guidance from the decision identified additional elements of the principles and methodology of a discipline to determine its probative evidentiary reliability:

- Whether the theory or technique in question can be (and has been) tested
- Whether it has been subjected to peer review and publication

- The known or potential rate of error
- Whether it has attracted widespread acceptance within a relevant scientific community, thus allowing that "general acceptance" can yet have bearing on the inquiry

The Court emphasized, "The inquiry is a flexible one, and its focus must be solely on principles and methodology, not on the conclusions that they generate" (p. 31).

Application of *Daubert* criteria and the FRE to mental health testimony was initially ambiguous. Mental health testimony about medical or psychological testing and drug therapies on groups of individuals with mental illness might pass muster with *Daubert*, but testimony about an individual did not easily fit into *Daubert's* metrics. This question about *Daubert's* applicability to psychiatry was specifically raised at the time of the *Daubert* decision by both Justice Stevens and Chief Justice Rehnquist. Two subsequent Supreme Court cases, *General Electric Co. v. Joiner* (1997) and ***Kumho Tire Co. Ltd. v. Carmichael*** (1999), answered this question.

Robert Joiner, a General Electric Company employee, developed small cell cancer of the lung and alleged that workplace exposure to polychlorinated biphenyls (PCBs) had been a substantial cause. In *General Electric Co. v. Joiner* (1997), plaintiff's experts were not admitted to testify about experiments in which large doses of PCBs injected into mice caused them to develop adenomas. The animal study was judged to be too different from the facts at trial. The court stated, "Experts commonly extrapolate from existing data. But nothing in either *Daubert* or the Federal Rules of Evidence requires a district court to admit opinion evidence which is connected to existing data only by the *ipse dixit* [Latin. he, himself, said it] of the expert" (*General Electric Co. v. Joiner* 1997, at 519). A mental health expert wanting to bolster the admissibility of testimony can include relevant, reliable references to the medical literature that directly bear on issues relevant to the facts being adjudicated.

In *Kumho Tire Co. Ltd. v. Carmichael* (1999), the Supreme Court clarified how the trial judge would apply criteria of admissibility from *Daubert* to experts such as mental health professionals who might offer testimony about facts and methods that were far from laboratory science.

> A federal trial judge's gatekeeping obligation under the Federal Rules of Evidence—to insure that an expert witness' testimony rests on a *reliable foundation* and is *relevant* to the task at hand—applies not only to testimony based on scientific knowledge, but rather to all expert testimony that is based on technical and other specialized knowledge. The Federal Rules of Evidence grant to all experts—not just to "scientific" ones—testimonial latitude unavailable to other witnesses on the assumption that an expert's opinion will have a reliable (trustworthy) basis in knowledge and experience of the expert's discipline. (*Kumho Tire Co. Ltd. v. Carmichael* 1999, at 138)

Mental health experts wanting to bolster the admissibility of testimony therefore also can cleave to the methods of diagnosis and treatment of the profession that have been proven reliable and to the methods of forensic examination endorsed by their professional discipline.

The Supreme Court continued that a federal judge may consider one or more of the factors articulated in *Daubert* where such factors are reasonable measures of the testimony's reliability. The trial judge may ask questions of this sort not only where an expert "relies on the application of scientific principles," but also where an expert relies "on skill- or experience-based observation" (*Kumho Tire Co. Ltd. v. Carmichael* 1999, p. 146).

Is Expert Testimony the Practice of Medicine?

The *practice of medicine* is more than a lay phrase. The term is used both in administrative law in reference to legal licensure and regulation and by professional societies that also have a role in establishing standards of ethical professional conduct. Other than medical professionals who practice as federal government employees, the legal definition and regulation of health care professionals are state specific, usually under the auspices of a state administrative board.

Some states require testifying physician experts to be licensed in the state in which they testify. Others do not. Still others require an outside expert to have an identified state-licensed colleague with whom to consult. Experts testifying in a state in which they are not licensed should check with that state's local medical board and also with Federation of State Medical Boards to determine the licensure requirements for providing testimony (see Chapter 2, "Introduction to the Legal System"). Local retaining counsel can be of assistance in clarifying this matter, although experts should not rely solely on retaining counsel's advice.

Legally, professional society codes of conduct are viewed as a legal contract between the society and the member. Those codes that have an enforcement arm are part of this contract. Since 1998, the AMA has defined *medical testimony* as the practice of medicine, thereby identifying testifying as an activity under the regulation of the AMA's ethical procedures, outlined as follows.

The AMA serves as an umbrella organization of state medical associations and national specialty societies. Because of this role, the AMA is not in a position to investigate allegations of unprofessional or unethical conduct at the local level. Instead, the AMA defers to state medical societies and national specialty societies to conduct fact-finding investigations when such allegations are made. If the physician in question is a member of the AMA, the investigative body will forward its findings to the AMA for review by the AMA's Council on Ethical and Judicial Affairs as set forth in the AMA Bylaws and Council on Ethical and Judicial Affairs Rules. The Council on Ethical and Judicial Affairs does not review complaints submitted by the general public. (American Medical Association 2004)

Both the AAPL's and the APA's ethical codes are silent about whether medical testimony is the practice of medicine. However, expert witnesses who are APA members can and have been the object of ethical complaints and sanctions when the more generic APA ethical principles are applied to judge the alleged misconduct. As discussed earlier, complaints submitted to AAPL regarding an AAPL member's conduct are referred to the member's APA district branch for investigation and adjudication. Codes and statements from the AMA and AAPL may have an advisory role in an APA ethics adjudication but cannot be used by themselves to determine whether a member has acted unethically.

Reviewing Opinions to Be Proffered Under Oath

An expert anticipating providing testimony at deposition or at trial typically reviews conclusions and opinions to be offered under oath, looking for strengths, weaknesses, and, especially, alternative views of the events in question. Cases that are litigated do not have all the sentinel facts on one side. Experts' beliefs in their own conclusions must not be a barrier to identifying those facts and conclusions that are most central or fundamental to the expert's argument. The opinion should then be re-reviewed both for fundamental weaknesses and for anticipatable avenues of impeachment.

Experts, their own opinions notwithstanding, should review the facts in question as if they were retained by the opposite side to identify counterarguments and alternative theories of the case. For example, if the expert's opinion about a plaintiff or a defendant rests on a conclusion that the individual was delusional, the expert can reasonably assume that this conclusion will come under scrutiny and attack. The expert should be prepared with evidence in the sources of information that both support the conclusion of delusion and argue against a different conclusion.

Experts also do well to observe a rule of parsimony in the number of conclusions they will attempt to assert. Which are essential? Which conclusions, although true, are not essential? Experts may want to leave no conclusion behind, but that may have the untoward effect of making the expert's testimony more vulnerable to impeachment. All conclusions are not equally defensible or equally necessary. Good opposing counsel will look for the weakest conclusion, even though it may not be central to the expert's argument, and then cross-examine that conclusion vigorously. An expert may unintentionally weaken the overall force of an argument by having to concede points that were not fundamental in the first place.

Experts should be prepared to concede points that reasonably should be conceded. An expert who has accepted the facts at trial is more likely to feel and appear settled and reasonable even in the face of challenges. Experts do not have the job of trying to be better than the facts. Attempting to do so will foreseeably lower credibility. When opposing counsel asks about an event in the case that does not conform with the expert's theory, the expert should concede quickly and without sounding or appearing ashamed. Experts should have reconciled themselves to the reality that not every element of the case is nicely lined up with their conclusions. Experts who overreach what they know to be their objective foundation are at risk for appearing unduly defensive.

Expert and retaining counsel should meet and discuss this material. An expert can help the attorney credential the expert by pointing to specific education or experience particularly relevant to the case being tried. The attorney may have actual knowledge of opposing counsel's style, which will aid in the expert's preparation. A discussion of the retaining attorney's and the expert's theory of the case and the relevant concepts and conclusions to be presented on direct examination is crucial. Counsel also can help prepare the expert for the likely form and substance of cross-examination. At the end of the meeting, counsel and expert should have a shared vision of the goals of direct examination while avoiding sounding rehearsed.

Experts are only in charge of what they write and say. That very circumscribed authority should be guarded zealously. Other parties will decide what may be asked and how, a process over which the expert has no authority. The expert's goals and the retaining attorney's goals may overlap or converge but not through a partisan alliance. In addition, the legal process is very socially interactive but not at all relational. The expert is required to

be objective in both ascertaining and representing an opinion to educate the trier of fact. Counsel is the client's zealous advocate. Both expert and attorney are constrained and directed by their respective job descriptions and their ethical duties, not by an interpersonal relationship.

Once testimony begins, the process shifts to the expert's being reactive to counsel's questions, strategy, and tactics being deployed. In a deposition, opposing counsel may want to probe certain facets of the theory of the case. Counsel also has the opportunity to see how the expert will handle challenges. Will the expert get ruffled or defensive? If opposing counsel sees a particular vulnerability in the expert's conclusions or qualifications, counsel may seek to have the expert crawl out further on a limb in order to set the expert up for revisiting this issue during cross-examination at trial.

Direct examination at trial is a direct product of the proactive preparation between expert and retaining counsel. Testimony should be coherent and not rehearsed. Save for a surprise motion from opposing counsel seeking to exclude the expert or bar admission of some aspect of the expert's anticipated testimony, direct examination should unfold as anticipated.

The language of testimony needs to be accessible to the audience. When technical terms are used, they must be defined in lay English. Simple and declarative language is more powerful than language in passive voice and sentences with multiple clauses and relative pronouns. Fewer words typically make for clearer, more authoritative statements. Visual aids may assist the trier of fact's retention of a series of assertions. High school language skills cannot be presumed of the average juror (Kirsch et al. 2002). Testimony crafted for people without a high school education will be more reliably accessible to every potential juror. Language can be more complex at a bench trial or a deposition because the listener and readers hold undergraduate and graduate degrees.

When answering a question posed by an attorney, whether retaining or opposing counsel, experts should try, as much as possible, to turn away from the questioner and address comments to the trier of fact. Expert witnesses should speak to a jury as individuals and make eye contact, if possible, without staring at any one juror. Visually locking in with the attorney posing the questions turns the trier of fact into a spectator of the interaction between the expert and the attorney rather than having the trier of fact feel addressed directly by the expert. Additionally, appearing friendly with retaining counsel can erode the expert's stance of independence.

Although the oath that begins the process of testimony gives hope to the idea that experts will tell the truth as best they know it, actual testimony involves answering only the question asked. Experts may reasonably believe that the question asked is not the best question, but if the judge allows it, the expert's job is to answer it if possible. Experts sometimes argue, squirm, or whine about questions they perceive to be unfair or wrongheaded. These responses are unseemly and lower the expert's hoped-for respect from the trier of fact. Retaining counsel may choose to readdress an issue on redirect examination, if counsel decides the expert has been unduly constrained by a question and the point is important enough to rehabilitate.

An attorney cross-examining a witness ideally likes to know in advance the answers to all questions asked and to control the witness. The witness is actively guarding against having his or her answers controlled. The expert is in charge of being an active listener and also of the

rate and rhythm of answering. Opposing counsel may have reason to speed the rate of questioning, rapidly beginning assertions with the interrogatory, "Isn't it a fact that...?" or "Doctor, you would agree with me that....." The expert will feel pressured to respond quickly and should resist that pressure. When asked "Isn't it a fact that the medical record shows...,?" experts should not answer unless and until they are sure. Attorneys are ethically permitted to take a comment out of context in an effort to have the expert agree with something that actually contradicts the expert's opinion.

At trial, opposing counsel also may ethically pose potentially demeaning questions. For example, if the expert failed board certification examinations, the expert should anticipate the possibility of being asked about this fact. If the expert has experienced professional difficulty, this too may be raised at trial. Experts may be asked about prior publications, prior testimony, and even personal questions (Gutheil et al. 2001). The judge, not the expert, decides if the question or answer is relevant to the trial. Experts often will be asked what they have been paid for their opinions in an attempt to imply that they are being paid to supply opinions helpful to the retaining counsel's client. Experts should be prepared to clearly and definitively respond that they were paid for their time, not for their opinions.

Experts often will be asked how many individuals they have treated and how many individuals they have examined with a diagnosis, conduct, or a legal issue similar to the defendant or examinee. If the expert has little experience, this will be used to challenge expertise on cross-examination. If the expert has a lot of testimonial experience, it may be used to infer monetary bias. Experts may be asked if they have typically testified for one side rather than both defense and prosecution or plaintiff and defense. If the figures are unbalanced, this may be used to suggest that the expert is partisan.

Mental health experts should expect questions about the sources of information on which they relied. If they chose not to review certain materials, they can anticipate being asked why. If they relied on psychological testing or neuroimaging, they should be prepared to explain what that testing is and why they relied on it. Psychiatrists may not be qualified to score a given psychological test or read a magnetic resonance image, but they should be prepared to explain how such testing works. Experts who cannot provide such explanations risk impeachment for relying on materials they do not understand.

Experts may be asked if they reviewed a given document, only to realize that the retaining counsel intentionally or mistakenly did not provide it. If asked, the expert should acknowledge, "I was not provided with this document." The expert also may be asked, "Would it change your opinion if you were to learn that the examinee…?" A candid, simple "yes," "no," or "possibly" is required.

As a rule, experts should avoid identifying any text as authoritative. An authoritative text is a legal term of art conferring on that text the broad authority to be dispositive about what is true on a subject. Instead of calling a text authoritative, an expert may acknowledge that the text is in wide use and commonly consulted.

Many experts will be asked the amount of time they spent with an examinee. The follow-up question typically will attempt to impeach how well the expert could expect to get to know the examinee in so short a time. The answer should indicate that the expert had enough time to reach the proffered conclusions within reasonable medical certainty. Questions should be anticipated about diagnostic terms and the method of diagnostic assessment, especially if an opposing expert has offered different diagnoses. Opposing counsel may ask, "Doctor, isn't it possible that…,?" thereby putting the expert in the position of agreeing with the attorney's hypothetical. The expert may be able to answer, "It's possible" or "Unlikely," thereby emphasizing that the hypothetical circumstances are a possibility, not a probability. Some judges will hold an expert to simple affirmatives or negatives, although some judges will allow the expert more latitude.

Conclusion

Psychiatrists are asked to participate at many levels of legal proceedings, from providing evaluations to providing courtroom testimony, and psychiatric expertise is frequently crucial for informed legal decision making. Nevertheless, providing testimony under oath always involves uncertainty and anxiety for the expert who may be challenged in very public settings over which he or she has little control. One definition of *forensic* is a narrative suitable for debate in a public forum. The uncertainty inherent in providing testimony can be substantially reduced by the expert's understanding what the adjudicatory process requires of an expert witness and why it does so.

Key Concepts

- Experts should be aware of rules that govern the admissibility of testimony.

- Experts should conduct a thorough review of the expected testimony, identifying and excluding unessential points.

- Experts should anticipate and prepare for potential vulnerabilities on cross-examination of essential conclusions.

- Experts should discuss with retaining counsel how the presentation of credentials and direct examination will proceed before the trier of fact.

- Experts and the retaining counsel should consider and prepare to respond to opposing counsel's introduction of alternative theories of the events in question.

- Experts should prepare to concede quickly those issues that are not consistent with the expert's conclusions.

References

American Academy of Psychiatry and the Law: Ethics Guidelines for the Practice of Forensic Psychiatry. May 2005. Available at: http://www.aapl.org/ethics.htm. Accessed December 19, 2016.

American Medical Association: Council on Ethical and Judicial Affairs: Report of the Council on Ethical and Judicial Affairs. CEJA Report 12-A-04: Subject: Medical Testimony. 2004.

American Medical Association: Medical ethics code frequently asked questions: what can the AMA do about a physician I believe is behaving unethically or unprofessionally? 2016. Available at: https://www.ama-assn.org/content/frequently-asked-questions-ethics. Accessed December 19, 2016.

American Psychiatric Association: The Principles of Medical Ethics With Annotations Especially Applicable to Psychiatry. 2013. Available at: https://www.psychiatry.org/psychiatrists/practice/ethics. Accessed December 19, 2016.

Austin v American Association of Neurological Surgeons, 253 F.3d 967 (7th Cir 2001)

Blanchard v Eli Lilly, 207 F.Supp.2d 308; LEXIS 16470 (U.S. Dist. 2002)

Commonwealth of Massachusetts v Barresi, 46 Mass. App. Ct. 907, 705 N.E.2nd 639 (1999)

Daubert v Merrell Dow Pharmaceuticals Inc., 509 U.S. 579, 113 S.Ct. 2786 (1993)

Federal Evidence Review: Federal Rules of Evidence 2015. [Federal Evidence Review Web site]. 2015. Available at: http://federalevidence.com/downloads/rules.of.evidence.pdf. Accessed December 21, 2016.

Frye v U.S., 54 App.D.C. 46, 293 F. 1013 (1923)

General Electric Co v Robert K. Joiner, 522 U.S. 136 (1997)

Gutheil TG, Commons ML, Miller PM: Personal questions on cross-examination: a pilot study of expert witness attitudes. J Am Acad Psychiatry Law 29(1):85–88, 2001 11302392

Gutheil TG, Hauser M, White MS, et al: "The whole truth" versus "the admissible truth": an ethics dilemma for expert witnesses. J Am Acad Psychiatry Law 31(4):422–427, 2003 14974796

Health Care Quality Improvement Act, Standards for Professional Review Actions, 42 U.S.C. 11112, 1986. Available at: https://www.npdb.hrsa.gov/resources/titleIv.jsp. Accessed December 19, 2016.

Kirsch IS, Jungeblut A, Jenkins L, Kolstad A: Adult Literacy in America: A First Look at the Findings of the National Adult Literacy Survey. April 2002. Available at: https://nces.ed.gov/pubs93/93275.pdf. Accessed December 19, 2016.

Kumho Tire Co., Ltd. v Carmichael, 526 U.S. 137, 119 S.Ct. 1167 (1999)

Meyer DJ, Price M: Peer review committees and state licensing boards: responding to allegations of physician misconduct. J Am Acad Psychiatry Law 40(2):193–201, 2012 22635290

Mossman D: "Hired guns," "whores," and "prostitutes": case law references to clinicians of ill repute. J Am Acad Psychiatry Law 27(3):414–425, 1999 10509941

CHAPTER 2

Introduction to the Legal System

Eric Y. Drogin, J.D., Ph.D.
Carol S. Williams, LL.B. (Hons.)

Landmark Cases

Frye v. U.S., 54 App.D.C. 46, 293 F. 1013 (1923)

Daubert v. Merrell Dow Pharmaceuticals, Inc., 509 U.S. 579, 113 S.Ct. 2786 (1993)

Jaffee v. Redmond, 518 U.S. 1; 116 S.Ct. 1923 (1996)

Kumho Tire Co., Ltd. v. Carmichael, 526 U.S. 137, 119 S.Ct. 1167 (1999)

Forensic psychiatrists are invaluable contributors to the functioning of the legal system in civil and criminal cases alike. As skilled as the court will be in interpreting laws, conducting trials, and ensuring appropriate verdicts or settlements, it has no real way to determine the presence or absence of required mental capacity, the degree of mental suffering, or the requirements for future medical treatment without resorting to the advice and consultation of qualified experts.

Familiarity with the legal system has a twofold benefit for forensic clinicians. It enables forensic psychiatrists to become more skilled and persuasive sources of mental health expertise and alerts them to the dangers that ignorance of key legal principles may pose for litigants and for the careers of expert witnesses themselves. In this chapter, we review sources of law, court jurisdiction, courtroom procedure, and evidentiary standards to inform and ensure effective and ethical forensic psychiatric practice.

Sources of Law

Statutes

The American legal system relies on three basic sources of law, each of which reflects, accommodates, and reinforces the others, within an overall scheme that the Constitution of the United States specifies in detail. The first of these, *statutes*, comprises the written laws passed by the U.S. Congress or any of the 50 state legislatures. Statutes provide codified guidance on the broadest range of legal issues. For example, a given state's statutes define who is a physician, delineates what activities are included in the practice of medicine, and establishes a medical board to set additional standards and provide oversight for the protection of the public. Statutory drafting and revision are complex, politically fraught, and time-consuming processes, especially because legislatures are typically not perpetually in session, convening every year or two for limited periods of just months or even weeks.

Regulations

Regulations, which some jurisdictions term *administrative rules*, may provide highly detailed guidance on what are often obscure, specialized technical matters. For this reason, regulations are often the responsibility of a legislatively appointed body, such as a medical board. Such bodies have a complement of professionals appointed by the governor along with laypersons to ensure that professionals do not promote guild interests over those of regular citizens. However, these laypersons are often attorneys whose lack of technical expertise is balanced by strong advocacy skills.

Fully "promulgated" regulations gain legislative approval after exposure to suggestions and challenges from all manner of stakeholders, including political action committees, consumer groups, and even rival boards seeking to gain previously restricted privileges for their own licensees. "Incorporation by reference" involves identifying an external source of guidance, such as an ethics code, and designating it as part of the law in order to "reap the significant benefits of collaborative governance through a public-private partnership in standards" (Bremer 2013, p. 135).

Case Law

Case law, often described as "common law," is a collection of appellate decisions in which higher courts interpret and settle legal issues that arise on appeal from lower court rulings. Appellate courts may address a final verdict rendered by the judge or jury, or they may intervene in a trial judge's decision in response to an interlocutory appeal in an active case.

Appellate judges do not second-guess the facts of a given case, focusing instead on matters of law. For example, they will not address whether a doctor did or did not commit a particular medical error, but they will address the legally recognized standard of practice in a given jurisdiction. An appellate decision may let the lower court's reasoning stand, it may sweepingly and conclusively overturn the lower court's reasoning, or it may intervene only to a limited extent and remand the case to the lower court for further proceedings.

Attorneys referring to an appealable ruling are not commenting on how egregious they think that decision might be; rather, they are describing a ruling sufficiently concrete and final to be the appropriate focus of a legal challenge. Appellate decisions apply to more than just the case at hand. They also provide guidance for lower courts that later address similar issues. The principle of *stare decisis* ("to stand by things decided") encourages appellate courts to respect and abide by prior appellate decisions, thus adhering to precedent when feasible (Waldron 2012, p. 2).

Court Systems and Jurisdiction

Ethical Obligations

Familiarity with the regulations of the jurisdiction in which the forensic expert is providing services is an ethical obligation. According to the *Ethics Guidelines for the Practice of Forensic Psychiatry* (American Academy of Psychiatry and the Law 2005), mastering "the appropriate laws of the jurisdiction" (p. 2) is a necessary task that requires a solid grounding in the "institutions, policies, procedures, values, and vocabulary" of the laws of the country, state, county, or municipality in question (p. 1). Additionally, *The Principles of Medical Ethics With Annotations Especially Applicable to Psychiatry* (American Psychiatric Association 2013) calls on forensic psychiatrists to "respect the law" and to "seek changes" to maladaptive legal rules (p. 4). These obligations require a solid grounding in the case law, statutes, and regulations for each jurisdiction in which clinical and forensic psychiatrists practice.

Court Hierarchies

The U.S. Supreme Court is the final arbiter of matters that make their way to the pinnacle of the legal system. Unlike lower appellate courts, which often have no choice but to hear certain types of appeals, the Supreme Court retains the right to decide which matters it will entertain, following a process called *granting certiorari*.

Cases may be appealed to the Supreme Court through one of two parallel judicial systems. The first of these is the federal system, dedicated specifically to set-tling matters of federal law. The federal system consists of 12 geographically determined Circuit Courts of Appeals that consider matters that arise from trials in whichever of the 94 federal district courts fall within their respective jurisdictions. A U.S. Court of Appeals for the federal circuit also reviews specialized matters such as patent disputes, international trade controversies, and lawsuits against the United States for damages.

The second legal route to the Supreme Court is the state judicial system, composed of 50 different constellations of trial, intermediate appellate, and state supreme courts dedicated specifically to state law. Trial-level matters are typically addressed by a two-tiered system in which district or magistrate courts handle misdemeanors and minor civil matters and circuit or superior courts handle felonies and major civil matters. State appellate courts retain a fair amount of discretion concerning which cases they decide to hear, although certain appeals, such as those involving application of the death penalty, will automatically be entertained as a "matter of right." A state supreme court's decisions are binding only in that particular jurisdiction but may offer useful guidance for judges in another state grappling with similar issues.

State court issues may make their way into federal courts under the notion of *diversity jurisdiction*, meaning that a civil lawsuit involves parties in different states. For diversity jurisdiction to be invoked, a sufficiently high *amount in controversy*, meaning damages, is necessary. The U.S. Congress statutorily sets this amount, which is currently $75,000 or more (see 28 USC §1332[a]). Forensic psychiatrists sometimes will be retained to address the same set of facts in parallel federal and state proceedings when attorneys attempt to pursue somewhat similar civil remedies in each system simultaneously.

Which Law Controls?

The assumption that Supreme Court decisions are the final, authoritative word on whatever legal matters they address is not necessarily correct. In fact, the justices are not required to settle every legal detail that lower courts cannot resolve to the satisfaction of one party or the other. Rather, a Supreme Court decision is supposed to focus primarily on Constitutional issues and interpretation of federal statutes. The extent to which individual justices adhere to this principle allows critics to place them on a spectrum that runs from strict constructionist to judicial activist.

In the landmark case of *Jaffee v. Redmond* (1996), for example, the Supreme Court endorsed, for the first time, the existence of a federal psychotherapist–patient privilege. Specifically, the Court held that "confidential communications between a licensed psychotherapist and a patient... in the course of diagnosis and treatment are protected from compelled disclosure under Rule 501 of the Federal Rules of Evidence" (*Jaffee v. Redmond* 1996, at 15). However, the Court's ruling does not prevent a psychiatrist's records from being subpoenaed in *state* court.

Persuasive Authority and Publication

Many of these jurisdictional and legal issues bedevil even experienced attorneys and their expert witness counterparts. Supreme Court opinions, even if they are not directly controlling for a given jurisdiction, are nonetheless given considerable weight when a trial court is struggling to find its way in a case of first impression for which no local or directly controlling appellate precedent can be identified. A trial court's decision-making process may be influenced by opinions from prominent appellate courts in other jurisdictions. This legal strategy

is known as invoking *persuasive authority* (Flanders 2009).

The legal weight given to appellate decisions may be confused even further by the fact that some appellate court decisions are *published*, whereas others are *unpublished*. This does not mean that only some of these decisions can be accessed and reviewed. Instead, the difference between a published and an unpublished decision is that the courts decide which of their opinions can formally be cited as precedent in *other* cases (published) and which of their opinions will be documented merely as a source of information on how the court ruled in a particular matter at a given point in time (unpublished).

Jurisdiction and Forensic Practice

A jurisdictional issue of considerable importance to forensic psychiatrists is whether local medical licensure is required to conduct evaluations or provide testimony in a given state. Each state has its own rules for deciding whether certain services fall within applicable definitions of medical practice, as defined by jurisdiction-specific statutes and regulations. State statutes and regulations also define each state's rules for determining which exceptions might be available.

For example, a state might provide a physician licensed in another state a waiver for a one-time (pro hac vice) visit to conduct an examination. Some states might allow physicians with an out-of-state license to practice for a limited number of days or might grant permission for the physician to practice as long as a "local" physician participates or agrees to supervise. Some states might require temporary licensure or might require that the out-of-state physician obtain a full medical license in order to provide expert witness testimony or to conduct a psychiatric examination for forensic purposes.

Before engaging in a case in a state in which the physician is not licensed, physicians are advised to contact the state medical board directly (Simon and Shuman 1999). State medical boards may have regulations that address the specific circumstances of the expert's activities, although many do not. Additionally, some state medical boards may have their own interpretations of their regulations that may or may not comport with what attorneys call the "black letter" or facially apparent meaning of codified licensure laws. In some states, the issue of out-of-state practitioners conducting forensic examinations and providing expert testimony has been addressed through case law rather than state statute.

Attorneys who retain a forensic psychiatrist can lend some insight but cannot advise the expert legally. The Federation of State Medical Boards (2016) provides references on a state-by-state basis to relevant state statutes or case law regarding out-of-state forensic practice but may not always reflect the most recent case law or state statutes. Local judge approval of out-of-state expert participation does not provide immunity to the expert against lawsuits and board complaints for practicing medicine without a license. The unauthorized practice of medicine is a felony in some states, which can result in heavy fines, incarceration, or both, in addition to eventual loss of licensure in the physician's home jurisdiction.

Civil and Criminal Procedure

Prior to Trial

In civil cases, formal proceedings commence with the filing of a complaint.

Forensic psychiatrists often profess surprise at the sweeping nature of these documents, which seem designed to vilify the defendant in every conceivable fashion. The plaintiff's counsel himself or herself is unlikely to believe all of these terrible things actually happened, but listing every misdeed to its fullest reasonably likely extent avoids forfeiting such issues later.

Criminal cases begin with an arrest. The nature and circumstances of obtaining the defendant's statement about what allegedly occurred often becomes the primary focus of the forensic psychiatrist's involvement. Evaluations of capacity to stand trial, criminal responsibility, and a *mens rea* defense (diminished capacity) also occur pretrial (see Chapter 18, "Evaluation of Competencies in the Criminal Justice System").

Attorneys settle most matters prior to trial. Civil and criminal case filings in state courts first surpassed the 100,000,000 mark, or approximately one for every three American citizens, in 2006 (Bureau of Justice Statistics 2013). The court system simply cannot bring more than a fraction of these disputes to a jury. Pretrial negotiations are an ongoing background factor in all but the most egregious of cases in order to "promote settlement and thus reduce the number of actual trials" (Kim and Ryu 2000, p. 286).

As a means of gaining the upper hand in negotiations or at a later trial, civil and criminal attorneys may file various motions. These motions *in limine* ("on the threshold") may include attempts to obtain a protective order to keep experts from being pressured to produce more documentation or to ensure the confidentiality of sensitive private information. In civil cases, motions may involve a request for summary judgment when defendants assert that the plaintiff has not offered enough evidence to satisfy the sufficient elements required to establish liability (Pfautz 2015).

During Trial

Determining which party must present its evidence first at trial will depend on who bears the burden of proof. Courts impose this burden on whichever party brought the action in the first place, based on the reasoning that those making complaints establish a basis for imposing civil penalties or criminal punishment. Specifically, this burden has two embedded components: the burden of persuasion, arguing the case for one decision over another, and the burden of production, providing sufficient tangible evidence to support that argument (Allen and Jehl 2003).

The standard of proof governs the degree of proof required. In most civil matters, this requires convincing the judge or jury by a preponderance of the evidence, by which, no matter how narrow the margin, "a defendant will be held liable if fact finders believe that the defendant has more likely than not engaged in the conduct giving rise to liability" (Chmielewski 2013, p. 150). Some weightier civil matters (such as termination of parental rights, civil commitment to a psychiatric hospital) as well as some issues embedded within criminal proceedings (such as determining whether to medicate nondangerous criminal defendants to assist them in becoming competent to stand trial) call for the evidentiary middle ground of clear and convincing evidence (Cochrane et al. 2013). Criminal convictions are so serious in nature that they require establishment of guilt beyond a reasonable doubt, calling for utmost certainty in this regard (Minhas 2003).

The certainty required when rendering a jury verdict is often confused with the reasonable degree of medical certainty forensic psychiatrists are frequently asked to endorse when rendering an expert opinion at trial. Uncertainty on the part of the legal profession concerning what *certainty* actually means in the latter context moved Gianelli (2010) to suggest that "experts could avoid the term altogether and testify how confident they are in their opinion" (p. 40). This uncertainty is rampant among mental health professionals as well, reflecting "ambivalence in both the legal and scientific literature" on the meaning of *reasonable medical certainty* "in civil and criminal cases" alike (Drogin et al. 2012, p. 351).

At the End of Trial

After presentation of all evidence, either party can move for a directed verdict, asking the judge to rule that whatever the jury may decide, the other side failed to meet its burden of proof (Lerner 2013). Once the jury has decided on a verdict, counsel for the losing party can request a judgment *non obstante veredicto* ("notwithstanding the verdict"), in which the judge rejects the jury's findings as unreasonable, unlawful, or both, as a measure to "control runaway verdicts" (Cavanagh 2015, p. 642). If the case was tried directly to a judge without a jury (a bench trial), then the losing party might simply move for the court to reconsider its verdict.

Either party, anticipating appellate proceedings that could take years, may make a settlement offer at the end of trial to curtail future ligation. If the victors think that they have proven their point and have misgivings about the number of errors that were "preserved" via objections for appellate review, they may be open to such entreaties. In criminal cases, there may be direct appeals related to trial error or postconviction relief proceedings that involve a claim of ineffective assistance of defense counsel. Either issue could come back to justify a different sentence or, on occasion, a new trial (Stephens 2013).

Evidence

Civil and criminal procedures make clear that without properly qualified evidence, nothing can be decided. The courtroom is not a place for guesswork or speculation, and its work constitutes more than a simple exchange of ideas or opinions about agreed-on circumstances. Instead, the courtroom is a venue where rival parties offer themselves up to the authority of the legal system to obtain a fact-based ruling on what constitutes the "truth" and to learn what the consequences of that truth will be. How does the legal system obtain these facts?

Interrogatories

In a legal matter, the "discovery," which refers not only to the act of seeking information but also to the obtained information, reflects various overlapping methods of inquiry. Experienced attorneys will seek out as much information as possible from other attorneys and trusted psychiatric colleagues about witnesses they want to hire and witnesses they wish to discredit. Paralegals, consultants, and investigators will track down additional details when the stakes are high enough and the opinions of a particular expert are central to the case. However, none of this information may be ultimately as useful as information that counsel can obtain directly from forensic psychiatrists themselves.

Interrogatories are exhaustive collections of searching inquiries that can suggest that legal services are billed by the pound instead of by the hour. As an example, forensic psychiatrists may be asked to identify every book, chapter, or article they have ever read that addressed the notion of anxiety. They could be asked and expected to calculate, with certainty, overall percentages for the sexual orientation, culture of origin, primary diagnosis, and amenability to treatment for all patients they have ever seen. Retaining counsel can advise which questions merit or require a response and which questions can be dismissed with a detailed and polite but firm written refusal. However, ignoring an interrogatory question is not an option (Wise 2013). Forensic psychiatrists may find it necessary to hire their own attorney if arguments about the contents of interrogatories escalate and important issues of confidentiality and privilege are at stake.

Depositions

Once counsel for both sides have had the opportunity to peruse the interrogatory responses, they typically will conduct a sworn deposition of every expert witness who may be called to testify at trial. Depositions are an opportunity to determine what forensic psychiatrists might say, how they claim to be able to back up their assertions, their level of experience, what they actually know about their chosen field, how well they can communicate, and how they hold up under adversarial questioning (Keleher 2015). If the expert is legitimately unavailable at trial, counsel may seek to have the recording of the deposition played to the jury during proceedings that in some cases could occur years later. Additionally, depositions may be used on cross-examination to catch forensic psychiatrists contradicting their testimony about facts, opinions, and the scientific underpinnings of various procedures and opinions.

The circumstances of the deposition can be a critical factor in ensuring that forensic psychiatrists can convey their knowledge accurately, effectively, and at the least inconvenience and expense. Some experts prefer to be deposed in their own offices to take advantage of familiar surroundings, access to resources, and avoidance of last-minute travel emergencies. On the other hand, at the end of a deposition, clearing attorneys, videographers, legal assistants, and litigants from one's own office is much more difficult than simply getting up and walking out of an attorney's office.

Forensic psychiatrists are within their rights to require nonrefundable payment in advance of a deposition for exactly as much time as opposing counsel claims to need. Opposing counsel pays for the time the expert spends in the deposition, and retaining counsel pays for the time the expert spends in preparation. If opposing counsel is not ready to start on time, that is opposing counsel's problem, and forensic psychiatrists may or may not decide to extend their participation. Under any circumstances, it is entirely reasonable to stop answering questions at the end of the agreed-on period of time. Opposing counsel can always request, and pay for, an additional session. Lawyers understand why these arrangements are necessary, even if they may profess otherwise. They devised these rules, and they can be expected to use them for their own purposes when needed.

At the end of a deposition, the court reporter will ask whether the expert wants to review and sign the deposition transcript or waive a review. Experts should always reserve the right to review the transcript. When a deposition transcript arrives, forensic psychiatrists must review it with care, no matter how time-consuming or reminiscent of a distasteful encounter that may be. Experts can charge the retaining attorney their usual fees for the time spent reviewing the deposition. Reviewing deposition testimony is especially important in jurisdictions that allow experts to offer amended answers instead of merely identifying outright errors in documentation. Reviewing a deposition also helps forensic psychiatrists reacquaint themselves with previously made assertions, an exercise absolutely critical in preparing for trial.

Subpoenas

Forensic psychiatrists should not be insulted when, before trial, either party insists on having the court issue a subpoena requiring that experts formally accept a document that requires their compliance with the court's demands. Issuing a formal demand is counsel's obligation to judges and clients alike, and counsel will have to answer to both if the expert does not follow through, even as a result of unforeseen or otherwise understandable circumstances. Sometimes forensic psychiatrists seek to be subpoenaed to guarantee that an employer or another court can receive documented proof of conflicting obligations.

Courts, or in some jurisdictions attorneys, may issue subpoenas primarily to ensure that forensic psychiatrists are present to testify in court. These documents may focus instead on the production of certain documents, such as reports, records, or other evidence. They also may take the form of a subpoena *duces tecum* ("bring with you"), which requires the expert to appear and hand over various forms of potentially admissible evidence at the same time. There is no acceptable alternative to reading through subpoenas with great care and to obtaining retaining counsel's clarification of any misunderstood or seemingly contradictory language.

Like interrogatories, subpoenas cannot simply be ignored, but they can sometimes be nullified ("quashed") with the help of retaining counsel or one's own attorney. This could occur if stated demands vary unreasonably from previously agreed-on locations or dates of availability, if forensic psychiatrists simply do not possess a particular source of information, or if forensic psychiatrists can offer a convincing argument that they are not legally required or even allowed to convey such material to the court or anyone else (Buchanan 2005).

Trial

Federal and state statutes and Supreme Court case law govern or influence the admissibility of forensic psychiatric evidence at trial in a given jurisdiction (see Chapter 1, "The Expert Witness"). In brief, *Frye v. U.S.* (1923) established the general acceptance rule for admissibility of expert testimony. The Supreme Court confirmed in *Daubert v. Merrell Dow Pharmaceuticals, Inc.* (1993) that the Federal Rules of Evidence (FRE), approved by Congress in 1975, had essentially replaced *Frye* in the federal courts almost 20 years earlier, although states employing the *Frye* standard remained free to do so. FRE 702 outlines requirements for a witness "qualified as an expert by knowledge, skill, experience, training, or education" to testify in federal court. In *Kumho Tire Co. Ltd. v. Carmichael* (1999), the Supreme Court clarified that *Daubert* requirements applied to *all* expert witness testimony, including "scientific," "technical," or some other form of "specialized" knowledge (p. 149).

The full FRE (Federal Evidence Review 2015), as widely adopted in whole or in part by various state jurisdictions (Evans 2011), comprises 68 rules, some with as many as two dozen subsections. Several of these include additional provisions relevant for forensic psychiatrists. Aspiring and experienced forensic psychiatrists alike are encouraged to review the complete list, along with whatever version exists for their home state and any other jurisdiction in which they testify. Without knowing what can and cannot be said in court, expert witnesses may commit unintentional errors that, in extreme cases, can bring legal proceedings to a complete halt and even require a costly retrial.

Conclusion

Forensic psychiatry is an exciting, demanding, and constantly evolving practice specialty that requires a working knowledge of the legal system for effective and ethical participation. Achieving and maintaining this knowledge will depend on monitoring critical source materials, consulting closely with retaining counsel, and on occasion seeking advice from one's own attorney. As complex and occasionally frustrating as this system may be, forensic psychiatrists can draw comfort from the fact that the legal system simply cannot function without them. This lends itself to an atmosphere of mutual respect and collegiality that can smooth out the inevitable stresses and strains of participating in an adversarial system.

Key Concepts

- The American legal system relies on three complementary sources of guidance: statutes, regulations, and case law.

- Forensic psychiatrists have an ethical and a practical obligation to master jurisdiction-specific legal issues.

- Decisions of the U.S. Supreme Court are often limited in scope, so it is important to determine whether its rulings actually address standards in state as opposed to federal proceedings.

- States have rules regarding physicians not licensed in that state providing expert services, and those rules are best identified by contacting that state's medical board directly.

- At trial, burden of proof attaches to the party bringing a civil or criminal action, and standard of proof addresses whether the jury needs to be convinced by a preponderance of the evidence, by clear and convincing evidence, or beyond a reasonable doubt.

- Interrogatories are written pretrial requests to obtain information, depositions are pretrial inquisitions designed to determine what forensic psychiatrists are likely to say and do on the witness stand, and subpoenas can require presence in the courtroom as well as the production of various forms of evidence. All of these may be finessed in some fashion, but none can simply be ignored.

- Admissibility of expert evidence at trial is governed either by the Federal Rules of Evidence or by state evidentiary rules. The judge determines whether an expert's evidence has the necessary relevance and scientific reliability to be admitted.

References

Allen RJ, Jehl SA: Burdens of persuasion in civil cases: algorithms v. explanations. Mich State Law Rev 2003:893–944, 2003

American Academy of Psychiatry and the Law: Ethics Guidelines for the Practice of Forensic Psychiatry. May 2005. Available at: http://www.aapl.org/ethics.htm. Accessed December 19, 2016.

American Psychiatric Association: The Principles of Medical Ethics With Annotations Especially Applicable to Psychiatry. 2013. Available at: https://www.psychiatry.org/psychiatrists/practice/ethics. Accessed December 21, 2016.

Bremer ES: Incorporation by reference in an open-government age. Harv J Law Public Policy 13:131–210, 2013

Buchanan JD: Subpoena duces tecum vs. HIPAA: which wins? FLA Bar J 79:39–44, 2005

Bureau of Justice Statistics: State court caseload statistics. [Bureau of Justice Web site]. 2013. Available at: https://www.bjs.gov/index.cfm?ty=tp&tid=30. Accessed December 21, 2016.

Cavanagh ED: Federal civil litigation at the crossroads: reshaping the role of the federal courts in twenty-first century dispute resolution. Oregon Law Rev 93:631–682, 2015

Chmielewski A: Defending the preponderance of the evidence standard in college adjudications of sexual assault. Brigham Young University Education and Law Journal 2013:143–168, 2013

Cochrane RE, Herbel BL, Reardon ML, et al: The Sell effect: involuntary medication treatment is a "clear and convincing" success. Law Hum Behav 37(2):107–116, 2013 22746284

Daubert v Merrell Dow Pharmaceuticals Inc., 509 U.S. 579, 113 S.Ct. 2786 (1993)

Drogin EY, Commons ML, Gutheil TG, et al: "Certainty" and expert mental health opinions in legal proceedings. Int J Law Psychiatry 35(5–6):348–353, 2012 23022469

Evans LH: Article Eight of the Federal Rules of Evidence: the hearsay rule. Valparaiso Univ Law Rev 8:261–301, 2011

Federal Evidence Review: Federal Rules of Evidence 2015. [Federal Evidence Review Web site]. 2015. Available at: http://federalevidence.com/downloads/rules.of.evidence.pdf. Accessed December 21, 2016.

Federation of State Medical Boards: Expert witness qualifications: board by board overview [FSMB Web site]. 2016. Available at: http://www.fsmb.org/Media/Default/PDF/FSMB/Advocacy/GRPOL_ExpertWitness.pdf. Accessed December 21, 2016.

Flanders C: Toward a theory of persuasive authority. Oklahoma Law Rev 62:55–88, 2009

Frye v U.S., 54 App.D.C. 46, 293 F. 1013 (1923)

Gianelli PC: "Reasonable scientific certainty": a phrase in search of a meaning. Criminal Justice 25(1):40–41, 2010

Jaffee v Redmond, 518 U.S. 1, 116 S.Ct. 1923 (1996)

Keleher CP: When a deposition will do: overcoming the hearsay bar to deposition testimony. Mich Bar J 94:34–37, 2015

Kim J, Ryu K: Pretrial negotiation behind open doors versus closed doors. Int Rev Law Econ 20:285–294, 2000

Kumho Tire Co., Ltd. v Carmichael, 526 U.S. 137, 119 S.Ct. 1167 (1999)

Lerner RL: The rise of directed verdict. George Washington Law Rev 81:448–525, 2013

Minhas AJ: Proof beyond a reasonable doubt: shifting sands of a bedrock? North Ill Univ Law Rev 23:109–130, 2003

Pfautz MW: What would a reasonable jury do? Jury verdicts following summary judgment reversals. Columbia Law Rev 115:1255–1293, 2015

Simon RI, Shuman DW: Conducting forensic examinations on the road: are you practicing your profession without a license? J Am Acad Psychiatry Law 27(1):75–82, 1999 10212028

Stephens R: Disparities in postconviction remedies for those who plead guilty and those convicted at trial: a survey of state statutes and recommendations for reform. J Crim Law Criminol 103:309–341, 2013

Waldron J: Stare decisis and the rule of law: a layered approach. Mich Law Rev 111:1–31, 2012

Wise RK: Ending evasive responses to written discovery. Bayl Law Rev 65:510–608, 2013

CHAPTER 3

Ethics in Forensic Psychiatry

James L. Knoll IV, M.D.

Landmark Cases

Estelle v. Smith, 451 U.S. 454, 101 S.Ct. 1866 (1981)

McKune v. Lile, 536 U.S. 24, 122 S.Ct. 2017 (2002)

Clark v. Arizona, 548 U.S. 735, 126 S.Ct. 2709 (2006)

Physicians have used the term *medical ethics* to refer to principles of professional conduct owed to their patients and fellow practitioners (Stedman's Medical Dictionary 2006). *Legal ethics* have been defined as "the standards of professional conduct applicable to members of the legal profession within a given jurisdiction" (Black's Law Dictionary 2014, p. 1031). The discipline of forensic psychiatry "operates at the interface" of these "disparate disciplines—law and psychiatry—with differing objectives, philosophies, values, approaches, and methods" (Weinstock et al. 2003, p. 56).

When providing forensic services as expert witnesses for the courts, psychiatrists remove their treating hats and don the hats of forensic scientists (Strasburger et al. 1997). Medical ethical principles such as beneficence and confidentiality yield their primacy in forensic legal settings to the principles of truth, honesty, and objectivity. Forensic psychiatrists "operate outside the medical framework" when they enter the legal realm, and the ethical principles that underlie and support their practice cannot be the same as those that underlie the practice of treating clinicians (Appelbaum 1990).

As psychiatric clinical science progresses, forensic psychiatrists will have more useful knowledge to offer the courts than ever before (Appelbaum 2008). The preamble of the American Academy of Psychiatry and the Law's (AAPL's) ethical guidelines emphasizes the importance of balancing competing obligations to the individual and to society. In seeking to maintain this balance, AAPL stresses that forensic psychiatrists should be bound by the following ethical principles: 1) respect for persons, 2) honesty, 3) justice, and 4) social responsibility (American Academy of Psychiatry and the Law 2005).

Development of American Forensic Psychiatric Ethics

In the early 1980s, former American Psychiatric Association (APA) President Alan Stone, M.D., took a distinctly critical view of forensic psychiatry and challenged the profession to reflect on and develop ethical guidelines. In his 1982 AAPL address on the "ethical boundaries" of forensic psychiatry, Dr. Stone articulated multiple issues that he believed rendered forensic psychiatry inherently unreliable and ethically untenable (Stone 1984). He raised issues that forensic psychiatrists still consider carefully, including those of dual agency and the adversarial system's direct and indirect biasing effects on psychiatrists and their testimony.

Stone and others forced forensic psychiatrists to ask the question: "Is it ethical to permit oneself to deviate from the physician/healer role at all?" (Diamond 1994, p. 239). On careful reflection, refusal to deviate from that role ultimately becomes an untenable position. The fact that our legal system has a clearly stated need for competent, objective psychiatric opinions makes failure to respond to that need "irresponsible" (Diamond 1994, p. 239). It can also be argued that forensic psychiatry is ethical insofar as it recognizes every evaluee's moral worth and human dignity and acts in accordance with its duty as part of a "moral community" (Pouncey 2015).

Dr. Paul Appelbaum took up Stone's challenge by laying out a well-reasoned ethical foundation on which American forensic psychiatry could rest. Appelbaum (1990) pointed out that psychiatrists operate outside the medical framework when they choose to work in the courtroom, and thus the ethical principles that guide their behavior cannot be the same. Appelbaum (2008) observed that when forensic psychiatrists follow a responsible set of ethics principles based on commitments to telling the truth and respecting persons, they are in a better position to offer reliable and valid testimony and avoid lapsing into an advocacy role.

Stone's criticisms also led AAPL to propose formal ethics guidelines for the practice of forensic psychiatry in 1987, most recently revised in 2005 (American Academy of Psychiatry and the Law 2005). In responding to Stone's critique, the efforts of AAPL and its leaders have played a fundamental role in the evolution of the field into its current status as "multidisciplinary science" (Sadoff 2015). The practice of forensic psychiatry "demands high ethical standards and sophisticated knowledge of many aspects of psychiatry, law, ethics and public policy" (Pinals 2005, p. 322).

Basic Principles and Guidelines

The principle of "respect for persons" has been described as having respect for the human dignity of an evaluee. This guideline proscribes engaging in "deception, exploitation, or needless invasion of the privacy of the evaluee" (Appelbaum 2008, p. 197). This fundamental ethical principle "is usually laid down without conditions, raising the question of what aspect of someone's 'personhood' might deserve our unconditional respect" (Buchanan 2015, p. 12). Buchanan suggests that human dignity should garner the forensic psychiatrist's respect. The principle of respect for human dignity has the advantage of its connotation with respect for the moral worth of the evaluee while also protecting the vulnerable. Respect for persons also may refer to "not capitalizing on [the evaluee's] misunderstanding of [the forensic psychiatrist's role] and by keeping information confidential, except to the degree required by the legal process to fulfill the forensic function" (Weinstock et al. 2003, p. 57).

AAPL's ethical guidelines (American Academy of Psychiatry and the Law 2005) can be broken down into four basic tenets: 1) confidentiality, 2) consent, 3) honesty and striving for objectivity, and 4) qualifications.

Confidentiality

Protecting and maintaining patient confidentiality has been a fundamental ethical duty of physicians since the time of Hippocrates. In contrast, confidentiality in the forensic-legal setting is inherently limited. The purpose of forensic evaluation is not to provide treatment but rather an assessment that is intended to be shared with lawyers, judges, and jurors (Simon and Shuman 2007). Nevertheless, the exception to confidentiality in forensic practice is tempered by the ethical obligation to keep information not relevant to the forensic-legal question confidential (American Academy of Psychiatry and the Law 2005). Ultimately, decisions regarding the extent of confidentiality are under the control of the court and legal rules and not the evaluating or testifying psychiatrist.

Forensic psychiatrists should begin all examinations by giving warnings to examinees about these limitations on confidentiality and about the differences between a forensic and a clinical examination. At the outset of the interview, the evaluee should be told the purpose of the evaluation, including the fact that no treatment will be provided, the identity of the attorney or person for whom the examination is being conducted, and what will be done with the information obtained (American Academy of Psychiatry and the Law 2005). Evaluees also should be advised that the forensic psychiatrist cannot guarantee confidentiality but will strive to maintain the confidentiality of nonrelevant information whenever possible. All of these warnings are intended to help the examinee understand that the encounter is not being conducted for therapeutic reasons and may potentially have harmful rather than helpful results for the evaluee. When a face-to-face or telephone interview of a defendant's or an evaluee's family member, friend, or employer is legally permissible, such discussions also will require a preliminary disclosure of the limits of confidentiality.

Forensic reports should contain a *statement of nonconfidentiality* to document that all of the required disclosures were made and understood (or not) by the evaluee as well as persons contacted as collateral sources of information. After completion of the forensic evaluation, information not relevant to the forensic-legal question, especially sensitive information, should be excluded from the report. Furthermore, such information should not be disclosed to colleagues or to the public, because it would constitute an ethical breach of confidentiality and may create legal liability for the forensic psychiatrist (Binder 2002).

Despite the nonconfidentiality warnings and explanations of the purpose of the forensic evaluation, some evaluees may have a tendency to "slip" back into relating to the examiner as a treating physician. Therefore, forensic evaluators may need to stop the interview periodically and repeat the warnings described earlier to reinforce the forensic nature of the evaluation. Ethical practice requires that forensic psychiatrists remain vigilant throughout the evaluation for signs that the evaluee is slipping away from a proper understanding of the forensic psychiatrist's role and reinforce the nature of the evaluation as often as necessary.

Concerns about an evaluee's slippage into a "therapeutic" manner of relating to a forensic evaluator raise the question of the proper interview style in a forensic evaluation. The quality and quantity of data obtained from the forensic evaluation may depend on the rapport established with the evaluee and the interview style of the examiner. Therefore, the question of type and degree of empathy in a forensic evaluation becomes a profound concern.

The concept of *forensic empathy* has been defined as a state of "awareness of the perspectives and experiences" of evaluees in order to allow them to express concerns appropriately during the evaluation (Appelbaum 2010, p. 44). Glancy et al. (2015, p. 12) observed, "Some support is necessary, for example, in ensuring the comfort of the evaluee. Likewise, empathy is not entirely off limits in a forensic assessment." Nevertheless, forensic interview style requires vigilance and balance. Clinical skills must be tempered by respect for the evaluee. For example, communicating too much empathy, giving interpretations, or offering advice risks implying a therapeutic relationship that may be misleading to the evaluee, even if inadvertent (Glancy et al. 2015).

Consent

The right to consent, an attribute of personal autonomy, is a fundamental principle of medical ethics. The doctrine of informed consent requires that the individual possess 1) voluntariness of choice, 2) understanding and access to the relevant information, and 3) mental competence to make the decision at issue (Appelbaum 2007). Breach of informed consent when evaluation and treatment are provided may be actionable as malpractice. In obtaining informed consent from a forensic evaluee, evaluators should assess whether the evaluee possesses the ability to

- Understand information relevant to the decision.
- Appreciate the situation and its consequences.
- Manipulate relevant information rationally.
- Express a stable, voluntary choice. (Appelbaum 2007)

The informed consent of forensic evaluees should be obtained when necessary and feasible. In the event that evaluees refuse to participate in the evaluation, they should be informed that this fact will be included in a report or testimony. If forensic examiners suspect an evaluee is not competent to give consent, they should follow the appropriate laws of the jurisdiction. In many court-ordered evaluations (such as competency to stand trial or involuntary commitment), neither the evaluee's assent nor his or her informed consent is required. Nevertheless, if the evaluee is too impaired to give consent, this should be documented in the forensic report.

In the absence of a court order, forensic psychiatrists retained by the prosecution should not evaluate defendants if they have not yet had the opportunity to consult with their defense attorneys. In the case of *Estelle v. Smith* (1981), the U.S. Supreme Court held that the defendant's Sixth Amendment rights were violated, in part, because he was evaluated by the prosecution expert before he had a chance to consult with counsel. This ethical principle becomes particularly important when a defendant 1) has been charged with a criminal act; 2) is being held in government custody or detention; or 3) is being interrogated for criminal or quasi-criminal conduct, hostile acts against a government, or immigration violations. In contrast, evaluations for the purpose of making diagnostic and treatment recommendations are not prohibited by these restrictions. Examples include civil commitment evaluations, risk management assessments, and conditional release evaluations from secure forensic facilities.

Honesty and Striving for Objectivity

Federal Rule of Evidence 702, which governs the admissibility of all types of evidence in federal cases, indicates that the role of expert witnesses is to "assist the trier of fact to understand the evidence or to determine a fact in issue" (Federal Criminal Code and Rules 1995). Forensic psychiatrists, as expert witnesses, subscribe to the principles of honesty and of striving for objectivity (American Academy of Psychiatry and the Law 2005). They are expected to use reliable methods, analyses, and reasoning to arrive at their opinions. As part of ongoing performance improvement, forensic psychiatrists should engage in continued monitoring of the quality and objectivity of their own work. For example, Appelbaum (2008) has recommended adoption of a peer review model, in addition to continuing training in ethics for forensic psychiatrists.

In *Clark v. Arizona* (2006), the U.S. Supreme Court recognized that forensic psychiatrists must move from methods and concepts designed for treatment to legal concepts such as those relevant to determinations of insanity. This "leap" from one discipline to another requires cautious, objective judgment. Facts should be distinguished from impressions, relevant collateral data should be reviewed, and opinions should be well supported with factual data.

A forensic psychiatrist's honesty and objectivity "may be called into question" if an expert opinion is given without the expert psychiatrist first performing a personal examination in cases that require one (Glancy et al. 2015). Although opinions in malpractice cases involving suicide may rely primarily on record reviews, examinations of competency or sanity generally require a face-to-face evaluation. In some cases, a personal evaluation may not be possible for a variety of legal or practical reasons. Nevertheless, reasonable efforts should be made to conduct a personal evaluation. When a personal evaluation cannot be conducted, the forensic psychiatrist is obligated to clearly state the lack of a personal evaluation as a limitation to his or her opinions.

Before formally beginning a case, the forensic examiner and retaining party should clearly understand the fee arrangements. Contingency fee arrangements are unethical for forensic psychiatrists, because they can exert a biasing pressure. Contingency fees make the forensic psychiatrist's financial remuneration dependent on the outcome of a case. This presents a scenario in which the forensic psychiatrist may easily become financially invested in the outcome, resulting in a loss of objectivity. To avoid this ethical pitfall, forensic psychiatrists charge fees based on the time spent on a case, and their opinions should not be or appear to be influenced by payment or final case outcome.

Similarly, forensic psychiatrists may become labeled, either rightly or wrongly, as either prosecution/plaintiff- or defense-oriented expert witnesses. The ethical expert witness should be open to working for either side. When the forensic psychiatrist is "offering an unbiased opinion (which we usually assume to be the case), then one can work for either side" (Sadoff and Dattilio 2008, p. 170). When forensic examiners recognize a personal bias that creates an ethical conflict, they should consider consultation with a colleague or declining to work on the case.

In the United States, trials are adversarial, and attorneys are taught and encouraged to be "zealous advocates" of the causes and clients they represent. Treating clinicians are also ethically required to be advocates for their patient's best mental health interests. Forensic psychiatry requires a transition from the partisan clinical stance (that may even be encouraged by the ethical and practical stance of the attorneys) to the neutral stance of the psychiatrist. To maintain ethical standards, the forensic psychiatrist must resist the temptation to accept an advocate's role (American Academy of Psychiatry and the Law 2005; McGarry and Curran 1980).

Two models have been proposed for ethical expert testimony: the *advocate for truth model* and the *honest advocate model* (Gutheil 1998). In the advocate for truth model, the expert becomes a completely neutral observer and adheres to absolute truth during testimony. In contrast, the honest advocate model holds that being a persuasive advocate, after forming an objective opinion, is acceptable when operating in an adversarial system. However, the expert must be honest about the limits of testimony and remain truthful on cross-examination. In actual practice, most experts adopt a combination of these two models.

Some forensic psychiatrists may take the position that advocacy is always unethical, whereas AAPL has followed the view that advocacy is permissible, and advocacy for an opinion may even be desirable. Identification with a cause and even bias are not always unethical in and of themselves, and some emotionality and bias may be inevitable. However, "bias must be openly acknowledged and must not lead to distortion, dishonesty, or failure to strive to reach an objective opinion" (Candilis et al. 2007, p. 47). The important distinction made here is that the expert is advocating "for an opinion, rather than a client" (Candilis et al. 2007, p. 88).

Novice forensic psychiatrists, attempting to achieve this neutral stance, may find that "attorneys frequently expect outright cheerleading from their expert" (Candilis et al. 2007, p. 88). Because attorneys are held to an ethic of active advocacy, they may not always appreciate a more objective perspective from their expert witness and may exert pressure on the forensic expert to adopt more of an advocacy role. The forensic psychiatrist's adherence to either the advocate for truth model or the honest advocate model in such situations shows his or her integrity and commitment to the ethics of the field.

The assumption that the forensic psychiatrist can be absolutely impartial is unrealistic. To guard against or minimize bias, the forensic psychiatrist should strive to approach a case with an impartial attitude. Once a comprehensive analysis has produced a well-reasoned, objective opinion, it becomes natural to identify with that opinion. On taking the witness stand, the expert must strive to impartially preserve the truth. Relevant information may not be kept secret (Halleck et al. 1984).

Experts also should guard against a sense of "loyalty" to the retaining attorney, which might cause a shift from objective expert to advocate. Blatant advocacy is easily recognized by the trier of fact, and experts should not go beyond the available data or the scholarly foundations of their testimony (Brodsky and Poythress 1985; Gutheil and Dattilio 2008). Ethical forensic psychiatrists can enhance their credibility by appropriately acknowledging facts of the case that are unfavorable to their opinions, the limitations of their opinions, and hypothetical situations under which their opinions would be different (Gutheil 1998).

Perhaps the most pejorative stigma associated with forensic psychiatry is the perception of the expert witness as a "hired gun," that is, an expert who, in exchange for large fees, is willing to testify to whatever opinion best serves the party paying those fees. This issue has long been considered one of the foremost problems associated with the practice of forensic psychiatry. At times, the perception of psychiatric expert witnesses as hired guns has seemed to threaten the credibility of the entire profession, especially when the term is raised in the wake of high-profile cases (Mossman 1999).

In certain cases, it may be "difficult to distinguish honest bias, sometimes even unconscious, from a 'hired gun'" (Weinstock et al. 2003, p. 64). For example, commonly observed reasons that psychiatrists intentionally or unintentionally express bias can include the desire for a "just" outcome or having an "agenda" of bringing public attention to the mental condition at issue. Nevertheless, under AAPL's ethical tenet of honesty and striving for objectivity, practices such as "selling opinions" and the deliberate distortion of data are clearly unethical. The forensic psychiatrist "must clearly distinguish between his own idiosyncratic views and that of the scientific community" (Diamond 1994, p. 124).

One primary concern about the ethics of forensic psychiatry involves the dilemma of dual agency, that is, the tension between the psychiatrist's obligation of beneficence toward patients and the conflicting obligations to the legal system (Stone 1984). Dual agency concerns inevitably arise in situations in which the psychiatrist acts as both treating physician and forensic evaluator (Strasburger et al. 1997). AAPL's ethical guidelines warn that treating psychiatrists should "generally avoid acting as an expert witness for their patients or performing evaluations of their patients for legal purposes" (American Academy of Psychiatry and the Law 2005).

Attorneys and judges often believe that the treating psychiatrist is in the best position to serve as an expert witness. This mistaken assumption rests on the notion that the treating psychiatrist has spent the most time with the individual and therefore would be expected to "best" explain a defendant's actions or mental status or causation and damages in a personal injury claim. However, this assumption contains many fallacies of which legal professionals are typically unaware.

Independent forensic evaluators are in fact generally better suited than treating psychiatrists to evaluate an individual for forensic-legal purposes. For example, treating psychiatrists must necessarily accept the patient's subjective psychic reality and work with it for the benefit of the patient. Treating psychiatrists usually will not threaten the therapeutic relationship by compromising confidentiality, which is easily breached by gathering collateral data from the patient's friends, family, and coworkers. In addition, treating psychiatrists see patients on multiple occasions over time but only in a clinical setting and know only what their patients tell them. In contrast, forensic psychiatrists have the opportunity to obtain data about the evaluee from many sources in varied settings and are not limited to the evaluee's perspective or the information the evaluee is willing to share. Table 3–1 summarizes the areas of role conflict that arises when a treating psychiatrist functions as an expert witness.

Attorneys sometime seek to have a treating psychiatrist who was to appear as a "fact" witness sworn in or "tendered" as an expert witness. The AAPL's ethical guidelines (American Academy of Psychiatry and the Law 2005) caution that treating psychiatrists should remain vigilant for this scenario, because it may result in the unnecessary disclosure of private information or the possible misinterpretation of fact testimony as "expert" opinion.

When a treating psychiatrist testifies in court, even as a fact witness, role conflict might be clinically detrimental to the patient (Strasburger 1999; Strasburger et al. 1997). The treating psychiatrist has formed a relationship with the patient based on the understanding that the information provided by the patient will be confidential. The treatment relationship may be seriously and irrevocably damaged should confidential information be revealed in court by the patient's treating psychiatrist (Perlin et al. 2008). Another potential adverse outcome can arise if the patient does not obtain a favorable outcome and blames the treating psychiatrist. In such a scenario, the therapeutic alliance is also likely to be damaged.

AAPL's ethical guidelines acknowledge that in some limited circumstances, the dual role may be unavoidable. For example, in certain areas, a lack of availability of forensic services may necessitate a forensic evaluation by the treating psychiatrist (American Academy of Psychiatry and the Law 2005). Other examples in which the dual role, although not ideal, may be permissible include workers' compensation cases, disability evaluations, civil commitment cases, and guardianship hearings. Nevertheless, the professional consensus of opinion and ethical guidelines indicate that dual roles, particularly that of treatment provider and expert witness, should be avoided whenever possible.

Qualifications

Before accepting a case, forensic psychiatrists should determine whether they have the proper knowledge, skill, experience, training, or education required for the particular forensic-legal question under consideration. An expert's qualifications can be, and often are, vigorously challenged during cross-examination by opposing counsel. In addition to the routine probing questions about the expert's curriculum vitae (CV), licensing, education, training, and publications, opposing counsel is likely to ask experts about their actual experience dealing with the subject matter at issue. This may present a significant problem if the expert's experience does not match the issues in question in the case at hand.

The expert should ask himself or herself some basic questions to determine whether he or she is qualified for a particular case:

- Is the case actually within the expert's area of expertise?
- How much clinical experience does the expert have with the subject matter under consideration?
- Does the expert have the proper training and certification?
- Does the expert understand the legal question and legal standards at issue?
- Has the expert published in the area under consideration?

TABLE 3–1.   **Treating psychiatrist versus expert witness: areas of potential role conflict**

Treating psychiatrist	Expert witness
Natural bias in favor of patient's best interests	Trained to maintain neutral position
Possible reduced objectivity because of bias in favor of patient	Maximized objectivity, as required by ethical guidelines
Unlikely to seek or to have access to multiple sources of data because of issues of confidentiality	Required to seek multiple sources of data
Less likely to challenge patient's self-report or version of events	More likely to challenge evaluee's self-report and version of events based on collateral data
More likely to lead to breach of patient confidentiality	Lack of confidentiality inherent; evaluee clearly informed about the lack of confidentiality
Adverse effects on therapeutic relationship	No therapeutic relationship to compromise

- Does the jurisdiction in which the expert is to testify have statutes outlining the percentage of time an expert is allowed to perform expert witness work, and does the expert meet the criteria?
- Does the expert have critical biases or conflicts of interest?

Psychiatrists should make certain that their credentials accurately reflect their expertise, as attorneys are advised to routinely 1) verify the accuracy of the expert's CV; 2) inquire about the expert's membership in professional organizations; 3) verify accreditation and reputation of any institution from which an expert's degree has been claimed; and 4) contact the state licensing board to verify the license issue date, status, and credentials (Sadoff and Dattilio 2008).

If a court finds a psychiatrist "not qualified" for a particular case, this becomes a matter of public record that may then be used against the expert in future cases. To avoid this problem and to abide by the AAPL ethical guideline of claiming expertise "only in areas of actual knowledge, skills, training, and experience" (American Academy of Psychiatry and the Law

2005), experts should take care to stay within their areas of expertise when accepting a case. This recommendation may be more obvious for cases that clearly involve special expertise, such as the evaluation of children, correctional mental health issues, or the evaluation of persons from other cultures. However, it may be less clear in cases in which the expert has had some limited amount of involvement with the issue in question. In such instances, referring the case to a colleague who does possess the necessary expertise may be the most prudent course of action.

Evolving Areas of Ethical Inquiry

Death Penalty Concerns

In 2001, the AAPL Executive Council formally endorsed a moratorium on the use of capital punishment

> at least until death penalty jurisdictions implement policies and procedures that: A) Ensure that death penalty cases are administered fairly and

impartially in accordance with basic due process; and B) Prevent the execution of mentally disabled persons and people who were under the age of 18 at the time of their offenses. (Norko 2004, p. 178)

Despite this position, diverse opinions exist about the ethical permissibility of psychiatrists' participation in death penalty cases (see Chapter 20, "Psychiatry and the Death Penalty").

Interrogations

AAPL's ethical guidelines are clear that a psychiatrist's participation in procedures that constitute torture is unethical. Both the APA and the American Medical Association have issued position statements that prohibit psychiatrists from "direct participation" in interrogations (American Medical Association 2015; American Psychiatric Association 2006). The APA defines participation as being present, asking or suggesting questions, or offering advice to interrogators. Military forensic psychiatrists may have different mandates on this issue according to the U.S. Department of Defense (Marks and Bloche 2008) and might consider consulting with colleagues and/or the AAPL ethics panel when military and APA ethical guidelines present a dilemma (see Chapter 31, "Military Forensic Psychiatry" for further discussion).

Corrections

In correctional settings, the restriction of liberty presents many complex ethical challenges (Trestman 2014). Indeed, the forensic psychiatrist may encounter many evolving ethical and human rights issues in correctional settings. These include the use of punitive isolation, reporting inmate abuse, and dual agency conflicts. The proposed purposes of incarceration are sometimes contradictory and ambig-

uous. The roles of forensic psychiatrists working in corrections also may be ambiguous, with conflict between forensic and treatment duties (see Chapters 21, "Correctional Settings and Prisoner Rights," and 22, "Psychiatric Treatment in Correctional Settings").

Isolation units in prisons remain the subject of contentious debate (Goode 2012). Although the degree of isolation usually varies, the most extreme form consists of near total sensory deprivation by lack of access to light, sound, or fresh air. The more standard form consists of single cells in which inmates spend 23 hours a day with limited access to outside light and air. No judicial decision has found that isolation, even long term, is unconstitutional per se. However, several decisions bar or limit its use for those with serious mental illness (*Austin v. Wilkinson* 2002; *Jones 'El v. Barge* 2001; *Madrid v. Gomez* 1995).

The American Bar Association Standards have described the isolation of inmates with serious mental illness as "simply inhumane" (American Bar Association 2011). Various states have adopted exclusionary rules for vulnerable populations, including those with serious mental illness, in their policy and procedures. However, such rules commonly fall short of being effective in real-world practice and conditions. The forensic psychiatrist working in a correctional setting may be confronted with the dilemma of whether to report inappropriate use of punitive isolation or may be asked to testify at a disciplinary hearing of a mentally ill inmate facing punitive isolation.

The National Commission on Correctional Health Care (2016) has issued a position statement that states that prolonged (greater than 15 consecutive days) solitary confinement is cruel, inhuman, and degrading treatment and harmful to an individual's health. The position statement also calls for mentally ill inmates to be excluded from solitary confinement altogether. Additionally, psychiatrists should evaluate individuals in solitary confinement on placement and on a daily basis and advocate for removal if individuals' medical or mental health deteriorates (National Commission on Correctional Health Care 2016).

The issue of how, and under what circumstances, a correctional psychiatrist should report inmate abuse has seldom been formally addressed (Knoll 2014). The issue may raise concerns about correctional staff morale, retaliation, and safety of the psychiatrist. In contrast, American Medical Association and APA ethical guidelines seem to be manifestly incompatible with ignoring the abuse of inmates, particularly inmate-patients, by another correctional mental health "team member." Yet the fact that psychiatrists may find themselves concerned about their physical safety for acting ethically and professionally suggests a more serious underlying issue: the correctional culture that embraces physical and mental abuse as a tolerable side effect of retribution.

Traditionally, correctional administrators and security staff have assumed full responsibility for the prevention of institutional violence (Pont et al. 2015). This has left psychiatrists out of the dialogue and problem-solving process. Because the forensic psychiatrist is uniquely qualified to assist in identifying and preventing violence, a future challenge will be for forensic psychiatrists to assume more of a leadership role in correctional multidisciplinary efforts to prevent violence.

Sex Offender Treatment

In *McKune v. Lile* (2002), the Supreme Court held that Kansas's Sexual Abuse Treatment Program did not violate inmate-patients' Fifth Amendment rights by requiring them to divulge details of all prior sexual offenses, even those for which they were not charged. This "admission of responsibility" was not privileged, and refusal to participate resulted in reduced privileges. Although the Court based its reasoning on the compelling interests of penological purposes, the ruling created a confusing dichotomy that pits beneficence and nonmalfeasance (in a treatment context) against community protection interests (Birgden and Cucolo 2011).

Sex offenders receiving treatment have obvious motivations for restricting or censoring themselves during therapy, and *McKune* has greatly accentuated these motivations. Furthermore, such patients' denial of their offenses may be a result of distorted cognitions and/or maladaptive defenses (Levenson 2011). These and other complexities of sex offender treatment have led some in the field to suggest that a separate set of ethical guidelines, outside of traditional psychotherapy, should be adopted (Mela and Ahmed 2014).

Conclusion

Since Stone's 1984 clarion call, forensic psychiatry has crafted a system of ethics, the evolution of which has been both disciplined and principled (Candilis et al. 2007). Indeed, "mindful and intelligent evolution is in the best tradition of academic scholarship. It is a method for fine-tuning arguments, receiving feedback, and contributing to the evolution of professional discourse" (Candilis et al. 2007, p. 176). In response to Stone's critique, the discipline of forensic psychiatry listened, analyzed, and deliberated before proceeding to outline a clear and reasonable set of ethical principles.

To practice forensic psychiatry is to engage in Stone's "moral adventure," while treading across the psychiatric razor's edge of sociolegal culture, a task that demands a vigilant concern for ethical principles.

Key Concepts

- Forensic psychiatrists should adhere to the following ethical principles, as outlined by the American Academy of Psychiatry and the Law (2005): 1) respect for persons, 2) honesty, 3) justice, and 4) social responsibility.

- Serious conflicts of interest may arise when a psychiatrist acts as both forensic evaluator and treating psychiatrist. If at all possible, this type of dual agency should be avoided.

- Forensic psychiatrists do not distort data and should concede the current limits of the psychiatric science at issue.

- Forensic examinations should begin with warnings to evaluees about limitations on confidentiality and about the differences between a forensic and a clinical examination.

- Before accepting a case, forensic psychiatrists should determine whether they have the proper knowledge, skill, experience, training, or education required for the particular forensic-legal question under consideration.

References

American Academy of Psychiatry and the Law: Ethics Guidelines for the Practice of Forensic Psychiatry. May 2005. Available at: http://www.aapl.org/ethics.htm. Accessed December 19, 2016.

American Bar Association: American Bar Association Standards for Criminal Justice: Treatment of Prisoners, 3rd Edition. Chicago, IL, American Bar Association, 2011

American Medical Association: The AMA Code of Medical Ethics' Opinion on Interrogation of Detainees. Opinion 2.068—Physician Participation in Interrogation. AMA Journal of Ethics 17(10):922–923, 2015. Available at: http://journalofethics.ama-assn.org/2015/10/coet1-1510.html. Accessed May 5, 2017.

American Psychiatric Association: Psychiatric participation in interrogation of detainees: position statement, 2006. Available at: http://archive.psych.org/edu/other_res/lib_archives/archives/200601.pdf. Accessed December 21, 2016.

Appelbaum KL: Commentary: the art of forensic report writing. J Am Acad Psychiatry Law 38(1):43–45, 2010 20305073

Appelbaum PS: The parable of the forensic psychiatrist: ethics and the problem of doing harm. Int J Law Psychiatry 13(4):249–259, 1990 2286491

Appelbaum PS: Clinical practice. Assessment of patients' competence to consent to treatment. N Engl J Med 357(18):1834–1840, 2007 17978292

Appelbaum PS: Ethics and forensic psychiatry: translating principles into practice. J Am Acad Psychiatry Law 36(2):195–200, 2008 18583695

Austin v Wilkinson, 4:01-CV-71 ND Ohio (2002)

Binder RL: Liability for the psychiatrist expert witness. Am J Psychiatry 159(11):1819–1825, 2002 12411212

Birgden A, Cucolo H: The treatment of sex offenders: evidence, ethics, and human rights. Sex Abuse 23(3):295–313, 2011 20937793

Black's Law Dictionary, 10th Edition. Edited by Garner B. St. Paul, MN, Thomson Reuters, 2014, p 1031

Brodsky SL, Poythress NG: Expertise on the witness stand: a practitioner's guide, in Psychology, Psychiatry, and the Law. Edited by Ewing CP. Sarasota, FL, Professional Resource Exchange, 1985, pp 389–411

Buchanan A: Respect for dignity and forensic psychiatry. Int J Law Psychiatry 41:12–17, 2015 25888501

Candilis P, Weinstock R, Martinez R: Forensic Ethics and the Expert Witness. New York, Springer Science, 2007

Clark v Arizona, 548 U.S. 735, 126 S.Ct. 2709 (2006)

Diamond B: The Psychiatrist in the Courtroom: Selected Papers of Bernard L. Diamond, M.D. Hillsdale, NJ, Analytic Press, 1994

Estelle v Smith, 451 U.S. 454, 101 S.Ct. 1866 (1981)

Federal Criminal Code and Rules: Testimony by Experts Rule 702. St. Paul, MN, West Publishing, 1995

Glancy GD, Ash P, Bath EP, et al: AAPL practice guideline for the forensic assessment. J Am Acad Psychiatry Law 43(2, suppl):S3–S53, 2015 26054704

Goode E: Prisons rethink isolation, saving money, lives and sanity. The New York Times, March 10, 2012. Available at: http://www.nytimes.com/2012/03/11/us/rethinking-solitary-confinement.html. Accessed December 21, 2016.

Gutheil T: The Psychiatrist as Expert Witness. Washington, DC, American Psychiatric Press, 1998

Gutheil T, Dattilio F: Practical Approaches to Forensic Mental Health Testimony. Philadelphia, PA, Lippincott Williams & Wilkins, 2008

Halleck SL, Appelbaum P, Rappeport JR, et al: Psychiatry in the Sentencing Process. Washington, DC, American Psychiatric Association, 1984

Jones 'El v Berge, 164 F Supp 2d 1096 (WD Wis 2001)

Knoll J: The psychiatrist's obligation: same as it ever was. Correctional Mental Health Report 15:69–70, 2014

Levenson JS: "But I didn't do it!": ethical treatment of sex offenders in denial. Sex Abuse 23(3):346–364, 2011 20937795

Madrid v Gomez, 889 F Supp 1146 (ND Cal 1995)

Marks JH, Bloche MG: The ethics of interrogation—the U.S. military's ongoing use of psychiatrists. N Engl J Med 359(11):1090–1092, 2008 18784097

McGarry AL, Curran WJ: Courtroom presentation of psychiatric and psychological evidence, in Modern Legal Medicine, Psychiatry, and Forensic Science. Edited by Curran WJ, McGarry AL, Petty CS. Philadelphia, PA, FA Davis, 1980, pp 963–987

McKune v Lile, 536 U.S. 24, 122 S.Ct. 2017 (2002)

Mela M, Ahmed AG: Ethics and the treatment of sexual offenders. Psychiatr Clin North Am 37(2):239–250, 2014 24877710

Mossman D: "Hired guns," "whores," and "prostitutes": case law references to clinicians of ill repute. J Am Acad Psychiatry Law 27(3):414–425, 1999 10509941

National Commission on Correctional Health Care: Position Statement on Solitary Confinement (Isolation). Adopted by the National Commission on Correctional Health Care Board of Directors April 10, 2016. Available at: http://www.ncchc.org/solitary-confinement. Accessed December 21, 2016.

Norko MA: Organized psychiatry and the death penalty: an introduction to the special section. J Am Acad Psychiatry Law 32(2):178–179, 2004 15281421

Perlin M, Bursztajn H, Gledhill K, et al: Psychiatric ethics and the rights of persons with mental disabilities in institutions and the community, in From Informed Consent to Conflicts of Interest to Informed Consent. Haifa, Israel, UNESCO Chair in Bioethics, 2008, pp 113–115

Pinals DA: Forensic psychiatry fellowship training: developmental stages as an educational framework. J Am Acad Psychiatry Law 33(3):317–323, 2005 16186194

Pont J, Stöver H, Gétaz L, et al: Prevention of violence in prison—the role of health care professionals. J Forensic Leg Med 34:127–132, 2015 26165671

Pouncey C: Forensic psychiatric ethics: a return to the ivory tower, in The Evolution of Forensic Psychiatry: History, Current Developments, Future Directions. Edited by Sadoff R. New York, Oxford University Press, 2015, pp 213–220

Sadoff R (ed): The Evolution of Forensic Psychiatry: History, Current Developments, Future Directions. New York, Oxford University Press, 2015

Sadoff R, Dattilio F: Crime and Mental Illness: A Guide to Courtroom Practice. Mechanicsburg, PA, PBI Press, 2008

Simon R, Shuman D: Clinical Manual of Psychiatry and Law. Washington, DC, American Psychiatric Publishing, 2007

Stedman's Medical Dictionary, 28th Edition. Baltimore, MD, Lippincott Williams & Wilkins, 2006

Stone AA: The ethical boundaries of forensic psychiatry: a view from the ivory tower. Bull Am Acad Psychiatry Law 12(3):209–219, 1984 6478062

Strasburger LH: The litigant-patient: mental health consequences of civil litigation. J Am Acad Psychiatry Law 27(2):203–211, 1999 10400429

Strasburger LH, Gutheil TG, Brodsky A: On wearing two hats: role conflict in serving as both psychotherapist and expert witness. Am J Psychiatry 154(4):448–456, 1997 9090330

Trestman RL: Ethics, the law, and prisoners: protecting society, changing human behavior, and protecting human rights. J Bioeth Inq 11(3):311–318, 2014 24996632

Weinstock R, Leong G, Silva J: Ethical guidelines, in Principles and Practice of Forensic Psychiatry, 2nd Edition. Edited by Rosner R. New York, Hodder Arnold, 2003, pp 56–72

CHAPTER 4

Forensic Evaluations and Reports

Graham D. Glancy, M.B., Ch.B., FRCPsych, FRCPC

The basic competencies of forensic psychiatry include conducting an evaluation, writing a forensic report, and testifying at trial. Each of these competencies has its own skill set, and the forensic psychiatrist must be competent in all three because poor performance at any stage will adversely affect the end product. In this chapter, I provide an overview of forensic evaluation and report writing and discuss concepts that can be applied to different types of civil and criminal forensic assessment.

Distinctiveness of the Forensic Evaluation and Report

Several distinctive characteristics characterize forensic evaluations and reports, distinguishing them from a general psychiatric assessment. First, the ethical foundation of the forensic evaluation differs from that of evaluations conducted for

treatment purposes (see Chapter 3, "Ethics in Forensic Psychiatry"). Second, forensic evaluators must be aware that evaluees' accounts of their histories may be inaccurate and therefore must carefully consider the possibility of dissimulation and malingering (see Chapter 6, "Evaluation of Malingering"). For this reason, greater emphasis is sometimes placed on gathering collateral information, as discussed later in this chapter (see subsection "Gathering Information"). Finally, attention to physical safety, interview style, and confidentiality and informed consent also differ somewhat from that in psychiatric evaluations conducted for treatment purposes.

Assessment Process

Style of Interview

Generally speaking, open-ended questions are preferable in forensic evaluations, bearing in mind that the evaluator is striving for objectivity and honesty (Glancy and Saini 2009; Glancy et al. 2015). Open-ended questions generally begin with who, what, why, how, or similar phrases such as "please tell me about" or "please explain." The use of open-ended questions ensures that the evaluator is not suggesting answers to the evaluee and thus enables a neutral exploration of the evaluee's narrative and state of mind. This style of inquiry also may make evaluees feel more comfortable and believe that their voice is being heard.

Leading questions requiring a yes or no answer may be used if no alternative appears likely to obtain specific information required in the assessment, such as a review of systems or some parts of the mental status examination. However, leading questions have certain disadvantages, in that they can give the appearance of suggesting or actually suggest an answer to the evaluee. More directive leading questions, such as "Was anyone with you when you assaulted Mr. Jones?," may cause the evaluee to feel threatened or cornered.

In contrast to the general psychiatric interview, forensic evaluators adopt a neutral approach toward evaluees (Wettstein 2010). Forensic evaluators are not unduly empathic, judgmental, or biased against the evaluee. Evaluators should guard against these stances by monitoring their emotional reactions to evaluees and ensuring that their manner is professional but not unduly empathic or challenging.

Some empathy and support in a forensic evaluation may be appropriate. Appelbaum (2010) described a type of forensic empathy, wherein evaluators are aware of the perspective and experience of the evaluee. For instance, when assessing physicians in relation to disciplinary proceedings from their licensing bodies, an acknowledgment of the evaluee's distress (e.g., "It must be very difficult to be sit-

ting on that side of the desk instead of on this side as you usually are") is sometimes appropriate. Overemotional responses in evaluators and preoccupations with an examinee may be indicators of inappropriate countertransference of which the examiner should be aware (Gutheil and Simon 2002).

Physical Setting

Forensic evaluations take place in multiple settings ranging from jails or detention centers to a psychiatrist's private office to, at times, an attorney's office. Forensic evaluators should prioritize their own comfort and safety because absence of these can affect the objectivity of the assessment. The evaluator therefore should consider strategies for ensuring his or her own comfort and safety, including having a colleague present, leaving the door open, or having a third party at hand.

Ideally, evaluators and evaluees should be seated at an equal distance from, and with clear access to, the door. This arrangement facilitates either the examiner's or the evaluee's safe exit from the room in the event that either party feels a precipitous need to leave. Correctional facilities may make this ideal arrangement more complicated, because the type of office available and the furniture arrangement may be out of the evaluator's control. Every effort should be made to ensure that the confidentiality of evaluees is preserved but not at the expense of the physical safety of evaluators.

Recording

Documenting the interview in some way is necessary, and attention should be paid to the presence and arrangement of a desk or table and of lighting, if possible. Detailed note taking during the interview is often considered sufficient. However, some evaluators use audio or video recording. The evaluator should be aware that notes and recordings may be requested by the referring attorney or the court and will constitute part of the record.

The American Academy of Psychiatry and the Law (AAPL) has indicated that recording an interview is acceptable but not mandatory (American Academy of Psychiatry and the Law 1999). Audio or video recording creates a complete record of the interview, which may be most useful in a criminal case when an evaluee with a disturbed mental state was seen immediately after the alleged crime. The recording can be reviewed sometime later, perhaps at a time when the evaluee has recovered from his or her mental illness, immediately prior to trial or at trial. The obverse situation also may occur, in which an evaluee who was not psychotic in an interview immediately after an incident becomes psychotic by the time of trial.

Video recording in these situations may significantly enhance the credibility of the testimony. The pros and cons of recording are discussed in the AAPL Task Force report (American Academy of Psychiatry and the Law 1999). Evaluators should be aware that recordings could demonstrate stylistic problems, such as the use of leading questions, which could damage evaluators' credibility. On the contrary, recordings can protect evaluators against claims of inappropriate behaviors. As a practical matter, recording may produce logistical problems, such as finding suitable interview locations, correcting inadequate lighting, and taking equipment into jails or prisons. Evaluees should give consent to recording as part of the informed consent process.

Assessments Without an Interview

Certain situations require that evaluators conduct assessments without an interview (e.g., suicide malpractice cases, psychological autopsies, and testamentary capacity cases in which the evaluee is deceased). At times, in criminal cases, evaluators are retained by the prosecution but are declined access to the evaluee and are limited to a record review. The AAPL ethics guidelines state that appropriate efforts should be made to conduct a personal examination, but if not possible, evaluators may nevertheless come to certain conclusions. In these cases, evaluators should state that no personal examination took place and note limitations, if any, to the opinions rendered (American Academy of Psychiatry and the Law 2005).

Gathering Information

Evaluators must decide, based on their own judgment and experience, whether to begin the interview by asking about the critical forensic issue. In some cases, delaying inquiry into this issue until later in the evaluation process may be a better strategy. This strategy allows the examiner to establish rapport before discussing more sensitive material. For instance, when asking an evaluee about a particular trauma in a psychiatric injury case, a delay in discussing this issue may be best so as not to cause the evaluee to become upset immediately. By asking other necessary questions first, such as those regarding personal history, the evaluee may feel a little more trusting and relaxed and thus be able to build up to talking about the particularly emotional issue. In other cases, beginning with the major issue, before the evaluee becomes bored and irritable, may be best.

When asking about a significant traumatic event, the duration and amount of trauma and the evaluee's perception of the event are generally discussed. Forensic evaluators may have to spend extra time discussing this subject in order to elicit significant details. When asking about the effect of the trauma, it may be helpful to ask about the immediate effects within the first month; the medium-term effects from 1 month to 1 year after the incident; and the long-term effects lasting longer than 1 year (Glancy et al. 2015).

Conceptualizing claims of emotional damage into categories of social functioning, occupational functioning, and psychological functioning can be helpful. Each domain of functioning may be covered and carefully asked about. Evaluators might question inconsistencies with collateral information and seek an explanation for these inconsistencies. Evaluators should inquire about regular activities such as the activities of daily living. Evaluators also should conduct a separate line of inquiry about other potential stressors and the effect of these on social, occupational, and psychological functioning.

In some criminal cases (e.g., insanity), forensic psychiatrists generally undertake careful questioning about the exact circumstances leading up to an offense. Asking about the evaluee's thoughts and feelings at the material time may be necessary to decide which particular psychological motive was operant. This may require patience and perseverance because the evaluee may try to avoid discussing unpleasant or emotionally charged topics.

The purpose of the insanity evaluation is to determine whether the defendant's thoughts and behaviors at the time of the alleged offense are consistent with the mental impairments necessary to meet the statutory definition of insanity particular to that jurisdiction. Evaluators may ask evaluees whether they knew the act was legally and morally wrong, whether they were laboring under a delusion, or whether they were capable of making a rational choice. Evaluators need to en-

courage evaluees to answer these questions, but evaluators should be certain not to suggest answers or ask leading questions in this crucial area.

Forensic evaluations need these details and very often take much longer than psychiatric consultations conducted for treatment purposes. Keeping evaluees on topic and concentrating on unpleasant issues is sometimes difficult. In other types of criminal evaluations, such as competency to stand trial, it may not be necessary to elicit details about the alleged crime. Evaluators may need to include only brief questioning about this area to ensure that evaluees understand the nature of the charges against them. In contrast, in an assessment regarding waiving *Miranda* rights, evaluators may need to take evaluees back to their thoughts and feelings pertaining to their mental state at the time that those rights were waived.

Psychiatric History

Evaluators generally elicit current psychiatric symptoms in a similar manner to the method of a general psychiatric examination conducted for treatment purposes. Current symptoms may be of primary importance when dealing with issues of competency, including competency to stand trial and civil competencies. These symptoms also may be relevant in various types of assessments such as psychiatric injury, disability, and fitness to practice. A retrospective analysis of symptoms is particularly relevant in assessing issues such as insanity, *mens rea* (the defendant's "guilty mind"), or fitness to waive *Miranda* rights.

Eliciting information about previous episodes of psychiatric illness is also helpful. This information can be checked against previous records gathered as collateral information. By examining the psychiatric history, psychiatrists may be able to formulate the effect of the specific event in question on the course of an illness as well as an evaluee's response to treatment and levels of impairment caused by illness at various times.

Types of treatment (e.g., pharmacological or psychological) and the relative success of each treatment modality may be especially important in cases of disability or alleged psychic harm. The adequacy of past treatments and complete information about the types of treatments may be important in recommending future treatment. In some cases, no history of psychiatric symptoms may exist, because first-episode psychosis may present with a criminal act (Bourget et al. 2004). In the absence of a psychiatric history, good supporting data may be necessary to establish that psychosis contributed to the current issue.

Personal History

The personal history is helpful in assessing the longitudinal course of an individual's development. Evaluators should ask about any particular delays or anomalies in development. The inquiry may begin with questions about the evaluee's mother's pregnancy and the evaluee's birth. Collateral information may be required to confirm this part of the history.

An informant may be able to provide a more detailed account of the attainment of developmental milestones. However, individuals' earliest memories are subjective, as are their perceptions of the atmosphere in the home. Evaluees' experience of parenting and discipline in the home may affect their future behavior. In particular, inquiry about the evaluee's exposure to violence or domestic violence in the home and the effect of emotional, physical, or sexual abuse may be particularly important in the genesis of future criminal, antisocial, or maladaptive behaviors and may be associated

with a range of psychopathology relevant to any formulation.

An educational history, especially if confirmed by collateral gathering of records, may give information about the possibility of developmental delays or learning disabilities, as well as attitudes toward authority. Forensic examiners can elicit the various symptoms of conduct disorder only by the use of leading questions, which are sometimes unavoidable during this part of the history. Academic performance and the highest level of education can be helpful in contributing to various forensic opinions. An occupational history is especially important in disability and other employment-related cases. In these cases, a more detailed occupational history, access to job descriptions if possible, and the evaluee's personnel file are also helpful.

Eliciting social, interpersonal, and relationship histories is also helpful in assessing the individual's ability to maintain intimate and other relationships. Care should be taken in eliciting a sexual history. In certain types of examinations, such as sex offender assessments, a detailed sexual history is appropriate. In other types of cases, such as assessing psychic trauma in some sexual assault cases, it may be inappropriate to take a detailed sexual history, unless the evaluee's sex drive and ability to enjoy sexuality are at issue. In these cases, the reason for exploring this area should be explained to the evaluee before asking these questions.

Previous Trauma

In many forensic evaluations, including those assessing claims of psychic injury, it is important to ask about previous trauma in detail. The evaluee's history of traumatic exposures and their effect and subsequent coping mechanisms may be related to future behaviors and to a range of subsequent psychopathology.

The effect of previous trauma must be placed in the context of the current legal claim. In some cases, previous victimization may make an evaluee sensitive or vulnerable to future victimization. For example, evaluees who have been victimized previously may have a tendency to misinterpret unintended acts by others and may claim sexual harassment or assault. Evaluators need to tease out and delineate these issues while striving for objectivity and honesty.

Medical and Surgical History

Medical disorders may have a relation to psychiatric symptomatology. A variety of comorbid medical conditions may cause decreased energy or apathy and may be related to significant impairment or disability. For example, endocrinological disorders, such as diabetes or thyroid disorders, have a close relation with psychiatric symptoms. Some of these may be directly related to a psycholegal issue such as the presence of an altered mental state resulting from hypoglycemia in a diabetic patient who is involved in a motor vehicle accident. Similarly, a seizure disorder may result in a postictal state that could have a relation to the evaluee's *mens rea* defense (diminished capacity). Questions about degenerative neurological diseases such as Huntington's disease or multiple sclerosis also may be related to an offense. Further investigation such as blood tests and consultation may be necessary to elucidate the connection between medical diseases and psychiatric symptoms.

Use of Adjunctive Tests

In addition to the psychiatric interview and collecting collateral information, forensic psychiatrists often use a range of adjunctive testing to augment their evaluations. Depending on the nature of the case, evaluators will make a decision about which types of tests are most relevant. Forensic assessment instruments are designed to measure specific forensic questions (see Chapter 5, "Psychological Testing in Forensic Psychiatry"). Any test used should be placed in the context of the specific psycholegal standard applicable to each specific jurisdiction. Whichever tests are used, the person administering and scoring the tests must have suitable qualifications and training.

Forensic psychiatrists oftentimes work within a multidisciplinary team that includes a forensic psychologist. When referring to a psychologist, psychiatrists should discuss the specific psycholegal question before the testing. Testing may be helpful in delineating the presence of psychosis or a personality disorder. Neuropsychological testing has a particular use in functional testing of cerebral performance, especially when a cognitive disorder or brain injury is suspected and may be the focus of the assessment. Psychological testing is also useful in contributing to the comprehensive assessment of malingering and dissimulation (Rogers 2012) (see Chapter 6).

Physical Examination

In the forensic evaluation, a physical examination may provide information relevant to the final formulation of psychiatric opinions. The presence of tattoos may indicate evidence of gang membership or other important relationships; therefore, the meaning of any tattoos to the evaluee should be explored. If forensic evaluators believe that a physical examination would be productive, then the most appropriate course of action is to discuss referring the evaluee to a medical colleague, after discussing the need for the referral with the retaining attorney or court. The findings of this physician then can be interpreted and, if appropriate, incorporated into the psychiatric formulation. Relevant physical examination findings could conceivably include evidence of exophthalmos, suggestive of hypothyroidism; evidence of hemiplegia, suggestive of a cerebrovascular accident; or pathognomonic neurological findings that may suggest a neurological disease such as multiple sclerosis. All of these conditions could be relevant to the forensic evaluation and conclusions.

Laboratory testing also may be helpful in formulating psychiatric opinions when these findings may bear on the psycholegal question, especially if psychiatric symptoms are suspected to be caused by an underlying medical condition. In persons with major or minor neurocognitive disorder, laboratory testing may identify an underlying reversible cause that is relevant to prognostic opinions contained in forensic reports.

Neuroimaging and Electroencephalography

In various types of forensic evaluations, neuroimaging (see Chapter 7, "Neuroimaging and Forensic Psychiatry") and electroencephalography may produce important findings. These tests must be interpreted by qualified clinical experts. However, forensic psychiatrists should be aware of the strengths and limitations of these types of data and be able to interpret their contribution to the forensic evaluation (David 2009). The relevance of the results from neuroimaging and other tests should be placed in the context of the overall forensic evaluation. Neuroimaging, if not carefully and reasonably put into context, can be erroneously interpreted and misused in the legal forum (Glancy et al. 2015; see also Chapter 7).

Mental Status Examination

Generally speaking, a forensic psychiatric assessment is incomplete without a mental status examination. This examination is based on general observations during the course of the clinical interview and direct inquiry into related aspects of functioning. If multiple interviews take place, then longitudinal observations should be noted. The mental status examination is similar to that performed in general psychiatry (American Psychiatric Association 2016). In certain forensic assessments, an emphasis on fantasies, thoughts, and urges related to violence or sexually violent behaviors becomes particularly relevant and should be pursued.

The presence of delusions is one aspect of the mental status examination that may be particularly difficult to elicit. Evaluees may present with no subjective symptoms, and objective examination may not detect the presence of obvious symptoms of formal thought disorder or hallucinations. Evaluees may not offer thoughts that show the presence of delusions unless asked a question specifically directed to the area. Sometimes collateral information provides indications of delusions that enable evaluators to ask about the particular beliefs. When inquiring about delusional beliefs, tact may be necessary to avoid upsetting or angering evaluees.

Cultural Considerations in Forensic Assessment

Mental health clinicians, including forensic psychiatrists, have been advised to take cultural contexts into consideration in their evaluations and conclusions (Tseng et al. 2004). Forensic psychiatrists, as well as other participants in the legal system, are influenced by preconceived notions, attitudes, and constructs in coming to conclusions (Tseng and Strelzer 2004). Cultural factors have been argued to produce disparities in diagnosing mental disorders in racial and ethnic minorities (Williams et al. 2007). Certain "culture-bound" syndromes may be relevant to psycholegal conclusions (Hicks 2004).

Different cultural attitudes that shape individuals' identities and concepts of themselves may influence their culturally subjective belief systems. Understanding these perspectives could help psychiatrists form a more complete understanding of an evaluee's thinking and behaviors (Aggarwal 2012). Situating the evaluee's behavior in its cultural context may aid in the process of understanding the evaluee's reasoning (Kirmayer et al. 2007). For example, culture may have a strong influence on a person's concept of boundaries (Miller et al. 2006). This may influence interactions with an evaluee, such as whether shaking hands with an evaluee is appropriate or in assessing the significance of an evaluee's tendency to avoid eye contact. In complicated cases, it may be helpful to consult colleagues who can provide additional advice about cultural influences (Hicks 2004).

Forensic Report

Some experts in the field of forensic psychiatry consider report writing the definitive forensic skill that establishes the evaluator's abilities, knowledge, experience, and training (Buchanan and Norko 2011). Forensic reports are often complex narratives that also require a performative element (Griffith and Baranoski 2007). The principles of crafting forensic reports are generally learned by the Socratic method. Guidelines for preparing reports generally are not formally stated. Some jurisdictions have specified a format for specific types of cases; evaluators practicing in those areas should be guided by these formats (Ontario 1990; Woolf 1996).

The American Academy of Psychiatry and the Law has not formally proposed or adopted guidelines for forensic reports and suggests that no one particular style or format for writing a report is correct (Giorgi-Guarnieri et al. 2002; Gold et al. 2008; Mossman et al. 2007). Thus, even within the broad guidelines required in particular jurisdictions, room exists for a variety of approaches in the writing of the forensic report. Buchanan and Norko (2011) acknowledge the differences in opinion and have attempted to develop principles of practice in writing forensic reports while acknowledging the range of practical approaches to this essential forensic psychiatric competency.

Purpose of the Report

The forensic report conveys the evaluator's opinions and the basis of those opinions. The forensic report also organizes the data for the evaluator and clarifies the forensic evaluator's opinions for the attorneys and the court (Reid 2013). In the event that the forensic evaluator has to give testimony, the report is a useful document to study before testifying. Attorneys often will use the forensic report for resolving or settling cases. Forensic reports also may be helpful in determining management and treatment of an evaluee. Psychiatrists should bear in mind while crafting their reports that any report ultimately may be read by all parties in the litigation, including the evaluee, as well as others not directly connected to the litigation.

Structure of the Report

The structure of a forensic report may depend on jurisdictional requirements, the type of report (civil, criminal, or administrative), and the particular psycholegal question addressed. Buchanan and Norko (2011) suggested a generic structure and showed how this standard structure can be applied to a variety of forensic situations. Greenfield and Gottschalk (2008) and Reid (2013) suggested a similar format and gave extensive examples of reports for a variety of forensic situations. An outline can be useful in imposing an organization on the writer. This outline also can be useful in organizing the interview, which then informs the basis of the report. Similarly, the use of headings related to the outline make a report more user friendly (Resnick and Soliman 2011). Table 4–1 lists the standard elements and provides a general structure of a forensic report.

A forensic psychiatric report also can be conceptualized as providing the basis for the examination in chief. In anticipation of the questions a lawyer will ask on the witness stand, beginning with "What is the basis for your opinions, Doctor?," the report will naturally and logically flow from the forensic expert's (metaphorical) pen. Facts contained in the body of the report should be clearly separated from inferences or opinions. The latter should appear in the opinion section (Melton et al. 2007).

Generally, forensic psychiatric reports begin with identifying information about the evaluee and, in some cases, a list of criminal charges or the date of the accident or injury at issue in a civil claim. The report then should specifically state its purpose and the reason for the psychiatric evaluation. In some cases, this might be followed by the specific legal standard relevant to the psycholegal ques-

TABLE 4–1. **General structure and elements of forensic reports**

Identifying data

Criminal charges/context/issue

Purpose of referral/psycholegal question(s)

Basis of forensic psychiatric opinion

    Dates and duration of interviews

    Sources of information

    Psychological testing

    Collateral interviews

    Materials reviewed

Confidentiality/warning

Caveat (if relevant)

Introduction (context)

Account of offense/circumstances of case

Delineated psychiatric problems

Family history

Personal history

    Psychiatric history

    Medical and surgical history

    Criminal history

    Substance abuse

    History of violence

    Previous trauma

Mental status examination

Adjunctive testing

Diagnostic formulation

Opinion

Signature

tion addressed. The basis of the forensic psychiatric opinions then can be listed, including all sources of information: interviews with the evaluee; the duration of these interviews; and other sources such as collateral interviews, documents reviewed (e.g., police reports, witness statements, medical records), and any other information reviewed. A clear list of all materials relied on alerts the reader to exactly which documents were reviewed and which were not available.

Most forensic evaluators include a statement regarding the discussion of the limitations of confidentiality with the evaluee. This statement typically documents that the forensic psychiatrist provided the evaluee with the information that anything the evaluee said may be included in a report that may be sent to the attorney and become part of litigation proceedings. This written statement also might include any possible mandatory and discretionary reporting requirements in that particular jurisdiction and that the evaluee was advised that he or she may refuse to answer any questions, may consult counsel at any time, and may terminate the evaluation at any time. This section should include whether the evaluee understood the information and consented to continue with the interview, either verbally or in writing.

The evaluee's narrative regarding the substantial issue is an important part of the report. This type of presentation has been described as a performative act that attempts to make sense out of behavior and persuades the reader that the argument is cogent, supported by data, and presented objectively. This kind of account demands the ability to present opinions and arguments that anticipate critical analysis, disagreement, and cross-examination (Griffith and Baranoski 2007). In a criminal case, for example, this may include the evaluee's thoughts, feelings, and behaviors immediately before, during, and after a crime. In civil cases, this may involve an account of the circumstances regarding the claimed tortious act, which also might include the evaluee's thoughts, feelings, and behaviors surrounding this act and subsequent alleged effects of the act on the evaluee's social, psychological, and occupational functioning.

Reports generally include a section on conclusions and recommendations (Ciccone and Jones 2011), summary and opinions (Greenfield and Gottschalk

2008), or opinions (Buchanan and Norko 2011; Resnick and Soliman 2011). The conclusions section is the crux of the report and will be most carefully read and scrutinized (Resnick and Soliman 2011). In some jurisdictions, the opinion section is traditionally placed at the start of the report, but in others, the opinion appears at the end of the report. No new material should be introduced in the opinion section; all the facts or issues used in the reasoning already should have appeared in the report (Melton et al. 2007).

Opinions should give clear answers to the psycholegal questions in the case. If this is not possible, the forensic evaluator should explain why a definitive answer cannot be provided. Importantly, the report should answer the legal question and not go beyond this question to address other matters (Melton et al. 2007; Reid 2013). For example, if the evaluation is related to the issue of criminal responsibility at the time of the specific act, the report should not address future dangerousness because this opinion may be prejudicial.

Forensic psychiatrists must create a nexus between the data and their conclusions. Opinions should have internal consistency and should follow logically and be founded on the data provided in the report (Arboleda-Flóréz 2000). Simply stating an opinion is not sufficient if the opinion is not supported by the data included in the report and the reasoning that naturally follows. Similarly, recording the data and then asserting a conclusion without explaining the reasoning also is not sufficient.

Style of the Report

The forensic psychiatric report should be easy to follow and written in plain language understandable to those without a medical background. Clarity, simplicity, and brevity are desirable qualities (Resnick and Soliman 2011). Reports should address the specifics of the case and be reasonably brief but complete (Arboleda-Floréz 2000). Use of the active voice and elimination of unnecessary information support these goals. Unnecessary words, redundancy, irrelevant detail, and editorial comments should be avoided because they complicate the report and may be used against the forensic psychiatrist in cross-examination.

Whether the forensic report should include direct opinions on the ultimate issue depends on the legal rules of the jurisdiction in which the case is heard. For example, in U.S. federal courts, evaluators can include opinions on the ultimate issue in their reports but cannot testify about the ultimate issue at a jury trial (Buchanan 2006). Forensic psychiatrists should clarify the jurisdictional requirements with the retaining attorney before including opinions on ultimate issues in their reports.

Conclusion

Performing forensic evaluations and writing a forensic report are key competencies in forensic psychiatry. Although no clear rules set out the content or style of forensic assessments or the structure of forensic reports, key concepts can guide the forensic psychiatrist in adapting a suitable evaluation and report to various types of cases and the goals and requirements of the report in any particular jurisdiction.

Key Concepts

- Conducting an ethical and complete forensic psychiatric evaluation and providing a well-written and thorough report are key competencies in forensic psychiatric practice.

- Forensic evaluations cannot rely solely on the subjective report of evaluees. Corroboration, whenever possible, should be obtained.

- Forensic psychiatrists should conduct face-to-face evaluations whenever possible. When it is not possible to do so, reports should indicate if and how this has affected opinions.

- Forensic examiners should maintain a neutral stance during a forensic examination, neither believing nor disbelieving an evaluee's report.

- Forensic reports should include the examiner's opinions, the basis of those opinions, and the reasoning underlying the opinions.

- Forensic opinions should be limited to the psycholegal question at issue and should not provide opinions on other matters that have not been raised.

- Reports should be clear, concise, and complete. Psychiatrists should avoid jargon and should bear in mind that the report will be read by the evaluee, attorneys, the court, and possibly others.

References

Aggarwal NK: Adapting the cultural formulation for clinical assessments in forensic psychiatry. J Am Acad Psychiatry Law 40(1):113–118, 2012 22396348

American Academy of Psychiatry and the Law: Videotaping of forensic psychiatric evaluations. AAPL Task Force. J Am Acad Psychiatry Law 27(2):345–358, 1999 10400441

American Academy of Psychiatry and the Law: Ethics Guidelines for the Practice of Forensic Psychiatry. May 2005. Available at: http://www.aapl.org/ethics.htm. Accessed December 19, 2016.

American Psychiatric Association: Practice Guidelines for the Psychiatric Evaluation of Adults, 3rd Edition, 2016. Available at: http://psychiatryonline.org/doi/pdf/10.1176/appi.books.9780890426760. Accessed December 22, 2016.

Appelbaum KL: Commentary: the art of forensic report writing. J Am Acad Psychiatry Law 38(1):43–45, 2010 20305073

Arboleda-Floréz J: Forensic Psychiatric Evidence. Oxford, UK, Butterworth-Heinemann, 2000

Bourget D, Labelle A, Gagne P, et al: First-episode psychosis and homicide: a diagnostic challenge. Can Psych Assoc Bull 36:6–9, 2004

Buchanan A: Psychiatric evidence on the ultimate issue. J Am Acad Psychiatry Law 34(1):14–21, 2006 16585229

Buchanan A, Norko MA (eds): The Psychiatric Report: Principles and Practice of Forensic Writing. Cambridge, UK, Cambridge University Press, 2011

Ciccone JR, Jones J: Criminal litigation, in The Psychiatric Report: Principles and Practice of Forensic Writing. Edited by Buchanan A, Norko MA. Cambridge, UK, Cambridge University Press, 2011, pp 98–111

David A: Lishman's Organic Psychiatry: A Textbook of Neuropsychiatry. New York, Wiley, 2009

Giorgi-Guarnieri D, Janofsky J, Keram E, et al; American Academy of Psychiatry and the Law: AAPL practice guideline for forensic psychiatric evaluation of defendants raising the insanity defense. J Am Acad Psychiatry Law 30(2 suppl):S3–S40, 2002 12099305

Glancy GD, Saini M: The confluence of evidence-based practice and Daubert within the fields of forensic psychiatry and the law. J Am Acad Psychiatry Law 37(4):438–441, 2009 20018992

Glancy GD, Ash P, Bath EP, et al: AAPL practice guideline for the forensic assessment. J Am Acad Psychiatry Law 43(2; suppl):S3–S53, 2015 26054704

Gold LH, Anfang SA, Drukteinis AM, et al: AAPL practice guideline for the forensic evaluation of psychiatric disability. J Am Acad Psychiatry Law 36(4; suppl):S3–S50, 2008 19092058

Greenfield DP, Gottschalk JA: Writing Forensic Reports: A Guide for Mental Health Professionals. New York, Springer, 2008

Griffith EE, Baranoski MV: Commentary: the place of performative writing in forensic psychiatry. J Am Acad Psychiatry Law 35(1):27–31, 2007 17389341

Gutheil TG, Simon RI: Mastering Forensic Psychiatric Practice: Advanced Strategies for the Expert Witness. Washington, DC, American Psychiatric Publishing, 2002

Hicks JW: Ethnicity, race, and forensic psychiatry: are we color-blind? J Am Acad Psychiatry Law 32(1):21–33, 2004 15497624

Kirmayer LJ, Rousseau C, Lashley M: The place of culture in forensic psychiatry. J Am Acad Psychiatry Law 35(1):98–102, 2007 17389351

Melton GB, Petrila J, Poythress NG, et al: Psychological Evaluations for the Courts: A Handbook for Mental Health Professionals and Lawyers, 3rd Edition. New York, Guilford, 2007

Miller PM, Commons ML, Gutheil TG: Clinicians' perceptions of boundaries in Brazil and the United States. J Am Acad Psychiatry Law 34(1):33–42, 2006 16585233

Mossman D, Noffsinger SG, Ash P, et al; American Academy of Psychiatry and the Law: AAPL Practice Guideline for the forensic psychiatric evaluation of competence to stand trial. J Am Acad Psychiatry Law 35(4; suppl):S3–S72, 2007 18083992

Ontario: Rules of Civil Procedure, RRO 1990, Reg 194. Available at: https://www.canlii.org//en/on/laws/regu/rro-1990-reg-194/latest/rro-1990-reg-194.html. Accessed April 29, 2017.

Reid WH: Developing a Forensic Practice: Operations and Ethics for Experts. New York, Routledge/Taylor & Francis Group, 2013

Resnick P, Soliman S: Draftsmanship, in The Psychiatric Report: Principles and Practice of Forensic Writing. Edited by Buchanan A, Norko MA. Cambridge, UK, Cambridge University Press, 2011, pp 81–92

Rogers R (ed): Clinical Assessment of Malingering and Deception, 3rd Edition. New York, Guilford, 2012

Tseng WS, Strelzer J: Introduction: culture and psychiatry, in Cultural Competence in Clinical Psychiatry. Edited by Tseng WS, Strelzer J. Washington, DC, American Psychiatric Publishing, 2004, pp 1–20

Tseng WS, Matthews D, Elwyn TS (eds): Cultural Competence in Forensic Mental Health: A Guide for Psychiatrists, Psychologists, and Attorneys. New York, Routledge, 2004

Wettstein RM: The forensic psychiatric examination and report, in The American Psychiatric Publishing Textbook of Forensic Psychiatry, 2nd Edition. Edited by Simon RI, Gold LH. Washington, DC, American Psychiatric Publishing, 2010, pp 175–203

Williams DR, González HM, Neighbors H, et al: Prevalence and distribution of major depressive disorder in African Americans, Caribbean blacks, and non-Hispanic whites: results from the National Survey of American Life. Arch Gen Psychiatry 64(3):305–315, 2007 17339519

Woolf TRHL: Access to Justice Final Report: Final Report to the Lord Chancellor on the Civil Justice System in England and Wales. London, HMSO, 1996

CHAPTER 5

Psychological Testing in Forensic Psychiatry

Madelon V. Baranoski, Ph.D.

Landmark Cases

***Daubert v. Merrell Dow Pharmaceuticals Inc.*, 509 U.S. 579, 113 S.Ct. 2786 (1993)**

***Atkins v. Virginia*, 536 U.S. 304, 122 S.Ct. 2242 (2002)**

Psychological testing is the administration and interpretation of standardized tests with acceptable psychometric properties. The tests are selected based on the functional area in question, including cognition and intelligence, learning styles and disabilities, memory, personality structure, and assessment of brain injury sequelae. The application of psychological testing in forensic cases has burgeoned since the 1970s. The measures of personality, the standardized testing, and specific assessments of function support the utility of psychological evaluations across the spectrum of forensic cases, including competency, criminal responsibility, disability, custody, and other questions in civil cases (Melton et al. 2007). The U.S. Supreme Court decision in *Atkins v. Virginia* (2002) prohibiting the execution of persons with mental retardation (now known as intellectual disability), for example, would require some IQ assessment to determine whether the individual is too intellectually impaired to be executed.

In this chapter, I present psychological evaluations as an adjunct to forensic psychiatric assessments. I define psychological testing and explore applications and advantages of psychological evaluations unique to forensic cases, describe categories of tests, and present the limits of psychological tests and caveats regarding their use.

Role of Psychological Testing in Forensic Assessments

Although not a required component of all forensic assessments, the absence of a psychological assessment weakens the formulation in certain evaluations. Cognitive and neurocognitive deficits cannot be accurately quantified without standardized testing that also assesses effort and malingering. Similarly, standardized measures offer additional information to support a psychiatric conclusion or to raise alternative hypotheses.

Characteristics of Psychological Testing

Standardized psychological tests are those with certain psychometric properties, including reliability (i.e., the capacity of a test to measure the same variable over time and across situations), validity (i.e., the capacity of a test to measure what it is designed to measure), the error rate, and the limitations to generalizability of the test. Psychological tests assess behavior to determine level of capacity, function, and symptoms compared with established norms. These tests are interpreted to answer the following question: How does this person compare with the populations tested; that is, where on the continuum or in which category does this person fall? The established continua and categories refer to function and characteristics, such as IQ, levels of depression, personality characteristics, and memory capacity. Similar to other medical tests such as blood tests, standard psychological tests have established norms and cutoffs that correlate with function in daily life.

In contrast to clinical interviews, psychological tests are not individualized to the person or the situation. Each test is administered, scored, and interpreted according to standard protocols. Although the administration of the tests is fixed, the selection of specific measures and the relevance of the findings are based on individual history, context, and purpose (Heilbrun 1992). The interpretation of psychological testing requires an individual assessment and collateral information that determine the applicability of the results of the testing (i.e., are the testing results supported by other data?). Just as with aberrant blood test results that do not coincide with the clinical picture or history, aberrant psychological testing results must not override what the history and individual assessment show.

Relevant testing results can augment clinical evaluations by providing functional assessments beyond those that can be determined by clinical interviews; by reconciling disparate historical, legal, and treatment data; and by identifying areas ripe for further assessment. Although clinical interviews can estimate intellectual range, formal testing can identify cognitive strengths and weaknesses, overall intellectual ability, and foundations for analyzing overall achievement. Because the results of most tests are normed by age and often by gender, test scores indicate how individuals compare with their referent groups.

Simulation of Relevant Situations

The standard battery of psychological tests includes measures of cognitive capacity, memory, attention, and concentration, as well as standard tests of personality characteristics and projective measures to elicit the individual's worldview and organizational capacity. An advantage of these tests is simulation of real-life demands. Sets of structured tasks can create conditions beyond those of usual clinical interviews. For example, visual-spatial tests create challenges similar to parking a car, sewing, eating, and organizing an apartment. In a disability case, the results can inform an assessment focused on the ability to return to work after a head injury. Similarly, cognitive testing evaluates concentration, attention, and effort in a way beyond what is assessed in a structured forensic interview. The testing procedures create emotional tension and distractions and then measure their effects on function.

Reconciling Disparate Data

Psychological testing can explain disparities within patients' histories and presentations and can suggest additional hypotheses for formulations. The testing provides information that can shape and strengthen the clinical opinion. When the psychological testing results do not support psychiatric formulations, they alert psychiatrists to weaknesses in their cases, the potential for missing data, and the need for further collateral information.

Special Relevance to Forensic Psychiatry

The utility of psychological testing applies to clinical, educational, and employment assessments as well as to forensic cases. Additional reasons for including psychological testing in a forensic assessment involve the nature of the psychiatric-legal interface.

Certainty and Time Limits

Critical questions about state of mind and function need to be answered in a relatively short time with reasonable medical or psychological certainty. Moreover, forensic opinions preclude speculation and hypothesis testing. Psychological

evaluations provide additional information and suggest areas for examination. When psychological testing is completed early in the evaluation and the results are available to the psychiatrist, the integration of results into both the evaluation itself and the formulation creates a solid and defensible opinion.

Due Diligence

For the court, the inclusion of psychological testing also gives the perception of due diligence and a comprehensive evaluation. Even when psychological testing results in contrary findings and requires explanation, the credibility of the forensic expert is enhanced by the documentation that shows that other hypotheses and opinions were considered and rejected.

Vulnerability Check

Psychological testing can identify weaknesses in formulations. In difficult forensic cases, differing opinions are common. Psychological testing helps the expert on either side to learn what the tests show and how those tests support or refute the opinion. Forewarned, the expert can decide how to address contrary findings.

Categories of Tests and Testing Procedures

Psychological tests vary in form, purpose, and foundation. Established psychological tests that would be acceptable in court and meet ***Daubert v. Merrell Dow Pharmaceuticals Inc.*** (1993), or other admissibility challenges (see Chapter 1, "The Expert Witness") have several characteristics in common: established reliability and validity, a known standard error rate for tests that are scored, standard scoring instructions, criteria for taking the test (such as age, language, and reading ability), and limits of interpretation and generalizability. These characteristics indicate who can take the test, how to score the test, how it can be interpreted, and how confident one is in the results.

Tests can be categorized in several different ways based on purpose and form. One system, based on the purpose of the testing and the characteristic evaluated, is relevant to forensic work.

Cognitive and Functional Tests

Cognitive and functional tests measure intelligence, capacity to learn, and function. The scores reflect a person's ability relevant to established population norms. Cognitive tests include intelligence tests, achievement tests, and tests to assess specific cognitive areas and deficits, such as attention deficits and dyslexia. These kinds of tests are included in educational assessments. Achievement tests, for example, track performance of students in different grades as well as competitiveness for placement in higher education (e.g., college boards, Medical College Admission Test, and Law School Admission Test).

Cognitive tests typically are included in a standard forensic battery of tests because of their diagnostic utility. The tests identify disorders in thinking, including formal thought disorders, attention and concentration impairments, and variation in capacity that can be pathognomonic of autistic spectrum and other developmental disorders. Performance on cognitive tests also can identify problem-solving style and obsessive-compulsive and paranoid characteristics.

Intelligence Tests

In forensic assessments, the most common cognitive tests are intelligence tests. These measure past learning, verbal skills, abstract reasoning, processing speed (how fast a person can think through a problem), perceptual organization, and working memory (how well a person can hold and manipulate information in mind while solving a problem). Intelligence tests are regularly updated and are designed to reflect a normal or bell-shaped distribution of intellectual ability. The scores roughly correlate with general adaptation and level of education and employment. In forensic evaluations, cognitive tests also serve as diagnostic tools in identifying psychosis, paranoid ideation, attention deficits, and malingering relevant to specific cases. Table 5–1 summarizes the most common standardized cognitive tests.

In intelligence tests, specific domains are assessed to measure two general categories of intelligence: *crystallized* (what is learned and recalled related to education) and *fluid* (active attention, concentration, and active problem solving). Index scores indicate the level of capacity in each domain: *Verbal Reasoning* (vocabulary, abstract reasoning); *Perceptual Integration* (pattern recognition, visual-motor integration); *Processing Speed* (rate and accuracy of problem solving); *Working Memory* (mental problem solving); and *General Ability* (blend of capacities). All IQ measures are correctly reported as a range of scores indicating the confidence limits of the score. Scores are based on a normal distribution with a mean of 100 and standard deviation of 15.

Beyond measuring the range of intelligence, the Wechsler Adult Intelligence Scale and the Wechsler Intelligence Scale for Children (through age 17 years) can provide valid indications of psychiatric symptoms and level of effort or malingering as shown in the following examples:

- *Flight of ideas, racing thoughts* (from the vocabulary test): Define the word

TABLE 5–1. Common cognitive tests

Test	Purpose of test	Target population (age, language)	Scoring	Forensic considerations
Wechsler series (Wechsler 2008)	Intelligence tests	Infants–adult English Spanish versions for some	Full Scale IQ Index scores	Gold standard, *Daubert*-tested Indicates psychosis, ADD Sensitive to ASD
Wechsler Preschool and Primary Scale of Intelligence, 4th Edition		Ages 2:6–7:7 English	Full Scale IQ Index scores: Verbal Ability Visual Spatial Working Memory Vocabulary Acquisition Nonverbal General ability	IQ indicative of failure to thrive, environmental deprivation Low scores not a reliable indicator of adult intelligence
Wechsler Intelligence Scale for Children, 5th Edition (WICS-V)		Ages 6–10 English (Spanish version under development)	Full Scale IQ Index scores: Verbal Comprehension Visual Spatial Fluid Reasoning Working Memory Processing Speed	Revised edition similar to the WISC-IV
Wechsler Adult Intelligence Scale, 3rd Edition (WAIS-III)		Ages 16–89 English	Verbal IQ Performance IQ Full Scale IQ	Still in use and included in past records Useful in assessing malingering
Wechsler Adult Intelligence Scale, 4th Edition (WAIS-IV)		Ages 16–90:11 English	Full Scale IQ Index scores: Verbal Comprehension Perceptual Reasoning Working Memory Processing Speed General Ability	Standard IQ measure with increased sensitivity to deficits in ASD

TABLE 5–1. Common cognitive tests *(continued)*

Test	Purpose of test	Target population (age, language)	Scoring	Forensic considerations
Wechsler series *(continued)*	Intelligence tests			
Wechsler Abbreviated Scale of Intelligence (original and 2nd Edition; WASI-and WASI-II)	Intelligence tests	Ages 6:0–90:11 English	Estimated Full Scale IQ	Used in lieu of WAIS when IQ score is repeated within 1 year
Stanford-Binet Intelligence Scales (Roid 2002)	Intelligence test	Ages 2–85	Verbal IQ Performance IQ Full Scale IQ	More precise for very low and very high IQs Less common in forensic assessment
Kaufman Brief Intelligence Test, 2nd Edition (KBIT-2; Kaufman and Kaufman 2004)	Intelligence test	Ages 4–90 English	Verbal and Nonverbal scores (mean=100; SD=15)	Used in educational settings WAIS preferred for forensic assessments
Peabody Picture Vocabulary Test, 4th Edition (PPVT-4; Dunn and Dunn 2007)	Receptive vocabulary	Ages 2:6–90+	Age-, grade-based scores based on normal curve equivalents	Estimates IQ, effective indicator of effort
Test of Nonverbal Intelligence, 4th Edition (TONI-4; Brown et al. 2010)	Assesses perceptive reasoning, concentration	Ages 6:0–89:11 Standard directions in Spanish, French, German, Chinese, Vietnamese, Korean, Tagalog	Standard scores, age based (mean=100; SD=15) Norms are based on the United States, Canada, and Western Europe	Useful in immigration cases Offers estimate of reasoning and problem solving Scores not reported as IQ

assemble: "That is an interesting word with ass right out front, which you could say is back-asswords [sic], pardon my French, which I did not major in; 'Take Spanish; it will help you get a job.' Thanks, mom! She didn't give that advice to my sister, her favorite."

- *Tangential, neologistic, and disorganized* (from the similarities abstract reasoning test): How are a bird and a starfish alike? "Fission and fusion confused, conbirded [sic] and bridled in sky."

- *Paranoid ideation* (from tasks): Put cards in order to make a specified design. "These other cards do not fit in, unless you are trying to trick me. The color on this card is lighter than the others. Unless this is a trick to get me to make a mistake. Am I being recorded?"

The concept of "scatter" is defined as higher than usual variation in scores within and among cognitive subtests. In cognitive testing, slight variation in scores across subtests is common and reflects relative strengths and weaknesses. In the presence of psychopathology, cognitive impairments, and learning disabilities, the difference in scores is greater, reaching statistically significant levels of difference. Excessive variation indicates a disrupted thought process like that found in attention-deficit/hyperactivity disorder and in the distractibility related to anxiety, trauma, depression, psychosis, and autism spectrum disorder.

The "Flynn effect" is another concept relevant to intelligence testing. First described by James Flynn (but first labeled by Herrnstein and Murray [1994]), the Flynn effect is the pattern of sustained increase in IQ scores within world populations since the 1930s when IQ was first measured (Flynn 1987). This general increase requires updates of the standardized testing to maintain the underlying construct that intelligence has a normal distribution within a population. As the Flynn effect occurs—that is, as increasing numbers of persons obtain higher scores—the meaningful distribution is disrupted; the higher IQ scores artificially inflate the estimate of intelligence. Although the statistical basis for and explanation of the Flynn effect are controversial, there is agreement that IQ testing must be updated to reflect changes in common experience and learning. For example, the Wechsler Adult Intelligence Scale is now in its fourth edition, and the fifth edition is being developed. Therefore, valid estimates of IQ require the use of current testing editions. DSM-5 notes the Flynn effect as one of the factors affecting IQ scores; testing with an earlier edition of the test will inflate the estimate of intelligence (American Psychiatric Association 2013). The Flynn effect has particular relevance in death penalty cases (see Chapter 20, "Psychiatry and the Death Penalty").

Achievement Tests

Achievement tests are a mainstay of educational assessments. They measure what was learned against standard expectations of performance. Different from IQ tests, which measure capacity to learn, achievement tests are a measure of what was learned and retained. Combining IQ test and achievement test results can identify under- and overachievers. Low achievement scores can be diagnostic of psychiatric disorders, attention and concentration disorders, poor attendance, substance and alcohol abuse, and poor education. The Wide Range Achievement Test–4 (Jastak and Wilkinson 1984; Wilkinson and Robertson 2006) and the Woodcock-Johnson III Tests of Achievement (Woodcock et al. 2001) are common achievement tests and tests of reading and reading comprehension.

Personality Tests

Personality tests are designed to measure the broadest definition of personality: orientation and style regarding social interactions, self-perception, worldview, coping mechanisms, vulnerability, resilience, capacity for intimacy, and management of anxiety. Standardized and projective tests are the two main categories of personality tests (see Table 5–2).

Unlike cognitive tests that rank individuals against a population norm, personality tests result in "profiles" that describe strengths, vulnerabilities, patterns of adjustment, and pathological conditions. Personality tests used in forensic assessments have established psychometric properties and formal rules for administration and scoring in order to pass evidentiary admissibility requirements.

Standardized Self-Report Measures

Standardized personality tests produce normative scores that define a profile correlated with personality styles and disorders. The most frequently used standardized personality tests in forensic assessments are the Minnesota Multiphasic Personality Inventory, 2nd Edition (MMPI-2; Hathaway and McKinley 1989), the Millon Clinical Multiaxial Inventory–III (MCMI-III; Millon 1994), and the Personality Assessment Inventory (PAI; Morey 2007). All of these tests have subscales that produce a profile of personality and symptom characteristics. The personality tests have embedded validity scales to indicate the attitude of the test taker. The tests are computer-scored through packaged programs that provide periodic updates, norms, and interpretive narratives based on the profile of scores. Frequently, the MMPI-2 or PAI is administered with the MCMI-III to provide data on personality and adaptive characteristics along with a profile of personality pathology.

Of all the structured personality tests, the MMPI-2 and the Restructured Form (MMPI-2-RF) have been researched and "normed" most extensively (Ben-Porath and Tellegen 2008a, 2008b; Tellegen and Ben-Porath 2008/2011). The tests have been used to screen applicants to police forces, astronaut candidates, and student resident advisers in college. The basis for this extensive use was the empirical nature of the tests: items distinguished between groups of those who were successful and those who were not. In addition, the test is easy to administer (often in groups), computer-scored, and viewed as less subject to bias by inexperienced interviewers.

The standard computer scoring also provides interpretive summaries of the results. These reflect group analyses and cannot be applied to the individual being testing without clinical correlation. That is, the summaries provide profiles based on aggregate statistics on samples of persons assessed during the development of the tests. The tests suggest hypotheses about personality structure and diagnostic indicators that require clinical validation.

Projective Tests

Projective tests are instruments that require the patient to interpret vague stimuli. The tests provide minimal direction, have no set form for the responses, and allow wide latitude in the way patients approach the task. The projective tests have been described as the "cocktail party" tests: that is, how would a person respond in a complex and unstructured setting? Projective tests include verbal reports and drawings. The results need to be reported with caution because standard scoring is not available for all of the tests. The lack of formal scoring and the vul-

TABLE 5–2. Common personality tests in forensic assessments

Test	Type	Objective	Scoring	Forensic considerations
Minnesota Multiphasic Personality Inventory–2 (MMPI-2; Hathaway and McKinley 1989)	Standardized personality trait inventories 567 T/F questions	Comparison to empirically based profiles related to employment categories, psychopathology, adjustment	Computer scored, clinician interpreted Validity and clinical scales enrich interpretation Subscales enrich interpretation	Extensive use and manualized administration and interpretation Computer scoring and interpretation guide Validity scales Useful for personality disorder assessments Computer scoring and interpretation guide preferred in forensic cases
Minnesota Multiphasic Personality Inventory–2 Restructured Form (MMPI-2-RF; Ben-Porath and Tellegen 2008a, 2008b; Tellegen and Ben-Porath 2008/2011)	338 T/F questions			
Personality Assessment Inventory (PAI; Morey 2007)	344 questions answered on a 4 point Likert scale (not true at all to very true) 22 scales including validity scales, clinical scales, treatment consideration scales, and interpersonal scales	Identification of personality disorders, psychosis, and depression; interpersonal styles and issues; and attitude toward treatment	Computer scored with standardized profile and interpretation	Strong psychometric properties Assessment of quality of symptoms Identifies cultural differences in psychosis Court-accepted test
Millon Clinical Multiaxial Inventory–III (MCMI-III; Millon 1994)	Personality checklist 175 T/F items 4 categories of scales: Validity Scales, Clinical Syndrome Scales, Personality Pattern Scales, and Grossman Personality Facet Scales	Identification of personality styles and disorders and clinical syndromes	Computer scored with standardized profile and interpretations	Strong psychometric properties More commonly used in clinical than in forensic cases

TABLE 5–2. Common personality tests in forensic assessments (continued)

Test	Type	Objective	Scoring	Forensic considerations
Rorschach Inkblot Test	Projective test 10 (6×8 inch) cards with black, red and black, and multicolored inkblots Presented by the examiner	Elicitation of themes and patterns of interpretation of ambiguous circumstances	Standard scoring through the Exner system identifies the organization of the percepts (Exner 1995)	Controversial test; available on the Internet Use in court should be limited to adjunctive test supported by other testing Useful as an evaluation and diagnostic tool
Thematic Apperception Test (Holmstrom et al. 1990)	Projective test Standard illustrations for which the patient is to tell a story	Elicitation of interpersonal themes and conflicts	No standard scoring; record themes of story and divergent interpretations	Useful as an evaluation and diagnostic tool
Sentence Completion Test	Projective test Patients are asked to complete sentence roots (e.g., *My mother…and I feel angry when…*)	Elicitation of expression of issues, values, and conflicts	No standard scoring	Useful as an evaluation and diagnostic tool
Human Figure Drawing/drawings	Projective test Drawings of a person and an inanimate object or of family interactions	Elicitation of representation of tangible environment	No formal scoring	Useful with children Useful as an evaluation and diagnostic tool

nerability of these tests to myriad influences unrelated to mental illness make these tests more likely to face admissibility challenges than would empirically established tests, such as the MMPI–2 (Grove and Barden 1999). Additionally, many of the projective tests were based on concepts no longer popular in psychiatry; for example, measures that were designed to elicit repressed thinking and the unconscious are hard to explain and justify with current theories of neuroscience. Despite these limitations, the tests are useful as one component of a complete battery. They also serve to alert examiners to areas for further exploration.

Neuropsychological Tests

From the 1940s through the 1980s, projective testing and research flourished. The current focus on psychological testing emphasizes neuropsychological tests and assessment of brain function. Corresponding to neuroimaging studies, neuropsychological testing has advanced and developed into a subspecialty that requires postdoctoral preparation.

Neuropsychological tests identify specific brain dysfunctions and allow the examiner to analyze the factors that result in disruptive behaviors, such as impulsivity, concentration deficits, and aggression. In forensic assessments, neuropsychological tests are most frequently involved in disability assessments after head trauma. The specialized testing can also complement cognitive and personality assessments in criminal cases that include an unexpected decline in function, chronic drug or alcohol use, or a history of head trauma.

A neuropsychological assessment requires a battery of tests that includes cognitive testing. The most common batteries are the Halstead-Reitan Neuropsychological Test Battery (Broshek and Barth 2000; Reitan and Wolfson 1993) and the Luria-Nebraska Neuropsychological Battery (Golden and Freshwater 2001; Golden et al. 1982, 2000). These are made up of individual tests to measure systematically discrete brain function.

Independent tests of brain function can be combined into different batteries based on the type of injury and the problems presented. In *A Compendium of Neuropsychological Tests*, Strauss et al. (2006) present a comprehensive description of various tests and highlight their uses, psychometric properties, and strengths and limitations. A common test used in screening for neuropsychological deficits is the Categories Test (in the Halstead-Reitan Battery), which is used to evaluate general brain dysfunction (Broshek and Barth 2000; Strauss et al. 2006).

The Rey-Osterrieth Complex Figure Test (Meyers and Meyers 2007; Osterrieth 1944) and the Draw-a-Clock Test (Freedman et al. 1994) are other screening tests that identify general brain dysfunction. Abnormal findings on either of these tests should be followed by a neurological examination and a full neuropsychological battery to determine the extent and severity of the disorder. These tests can also help to distinguish among diagnoses of cognitive deficiency, dementias, and psychoses.

Memory Assessments

Tests for memory are included as part of neuropsychological batteries and cognitive batteries. In forensic psychiatry, assessment of memory and of feigned memory impairments are required in both civil and criminal cases. For example, when a defendant reports no recollection of an alleged criminal behavior, a referral to assess memory is often the primary request. Memory assessments include a standard battery of discreet tests to assess verbal, figural, and association memory as well as immediate and intermediate memory. The most common memory battery is the Wechsler Memory Scale, 4th Edition (Pearson Education 2008).

The distinction between immediate and intermediate memory is important in understanding memory deficit etiology and treatment. Immediate memory is a loose term for the incorporation of information into awareness. In a mental status examination, immediate memory is also termed *registration*, referring to the patient's ability to repeat words when they are spoken. Intermediate memory is the capacity to retrieve stored material. Long-term memory is hard to assess in a testing session, because insufficient time has passed; usually, long-term memory is assessed, crudely, through the report of history.

Memory assessments cannot measure the effects of past interference on either short-term or intermediate memory. For example, in one case, a college student who had been drinking heavily got into a fist fight at a bar and severely beat another patron. He had spotty recollections of the evening but no organized recall of the fight and no recall of why he was fighting or what he thought at the time. Memory testing on the young man identified above average recollection on both immediate and intermediate memory. The results of the testing had limited bearing on the psychiatrist's report except to determine that the student did not have a primary memory deficit and did not malinger memory deficits. However, the normal memory testing did not preclude a blackout (Hartzler and Fromme 2003), and the lack of malingering did not ensure that he was truthful about his lack of recall.

In a general way, memory assessments show effects of attention and concentration deficits, obsessive intrusions, psychosis, dementia, and brain dysfunction.

The tests are most helpful in determining differential impairments between verbal and figural memory and in making recommendations for improving recall. In forensic work, this could be useful in designing restoration-to-competency curricula for those with memory loss.

Psychological Assessment of Malingering

Assessment of malingering is a frequent referral question for psychological testing. In forensic work, the identification of malingering has particular significance. DSM-5 (American Psychiatric Association 2013) advises that malingering be "strongly suspected" (p. 727) if any combination of four conditions is present. The first is an examination in the medicolegal context, thus covering nearly all forensic evaluations. The others, a notable discrepancy between the person's report of symptoms and impairment and the objective facts, lack of cooperation in the evaluation and noncompliance with treatment, and presence of antisocial personality disorder, are also found frequently in forensic evaluations.

The assessment of malingering is complicated and requires the triangulation of data from a comprehensive clinical assessment, psychological testing, and reliable collateral information (see Chapter 6, "Evaluation of Malingering"). Malingering instruments, more properly termed *feigning tests*, are specific psychological tests to assess the credibility of symptoms and disabilities. No psychological test is available for global malingering; tests are designed to assess the quality and nature of symptoms in reference to the usual manifestations of illness. The tests are designed around the assumptions that each major mental disorder has common presentations of major signs and symptoms and that the severity of the illness will have concomitant manifestations in function. Tests for feigning target specific areas that correlate with the presented symptoms. Common tests used to evaluate feigning of psychiatric symptoms or cognitive impairments are listed in Table 5–3.

Psychiatric-Psychological Collaboration

The forensic psychiatrist–psychologist team can be an effective unit for forensic assessments. Choosing a psychologist is similar to choosing any other specialist in circumstances for which qualifications, collegiality, and appreciation of forensic issues are desired. Minimally, the psychologist must be licensed in the state where the evaluation will be conducted and, if in private practice, preferably have diplomate status granted by the American Board of Professional Psychology. Diplomate status is afforded only after expertise is demonstrated. An effective collaboration between psychiatrist and psychologist depends on the appreciation of forensic work, particularly the understanding that results of the testing must be relevant and understandable in a legal arena. The psychiatrist can ask for past (redacted) reports by the psychologist to get an idea of what to expect. Recommendations from other experts are also helpful.

A framework to build effective collaboration includes ongoing communication, as described in these six steps (Campbell and Baranoski 2008):

1. *Formulation of the referral question.* Why is testing requested? What are the areas that raise evaluation issues: cognition, psychosis, malingering?

2. *A review of what testing can offer and possible results.* This step is critical. Unless the psychiatrist is already familiar with the psychologist's work and reports, an early discussion about how the psychiatrist works, the fee schedule, and the organization of the report will avoid later conflict and confusion.

3. *Provision of collateral data and clinical impressions to the psychologist.* Some psychologists review data before meeting the patient; others prefer a meeting first. The psychologist must know the legal parameters of the case (e.g., is the testing at the behest of the defense or the prosecution?) to determine how to introduce the testing and whether it is confidential. To complete a psychological assessment, the psychologist must conduct a clinical interview, collecting history of early development, education and employment, and head trauma and physical illness that may affect test results, as well as medication, social circumstances, and current function. Tests can be administered in a vacuum, but they cannot be interpreted without background data.

4. *Choice of tests made by the psychologist.* When psychiatrists or attorneys dictate to the psychologist what tests to perform, they hobble the usefulness and credibility of the evaluation. The referrer asks the question; the psychologist chooses and then defends the methods to answer it. An area of conflict for the psychologist concerns death penalty cases in which defense attorneys at sentencing request an assessment for mitigation. A frequent practice is to instruct the psychologist not to administer the MMPI-2 because of the risk that it will show antisocial characteristics. The psychologist in

TABLE 5–3. Common tests for feigning psychiatric impairments

Test	Target	Procedure	Advantages	Limitations
Miller Forensic Assessment of Symptoms (M-FAST; Miller 2001)	General malingering	Face-to-face mental status format	Short Easily administered and incorporated in clinical examination	Requires cooperation Risk of false-positive results in unusual or guarded presentation
Structured Interview of Reported Symptoms (SIRS; Rogers 1992; Rogers et al. 2002)	Feigned psychosis	Face-to-face structured interview	Strong psychometric properties Score includes assessment of quality of symptoms Useful in identifying cultural differences in psychosis Established as a court-accepted test	Lengthy assessment Training for administration preferred Complex scoring Most reliable in English or Spanish
Test of Memory Malingering (TOMM; Tombaugh 2009)	Feigned memory deficit	Face-to-face administration with booklets of simple line drawings	Strong psychometric properties No language or literacy requirement Useful in cross-cultural work	Overestimates feigning in ADD No norms established for those with PTSD
Validity Indicator Profile (VIP; Frederick 1997)	Lack of effort Feigned cognitive deficit	Pencil-and-paper test Vocabulary and geometric subtests	Computer scoring Strong psychometric properties Report includes estimate of range of IQ Literacy and language requirement for only one subtest Distinguishes between deception and careless responding	Limited usefulness with developmentally disabled Lengthy test Modest refusal rate

Note. ADD=attention-deficit disorder; PTSD=posttraumatic stress disorder.

that situation has the obligation to identify the risk of excluding a particular test on the attorney's request.

5. *Discussion of results before writing a report.* The psychologist usually writes an independent report, but a discussion of the results with the psychiatrist, who has additional clinical and forensic data, will help the psychologist frame the validity and applicability of the results. In some cases, the discussion will result in further testing.

6. *Reconciling of discrepancies.* When the results of psychological testing are in conflict with the psychiatric formulation, the psychiatrist and psychologist should work together to explain the discrepancy. Valid results cannot be ignored out of hand; that approach will leave the psychiatrist vulnerable on cross-examination. A discussion of the discrepancies in both reports is more effective.

The more explicit the communication about the role of the psychologist in the case, the smoother the collaboration will be. A contract in the form of a letter can clarify the question, method of payment, expectations about the report (separate reports or the psychological testing report included in the psychiatric report), and expectations about testimony. If the psychiatrist writes the letter and does the hiring, then contact between the attorney and the psychologist may be minimal. However, if the psychologist is hired by the attorney as a second or adjunct expert, then communication between the attorney and the psychologist will occur. In that case, three-way meetings (psychiatrist, psychologist, and attorney) can reduce confusion and conflict.

Psychologists practice under ethical and practice guidelines that address assessments, reporting, testifying, remuneration, and collaboration. These guidelines are available through the American Psychological Association (2017).

Common Pitfalls in Psychological Testing

As useful as psychological testing can be in case formulations, the testing can create substantial difficulties when misapplied, especially in forensic situations. Three of the most common errors in forensic psychological assessments are a lack of testing coherence, overtesting, and use of novel testing. Additionally, some courts may be unfamiliar with the role of psychological testing in forensic evaluations and may be less inclined to admit testing results as evidence. Finally, sometimes psychological testing is misapplied and therefore not relevant to the legal issue.

Lack of Coherence

Assessments generally follow a routine in the order and type of tests administered; when followed, that routine can help to ensure a coherent and meaningful report. A lack of coherence occurs when the report presents the result of one test as contrary to the result of another without reconciliation. Consider this example: in a presentence evaluation, the psychologist described a 24-year-old man in federal court on charges of participating in narcotic distribution as "extremely low in cognitive function with an IQ of 65" and as "faking symptoms on the MMPI-2." These findings are contradictory and uninformative: either the man had feigned cognitive deficits or he should not have been administered the MMPI-2, which requires a level of reading comprehension precluded by such a low IQ.

Overtesting

Overtesting occurs in two ways: through administration of redundant tests and by testing when no question has been asked. An example of the first is administration of tests that address the same question in different ways; for example, administering two different IQ tests when the first was seen as valid. More common is the administration of two similar standard tests such as the MMPI-2 and the PAI. Although the tests are similar, they provide different narrative and scales. If the goal is to raise clinical hypotheses, fishing for different perspectives can be productive. But in the forensic context, varying results muddy opinions and erode credibility.

The second form of overtesting is more problematic. When there is no question for psychological testing to answer, testing should not be done. Testing done to confirm the lack of a disorder is particularly risky. If the psychiatrist asks for testing so that he or she can be certain that nothing is missed, then testing is appropriate; but if the psychiatrist is comfortable with the finding of no diagnosis, administering tests raises the possibility of a finding that may complicate the forensic work.

Novel Testing

Federal and state courts are familiar with the incorporation of psychological evaluations in forensic cases. In some cases, testing is required to establish the elements of the case, such as the need for cognitive testing in death-eligible cases or neuropsychological evaluations for loss of cognitive capacity and memory in civil cases. Psychological assessments are vulnerable, however, to admissibility challenges. Although these challenges can be raised even when the most standard of batteries are used, certain situations are more likely to result in exclusion of testing results as evidence.

Post *Daubert*, the use of new tests or new twists on old tests has diminished but still occurs. Novel testing is not erroneous per se, even when the new tests have not successfully met an admissibility challenge. Over time, new tests establish precedent of use that makes them part of standard testing. Nevertheless, new tests run the risk, if an admissibility challenge is raised, of being rejected by the court (see, e.g., *State of Connecticut v. Cyrus Griffin* 2005). So many factors influence the decision to grant an admissibility hearing that even meritorious and reasonable tests can be scrutinized. The decision to use a new test requires a cost-benefit analysis of what the test will add and the potential cost of a successful admissibility challenge excluding the results.

Novel to Courts

Acceptance of psychological tests in forensic reports and testimony can vary across courts. Courts less familiar with the role of psychological testing and its relevance to legal questions are more likely to preclude admission. For example, judicial orders for presentence evaluations in the federal courts in Connecticut often include a request for psychological testing. In other federal districts, the acceptance of psychological testing is limited.

Misapplication of the Testing

Testing that does not appear relevant to the legal circumstance appropriately raises questions of acceptability. For example, the center of controversy around the use of the Rorschach inkblot test in custody cases has been its relevance. To meet an admissibility challenge, the psychologist must be able to defend both the test and its applicability in the specific case. In general, the standard psychological tests and their use can be supported by their psychometric properties and their frequent use in courts. Because psychological testing can be replicated and has standard methods, scoring, and interpretation, it can increase the court's confidence in the objectivity of a forensic evaluation.

Risks of Forensic Psychiatrists Using Psychological Tests

In clinical practice, psychiatrists sometimes use psychological tests, including brief intelligence tests and personality inventories that are computer-scored and provide profile summaries. Unavailability of psychologists and the desire to reduce patient costs contribute to the practice. The results suggest or confirm diagnostic impressions, the accuracy of which can be evaluated over time. Therefore, the limitations of tests and issues of reliability and validity are not as critical as they are in forensic evaluations in which opinions to a reasonable degree of medical certainty are treated as conclusions, not hypotheses. In forensic work, specialized expertise in testing is required.

Psychological testing comprises knowledge about and choice of tests, skill in administration, appreciation for sensitivity and specificity of results, the influences of demographic characteristics, and the strategies for collecting clinical corroboration to support or refute test results. The expertise is needed to defend the results on cross-examination, to address challenges to acceptability, and, most important, to protect against wrong and harmful conclusions.

Dattilio et al. (2011), in an analysis of the risks of administration of psychological tests by forensic psychiatrists, concluded that the conduct of psychological testing requires specialized training to understand test construction and the interpretation of test results. The issue of translating results based on group outcomes to individuals is especially challenging. Psychological testing is a specialty with its own knowledge base, training requirements, and jargon. In court, forensic psychiatrists without that specialized training may find themselves challenged for testifying beyond their expertise. Partnering with qualified psychologists for psychological testing protects forensic psychiatrists from attacks on credibility and admissibility of their opinions.

Conclusion

Psychological testing is a valuable adjunct to forensic psychiatric assessments. Standard tests, through research, have established psychometric properties that can meet an admissibility challenge. Testing offers an objective source of data and, thus, can aid in diagnostic and functional assessments for all phases of criminal and civil proceedings. Testing is a specialty of the field of psychology, supported by science. Clear formulation of the forensic question; careful selection of the tests; strict adherence to administration, scoring, and ethics; and research-backed interpretation maximize the applicability and success of psychological testing in the courts. A successful collaboration between the forensic psychiatrist and the psychologist offers a convergence of expertise in analysis and formulation of complex cases. As long as the limitations of testing are recognized, psychological testing has a place in the legal arena.

Key Concepts

- Psychological consultation can bolster the credibility and reliability of forensic opinions and show due diligence on the part of a forensic psychiatric expert.

- The consulting psychologist should be provided with a clear referral question and should be allowed to choose the particular tests that will most likely contribute to answering the questions(s).

- Communication between the psychiatrist and the consulting psychologist is crucial, and clarification of the roles of each expert before consultation is needed.

- Appropriate psychological tests in the forensic arena are those with established psychometric properties, including reliability (the capacity of a test to measure the same variable over time and across situations), validity (the capacity of a test to measure what it is designed to measure), the error rate, and the limitations to generalizability of the test.

- Psychological tests include measures of cognitive capacity, memory, attention, and concentration, as well as standard tests of personality characteristics and projective measures that elicit the individual's worldview and organizational capacity.

- Specific tests have been designed to detect feigning of psychiatric symptoms and cognitive deficits. These are very useful in the assessment of malingering.

References

American Psychiatric Association: Diagnostic and Statistical Manual of Mental Disorders, 5th Edition. Arlington, VA, American Psychiatric Association, 2013

American Psychological Association: Ethical principles of psychologists and code of conduct. 2017. Available at: www.apa.org/ethics/code. Accessed January 2, 2017.

Atkins v Virginia, 536 U.S. 304, 122 S.Ct. 2242 (2002)

Ben-Porath YS, Tellegen A: Minnesota Multiphasic Personality Inventory–2 Restructured Form: Manual for Administration, Scoring, and Interpretation. Minneapolis, University of Minnesota Press, 2008a

Ben-Porath YS, Tellegen A: Minnesota Multiphasic Personality Inventory–2 Restructured Form: User's Guide for Reports. Minneapolis, University of Minnesota Press, 2008b

Broshek DK, Barth JT: The Halstead-Reitan Neuropsychological Test Battery, in Neuropsychological Assessment in Clinical Practice: A Guide to Test Interpretation and Integration. Edited by Groth-Marnat G. New York, Wiley, 2000, pp 223–262

Brown L, Sherbenou RJ, Johnsen SK: Test of Nonverbal Intelligence, 4th Edition (TONI-4). San Antonio, TX, Pearson Corporation, 2010

Campbell WH, Baranoski MVB: Psychological testing for forensic psychiatrists. Article presented at the 39th Annual Meeting of the American Academy of Law and Psychiatry, Seattle WA, October 23–26, 2008

Dattilio FM, Sadoff RL, Drogin EY, et al: Should forensic psychiatrists conduct psychological testing? J Psychiatry Law 39:477–491, 2011

Daubert v Merrell Dow Pharmaceuticals, Inc., 509 U.S. 579, 113 S.Ct. 2786 (1993)

Dunn LM, Dunn DM: Peabody Picture Vocabulary Test, 4th Edition (PPVT™-4). San Antonio, TX, Pearson Corporation, 2007

Exner JE: The Rorschach: A Comprehensive System, Vol 1: Basic Foundations. New York, Wiley, 1995

Flynn JR: The mean IQ of Americans: massive gains 1932 to 1978. Psychol Bull 101:171–191, 1987

Frederick RI: Validity Indicator Profile Manual. Minneapolis, MN, National Computer Services, 1997

Freedman M, Leach L, Kaplan E, et al: Clock Drawing: A Neuropsychological Analysis. New York, Oxford University Press, 1994

Golden CJ, Freshwater SM: Luria-Nebraska Neuropsychological Battery, in Understanding Psychological Assessment: Perspectives on Individual Differences. Edited by Dorfman WI, Hersen M. New York, Kluwer Academic/Plenum, 2001, pp 59–75

Golden CJ, Hammeke TA, Purisch AD, et al: Item Interpretation of the Luria-Nebraska Neuropsychological Battery. Lincoln, University of Nebraska Press, 1982

Golden CJ, Freshwater SM, Vayalakkara J: The Luria-Nebraska Neuropsychological Battery, in Neuropsychological Assessment in Clinical Practice: A Guide to Test Interpretation and Integration. Edited by Groth-Marnat G. New York, Wiley, 2000, pp 223–262

Grove WM, Barden RC: Protecting the integrity of the legal system: the admissibility of testimony from mental health experts under Daubert/Kumho analyses. Psychol Public Policy Law 5:224–242, 1999

Hartzler B, Fromme K: Fragmentary and en bloc blackouts: similarity and distinction among episodes of alcohol-induced memory loss. J Stud Alcohol 64(4):547–550, 2003 12921196

Hathaway SR, McKinley JC: Minnesota Multiphasic Personality Inventory–2. Minneapolis, University of Minnesota Press, 1989

Heilbrun K: The role of psychological testing in forensic assessment. Law Hum Behav 16:252–272, 1992

Herrnstein RJ, Murray C: The Bell Curve: Intelligence and Class Structure in American Life. New York, Free Press, 1994

Holmstrom RW, Silber DE, Karp SA: Development of the Apperceptive Personality Test. J Pers Assess 54:252–264, 1990

Jastak J, Wilkinson G: Wide Range Achievement Test-Revised. Wilmington, DE, Jastak Associates, 1984

Kaufman AS, Kaufman NL: Kaufman Brief Intelligence Test, 2nd Edition (K-BIT-2). San Antonio, TX, Pearson Corporation, 2004

Melton GB, Petrila J, Poythress NG, et al: Psychological Evaluations for the Courts: A Handbook for Mental Health Professionals and Lawyers, 3rd Edition. New York, Guilford, 2007

Meyers JE, Meyers KR: Rey Complex Figure Test and Recognition Trial. Lutz, FL, Psychological Assessment Resources, 2007

Miller HA: The Miller Forensic Assessment of Symptoms Test (M-FAST): Professional Manual. Odessa, FL, Psychological Assessment Resources, 2001

Millon T: Millon Clinical Multiaxial Inventory–III. Minneapolis, MN, National Computer Systems, 1994

Morey LC: The Personality Assessment Inventory: Professional Manual. Lutz, FL, Psychological Assessment Resources, 2007

Osterrieth PA: The test of copying a complex figure: a contribution to the study of perception and memory. Arch Psychol 30:286–356, 1944

Pearson Education: Wechsler Memory Scale, 4th Edition. San Antonio, TX, Pearson Education, 2008

Reitan RM, Wolfson D: The Halstead-Reitan Neurological Test Battery: Theory and Clinical Interpretation, 2nd Edition. Tucson, AZ, Neuropsychology Press, 1993

Rogers R: Structured Interview of Reported Symptoms. Odessa, FL, Psychological Assessment Resources, 1992

Rogers R, Bagby M, Dickens SE: Structured Interview of Reported Symptoms. Lutz, FL, Psychological Assessment Resources, 2002

Roid GH: Stanford-Binet Intelligence Scale, 5th Edition. Rolling Meadows, IL, Riverside, 2002

State of Connecticut v Cyrus Griffin, 869 A.2d 640 (Conn. 2005)

Strauss E, Sherman EMS, Spreen O: A Compendium of Neuropsychological Tests. New York, Oxford University Press, 2006

Tellegen A, Ben-Porath YS: Minnesota Multiphasic Personality Inventory-2 Restructured Form Technical Manual. Minneapolis, University of Minnesota Press, 2008/2011

Tombaugh TN: Test of Memory Malingering. Princeton, NJ, Pearson Education, 2009

Wechsler D: Wechsler Adult Intelligence Scale—Fourth Edition (WAIS-IV). San Antonio, TX, Pearson Corporation, 2008

Wilkinson GS, Robertson GJ: Wide Range Achievement Test 4: Professional Manual. Lutz, FL, Psychological Assessment Resources, 2006

Woodcock RW, McGrew KS, Mather N: Woodcock-Johnson Tests of Achievement–III. Itasca, IL, Riverside Publishing, 2001

CHAPTER 6

Evaluation of Malingering

Barbara E. McDermott, Ph.D.

The assessment of malingering is critical in forensic psychiatry and psychology. DSM-5 (American Psychiatric Association 2013) indicates that malingering should be considered when any combination of the following is noted: a medicolegal context, discrepancy between reported and objective findings, uncooperativeness with the evaluation or recommended treatment, or the presence of antisocial personality disorder. However, given the substantial external incentives in forensic evaluations (medicolegal context), most experts agree that malingering always should be considered (Chesterman et al. 2008).

Estimates of the prevalence of malingering in forensic evaluations vary considerably, dependent largely on context, with estimates as low as 8% for competence to stand trial evaluations (Cornell and Hawk 1989) and up to 50% for personal injury litigation (Greve et al. 2009, Schmand et al. 1998). Methods for evaluating malingering also vary substantially, depending on the illness feigned. In 1838, Beck and Beck noted that illnesses most easily feigned include those with little to no physical manifestations or those based on self-report, suggesting that diseases most amenable to feigning include "insanity, epilepsy, and pain" (p. 26). This chapter provides an overview of malingering, including a review of the illnesses most typically feigned and possible methods for detection.

Motivations and External Incentives

The feigning of mental illness motivated by an external incentive has been recognized for centuries. For example, in Shakespeare's classic tragedy, Hamlet "put an antic disposition on" to avenge the murder of his father. In a more contemporary example demonstrating an external incentive commonly seen in criminal forensic evaluations, Randle McMurphy, the protagonist in *One Flew Over the Cuckoo's Nest*, feigned insanity in order to serve his sentence for statutory rape in a psychiatric hospital.

Although the term *feigning* is often used interchangeably with *malingering*, the two concepts are different. Feigning simply means to represent falsely in order to deceive. In contrast, malingering requires feigning *and* an identified external incentive. Some authors describe the distinction between feigning and malingering in terms of the difference between detection and diagnosis (Heilbronner et al. 2009; McCullumsmith and Ford 2011). A clinician may know that a symptom is falsely produced (detection), but to diagnose malingering, an external incentive must be identified.

According to DSM-5 (American Psychiatric Association 2013), only two disorders involve the intentional production of false symptoms: malingering and factitious disorder. Malingering is a "V code" in DSM-5 (i.e., not a mental disorder) and is distinguished from factitious disorder by the presence of an external incentive. DSM-5 states that factitious disorder "emphasizes the objective identification of falsification of signs and symptoms of illness, rather than an inference about intent or possible underlying motivation" (p. 326). It further emphasizes, "In contrast [to malingering], the diagnosis of factitious disorder requires the absence of obvious rewards" (p. 326). In DSM-5, malingering was removed from the differential diagnoses in all other somatic symptom and related disorders with the exception of conversion disorder.

Several theories have been proposed as explanations for malingering, although the theory that has garnered the most acceptance is the adaptational model proposed by Rogers (2008). In this model, the malingerer is confronted with an adverse situation (e.g., an arrest for a serious crime). The adaptational model suggests that under these circumstances, individuals weigh their options and determine that malingering mental illness is the optimal method for achieving the desired outcome (in the previous example, avoiding criminal responsibility).

The adaptational model is appealing because of its ability to provide explanations for malingering under a wide variety of contexts. However, even though this model provides an explanation for the behavior, it does not describe specific motivations. In a forensic psychiatric context, incentives can include avoidance of criminal responsibility (as in the previous example), reduction in sentences, financial compensation, and workplace accommodations.

In 1972, Miller and Cartlidge outlined methods for detecting malingering, as well as the various types of malingering. They noted that ailments most likely to be malingered include cognitive deficits after head trauma, blackouts, visual complaints, speech disturbances, loss of smell, and most psychiatric disorders. They also discussed three types of malingering: simulation, exaggeration, and false attribution. In a similar trichotomy, Resnick (1997) defined three types of malingering: 1) *pure malingering*, which he described as a complete fabrication of symptoms; 2) *partial malingering*, defined as an amplification of existing symptoms; and 3) *false imputation*, inappropriately assigning causal blame for symptoms.

Miller and Cartlidge (1972) recommended several factors to consider when faced with possible simulation. First and foremost is establishing an external incentive. Other evidence included severe disability following a trivial injury and a symptom pattern inconsistent with an organic cause. They also suggested that the patient's attitude toward the evaluation is telling. Almost 50 years later, these recommendations for evaluating malingering still apply and are included in DSM-5.

Costs of Malingering

The costs of malingering vary as widely as the prevalence. In the criminal justice system, costs are related primarily to delays in trial or plea agreements or to the very real costs of unnecessary mental health treatment. Costs in civil litigation are typically financial and can include loss of workdays (for malingered injuries), inappropriate awarding of disability payments, or financial awards associated with claims of emotional distress.

A noteworthy example of an unexpected cost of malingering was seen in the case of *United States v. Greer* (1998). Charles Greer was arrested for kidnapping and possession of a stolen weapon. During a hospitalization for restoration of his competence to stand trial, Greer was found to be malingering psychosis. At trial, Greer behaved bizarrely, prompting the judge to tell him, "get with the program, and stop acting like a fool" (p. 232). After conviction, Greer received an enhanced sentence (2 additional years) for obstruction of justice because of his malingering.

Prevalence of Malingering

Malingering in the Criminal Justice System

Incentives to malinger vary greatly depending on the context, as does the prevalence. Malingering in the context of the criminal courts is generally for one of three purposes: to present as incompetent to stand trial, to plead not guilty by reason of insanity, or to obtain a sentence reduction once found guilty. For individuals seeking an incompetent to stand trial or not guilty by reason of insanity finding, feigning a psychotic disorder is the most likely method of success, although feigned cognitive deficits is another effective strategy.

Estimates for malingering in incompetence to stand trial evaluations have varied from a low of 8% (Cornell and Hawk 1989) to a high of 17.4% (Rogers et al. 1998). More recently, one group of investigators (Vitacco et al. 2007) found a malingering rate of 21% in a sample of individuals evaluated for competence to stand trial. A group of forensic psychologists estimated that malingering occurred in almost 16% of forensic patients and more than 7% of nonforensic patients (Rogers et al. 1994). Additionally, almost 21% of the defendants undergoing evaluations of criminal responsibility engaged in or were suspected of engaging in malingering (Rogers et al. 1986).

Recent study data (McDermott et al. 2009) indicated that more than 18% of the patients found incompetent to stand trial were malingering their psychiatric symptoms on admission for restoration. The prevalence of malingering in these patients was significantly related to severity of the offense, with defendants found incompetent to stand trial for murder and robbery having prevalence rates three times those of other offenders (37% and 38%, respectively, compared with 13% for all other offenses) (McDermott et al. 2013).

Malingering in Civil Proceedings

In civil proceedings, estimates of malingering are generally much higher than in criminal medicolegal contexts. Financial incentives appear to drive this difference. Greiffenstein and Baker (2006) found a 37% base rate of malingering in individuals with mild head injury who were seeking financial compensation. Larrabee (2003), in a review of 11 studies, found a prevalence rate of 40% in 1,363 patients seeking compensation for a mild head injury. In fact, Larrabee (2000) opined that the incidence of exaggeration of deficits in mild head injury patients who were seeking compensation was 10 times higher than the base rate for actual deficits.

Although prominent in the literature, mild head injury is not the only disorder malingered for financial gain. Greve and colleagues (2009) found a malingering rate between 20% and 50% for 508 patients complaining of chronic pain who were also seeking financial compensation. Schmand and colleagues (1998) found exaggeration of memory deficits in 61% of postwhiplash patients involved in litigation, as compared with 29% in an outpatient clinic. A study conducted by Frueh and colleagues (2000) indicated that approximately 30% of veterans seeking disability compensation for posttraumatic stress disorder (PTSD) feign the disorder.

In other types of disability claims, Griffin and colleagues (1996) found that nearly 20% of Social Security disability claimants were malingering. Wierzbicki and Tyson (2007) determined that 43.5% of college students seeking a diagnosis of attention-deficit/hyperactivity disorder (ADHD), learning disability, or both in order to receive special accommodations under the Americans with Disabilities Act did not meet criteria for either diagnosis. This suggests that money is not the only incentive in disability claims. The prevalence of malingering seems directly related to the strength of the incentive (Binder and Rohling 1996; Rohling et al. 1995).

Assessment of Malingering

The prevalence rates of malingering in forensic evaluations support the commonly accepted axiom that regardless of the type of forensic assessment, malingering always should be considered. The optimal assessment of malingering is multifaceted and should include three components: 1) a clinical interview to clearly document the complaint as well as any discrepancies between the complaint and the observed behavior; 2) a review of relevant collateral information for corroborating evidence of the complaint or significant inconsistencies; and 3) psychological testing to assess response bias and to provide structured assessments of malingering.

Response bias may be defined as an individual responding in a manner unrelated to item content (McGrath et al. 2010). *Negative impression management* is one type of response bias, defined as "responding in an excessively aberrant manner" (p. 451). In contrast, *positive impression management* is defined as "the failure to report aberrant tendencies" (p. 451). Response bias also can include styles that are independent of intentional effort. Inconsistent (or random) responding, acquiescence, and negativism (yay or naysaying) are examples of response biases that may not necessarily be purposeful.

In addition to these response biases, several authors discuss the need to detect lack of effort (e.g., Boone 2017). The concept of effort has been almost exclusively associated with the assessment of neurocognitive function. Symptom validity tests were designed specifically to evaluate the credibility of neurocognitive dysfunction. A less than chance performance on these instruments is indicative of lack of effort or a deliberate effort to fail. Recently, Larrabee (2012) has contended that the term *performance validity* provides more accuracy than the terms *response bias*, *effort*, or *symptom validity*.

Clinical Assessment

A clinical interview is an essential component of the assessment, and the evaluator's style is critical when considering malingering. The interviewer should avoid providing verbal or nonverbal communications to the evaluee (e.g., smiling at absurd questions; McDermott and Sokolov 2009). The evaluator should always attempt to ask open-ended questions to minimize the chance that the evaluee will learn about specific diagnostic criteria (Soliman and Resnick 2010). Unfortunately, the Internet provides abundant descriptions of the symptoms of actual disorders, supplying detailed information to potential malingerers (Hall and Hall 2006).

"If you tell the truth, you don't have to remember anything," a quote attributed to Mark Twain, eloquently summarizes one hallmark of malingering: inconsistency, both between reported symptoms and those observed or documented and in reporting symptoms over time. The evaluator should carefully record inconsistencies during the course of the evaluation and reviews of collateral information. Inconsistencies that may indicate malingering include the following (McDermott et al. 2008):

- The evaluee's presentation is inconsistent with his or her alleged symptom(s).
- The individual behaves in a dramatically different way depending on who is observing him or her.
- The individual reports symptoms that are inconsistent with how genuine symptoms normally manifest.

- The individual's report significantly contradicts records and other collateral information.

Psychological Assessment

Psychological testing is particularly useful in evaluating any type of response bias. Various types of tests can prove useful, depending on the deficit or illness feigned. The most common testing methods are described in the following subsections. One caveat with all these described assessments: individuals unable to concentrate because of severe psychosis should be evaluated when their psychosis remits.

Broad-Based Tests of Psychological Functioning and Symptom Validity Testing

Perhaps the most researched strategy in the detection of response bias is to use self-report instruments evaluating general psychological functioning that also include validity scales. The two instruments most often used in this regard are the revised version of the Minnesota Multiphasic Personality Inventory, the MMPI-2 (Butcher et al. 1989); and the Personality Assessment Inventory (PAI; Morey 1991).

The MMPI-2 is a 567-item self-report instrument designed as a measure of general psychopathology. It has been cited as being "the mostly widely administered objective personality test in forensic evaluations" (Wygant 2007, p. 8), largely because of the substantial body of research conducted on its ability to detect response bias via the embedded validity scales. On the original MMPI, various configurations of the validity scales were extensively researched to detect both positive and negative impression management ("faking good" or "faking bad") (Greene 1980). When the MMPI was revised, many more validity scales were developed that allow the examiner to distinguish between, for example, random responding and feigning.

The MMPI-2 is efficient at measuring at least two types of feigning: feigned severe psychopathology and feigned somatic and neurocognitive complaints (Larrabee 2005). Feigning of severe psychopathology (often associated with the feigning of psychosis in criminal cases or PTSD in civil litigation) is most often identified by elevations on the family of F (Infrequency) scales (F, Fb [F Back], Fp [F Psychopathology]).

The feigning of somatic, neurocognitive complaints or emotional distress often seen in civil litigation has led to the development of other composite validity scales. One such scale, termed the *Fake Bad Scale* (FBS) and renamed the *Symptom Validity Scale* when it was included in the standard MMPI-2 report, was developed to detect feigned emotional distress often claimed in civil litigation. This scale was developed by selecting items that distinguished simulators (individuals instructed to feign a disorder), litigants with clear evidence of feigning, and litigants with legitimate injury (Lees-Haley et al. 1991). The scale purports to capture two facets of feigned emotional distress: items that suggest the plaintiff is honest and trustworthy and items indicating that but for the alleged stressor, the individual would not have mental health symptoms (Greiffenstein et al. 2007). The FBS is capable of detecting feigning of much more subtle symptoms, unlike the F scales, which detect feigned severe psychopathology. Larrabee (1998) described the FBS as a measure of "somatic malingering," although others have described it as a measure of general maladjustment (Butcher et al. 2003).

The FBS has received criticism in the literature (Butcher et al. 2008), largely because of its application to inappropriate samples (Greiffenstein et al. 2007). The FBS has been criticized as overidentifying feigning, especially in women (Bury and Bagby 2002), although evidence suggests that a score of 30 or greater on the FBS is strongly suggestive of feigned disability, regardless of gender (Greiffenstein et al. 2007). In fact, Greiffenstein et al. (2007, p. 223) suggested that with scores greater than 29, "virtually 100%" of individuals are feigning symptoms.

A scale to assess feigned cognitive issues (Response Bias Scale; RBS) was developed by examining the endorsement of items in individuals both passing and failing performance validity tests (Gervais et al. 2007). The authors suggested that the RBS improves accuracy above the F scales or the FBS (Wygant et al. 2010). However, elevations on the RBS are more associated with cognitive complaints and failure on performance validity testing; the FBS is most associated with feigned somatic complaints or emotional distress; and the F scales are most associated with severe psychiatric symptom exaggeration.

The PAI (Morey 1991) is a 344-item self-report instrument designed to assess general psychopathology. As with the MMPI, inclusion of validity scales to assess response bias was a critical component of its development. The validity scale most relevant in malingering is the Negative Impression Management scale, which quantifies the endorsement of bizarre or unlikely symptoms.

More recently, two additional scales have shown promise in the detection of malingering. The Malingering Index (Morey 1996) was constructed on the basis of profile characteristics often associated with the feigning of psychiatric disorders. The Rogers Discriminant Function was created with information from three groups: a clinical group (patients with schizophrenia, major depression, and generalized anxiety disorder) and nonclinical participants categorized as either naïve or sophisticated (Rogers et al. 2012). The results of the discriminant analysis indicated that the weighted combination of scales produced a hit rate of 92% (accurately identifying malingerers). Furthermore, the Rogers Discriminant Function performed well even with the sophisticated malingerers, with a hit rate of 73%. However, the Negative Impression Management scale showed the strongest associations with malingering, at least of severe psychopathology (Kucharski et al. 2007).

Floor Effect

The concept known as the *floor effect* involves the incorporation of extremely easy questions or tasks in the testing methodology. Such items generally tap overlearned information or easily retained simple skills, even in those with limited intellectual functioning. Examples of such items include requests to perform simple arithmetic calculations (e.g., 2+2= ____?), questions about basic common information (e.g., Who is president of the United States?), and queries about basic autobiographical information (such as one's age or birthday). The Rey Fifteen-Item Test (FIT; Rey 1964) is an example of a floor effect assessment. The FIT requires that individuals remember a set of 15 letters, numbers, and geometric shapes that are in fact quite simple because of their redundancy (Figure 6–1).

A meta-analysis of the FIT indicated that its specificity was much higher than its sensitivity (92% vs. 43%), with an overall hit rate of 70% (Vickery et al. 2001). A score lower than 9 achieves reasonable sensitivity (58%–89%) and high specificity (96%–98%) (Frederick 2002). In an effort to improve the sensitivity in particular,

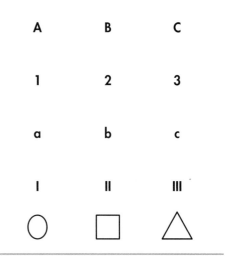

FIGURE 6–1. Rey Fifteen-Item Test stimulus.
Source. Rey 1964.

Griffin et al. (1997) modified the FIT by increasing its redundancy, providing standardized administration instructions, and outlining a method of qualitative scoring. In a clinical population, they used qualitative scoring to estimate the sensitivity at 71%, although the specificity declined to 75% with this scoring system.

Performance Validity Testing (Symptom Validity Testing)

The concept of symptom validity testing was initially described in the context of the assessment of sensory loss (Pankratz 1979). In this procedure, the individual is presented with a stimulus and instructed to guess whether the stimulus is present. If the individual performs worse than chance over several trials, it is presumed that he or she actually knows the correct response and purposefully selected the wrong response. In a two-alternative forced-choice task, below-chance performance is less than 50%.

These forced-choice tests, many of which are designed to assess feigned cognitive dysfunction, are more accurately termed *performance validity tests*, because most are developed to evaluate below-chance *performance* (Larrabee

2012). Larrabee proposed that the term *symptom validity testing* should be reserved for assessments evaluating psychiatric *symptoms*. Multiple assessments of feigned memory and cognitive deficits have been developed with this paradigm, often coupled with the floor-effect paradigm. One example is the Test of Memory Malingering, a visual recognition test that presents the individual with 50 different picture drawings (Tombaugh 1996). Two learning trials are conducted, followed by a retention trial. Scores less than chance or based on criteria developed from individuals with head injury or cognitive impairment are indicative of feigned memory impairment.

Unusual Pattern of Responses: Symptom Validity Testing

This paradigm is particularly effective in identifying individuals feigning psychiatric symptoms. Detection of feigned psychiatric symptoms historically has been based on the premise that malingerers "throw in a little extra" to convince examiners of the gravity of their symptoms. For example, the M test (Beaber et al. 1985) is a malingering assessment consisting of 33 items related to psychiatric illness. Endorsing three or more symptoms on one of the three subscales is suggestive of malingering.

Several psychological tests evaluate whether the examinee is providing atypical responses to questions about mental health symptoms. Examples include the endorsement of symptoms rarely presented by those with a genuine mental disorder or to the degree endorsed by malingerers or that are highly improbable. The most widely used assessment for the detection of feigned psychiatric symptoms with this paradigm is the Structured Interview of Reported Symptoms (SIRS; Rogers et al. 1992).

A broad range of strategies in the detection of feigning was used in the development of the SIRS. This 172-item structured interview takes approximately 30–45 minutes to administer. The original SIRS contained eight primary and five supplementary scales. The supplementary scales were used only if the respondent did not endorse symptoms in sufficient quantity to make a definitive determination of feigning. Responses on the primary scales were classified as honest, indeterminate, probable feigning, or definite feigning. An individual was considered to be feigning psychiatric symptoms if he or she scored in the definite range on at least one primary subscale or in the probable range on three or more primary subscales. Studies indicated that these criteria optimized both sensitivity and specificity (Rogers et al. 1992).

The SIRS was revised (SIRS-2; Rogers et al. 2010) because of high false-positive rates, most notably with individuals with a significant trauma history (Rogers et al. 2009). Although the item content remained the same, the SIRS-2 provides an algorithm for decision making that includes the use of composite scores and the primary scales. In a recent study comparing the SIRS with the SIRS-2, Tarescavage and Glassmire (2016) reported that the SIRS-2 had significantly poorer sensitivity (0.54 for the SIRS-2 vs. 0.87 for the SIRS). They found that the SIRS-2 underestimated feigning and concluded that clinicians should not rule out feigning based on SIRS-2 indeterminate results.

Assessment of Malingering in Specific Disorders

Almost any illness that relies on self-report can be feigned. Psychiatric disorders, the symptoms of which are based almost entirely on self-report, are easily feigned. Head injury and pain are the most commonly feigned medical disorders. Although describing the assessment of all potentially malingered disorders is beyond the scope of this chapter, this section reviews procedures for evaluating malingering in the most commonly feigned disorders in psychiatry and psychology: psychotic disorders; neurocognitive impairment, which can include both intellectual and memory deficits; and PTSD.

Malingered Psychosis

In 1944, Ossipov outlined various clinical indices of feigned psychosis, although he ultimately noted that "it is often impossible to differentiate between a psychosis and malingering on the basis of symptoms alone" (p. 41). Individuals who present as psychotic with an identifiable external incentive should be carefully observed to evaluate whether their behavior is consistent with the type and severity of reported symptoms, especially if the onset of symptoms is sudden (Chesterman et al. 2008).

Characteristics of malingered psychosis include continuous hallucinations, vague hallucinations, hallucinations not associated with delusions, an inability to state strategies to diminish voices, and a report that all command hallucinations are obeyed (Resnick 1999). Malingering should be suspected if reported delusions have an abrupt onset (similar to Chesterman et al. 2008), if the patient has an eagerness to call attention to the delusions, if behavior is inconsistent with reported delusions, or if the delusions are considered bizarre in the absence of disordered thinking (Resnick 1999).

"Successful malingerers" (i.e., individuals who simulated mental illness but scored below the cut points on structured assessments of malingering) differ from unsuccessful malingerers in specific ways. Successful malingerers endorse significantly fewer numbers of legitimate symptoms and avoid endorsing absurd or bizarre symptoms (Edens et al. 2001).

Psychological testing can be extremely useful in the detection of feigned psychosis. Several screening instruments can be useful in identifying individuals who are possibly malingering, including the Miller Forensic Assessment of Symptoms Test (Miller 2001) and the Structured Inventory of Malingered Symptomatology (Widows and Smith 2005). Because both of these instruments are brief screening tools, they should be followed by a more comprehensive assessment. The SIRS can provide confirmation of feigned psychosis and is recommended if the screening tool suggests the possibility of feigning. However, as noted previously, the SIRS-2 lacks the sensitivity of the SIRS and should not be used as definitive proof of honest responding (Tarescavage and Glassmire 2016).

Malingered Neurocognitive Impairment and Intellectual Deficiencies

In contrast to the production of psychiatric symptoms, feigning cognitive impairments typically requires a demonstration of absence of functioning. Slick and colleagues (1999) coined the term "malingering of neurocognitive dysfunction," which they note is characterized by the intentional exaggeration or fabrication of cognitive dysfunction for the purpose of obtaining some external incentive or avoiding responsibility.

The use of structured, standardized assessments is a critical component when evaluating the validity of neurocognitive dysfunction. Performance validity testing in particular has been described as the "evidentiary gold standard" for feigned cognitive impairment (Slick et al. 1999). In a meta-analysis of 32 studies of the most commonly used testing, Vickery and colleagues (2001) found that individuals feigning cognitive deficits achieved scores more than 1 standard deviation lower than honest responders on performance validity tests. In a survey of neuropsychologists who consistently practice in the area of compensation claims (Slick et al. 2004), more than 45% indicated that they routinely use the Test of Memory Malingering (Tombaugh 1996), a widely known performance validity test, and more than 33% indicated that they use the FIT (Rey 1964).

Unfortunately, individuals can successfully feign deficits on tests designed to measure intelligence. For example, Graue et al. (2007) showed that community volunteers were able to feign a lowered IQ on the Wechsler Adult Intelligence Scale, 3rd Edition, when instructed to do so, and embedded tests of malingering (e.g., Digit Span scaled score and Reliable Digit Span) did not reliably identify such feigning. Currently, DSM-5 places more emphasis on adaptive skills deficits than IQ score for the diagnosis of intellectual disability. However, measures of adaptive behavior, such as the Adaptive Behavior Assessment System, 2nd Edition (Harrison and Oakland 2000), are also susceptible to manipulation (Doane and Salekin 2009). The Validity Indicator Profile (Frederick and Foster 1997) was developed specifically to identify feigned intellectual deficits. This assessment consists of verbal and nonverbal subtests, both using a two-alternative forced-choice paradigm. Item difficulty is randomly distributed throughout the test to prevent a test taker from adopting a strategy of answering easy items accurately. After scoring is completed, response styles are categorized as compliant, careless, irrelevant, and malingered. One concern with the Validity Indicator Profile is that in order to be classified as malingering, the examinee has to exert effort; otherwise, responses are classified as either careless or irrelevant.

Malingered Posttraumatic Stress Disorder

PTSD is especially easy to feign, because the diagnosis is based almost entirely on self-report, and financial incentives are often associated with receiving the diagnosis. Estimates of feigning PTSD ranged from 14% to 30% for individuals in the military seeking disability benefits (Frueh et al. 2000; Gold and Frueh 1999), although one study reported a considerably higher prevalence (53%) for veterans seeking treatment (Freeman et al. 2008). This suggests that malingering is a significant problem and should always be considered in a thorough assessment of PTSD.

In DSM-IV-TR (American Psychiatric Association 2000), clinicians were cautioned to rule out malingering when financial matters were involved, although this cautionary statement was removed from DSM-5. Unfortunately, information about PTSD criteria is readily available on the Internet: more than 22 million sources describing symptoms of PTSD were noted in a 2016 Google search (https://www.google.com/?safe=active-andssui=on#safe=activeandq=PTSD; accessed September 5, 2016). Additionally, many standard instruments developed to assess PTSD use a structured interview format with questions that describe PTSD symptoms. Asking questions specifically about the symptoms and diagnostic criteria of the disorder may provide information that could increase the possibility of successful feigning.

Various authors have outlined procedures for evaluating PTSD, all of which include an assessment of malingering (e.g., Knoll and Resnick 2006). They recommend conducting a comprehensive review of records, preferably before the evaluation, so that inconsistencies can be questioned. Contact with collateral informants to corroborate self-report is also critical. Knoll and Resnick (2006) proposed several clinical signs of feigned PTSD, including inconsistencies in symptom presentation over time, recurrent nightmares that are invariant, an ability to enjoy recreational activities coupled with an inability to work, and vagueness in the description of symptoms. Extreme reports of symptoms are also more likely to be identified as malingering (Gold and Frueh 1999).

Broad-based tests of psychological functioning have proved to be the most fruitful in detecting malingered PTSD. The MMPI-2 in particular has shown utility in this regard, although this is complicated by the fact that individuals with genuine PTSD can experience substantial distress and may have legitimately elevated scores on some MMPI-2 validity scales. In a study of veterans seeking disability compensation who were instructed to feign, the family of F scales—most notably, F, Fb, and Fp—were most effective in discriminating between honest reporters and feigners (Arbisi et al. 2006). Fp in particular was superior in discriminating the two groups. The authors suggested using a cut score of Fp greater than 99 (T score) for identifying individuals feigning PTSD. The FBS initially showed promise in identifying malingered PTSD in personal injury claims (Lees-Haley 1992), but further research was mixed in this regard (Efendov et al. 2008; Elhai et al. 2001). The FBS has more utility in detecting feigned emotional distress, which was the goal when developed (Lees-Haley et al. 1991).

Elhai and colleagues (2002) developed a scale specifically to detect feigned PTSD, Fptsd (Infrequency-Posttraumatic Stress Disorder scale), which includes items from the MMPI-2 that were infrequently endorsed by veterans with legitimate PTSD. In the development sample, this scale was found to improve the accuracy of detection of feigned PTSD above other F scales. Subsequent research indicated that the Fptsd scale did not improve the accuracy of detection (above the traditional F scales) when used in a sample of civilians with PTSD (Elhai et al. 2004). In a study with veterans seeking compensation for PTSD, the study authors found that the Fptsd only minimally improved detection beyond the family of F scales, with the Fp providing the best discrimination (Arbisi et al. 2006).

The Morel Emotional Numbing Test (MENT; Morel 1998) for PTSD has been described as a symptom validity test specific to PTSD. This instrument assesses the recognition of various emotions in a two-alternative forced-choice format. The evaluee is told, "Some individuals with PTSD may have difficulty recognizing facial expressions," and they are then asked to note the emotion associated with the facial expressions shown. According to Morel (1998), any adult who puts forth a reasonable amount of effort (except for the visually impaired or those with less than a third-grade reading level) can complete the task with 90%–100% accuracy, even if they have PTSD, recommending that a total of more than nine errors is suggestive of malingering. In a study investigating the use of the MENT with Croatian war veterans, a cut score of nine produced a sensitivity of 92% and specificity of 96% (Geraerts et al. 2009). This finding suggests that the MENT may be useful as one component of an assessment of malingered PTSD.

The Atypical Response (ATR) scale of the Trauma Symptom Inventory, 2nd Edition (Briere 2010), also has been described as useful in distinguishing genuine symptoms of PTSD from simulated PTSD. In their study of 75 undergraduate students trained to simulate PTSD and 49 undergraduate students with genuine PTSD, Gray and colleagues (2010) determined that the ATR scale correctly classified 75% of genuinely distressed individuals and 74% of PTSD simulators. This scale is a revised version of the ATR scale from the original Trauma Symptom Inventory, which had shown unimpressive classification rates (Elhai et al. 2005).

Special Topics

Two scales have been developed to assess malingering in competency evaluations, both of which use the forced-choice format. The Inventory of Legal Knowledge (Musick and Otto 2006) is a 61-item true/false instrument designed to detect feigning of legal knowledge. Any score below 48 is suggestive of feigning. The authors caution that high scores on the Inventory of Legal Knowledge do not suggest competence and should not be interpreted as such. The Test of Malingered Incompetence (Colwell et al. 2008) is an assessment developed to identify feigned cognitive deficits in competency evaluations. The instrument contains two scales with 25 items each: general knowledge and legal knowledge. The authors suggest that scores less than 21 are suggestive of feigning.

Conclusion

The assessment of malingering is a critical component of a forensic evaluation. Virtually all psychiatric disorders rely on accurate self-report, which is obviously subject to extreme distortion in some cases. With the powerful motivator of money included, prevalence rates are remarkably high. In criminal cases, feigning rates are as high as 21% in competence to stand trial and criminal responsibility evaluations and greater than 60% in civil litigation. Considering response styles in forensic evaluations should be the standard of practice. Although DSM-5 suggests that an evaluation conducted in a medicolegal context, coupled with at least one other factor, should raise suspicions for malingering, a medicolegal context by itself should be sufficient to trigger a consideration of malingering.

Key Concepts

- Feigning is prevalent in both criminal and civil contexts, with higher rates in civil forensic evaluations likely related to the presence of financial incentives.

- Although DSM-5 suggests that medicolegal context is only one of a necessary two criteria to raise suspicions of feigning, it appears that one criterion (medicolegal) is sufficient to raise concerns.

- Establishing an external incentive is a necessary component of a malingering assessment.

- Evidence of feigning includes inconsistencies in reported versus observed behavior or inconsistencies in behavior over time or overendorsement of symptoms and deficits.

- Although validity scales in commonly used psychological instruments (e.g., Minnesota Multiphasic Personality Inventory, Personality Assessment Inventory) can be helpful in the assessment of malingering, specific performance validity testing is important in the assessment of malingered neurocognitive deficits, and symptom validity testing is most useful in the assessment of malingered psychiatric symptoms.

- Psychological assessment alone is not adequate to determine malingering, and a comprehensive evaluation should include interviewing and obtaining collateral information.

References

American Psychiatric Association: Diagnostic and Statistical Manual of Mental Disorders, 4th Edition, Text Revision. Washington, DC, American Psychiatric Association, 2000

American Psychiatric Association: Diagnostic and Statistical Manual of Mental Disorders, 5th Edition. Arlington, VA, American Psychiatric Association, 2013

Arbisi PA, Ben-Porath YS, McNulty J: The ability of the MMPI-2 to detect feigned PTSD within the context of compensation seeking. Psychol Serv 3:249–261, 2006

Beaber RJ, Marston A, Michelli J, et al: A brief test for measuring malingering in schizophrenic individuals. Am J Psychiatry 142(12):1478–1481, 1985 4073316

Beck TR, Beck JB: Elements of Medical Jurisprudence. Philadelphia, PA, Thomas, Cowperthwait, & Co. 1838

Binder LM, Rohling ML: Money matters: a meta-analytic review of the effects of financial incentives on recovery after closed-head injury. Am J Psychiatry 153 (1):7–10, 1996 8540596

Boone K: Forensic neuropsychology, in Principles and Practice of Forensic Psychiatry, 3rd Edition. Edited by Rosner R, Scott CL. Boca Raton, FL, CRC Press, 2017, pp 739–748

Briere J: Trauma Symptom Inventory, 2nd Edition (TSI-2): Professional Manual. Odessa, FL, Psychological Assessment Resources, 2010

Bury AS, Bagby RM: The detection of feigned uncoached and coached posttraumatic stress disorder with the MMPI-2 in a sample of workplace accident victims. Psychol Assess 14(4):472–484, 2002 12501573

Butcher JN, Dahlstrom WG, Graham JR, et al: MMPI-2: Manual for Administration and Scoring. Minneapolis, University of Minnesota Press, 1989

Butcher JN, Arbisi PA, Atlis MM, et al: The construct validity of the Lees-Haley Fake Bad Scale: does this scale measure somatic malingering and feigned emotional distress? Arch Clin Neuropsychol 18(5):473–485, 2003 14591444

Butcher JN, Gass CS, Cumella E, et al: Potential bias in MMPI-2 assessments using the Fake Bad Scale (FBS). Psychol Inj Law 1:191–209, 2008

Chesterman LP, Terbeck S, Vaughan F: Malingered psychosis. J Forensic Psychiatry Psychol 19:275–300, 2008

Colwell K, Colwell LH, Perry AT, et al: The Test of Malingered Incompetence (TOMI): a forced-choice instrument for assessing cognitive malingering in competence to stand trial evaluations. Am J Forensic Psychol 26:17–42, 2008

Cornell DG, Hawk GL: Clinical presentation of malingerers diagnosed by experienced forensic psychologists. Law Hum Behav 13:375–383, 1989

Doane BM, Salekin KL: Susceptibility of current adaptive behavior measures to feigned deficits. Law Hum Behav 33(4): 329–343, 2009 18821005

Edens JF, Guy LS, Otto RK, et al: Factors differentiating successful versus unsuccessful malingerers. J Pers Assess 77(2):333–338, 2001 11693862

Efendov AA, Sellbom M, Bagby RM: The utility and comparative incremental validity of the MMPI-2 and Trauma Symptom Inventory validity scales in the detection of feigned PTSD. Psychol Assess 20(4):317–326, 2008 19086755

Elhai JD, Gold SN, Sellers AH, et al: The detection of malingered posttraumatic stress disorder with MMPI-2 fake bad indices. Assessment 8(2):221–236, 2001 11428701

Elhai JD, Ruggiero KJ, Frueh BC, et al: The Infrequency-Posttraumatic Stress Disorder scale (Fptsd) for the MMPI-2: development and initial validation with veterans presenting with combat-related PTSD. J Pers Assess 79(3):531–549, 2002 12511019

Elhai JD, Naifeh JA, Zucker IS, et al: Discriminating malingered from genuine civilian posttraumatic stress disorder: a validation of three MMPI-2 Infrequency scales (F, Fp, and Fptsd). Assessment 11(2):139–144, 2004 15171461

Elhai JD, Gray MJ, Naifeh JA, et al: Utility of the trauma symptom inventory's atypical response scale in detecting malingered post-traumatic stress disorder. Assessment 12(2):210–219, 2005 15914722

Frederick RI: A review of Rey's strategies for detecting malingered neuropsychological impairment. J Forensic Neuropsychol 2(3):1–25, 2002

Frederick RI, Foster HG: The Validity Indicator Profile. Minneapolis, MN, National Computer Systems, 1997

Freeman T, Powell M, Kimbrell T: Measuring symptom exaggeration in veterans with chronic posttraumatic stress disorder. Psychiatry Res 158(3):374–380, 2008 18294699

Frueh BC, Hamner MB, Cahill SP, et al: Apparent symptom overreporting in combat veterans evaluated for PTSD. Clin Psychol Rev 20(7):853–885, 2000 11057375

Geraerts E, Kozaric-Kovacic C, Merckelbach H: Detecting deception of war-related posttraumatic stress disorder. J Forensic Psychiatry Psychol 20:278–285, 2009

Gervais RO, Ben-Porath YS, Wygant DB, et al: Development and validation of a Response Bias Scale (RBS) for the MMPI-2. Assessment 14(2):196–208, 2007 17504891

Gold PB, Frueh BC: Compensation-seeking and extreme exaggeration of psychopathology among combat veterans evaluated for posttraumatic stress disorder. J Nerv Ment Dis 187:680–684, 1999 10579596

Graue LO, Berry DTR, Clark JA, et al: Identification of feigned mental retardation using the new generation of malingering detection instruments: preliminary findings. Clin Neuropsychol 21(6):929–942, 2007 17886151

Gray MJ, Elhai JD, Briere J: Evaluation of the Atypical Response scale of the Trauma Symptom Inventory-2 in detecting simulated posttraumatic stress disorder. J Anxiety Disord 24(5):447–451, 2010 20347258

Greene RL: The MMPI: An Interpretive Manual. New York, Grune & Stratton, 1980

Greiffenstein MF, Baker WJ: Miller was (mostly) right: head injury severity inversely related to simulation. Leg Criminol Psychol 11:131–145, 2006

Greiffenstein MF, Fox D, Lees-Haley PR: The MMPI-2 Fake Bad Scale, in Detection of Noncredible Brain Injury Claims. Edited by Boone K. New York, Guilford, 2007, pp 210–235

Greve KW, Ord JS, Bianchini KJ, Curtis KL: Prevalence of malingering in patients with chronic pain referred for psychologic evaluation in a medico-legal context. Arch Phys Med Rehabil 90(7):1117–1126, 2009 19577024

Griffin GA, Normington J, May R, et al: Assessing dissimulation among Social Security disability income claimants. J Consult Clin Psychol 64(6):1425–1430, 1996 8991329

Griffin GAE, Glassmire DM, Henderson EA, et al: Rey II: redesigning the Rey screening test of malingering. J Clin Psychol 53(7):757–766, 1997 9356906

Hall RC, Hall RC: Malingering of PTSD: forensic and diagnostic considerations, characteristics of malingerers and clinical presentations. Gen Hosp Psychiatry 28(6):525–535, 2006 17088169

Harrison PL, Oakland T: Adaptive Behavior Assessment System. San Antonio, TX, Psychological Corporation, 2000

Heilbronner RL, Sweet JJ, Morgan JE, et al: American Academy of Clinical Neuropsychology Consensus Conference Statement on the neuropsychological assessment of effort, response bias, and malingering. Clin Neuropsychol 23(7):1093–1129, 2009 19735055

Knoll J, Resnick PJ: The detection of malingered post-traumatic stress disorder. Psychiatr Clin North Am 29(3):629–647, 2006 16904503

Kucharski LT, Toomey JP, Fila K, et al: Detection of malingering of psychiatric disorder with the personality assessment inventory: an investigation of criminal defendants. J Pers Assess 88(1):25–32, 2007 17266411

Larrabee G: Somatic malingering on the MMPI and MMPI-2 in litigating subjects. Clin Neuropsychol 12:179–188, 1998

Larrabee GJ: Forensic neuropsychological assessment, in Clinician's Guide to Neuropsychological Assessment, 2nd Edition. Edited by Vanderploeg AD. Mahwah, NJ, Erlbaum, 2000, pp 301–335

Larrabee GJ: Detection of malingering using atypical performance patterns on standard neuropsychological tests. Clin Neuropsychol 17(3):410–425, 2003 14704892

Larrabee GJ: Forensic Neuropsychology. New York, Oxford University Press, 2005

Larrabee GJ: Assessment of malingering, in Forensic Neuropsychology: A Scientific Approach, 2nd Edition. Edited by Larrabee GJ. New York, Oxford University Press, 2012, pp 116–159

Lees-Haley PR: Efficacy of MMPI-2 validity scales and MCMI-II modifier scales for detecting spurious PTSD claims: F, F-K, Fake Bad Scale, ego strength, subtle-obvious subscales, DIS, and DEB. J Clin Psychol 48(5):681–689, 1992 1401155

Lees-Haley PR, English LT, Glenn WJ: A Fake Bad Scale on the MMPI-2 for personal injury claimants. Psychol Rep 68(1):203–210, 1991 2034762

McCullumsmith CB, Ford CV: Simulated illness: the factitious disorders and malingering. Psychiatr Clin North Am 34(3):621–641, 2011 21889683

McDermott BE, Sokolov G: Malingering in a correctional setting: the use of the Structured Interview of Reported Symptoms in a jail sample. Behav Sci Law 27(5):753–765, 2009 19743514

McDermott BE, Leamon M, Feldman MD, et al: Factitious disorder and malingering, in The American Psychiatric Publishing Textbook of Psychiatry, 5th Edition. Edited by Hales RH, Yudofsky SC. Washington, DC, American Psychiatric Publishing, 2008, pp 643–654

McDermott BE, Rabin A, Scott CL, et al: Triaging the IST patient: a brief screen to reduce LOS. Paper presented at the 40th annual meeting of the American Academy of Psychiatry and the Law, Baltimore, MD, October 26–28, 2009

McDermott BE, Dualan IV, Scott CL: Malingering in the correctional system: does incentive affect prevalence? Int J Law Psychiatry 36(3–4):287–292, 2013 23664364

McGrath RE, Mitchell M, Kim BH, et al: Evidence for response bias as a source of error variance in applied assessment. Psychol Bull 136(3):450–470, 2010 20438146

Miller HA: The Miller Forensic Assessment of Symptoms Test (M-FAST): Professional Manual. Odessa, FL, Psychological Assessment Resources, 2001

Miller H, Cartlidge N: Simulation and malingering after injuries to the brain and spinal cord. Lancet 1(7750):580–585, 1972 4110060

Morel KR: Development and preliminary validation of a forced-choice test of response bias for posttraumatic stress disorder. J Pers Assess 70(2):299–314, 1998 9697332

Morey LC: Personality Assessment Inventory: Professional Manual. Odessa, FL, Psychological Assessment Resources, 1991

Morey LC: An Interpretive Guide to the Personality Assessment Inventory (PAI). Odessa, FL, Psychological Assessment Resources, 1996

Musick JE, Otto RK: Inventory of Legal Knowledge. Columbia, SC, Authors, 2006

Ossipov VP: Malingering; the simulation of psychosis. Bull Menninger Clin 8:39–42, 1944

Pankratz L: Symptom validity testing and symptom retraining: procedures for the assessment and treatment of functional sensory deficits. J Consult Clin Psychol 47(2):409–410, 1979 469093

Resnick PJ: Malingered psychosis, in Clinical Assessment of Malingering and Deception, 2nd Edition. Edited by Rogers R. New York, Guilford, 1997, pp 47–67

Resnick PJ: The detection of malingered psychosis. Psychiatr Clin North Am 22(1):159–172, 1999 10083952

Rey A: [The Clinical Examination in Psychology]. Paris, Presses Universitaire de France, 1964

Rogers R: Clinical Assessment of Malingering and Deception, 3rd Edition. New York, Guilford, 2008

Rogers R, Seman W, Clark CR: Assessment of criminal responsibility: initial validation of the R-CRAS with the M'Naghten and GBMI standards. Int J Law Psychiatry 9(1):67–75, 1986 3793347

Rogers R, Bagby RM, Dickens SE: Structured Interview of Reported Symptoms: Professional Manual. Odessa, FL, Psychological Assessment Resources, 1992

Rogers R, Sewell KW, Goldstein AM: Explanatory models of malingering: a prototypical analysis. Law Hum Behav 18:543–552, 1994

Rogers R, Salekin RT, Sewell KW, et al: A comparison of forensic and nonforensic malingerers: a prototypical analysis of explanatory models. Law Hum Behav 22(4):353–367, 1998 9711139

Rogers R, Payne JW, Correa AA, et al: A Study of the SIRS with severely traumatized patients. J Pers Assess 91(5):429–438, 2009 19672749

Rogers R, Sewell KW, Gillard ND: Structured Interview of Reported Symptoms, 2nd Edition: Professional Manual. Odessa, FL, Psychological Assessment Resources, 2010

Rogers R, Gillard ND, Wooley CN, et al: The detection of feigned disabilities: the effectiveness of the Personality Assessment Inventory in a traumatized inpatient sample. Assessment 19(1):77–88, 2012 21954300

Rohling ML, Binder LM, Langhinrichsen-Rohling J: Money matters: a meta-analytic review of the association between financial compensation and the experience and treatment of chronic pain. Health Psychol 14(6):537–547, 1995 8565928

Schmand B, Lindeboom J, Schagen S, et al: Cognitive complaints in patients after whiplash injury: the impact of malingering. J Neurol Neurosurg Psychiatry 64(3):339–343, 1998 9527145

Slick DJ, Sherman EM, Iverson GL: Diagnostic criteria for malingered neurocognitive dysfunction: proposed standards for clinical practice and research. Clin Neuropsychol 13(4):545–561, 1999 10806468

Slick DJ, Tan JE, Strauss EH, et al: Detecting malingering: a survey of experts' practices. Arch Clin Neuropsychol 19(4):465–473, 2004 15163448

Soliman S, Resnick PJ: Feigning in adjudicative competence evaluations. Behav Sci Law 28(5):614–629, 2010 20687120

Tarescavage AM, Glassmire DM: Differences between Structured Interview of Reported Symptoms (SIRS) and SIRS-2 sensitivity estimates among forensic inpatients: a criterion groups comparison. Law Hum Behav 40(5):488–502, 2016 27077677

Tombaugh TN: Test of Memory Malingering (TOMM). New York, Multi-Health Systems, 1996

United States v Greer, 158 F.3d 228 (5th Cir. 1998)

Vickery CD, Berry DTR, Inman TH, et al: Detection of inadequate effort on neuropsychological testing: a meta-analytic review of selected procedures. Arch Clin Neuropsychol 16(1):45–73, 2001 14590192

Vitacco MJ, Rogers R, Gabel J, et al: An evaluation of malingering screens with competency to stand trial patients: a known-groups comparison. Law Hum Behav 31(3):249–260, 2007 17058121

Widows MR, Smith GP: Structured Inventory of Malingered Symptomatology: Professional Manual. Odessa, FL, Psychological Assessment Resources, 2005

Wierzbicki MJ, Tyson CM: A summary of evaluations for learning and attention problems at a university training clinic. J Postsecond Educ Disabil 20:16–27, 2007

Wygant DB: Validation of the MMPI-2 infrequent somatic complaints (Fs) scale. Unpublished doctoral dissertation, Kent State University, Kent, OH, 2007

Wygant DB, Sellbom M, Gervais RO, et al: Further validation of the MMPI-2 and MMPI-2-RF Response Bias Scale: findings from disability and criminal forensic settings. Psychol Assess 22(4):745–756, 2010 20919770

CHAPTER 7

Neuroimaging and Forensic Psychiatry

Judith Edersheim, J.D., M.D.

Marlynn Wei, J.D., M.D.

Landmark Cases

Frye v. U.S., 54 App.D.C. 46, 293 F. 1013 (1923)

Daubert v. Merrell Dow Pharmaceuticals Inc., 509 U.S. 579, 113 S.Ct. 2786 (1993)

Roper v. Simmons, 543 U.S. 551, 125 S.Ct. 1183 (2005)

Graham v. Florida, 560 U.S. 48, 130 S.Ct. (2011)

Miller v. Alabama, 567 U.S. 460, 132 S.Ct. 2455 (2012)

Over the past 15 years, neuroscience and neuroimaging have made an accelerated foray into the courtroom. Conservative estimates indicate that neurobiological evidence is introduced in approximately 5%–6% of murder trials in the United States and in 1%–4% of an array of felony cases. Although methodological barriers in legal research cause a significant underestimation of these numbers, approximately 15% of recorded cases that discuss neuroscience also discuss brain scans as part of the analysis (Farahany 2016). Responsible legal scholars and neuroscientists have cautioned against the overuse of neuroimaging and other modalities in the determination of individual civil or criminal cases but also acknowledge that a deeper understanding of human cognition and motivation might assist fact finders in determining guilt and innocence and in tailoring sentences and other legal interventions (Presidential Commission for the Study of Bioethical Issues 2015).

Foundations of Neuroimaging in Forensic Psychiatry

Modalities of Neuroimaging Scans

Both structural and functional neuroimaging have an increased presence in the courtroom. Structural brain imaging, including computed tomography (CT) and magnetic resonance imaging (MRI), provides a static snapshot of the brain. CT uses multiple X-ray beams to acquire images quickly and provides cross-sectional images based on density. CT is fast and easy to use and can show fractures, hemorrhage, and mass effect. CT is valuable in acute care settings for disorders such as traumatic brain injury or stroke to capture the mechanism, severity, and timing of the injury and is often used to establish the initial diagnosis or baseline (Bigler et al. 2012). CT is limited in resolution and ability to determine structures of different composition, so most nonemergent clinical neuroimaging uses MRI.

MRI uses a powerful magnet to obtain images based on electromagnetic signals from hydrogen nuclei and shows the density and magnetic environment of tissue. Brain MRI is used to track lesions or injuries over time, including follow-up imaging of stroke or head trauma, and can be used to detect shear lesions or atrophic changes associated with degenerative diseases. Structural MRI measures the actual size, shape, and density of brain structures. Quantitative MRI compares an individual's MRI with a normative sample, including volume and cortical thickness. Given the strength of the magnetic and radiofrequency fields,

metallic foreign bodies, pacemakers, defibrillators, and other implanted devices such as deep brain stimulators or neurosurgical clips can contraindicate the use of MRI. Therefore, the decision about use of MRI should be made on a case-by-case basis.

Diffusion MRI is based on the signal related to the micromovement of water molecules. Diffusion tensor imaging (DTI) examines neural connectivity by mapping three-dimensional diffusion of water and describes white matter connectivity patterns in the brain. DTI is highly sensitive to detecting tissue microstructural and organizational changes that occur in developmental, aging, and pathological processes. Fiber tracking, or tractography, is one method of analyzing DTI data in order to map neural fibers (Mukherjee et al. 2008). DTI findings have played a role in mild traumatic brain injury cases when no abnormalities were seen on CT or conventional MRI.

Many functional imaging modalities exist, but the most widely available are functional MRI (fMRI), positron emission tomography (PET), and single-photon emission computed tomography (SPECT). These methods are able to provide dynamic images of brain activity over time. fMRI is a noninvasive method that detects blood oxygen level–dependent signal to measure blood flow to areas of the brain and monitors real-time brain metabolic activity. PET and SPECT are clinical nuclear imaging techniques that detect photons emitted by radioactive tracers that are injected to detect metabolic activity in the brain. PET can be used to show cerebral abnormalities, such as reduced tissue perfusion. PET is more sensitive but less specific than SPECT. SPECT is less expensive and technically simpler but offers lower spatial and temporal resolution (Rushing et al. 2012).

History of Neuroimaging in the Courtroom

One of the first cases of neuroimaging presented as "objective" evidence in the courtroom was in *United States v. Hinckley* (1982). The defense expert suggested that Hinckley's CT brain scan demonstrated widened sulci, which he testified was evidence of schizophrenia. The jury rendered a verdict of not guilty by reason of insanity. In *McNamara v. Borg* (1991), the court admitted PET scans as evidence used to show that the defendant had schizophrenia. A few jurors reported that the scans influenced their decision to grant leniency in their verdict of a life sentence instead of the death penalty (Edersheim et al. 2012).

Brain MRI and PET scans were presented in *People of New York v. Weinstein* (1992), involving an executive charged with second-degree murder of his wife. The MRI scan identified an arachnoid cyst, and two PET scans found decreased glucose metabolism in the left frontal, temporal, and parietal lobes. The court determined that testimony regarding PET data was admissible but prohibited experts from suggesting that the findings were direct causes of violent behavior.

Functional neuroimaging is also increasingly offered as evidence in the courtroom and often has a high rate of acceptance as reliable evidence. A 2006 study found approximately 130 court opinions involving PET or SPECT evidence, which has been admitted in more than four-fifths (82.0%) of cases in which it has been introduced (Feigenson 2006). The first reported case of fMRI being admitted was in the 2009 capital sentencing phase of serial killer Brian Dugan. The defense could not show actual scans, but defense expert witnesses were allowed to discuss fMRI and structural MRI findings to sup-port the diagnosis of psychopathy as a mitigating factor (Hughes 2010). However, evidentiary rules are less restrictive in the sentencing phase of capital crimes, so it is unclear whether courts will determine that fMRI results meet evidentiary gatekeeping standards when applied to determine responsibility in civil or criminal cases using strict *Daubert v. Merrell Dow Pharmaceuticals Inc.* (1993) and *Frye v. U.S.* (1923) criteria.

Ethical Considerations of Forensic Neuroimaging

The use of neuroimaging in the courtroom raises several ethical concerns, including the validity and reliability of imaging modalities, limitations of what neuroimaging can detect, and potential prejudicial influence of brain images. Proper interpretation of neuroimaging requires an understanding of its limitations. Neuroimaging cannot reflect the intention behind a criminal act or allocate personal responsibility. Scientific theories of cognition do not map directly onto legally defined mental states and require thoughtful translation in order to be accurate and relevant. Most neuroimaging studies are small and unreplicated and use healthy volunteers in controlled research settings. Because these studies deal with averages across groups, conclusions are difficult to draw for individuals. Also, abnormal findings on a scan do not necessarily indicate irreversible disability.

Neuroimaging also can potentially have a "seductive allure" that might mislead the jury and inflate the scientific credibility of pathology, making neuroimaging evidence appear more objective than is scientifically accurate, an issue termed *neurorealism*. Concerns exist that juries might overvalue and overweigh vividly colored brain scans that purport to reflect human thought (Baskin et al. 2007). Studies have shown that brain images can be convincing, even when accompanied by nonsensical text (McCabe and Castel 2008). As research has progressed, however, jurors appear to have a more nuanced understanding than was originally feared, although in some contexts they are nevertheless unduly swayed by brain scans (Roskies et al. 2013; Schweitzer et al. 2011). Finally, judges and jurors may come to expect neuroimaging evidence and make assumptions when such evidence is absent, a bias termed the *CSI effect* (Perlin 2009). This may lead to inequitable results because neuroimaging technology is costly.

Neuroimaging and Mental States

Despite the ethical and technological cautions discussed earlier, neuroimaging has been used to support mental state claims at all stages of criminal proceedings (Presidential Commission for the Study of Bioethical Issues 2015).

Neuroimaging and Criminal Competencies

Attorneys and judges are increasingly relying on neuroimaging techniques to supplement the more traditional psychological and neuropsychological metrics used in competency to stand trial evaluations. Challenges to competency are the second most common use of neurobiological evidence in criminal cases (Farahany 2016). This is not surprising, because competency inquiries are concerned with the measurement of current mental capacities rather than the retrospective reconstruction of mental states.

Neuroimaging techniques, particularly when combined with collateral psychological and neuropsychological testing, can help identify the existence of structural or functional brain abnormalities that might cause deficits in the fundamental abilities associated with competence to stand trial. It is increasingly common to see that fluorodeoxyglucose-PET scans have been offered to bolster the diagnosis of dementia when it forms the basis of assertions that a litigant is unable to work with his or her defense attorneys (Rushing 2014). However, abnormalities found on neuroimaging alone are likely irrelevant if the defendant possesses the requisite cognitive abilities, because competency is related to functional and not diagnostic findings (Morse and Newsome 2013).

One of the earliest attempts to use neuroimaging to bolster claims of incompetency occurred in *United States v. Gigante* (1998), the trial of an alleged organized crime family leader in New York City. Mr. Gigante presented experts who concluded that he had dementia and used both neuropsychological test results and PET scans to support this diagnosis. Despite this evidence, Mr. Gigante was found competent to stand trial and guilty of the charges (Baskin et al. 2007). In contrast, in *United States v. Kasim* (2008), various forms of neuroimaging evidence (electroencephalogram [EEG], MRI, SPECT) were used to evaluate a defense claim of incompetence to stand trial. In the face of conflicting expert testimony on whether the defendant had dementia, the court determined that the behavioral evidence of impaired capacity, the deficits found on neuropsychological and psychological testing, and the functional neuroimaging supported a diagnosis of dementia and a finding of incompetency (Shafi 2009).

Neuroimaging and Insanity Defenses

Despite the concerns about the mismatch between neuroimaging studies and courtroom testimony (Schauer 2010), neuroimaging is frequently presented in insanity defense cases, with mixed results. The most frequent use is to support psychiatric diagnoses made with traditional clinical interviews and psychological and neuropsychological testing, with functional neuroimaging offered to support frontal lobe dysfunction in primary psychotic illnesses (Farahany 2016). Insanity defenses involving the assertion of a brain injury or neurodegenerative disorder seem to offer the greatest opportunity for the contribution of structural and functional neuroimaging. Images that present focal brain damage, evidence of progressive dementia, anoxic brain injuries, and mass lesions may play a central evidentiary role, particularly when they correlate with behavioral evidence and neuropsychological test results showing deficits in cognition and control functions (Morse and Newsome 2013).

In certain circumstances, courts have rejected structural and functional brain images even as supporting evidence during the guilt phase of an insanity case. One such circumstance occurs when the scan is so remote in time from the event in question that its ability to shed light on the defendant's state of mind during the crime is questionable. A second circumstance occurs when the scan is offered to show the defendant's general inclination without offering a specific link to the mental state in question (Presidential Commission for the Study of Bioethical Issues 2015). Functional neuroimaging has come under particular scrutiny, and courts have rejected its use when

- The modality in question is not typically used to diagnose the condition at issue.
- The abnormality shown has no articulated link to disproving cognitive or control abilities.
- The scans might mislead juries because they are temporally remote from the date of the events in question. (Rushing 2014)

Neuroimaging, Diminished Capacity, and Diminished Responsibility

Defense attorneys increasingly use neuroimaging to support assertions that because of a mental abnormality, the defendant could not form the specific mental state required for the charged offense. Formulations of diminished capacity are idiosyncratic and vary widely by jurisdiction. Nevertheless, the typical assertion is that because of a mental illness or brain injury, the defendant could not or did not premeditate, deliberate, or have a willful or wanton state of mind (Edersheim et al. 2012). In other words, the defendant lacked specific intent to be found guilty of the legal charge, although he or she may be guilty of a lesser included offense. For example, the defendant might be found guilty of manslaughter but lacked the mental state required to be guilty of murder. Structural and functional neuroimaging findings, as well as EEG and neuropsychological abnormalities, have been combined to assert that defendants have prefrontal cortical deficits or deficits in other brain regions and networks that undermine cognitive and volitional control.

Military tribunals are also seeing an increasing use of neuroimaging to support *mens rea* defenses. This phenomenon likely represents the confluence of an influx of returning veterans with traumatic brain injury (TBI) and posttraumatic stress disorder (PTSD) and the increasing sophistication of neuroimaging with respect to these conditions (Elbert 2012). Once again, this increase has occurred against a backdrop of scientific and scholarly caution regarding the use of indirect measures of blood flow or metabolic activity as a proxy for reconstructing individual intent (Snead 2007).

Litigants have had some success in admitting neuroimaging in these cases but have had only rare success convincing juries and judges that the abnormalities alleged have prevented them from premeditating, forming murderous intent or planning, and carrying out complex criminal enterprises (Edersheim et al. 2012). This is partly the product of legal doctrine, as defeating *mens rea* (as opposed to proving insanity) requires substantial negation of the building blocks of intentionality. This high level of mental impairment is often belied by the behavioral circumstances of the crime (Farahany and Coleman 2009). The outright exclusions follow a pattern similar to those observed in the context of insanity defenses and appear to appropriately reflect the current technological and inferential limitations of the modalities themselves. Neuroimages are excluded in diminished capacity cases when

- They fail to meet **Daubert** or **Frye** admissibility standards.
- An insufficient causal link exists between the brain abnormality presented and its ability to negate specific intent.
- The scan is temporally irrelevant to the offense.
- The modality proposed is not clinically reliable in diagnosing the condition at issue. (Edersheim et al. 2012)

Neuroimaging in Sentencing

The single most frequent use of neuroimaging in the courtroom has been in the context of the presentation of mitigation evidence during the sentencing phase of capital trials. The goal is to prove that neurological deficits rendered the defendant less able to control violent or aggressive behaviors or less able to make socially appropriate choices (Edersheim et al. 2012). These mitigation arguments have been premised on a wide array of underlying abnormalities, including frontal lobe dysfunction, mass lesions, TBI, psychiatric disorders, developmental disorders, and substance use disorders.

The evidentiary success for brain scans during the penalty phase of proceedings is not surprising, because the U.S. Supreme Court has repeatedly given defendants the widest berth to introduce evidence that pertains to underlying cognitive, neuropsychological, or psychiatric abnormalities (*Lockett v. Ohio* 1978; *Tennard v. Dretke* 2004). Many jurisdictions also allow defendants to present any "other factor" in their backgrounds that mitigates against a death sentence (Rushing 2014). Several courts have ruled that failure to obtain or admit probative neuroimaging evidence may be reversible trial error or might form the basis of an ineffective assistance of counsel claim (Edersheim et al. 2012).

That said, experts on death penalty mitigation caution that the single greatest risk in procuring neuroimaging evidence is that a so-called normal brain scan may undermine or negate other clinically sound evidence of neurological or psychological abnormality (Blume and Paavola 2011). Finally, neuroimaging evidence presented for mitigation should be strategically evaluated for its possible use as an aggravating factor. Scans offered to support the argument that a defendant is less blameworthy because of a neurobiological predilection for violence are sometimes used by prosecutors to argue in favor of the death penalty because they emphasize the defendant's future dangerousness and poor rehabilitation potential (Denno 2015).

Special Topics

Detection of Truth and Deception

Advances in neuroimaging technology are also offering the promise of enhancing methods of lie detection in both civil and criminal contexts. The early importation of these technologies into the legal arena has been met with appropriate caution, given the current limitations of the modalities and their lack of congruence with respect to real-world determinations of truth and deception (Greely and Illes 2007). Despite these critiques, novel neuroimaging-based lie detection technologies have expanded in the wake of the general inadmissibility of contested polygraph examinations and the lack of general acceptance in the scientific community (Pivovarova et al. 2014).

These new central nervous system lie detection methods rest on differential event-related brain potential measurements for EEG-based lie detection (Greely and Illes 2007) or differential brain blood flow or metabolic demands in lying versus truth telling conditions with fMRI-based lie detection (Wagner 2010). Lie detection that uses fMRI technology has received the most attention from legal scholars, the scientific community, and the courts (Rusconi and Mitchener-Nissen 2013). The premise underlying fMRI use is that deception is an effort that taxes working memory and that the metabolic demands of this task will differentially engage specific prefrontal cortical and parietal regions (Langleben 2008).

Attempts to use fMRI lie detection in court have failed in both criminal and civil contexts. In *United States v. Semrau* (2010), the defendant was charged with improperly billing Medicare and was convicted of three counts of federal health care fraud. Dr. Semrau's trial expert wished to opine that, pursuant to the results of his fMRI lie detection protocol, Dr. Semrau lacked the intent to deceive. The court concluded that the evidence failed to meet *Daubert* gatekeeping standards and that the probative value of the evidence was substantially outweighed by its potential to mislead or confuse the jury. The admissibility of fMRI has been banned in *Frye* jurisdictions as well (e.g., *State of Maryland v. Gary James Smith* 2012).

fMRI lie detection also has been rejected in civil contexts. In *Wilson v. Corestaff Services* (2010), the plaintiff sued an employment agency, asserting that its employees retaliated against her after she reported sexual harassment. The fMRI lie detection evidence was offered to support the truthfulness of the testimony of a Corestaff employee who confirmed this retaliatory practice. The New York State trial court judge excluded fMRI lie detection evidence under the *Frye* standard, holding that the expert testimony was equivalent to a credibility determination, which was well within the province of the typical juror. The judge also opined that the use of fMRI for these purposes generally was not accepted in the scientific community.

Neuroimaging and Developmental Neuroscience

In a trilogy of cases between 2005 and 2012, the U.S. Supreme Court cited neuroscientific and psychological evidence regarding the adolescent brain in finding it unconstitutional under the Eighth Amendment to execute juveniles (*Roper v. Simmons* 2005), to impose a life sentence without the possibility of parole for nonhomicide offenses (*Graham v. Florida* 2011), and to have a scheme of mandatory life imprisonment without the possibility of parole (*Miller v. Alabama* 2012). In these cases, the Court drew on scientific studies of the adolescent brain showing that neuronal systems responsible for impulse control, reward processing, and emotional regulation were incompletely developed until the early 20s. The Court used these studies to support a determination that adolescents, by virtue of their inherent psychological and neurobiological immaturity, were both less responsible and more amenable to long-term rehabilitation than similarly charged adults (Steinberg 2013).

While the Supreme Court used the neuroscientific insights regarding the adolescent brain to develop procedural rules for the treatment of adolescents as a class, attorneys began attempting to apply the principles behind these policy determinations to individual cases. This has presented a considerable challenge for trial courts, which have had to determine whether group data regarding adolescent immaturity and neuroplasticity can be relevant and probative for determinations of individual guilt or degrees of culpability (Faigman et al. 2014).

Attorneys who practice in juvenile justice settings routinely attempt to include these concepts as so-called framework evidence for a variety of proceedings, including transfer or certification, accomplice liability, Miranda waivers, and sentencing guidelines (Shen 2013). The greatest effect of this evidence in individual cases appears to be with respect to juvenile sentencing: defense attorneys argue that juvenile brains are not yet fully matured, that juveniles have less-well-developed capacities for self-restraint, and that they should be punished less harshly than similarly situated adults (Farahany 2016). If neuroimaging techniques advance to the point at which individual adolescents might be located on a continuum of developmental maturity, the courts will face a new set of challenges regarding use of these images as *mens rea* evidence (Maroney 2010).

Neuroimaging and Psychopathy

Researchers have sought neural correlates for antisocial behavior and psychopathy because of the hypothesis that such behavior may be the result of a disruption in regions or networks related to moral judgment and emotional and social processing. The most replicated findings are structural and functional abnormalities in the prefrontal cortex, including a reduction in gray matter volume and reduced blood flow, and the paralimbic system (Glenn et al. 2012). Studies also have reported reduced activity in the amygdala during emotional stimuli and the angular gyrus, which is associated with the experience of guilt and embarrassment. Reduced volume and activity of the posterior cingulate, a region involved in emotional recall and experience, self-reflection, and sense of duty, also have been observed in psychopathic groups. Whether these brain abnormalities lead to the development of psychopathy or whether environmental factors and behaviors of psychopathic persons make them more likely to have these abnormalities is not yet clear.

Despite these ambiguities, the associations between psychopathy and functional and structural brain abnormalities have been used at trial to assert that a defendant has underlying deficits in affective regulation that should be mitigating for sentencing purposes (Gaudet et al. 2014). Although this use of neuroimaging has been highly controversial (Mayberg 2010), recent mock-juror studies have concluded that neuroimages presented in the penalty phase for the purpose of demonstrating the neural correlates of psychopathy tend to reduce judgments of responsibility and decrease the number of death sentences meted out by juries (Saks et al. 2014).

For example, in the sentencing hearing of a capital murder case, a defense expert was permitted to discuss structural and functional MRI analyses, which he presented to support a claim that the defendant shared abnormalities with other psychopathic patients (Hughes 2010). The defense was not, however, permitted to show actual scans. The neuroimaging of psychopathy also may play a future role in the assessment of dangerousness, alongside conventional psychometric testing, but it is not yet reliable enough to be used for conclusions about dangerousness.

Neuroimaging and Civil Litigation

Neuroimaging of Traumatic Brain Injury

Neuroimaging has been admitted in several cases to support claims of TBI and is given greater weight when obtained at the time the individual is evaluated in an acute care setting. In a work-related injury case, *Blodgett-McDeavitt v. University of Nebraska* (2004), PET scan findings were found admissible to support a claim of electric shock brain injury. In *Lanter v. Kentucky State Police* (2005), MRI and SPECT scans were found admissible, but disability claims were denied based on lack of established causation. In *McCor-*

mack v. Capital Electric Construction Company (2005), the plaintiff's PET brain scans were found admissible, but the court ruled in favor of the plaintiff based on other clinical evidence.

DTI has played an emerging role for plaintiffs in personal injury cases to detect TBIs not detected by other forms of neuroimaging. However, studies of mild TBI with DTI have yielded inconsistent and conflicting results, leading to a lack of consensus on whether mild TBI can be detected on DTI in a reliable manner for use in the courtroom (Berlin 2014).

Earlier courts tended to exclude DTI evidence. However, courts have more recently admitted DTI as evidence for TBI. One court held that DTI was a reliable method that was "FDA approved, peer reviewed and approved, and a commercially marketed modality which has been in clinical use for the evaluation of suspected head traumas including mild traumatic brain injury" (*Hammar v. Sentinel Ins. Co., Ltd.* 2010 at 2). Another court found DTI "a generally accepted method for detecting TBI" (*Andrew v. Patterson Motor Freight* 2014). In another case, the court determined that the plaintiff had met the burden of showing that "DTI is a reliable technology" (*White v. Deere and Company* 2016). Neuroimaging in mild TBI cases is becoming common enough that one court denied a plaintiff's claims of injury based on the lack of neuroimaging, despite available neuropsychological testing (*Harris and Harris v. United States* 2005).

Neuroimaging of Dementia

Neuroimaging has been used to support the diagnosis of dementia in civil cases, including cases in which mental capacity is at issue. In In re Estate of Meyer (2001), appellants challenged a trust, claiming the decedent lacked mental capacity. The court allowed an expert witness affidavit describing brain CT scans that indicated brain atrophy and evidence suggestive of vascular dementia. Although neuroimaging can help diagnose and distinguish neurodegenerative conditions, dementia is ultimately diagnosed clinically. Therefore, clinical expert evidence is still needed to support the diagnosis of dementia.

Emerging Areas

Neuroimaging and Addictions

Voluntary intoxication alone almost never supports an insanity or automatism defense and is rarely successful even when offered for the limited purpose of negating *mens rea*. This settled legal doctrine reflects the public policy and safety concern that allowing voluntary intoxication to serve as an excuse for antisocial behavior would threaten public safety and potentiate criminality (Melton et al. 2007). Advances in the neuroscience of addiction may, however, pose a future challenge to this paradigm, because they may undermine the notions of voluntariness that justify this categorical exclusion.

Current neurobiological models of addiction posit that drugs of abuse usurp the brain's normal systems of reward-related learning and memory, which under optimal circumstances serve to direct behavior toward the pursuit of survival-related cues and rewards (Hyman 2005). Drug use becomes both compulsive and self-reinforcing, and its persistence appears to depend on both genetic predisposition and the environmental exposures that potentiate use (Hyman et al. 2006). Neuroimaging studies have played a central role in identifying biomarkers for relating neural circuits to molecular mechanisms and behaviors (Garrison and Potenza 2014).

Despite this neuroscientific consensus, whether the neuroscience of addiction should or will play a central role in determinations of legal responsibility is not clear. For the neuroscience of addiction to be dispositive, it would have to begin to quantify degrees of volitional impairment in order to shed light on the legal question of whether a defendant could have acted otherwise (Hyman 2007). Any theory of lack of criminal responsibility based on addictive compulsion would have to take into account the foreseeability of the consequences of initial use and the dynamic and temporal fluctuations in addiction-related mental states. Similarly, it would have to elucidate the brain's ability to compensate for damage to areas that subsume executive functions with redundant neural pathways (Husak and Murphy 2013).

Nevertheless, addiction neuroscience is likely to play a significant role with respect to sentencing determinations and legal policy. Addiction is cautiously offered as a mitigating factor in death penalty sentencing hearings. However, juries appear to give this little weight in determining a life or death sentence. In the setting of capital crimes, the same evidence of drug use might be considered an indicator of future dangerousness, rendering it a de facto statutory aggravator (Bjerregaard et al. 2010). With respect to legal policy, advancements in the neuroscience of addiction have provided support for the expansion of drug treatment courts. Approximately 3,400 diversionary specialty drug courts exist today and operate on a collaborative model of therapeutic jurisprudence (Wilson et al. 2006).

Neuroimaging and Posttraumatic Stress Disorder

The diagnosis of PTSD has played a significant role in both civil and criminal litigation since its codification in DSM-III (American Psychiatric Association 1980). Its most prominent role has been in civil litigation because the diagnosis explicitly provides a causal link between the injurious event and the resulting psychological injury (Melton et al. 2007). PTSD also has been used by criminal defendants to support claims of automatism, insanity, diminished capacity, and self-defense, as well as mitigation in sentencing. With respect to criminal cases, the success or failure of PTSD-related claims depends on two general factors: the quality and reliability indicators in the diagnostic evaluation and the direct connection between the PTSD symptoms and the criminal act (Berger et al. 2012).

Although courts initially were reluctant to give weight to a PTSD diagnosis because of concerns about malingering and the potential ubiquity of the claim, this appears to be changing. Federal and state courts are increasingly recognizing PTSD as a penalty mitigator in two particular contexts: in cases involving military veterans and in the context of a "battered woman syndrome" defense (Gray 2012). The most significant hurdle for PTSD in the courtroom has been the subjective nature of the articulated symptoms. In recent years, however, research clinicians have begun trying to use functional neuroimaging to elucidate the brain circuitry involved in the development of PTSD. If researchers could conclusively prove that the psychological trauma underpinning PTSD induces neurological damage, it would dramatically increase the influence of this disorder in both civil and criminal contexts.

A review of the literature makes it clear, however, that no current scientific consensus around reliable neuroimaging biomarkers for PTSD exists. In general terms, much of the burgeoning work in this area has yet to disambiguate whether the findings signify preexisting genetic risk factors or acquired abnormalities. The most common structural findings in PTSD neuroimaging have been decreased hippocampal volumes, although several studies have not replicated these results. Other investigators have found decreased anterior cingulate and ventromedial prefrontal cortical volumes in PTSD (Dekel et al. 2016).

With respect to functional neuroimaging of PTSD, a review of current research concluded that the most support is for hyperresponsivity in the amygdala and hyporesponsivity in the rostral and ventral portions of the medial prefrontal cortex. The hippocampus appears to function abnormally in PTSD, although the direction of this abnormality seems to vary depending on the study methods used (Hughes and Shin 2011). In short, although neuroscientists are beginning to identify certain functional and structural abnormalities in the brain regions associated with fear, emotional processing, and memory, they have not established biomarkers for PTSD.

Conclusion

Both structural and functional neuroimaging are increasingly used in both civil and criminal cases. Although some courts have admitted neuroimaging evidence, others have been more cautious as the state of the science is still relatively new and often does not meet legal evidentiary standards. More research and clinical correlation are needed and are likely to become available as neuroimaging continues to offer clinical and forensic tools for clinical and forensic evaluation, treatment, and testimony.

Key Concepts

- The use of neuroimaging in the courtroom raises both scientific and ethical limitations, including the potential for prejudicial bias.

- Neuroimaging evidence is most commonly offered during the sentencing phase of criminal trials, when evidentiary restrictions on novel scientific evidence are less stringent.

- The presentation of neuroimaging evidence should be handled with caution, because it may be perceived as both mitigating and aggravating and may undermine other reliable forms of relevant evidence.

- The use of neuroimaging in civil cases involving traumatic brain injury and dementia is increasing.

- The most pervasive effect of neuroimaging data has been at the legal policy level, where developmental neuroscience and addictions research have influenced determinations of responsibility and appropriate legal triage.

- Some novel uses for functional neuroimaging in legal contexts are not widely accepted, because they do not yet represent scientific consensus. These include functional magnetic resonance imaging–based lie detection and the neuroimaging of biomarkers for psychopathy and posttraumatic stress disorder.

References

American Psychiatric Association: Diagnostic and Statistical Manual of Mental Disorders, 3rd Edition. Washington, DC, American Psychiatric Association, 1980

Andrew v Patterson Motor Freight, 2014 U.S. Dist. LEXIS 151234 (W.D. La. Jun 06, 2014)

Baskin JH, Edersheim JG, Price BH: Is a picture worth a thousand words? Neuroimaging in the courtroom. Am J Law Med 33(2–3):239–269, 2007 17910159

Berger O, McNiel DE, Binder RL: PTSD as a criminal defense: a review of case law. J Am Acad Psychiatry Law 40(4):509–521, 2012 23233473

Berlin L: Neuroimaging, expert witnesses, and ethics: convergence and conflict in the courtroom. AJOB Neurosci 5:3–8, 2014

Bigler ED, Allen M, Stimac GK: MRI and functional MRI, in Neuroimaging in Forensic Psychiatry. Edited by Simpson JR. Oxford, UK, Wiley-Blackwell, 2012, pp 27–40

Bjerregaard B, Smith MD, Fogel SJ, et al: Alcohol and drug mitigation in capital murder trials: implications for sentencing decisions. Justice Q 27:517–537, 2010

Blodgett-McDeavitt v University of Nebraska, No. A-04–211, 2004 Neb. App. LEXIS 329 (Neb. Ct. App. Dec. 7, 2004)

Blume JH, Paavola EC: Life, death and neuroimaging: the advantages and disadvantages of the defendant's use of neuroimages in capital cases. Mercer Law Rev 62:909–931, 2011

Daubert v Merrell Dow Pharmaceuticals Inc., 509 U.S. 579, 113 S.Ct. 2786 (1993)

Dekel S, Gilbertson MW, Orr SP, et al: Trauma and posttraumatic stress disorder, in Massachusetts General Hospital Comprehensive Clinical Psychiatry. Edited by Stern TA, Fava M, Wilens TE, et al. New York, Elsevier, 2016, pp 380–394

Denno DW: The myth of the double edged sword: an empirical study of neuroscience evidence in criminal cases. Boston Coll Law Rev 56:493–552, 2015

Edersheim JG, Brendel RW, Price BH: Neuroimaging, diminished capacity and mitigation, in Neuroimaging in Forensic Psychiatry. Edited by Simpson JR. Oxford, UK, Wiley-Blackwell, 2012, pp 163–193

Elbert JM: A mindful military: linking brain and behavior through neuroscience at court-martial. Army Lawyer (September):4–24, 2012

Faigman DL, Monahan J, Slobogin C: Group to individual (G2i) inference in scientific expert testimony. Univ Chic Law Rev 81(12):417–480, 2014

Farahany NA: Neuroscience and behavioral genetics in US criminal law: an empirical analysis. J Law Biosci 2(3):485–509, 2016 27774210

Farahany NA, Coleman JE: Genetics, neuroscience, and criminal responsibility, in Impact of Behavior Science on Criminal Law. Edited by Farahany NA. New York, Oxford University Press, 2009, pp 183–239

Feigenson N: Brain imaging and courtroom evidence: on the admissibility and permissiveness of fMRI. Int J Law Context 2:233–255, 2006

Frye v U.S., 54 App.D.C. 46, 293 F. 1013 (1923)

Garrison KA, Potenza MN: Neuroimaging and biomarkers in addiction treatment. Curr Psychiatry Rep 16(12):513, 2014

Gaudet LM, Lushing JR, Kiehl KA: Functional magnetic resonance imaging in court. AJOB Neurosci 5:43–45, 2014

Glenn AL, Yaling Y, Raine A: Neuroimaging in psychopathy and antisocial personality disorder: functional significance and a neurodevelopmental hypothesis, in Neuroimaging in Forensic Psychiatry. Edited by Simpson JR. Oxford, UK, Wiley-Blackwell, 2012, pp 81–98

Graham v Florida, 560 U.S. 48, 130 S.Ct. (2011)

Gray BJ: Neuroscience, PTSD and sentencing mitigation. Cardozo Law Rev 34:53–103, 2012

Greely HT, Illes J: Neuroscience-based lie detection: the urgent need for regulation. Am J Law Med 33(2–3):377–431, 2007 17910165

Hammar v Sentinel Ins. Co., Ltd., No. 08–019984 (Fla. Cir. Ct. 2010)

Harris and Harris v United States, Civil Action No. 03–6430 in Eastern District of Pennsylvania (Nov. 2, 2005)

Hughes KC, Shin LM: Functional neuroimaging studies of post-traumatic stress disorder. Expert Rev Neurother 11(2):275–285, 2011 21306214

Hughes V: Science in court: head case. Nature 464(7287):340–342, 2010 20237536

Husak D, Murphy E: The relevance of the neuroscience of addiction to criminal law, in A Primer on Criminal Law and Neuroscience. Edited by Morse SJ, Roskies AL. New York, Oxford University Press, 2013, pp 216–239

Hyman SE: Addiction: a disease of learning and memory. Am J Psychiatry 162(8):1414–1422, 2005 16055762

Hyman SE: The neurobiology of addiction: implications for voluntary control of behavior. Am J Bioeth 7(1):8–11, 2007 17366151

Hyman SE, Malenka RC, Nestler EJ: Neural mechanisms of addiction: the role of reward-related learning and memory. Annu Rev Neurosci 29:565–598, 2006 16776597

In re Estate of Meyer, 747 N.E.2d 1159 (Indiana 2001)

Langleben DD: Detection of deception with fMRI: are we there yet? Legal and Criminological Psychology 13:1–9, 2008

Lanter v Kentucky State Police, 171 S.W. 3d 45 (Ky. 2005)

Lockett v Ohio, 438 U.S. 586, 98 S.Ct. 2954 (1978)

Maroney TA: The false promise of adolescent brain science. Notre Dame Law Rev 85:89–176, 2010

Mayberg HS: Does neuroscience give us new insights into criminal responsibility? in A Judge's Guide to Neuroscience: A Concise Introduction. Edited by Gazzaniga M. Santa Barbara, University of California, Santa Barbara, 2010, pp 37–41

McCabe DP, Castel AD: Seeing is believing: the effect of brain images on judgments of scientific reasoning. Cognition 107(1):343–352, 2008 17803985

McCormack v Capital Elec. Constr. Co., 159 S.W. 3d 387 (Mo. App. W.D. 2005)

McNamara v Borg, 923 F.2d 862, 862 (9th Cir. 1991)

Melton GB, Petrila J, Poythress NG, et al: Psychological Evaluations for the Courts: A Handbook for Mental Health Professionals and Lawyers, 3rd Edition. New York, Guilford, 2007, pp 229–231

Miller v Alabama, 567 U.S. 460, 132 S.Ct. 2455 (2012)

Morse SJ, Newsome WT: Criminal responsibility, criminal competence and prediction of criminal behavior, in A Primer on Criminal Law and Neuroscience. Edited by Morse SJ, Roskies AL. New York, Oxford University Press, 2013, pp 150–178

Mukherjee P, Berman JI, Chung SW, et al: Diffusion tensor MR imaging and fiber tractography: theoretic underpinnings. AJNR Am J Neuroradiol 29(4):632–641, 2008 18339720

People of New York v Weinstein, 591 N.Y.S. 2d 715 (Sup. Ct. 1992)

Perlin ML: "His brain has been mismanaged with great skill": how will jurors respond to neuroimaging testimony in insanity defense cases? Akron Law Rev 42:886–916, 2009

Pivovarova E, Edersheim JG, Baker JT, Price BH: A polygraph primer: what litigators need to know. The Jury Expert 26:1, 2014

Presidential Commission for the Study of Bioethical Issues: Neuroscience and the legal system, in Gray Matters: Topics at the Intersection of Neuroscience, Ethics, and Society, Vol 2. Washington, DC, Presidential Commission for the Study of Bioethical Issues, March 2015, pp 85–116. Available at: http://bioethics.gov/sites/default/files/GrayMatter_V2_508.pdf. Accessed December 28, 2016.

Roper v Simmons, 543 U.S. 551, 125 S.Ct. 1183 (2005)

Roskies AL, Schweitzer NJ, Saks MJ: Neuroimages in court: less biasing than feared. Trends Cogn Sci 17(3):99–101, 2013 23428934

Rusconi E, Mitchener-Nissen T: Prospects of functional magnetic resonance imaging as lie detector. Front Hum Neurosci 7:594, 2013 24065912

Rushing SE: The admissibility of brain scans in criminal trials: the case of positron emission tomography. Court Review 50(2):62–69, 2014

Rushing SE, Pryma DA, Langleben DD: PET and SPECT, in Neuroimaging in Forensic Psychiatry. Edited by Simpson JR. Oxford, UK, Wiley-Blackwell, 2012, pp 3–25

Saks MJ, Schweitzer NJ, Ahroni E, et al: The impact of neuroimages in the sentencing phase of capital trials. J Empir Leg Stud 11:105–131, 2014

Schauer F: Can bad science be good evidence? Neuroscience, lie detection, and beyond. Cornell Law Rev 95(6):1191–1220, 2010 20939147

Schweitzer NJ, Saks MJ, Murphy ER, et al: Neuroimages as evidence in a mens rea defense: no impact. Psychol Public Policy Law 17:357–393, 2011

Shafi N: Neuroscience and law: the evidentiary value of brain imaging. Graduate Student Journal of Psychology 11:27–39, 2009

Shen FX: Legislating neuroscience: the case of juvenile justice. Loyola of Los Angeles Law Review 46:985–1018, 2013

Snead OC: Neuroimaging and the "complexity" of capital punishment. NYU Law Review 82:1265–1339, 2007

State of Maryland v Gary James Smith, Memorandum Opinion & Order No. 106589C (Montgomery County Cir. Ct., M.D. Oct. 3, 2012)

Steinberg L: The influence of neuroscience on US Supreme Court decisions about adolescents' criminal culpability. Nat Rev Neurosci 14(7):513–518, 2013 23756633

Tennard v Dretke, 542 U.S. 274, 124 S.Ct. 2562 (2004)

United States v Gigante, 996 F.Supp. 194 (2d Cir. 1998)

United States v Hinckley, 525 F.Supp. 1342 (D.D.C. 1981), clarified, 529 F.Supp. 520 (D.D.C.), affirmed 672 F.2d 115 (D.C. Cir. 1982)

United States v Kasim, No. 2:07 CR 56 U.S. Dist. LEXIS 89137 (N.D. Ind. Nov. 2008)

United States v Semrau, No. 07–10074 MI/P, 2010 WL 6845092 (W.D. Tenn. May 31, 2010)

Wagner A: Can neuroscience identify lies?, in A Judge's Guide to Neuroscience: A Concise Introduction. Edited by Gazzaniga M. Santa Barbara, University of California, Santa Barbara, 2010, pp 13–23

White v Deere and Company, District Court of Colorado, 2016 U.S. Dist. LEXIS 15644

Wilson v Corestaff Services, 900 N.Y.S. 2d 639, 642 (N.Y. Sup. Ct. 2010)

Wilson DB, Mitchell O, MacKenzie DL: A systematic review of drug court effects on recidivism. J Exp Criminol 2:459–487, 2006

PART II

Legal Regulation of Psychiatry

CHAPTER 8

Physician–Patient Relationship in Psychiatry

Annette Hanson, M.D.

Landmark Cases

Canterbury v. Spence, 150 U.S. App. D.C. 263, 464 F.2d 772 (1972)

Kaimowitz v. Michigan Dept. of Mental Health, 1 MDLR 147 (1973)

Tarasoff v. Regents of University of California,
17 Cal. 3d 425, 551 P.2d 334, 131 Cal. Rptr. 14 (1976)

Roy v. Hartogs, 381 N.Y.S. 2d 587 (1976)

Lipari v. Sears, 497 F.Supp. 185 (D. Neb. 1980)

Jablonski v. U.S., 712 F.2d 391 (1983) (ABPN only)

Cruzan v. Director, Missouri Dept. of Mental Health, 497 U.S. 261, 110 S.Ct. 2841 (1990)

Washington v. Glucksberg, 521 U.S. 702, 117 S.Ct. 2258 (1997)

Hargrave v. Vermont, 340 F.3d 27 (2003) (AAPL only)

The regulation of medicine is a complex process that must be imposed on the moving target of evolving medical knowledge and practice. State governments regulate the practice of professions that involve public health or safety, but these regulations differ from state to state. Legislators condense a seemingly infinite list of treatment and practical issues into the state's statutory codes and then must designate systems to monitor and enforce compliance with state code.

109

The regulation of psychiatric practice is particularly complex. Many factors shape the duration, purpose, and nature of psychiatric care. Each patient is unique, and psychiatrists treat patients in a variety of settings and conditions. A therapeutic contact can be as limited as a single telephone call in the middle of a night or as complicated as several years of individual therapy. The setting where care is provided can be a crowded and noisy emergency department or the quiet solitude of a psychiatrist's office. Legislators condense an endless list of hypothetical treatment scenarios into a single body of core legal principles, all of which are enforceable and monitored.

Additionally, the practice of psychiatry differs in significant ways from the practice of general medicine. Psychiatric care often requires that patients reveal intimate, embarrassing, or distressing information. Such information could be personally damaging if disclosed inadvertently or if discovered in the course of litigation. Even when confidentiality is breached for benevolent purposes and with the patient's permission, such as when a patient applies for disability benefits or insurance reimbursement, the therapeutic alliance potentially can be strained or damaged. For these reasons, the requirements of the psychiatric physician–patient relationship are often held to a higher standard, in some respects, than in general medicine.

The Fiduciary Relationship

The threshold condition of any medicolegal issue is the formation of a physician–patient relationship. The patient's clinical condition and willingness to participate in treatment and the physician's ability to provide care determine how this relationship begins, what obligations the relationship places on both the physician and the patient, and how the relationship ends. Throughout the relationship, the physician has a legal duty to provide care to the patient. How the physician fulfills that duty is determined by prevailing practices within the specialty as well as by community standards and laws.

Regardless of medical specialty, the physician–patient relationship is considered a legal, fiduciary relationship (Bartlett 1997). Derived from the Latin *fiducia* or *trust*, the term *fiduciary* is used in civil law to describe the relationship between estate administrators, bankers, public officials, corporate executives, and other professionals to whom people turn for advice. The term implies an imbalance of knowledge and authority; the person who relies on the fiduciary is known as the *beneficiary* because he or she benefits from the knowledge of the fiduciary. The fiduciary, with his or her superior knowledge and skill, is obliged to act solely in the beneficiary's interests and must be careful to avoid conflicts in carrying out this duty.

In medicine, a fiduciary relationship is established when a physician takes some affirmative action that creates a reasonable expectation on the part of the patient that the physician is providing treatment (Blake 2012). Such actions include conducting an examination of a patient, making a diagnosis, making a treatment recommendation, or beginning treatment. Generally, some affirmative action is required on the part of the physician; an inquiry for information alone is not sufficient to create a duty. For example, a potential patient who calls to check on available appointments, or who asks about the physician's area of specialization or qualifications, is not a beneficiary of the physician's specialized knowledge. However, a forensic consultant who suggests a change in medication dosage to an evaluee may create a reasonable expectation of treatment and may be found to have created a fiduciary relationship with the patient.

Once the relationship is established, the specific obligations of both patient and physician will be shaped by the nature of the treatment and the treatment setting. In a psychotherapy practice, this might involve issues such as consistent appointment times, length of sessions, goals and methods of treatment, and expectations for behavior on the part of both the physician and the patient. The patient's obligation includes a responsibility to keep scheduled appointments, disclose pertinent and truthful information, and provide timely payment for services. The American Medical Association's (AMA's) Code of Medical Ethics (American Medical Association 2016a) states, "The relationship between a patient and a physician is based on trust, which gives rise to physicians' ethical responsibility to place patients' welfare above the physician's own self-interest or obligations to others, to sound medical judgment on patients' behalf, and to advocate for their patients' welfare" (AMA Opinion 1.1.1). The physician's obligations include the duties to practice competently within one's scope of training, to practice ethically, to maintain professional skills with ongoing medical education and training, and to practice within the standard of care.

Informed Consent

Before treatment is initiated, physicians should provide patients with enough relevant information for patients to give informed consent for care. Undertaking treatment without obtaining informed consent could leave the physician liable to a claim of battery (Shultz 1985). The patient's consent for care must be made competently. In other words, the patient must have the mental capacity to understand the nature of the proposed treatment, the risks and benefits of proposed treatment, and the risks and benefits of other treatment options (Vars 2008).

The extent and type of information disclosed varies according to the proposed procedure and the seriousness of the risks involved but must include any information that might be material to a patient's decision to accept or reject the treatment. Some jurisdictions use a *reasonable practitioner standard* (i.e., what information most reasonable practitioners disclose to patients in that particular jurisdiction). However, many jurisdictions have moved to a *materiality of the information standard* (i.e., what a reasonable patient would want to know before consenting).

In **Canterbury v. Spence** (1972), a 19-year-old man with back pain was referred to a neurosurgeon who recommended a laminectomy. The patient's mother was told that the risks of the procedure were "no more than any other operation," and she gave consent for the operation. The day after the operation, the patient fell and sustained paralysis in the lower half of his body. At the ensuing malpractice trial, the surgeon acknowledged that paralysis was a rare potential complication of the surgery but that communication of this risk was contraindicated because it could cause an adverse psychological reaction that would affect the patient's treatment response. The surgeon also believed that disclosure of all possible risks might have deterred the patient from treatment.

The trial court found in favor of the physician, but the District of Columbia Court of Appeals held that failure to disclose the risk of paralysis was a violation of the physician's duty to provide informed consent. The appellate opinion quoted Justice Benjamin Cardozo's opinion in *Schloendorff v. Society of New York Hospital* (1914): "Every human being of adult years and sound mind has a right to determine what shall be done with his own body." Under *Canterbury*, a physician is required to disclose the "material risks" of a procedure—that is, those risks that might influence a patient to accept or reject treatment.

In *Kaimowitz v. Michigan Dept. of Mental Health* (1973), the issue of informed consent was addressed from a different perspective. "John Doe" was committed to a state hospital as a sexual psychopath. He was subsequently transferred to a facility to be a research subject in the use of psychosurgery for uncontrollable aggression. John Doe gave written consent for the procedure, and two separate review committees also approved the procedure after reviewing his consent.

Plaintiff Kaimowitz, a Michigan Legal Services lawyer, filed a writ of habeas corpus on John Doe's behalf, alleging that Doe was being held illegally at the research facility for the purpose of psychosurgery. The question before the court was "whether legally adequate consent could be obtained from adults involuntarily confined in the state mental health system for experimental or innovative procedures on the brain to ameliorate behavior, and, if it could be, whether the State should allow such experimentation on human subjects to proceed" (*Kaimowitz v. Michigan Dept. of Mental Health* 1973).

In *Kaimowitz v. Michigan*, the trial court held that for involuntarily committed patients, true informed consent was impossible when the procedure involved a high-risk, low-benefit ratio. Experimen-

tal psychosurgery, which met these conditions, required an even higher level of decision-making capacity than that required for routine or low-risk procedures. Therefore, capacity to give informed consent is dependent, among other factors, on the nature of the proposed intervention. Furthermore, the court held that to be legally valid, consent must be uncoerced as well as both "competent" and "knowing."

In addition to disclosing the benefits and risks of treatment, physicians are required to disclose material risks related to declining treatment. In *Truman v. Thomas* (1980), a physician failed to perform a Papanicolaou test on a woman who eventually died of cervical cancer. The physician testified that he had offered to perform the test, but she declined. The plaintiff alleged wrongful death, arguing that the woman should have been warned about the risks of refusing the procedure. The court heard contradictory expert testimony about the existing standard of care for informed refusals. The physician was found not liable at trial, but the appellate court reversed the decision, stating that a test that could detect a fatal disease required more disclosure by the physician than a mere blood test.

Informed consent also should be obtained for most evaluations performed for purposes other than treatment, including forensic evaluations. The American Academy of Psychiatry and the Law's (2005) *Ethics Guidelines for the Practice of Forensic Psychiatry* state that

> notice should be given to the evaluee of the nature and purpose of the evaluation and the limits of its confidentiality. The informed consent of the person undergoing the forensic evaluation should be obtained when necessary and feasible. If the evaluee is not competent to give consent, the evaluator should follow the appropriate laws of the jurisdiction.

Forensic consultation and court-ordered evaluations also require that the evaluee understand why the information is being requested, how it will be used, and who will have access to it.

The physician's duty to obtain informed consent has some exceptions. For example, consent is not required in emergency situations when the patient is mentally or physically incapable of agreeing to treatment. If a patient is a minor or has been legally adjudicated unable to make treatment decisions, consent must be obtained from a designated proxy or guardian (see Chapter 13, "Competencies in Civil Law"). Patients also may decline to engage in a risk–benefit discussion, a process known as a *therapeutic waiver* of consent. A patient who does not want to hear about possible risks and states, "I trust you doc, do whatever you think is best," is exercising a waiver of a risk–benefit discussion. In this case, the patient is in effect deciding that he or she does not want to hear about material risks. The physician should document the attempt to disclose risks as well as the patient's waiver.

The term *therapeutic privilege* refers to another set of circumstances that have been deemed an exception to obtaining informed consent. Therapeutic privilege may be invoked when a physician intentionally withholds information normally considered important for informed consent out of the belief that disclosure of the information would cause the patient harm or suffering. Therapeutic privilege is a controversial practice; although legal in some circumstances, it should rarely be used.

Duty to Warn or Protect

In tort law, an injured party can sue for damages if the injury is a direct result of a defendant's negligent act. A third party, such as a parent or an employer, could be liable for damages if the negligence was committed by someone the third party had an obligation to supervise or control (Lennon 2004). In some circumstances, psychiatrists may be held liable for an injury committed by patients under their care.

Psychiatrists generally were not considered responsible for the actions of their patients prior to the opinion in *Tarasoff v. Regents of University of California* (1976). In this case, Prosenjit Poddar killed Tatiana Tarasoff. Poddar had told his therapist 2 months earlier that he planned to kill the victim. The therapist sent the police to take Poddar into custody for hospitalization, but the police failed to transport him because Poddar appeared rational. The victim's parents sued the police, the Regents of the University of California, Poddar's therapist, and the supervising psychiatrist. The basis of the claim was that the defendants failed to warn the victim of impending danger and failed to hospitalize Poddar. The trial court issued summary judgment for the defendants.

On appeal, the issue under consideration was whether a physician–patient relationship required the physician to protect others from the acts of a dangerous patient. The California Supreme Court held that there was a duty to act "when a therapist determines, or pursuant to the standards of his profession should determine, that his patient presents a serious danger of violence to another" (*Tarasoff v. Regents of University of California* 1976 at 431). The court further held that warning an intended victim does not violate the physician–patient privilege because "the protective privilege ends where the public peril begins" (at 442).

Once the duty to protect third parties was established, a series of subsequent cases addressed the boundaries of the duty and the threshold criteria for establishing a duty. In *Lipari v. Sears* (1980), a Veterans Administration (VA) patient was referred for treatment in a hospital program. In spite of a previous civil commitment, he was able to purchase a shotgun. After dropping out of treatment, he walked into a crowded nightclub and opened fire, killing Dennis Lipari and wounding his wife. She sued for damages, alleging that the VA failed to protect her and her husband from harm. The district court held that a therapist was liable only for injuries to "those persons foreseeably endangered by the VA's negligent conduct" (*Lipari v. Sears* 1980 at 194). In other words, a psychiatrist had no duty to protect the general public.

The foreseeability of harm is determined by the nature of the target and also by the actions of the patient. In *Jablonski v. U.S.* (1983), the Ninth Circuit Court of Appeals held that the history and behavior of the patient were enough evidence of dangerousness to trigger a duty to warn, even though the patient made no specific threats to the victim in this case.

Phillip Jablonski underwent a voluntary psychiatric evaluation at a VA hospital after he threatened his girlfriend's mother. The police officer who transported Jablonski informed one of the VA psychiatrists of Jablonski's history of violence and recommended admission. This information was not communicated to the evaluator, and Jablonski was not admitted. During a second appointment, Jablonski was assessed as dangerous because of his antisocial personality disorder, but again, he was not admitted. The evaluating psychiatrist warned Jablonski's girlfriend that Jablonski was potentially dangerous and advised her to leave the home. Jablonski later killed his girlfriend.

The VA was sued on behalf of the victim's minor child. The court held that the VA psychiatrists had failed to warn the victim adequately and that they had failed to obtain the patient's past treatment records, which documented his history of violence. The court also found that the physician had failed to document and communicate pertinent risk assessment information provided by police. The court concluded that the patient's girlfriend was a foreseeable victim considering his history and that the warning given by the psychiatrist was insufficient.

Almost all states have a *Tarasoff*-derived duty to warn or protect, although many variations on this duty exist nationwide. In 33 states, the duty to warn or protect is mandated by statute or case law. In 11 states, a breach of confidentiality is permitted but not mandated, and 6 states are silent on the issue (Johnson et al. 2014; National Conference of State Legislatures 2015). Federal law has not established a duty to warn or protect.

Following several mass shooting incidents, some states have sought to broaden mandatory reporting laws. For example, the New York Secure Ammunition and Firearms Enforcement (SAFE) Act of 2013 mandates that clinicians report to the government any patient who is "likely to engage in conduct that will cause serious harm to self or others" (New York State Office of Mental Health 2013). Once such a report is made, the SAFE Act authorizes local law enforcement to confiscate any weapons in the patient's possession and to revoke the individual's firearms license. However, the SAFE Act has been controversial, in part because of both the mandatory reporting requirements and the breach of patient confidentiality (Price et al. 2015).

Boundary Violations

The term *boundary* in the physician–patient relationship refers to the parameters of appropriate physician behavior and professional conduct. In the context of a fiduciary relationship, physicians are obligated to refrain from misusing that relationship for their own personal gain or for the benefit of someone other than the patient. The term *boundary violation* refers to any behavior that misuses the relationship and that can potentially cause harm to the patient or damage to the patient's treatment. As noted earlier, the psychiatrist–patient relationship is often held to a higher standard than that of general physicians. For example, benign practices such as receiving a gift from a patient or revealing innocuous personal information may carry more import for psychiatrists than such actions do for general practitioners. Therefore, psychiatrist–patient relationships require more strictly circumscribed boundaries.

Gutheil and Simon (2002) have distinguished between boundary violations and *boundary crossings*—that is, behaviors that go beyond the traditional boundaries of the physician–patient relationship in psychiatry but that are in the patient's best interest and enhance the therapeutic alliance. Examples of boundary crossings include behaviors such as phoning or texting patients to remind them of an upcoming appointment or expressing personal grief at a patient's loss. A boundary crossing is a socially appropriate expression of concern or encouragement, whereas a boundary violation has no therapeutic purpose and should be strictly avoided.

Over time, boundary violation has become synonymous with sexual contact, but many other potentially damaging types of behavior also constitute serious boundary violations. Therapists who disclose personal information about their marriages or financial situations; who continue a personal relationship with a patient beyond the end of treatment; or

who prescribe medication for family, friends, and others may be entering a gray area of ethical conduct.

In one study, Brooks et al. (2012) reviewed the records of physicians monitored by a physician's health program over a 19-year period. The authors described the behavior and characteristics of 120 physicians referred to the program as a result of boundary violations. Compared with other physicians in the physician's health program, physicians who committed boundary violations were more likely to be male psychiatrists between ages 40 and 49. Examples of nonsexual boundary violations included prescribing narcotics to patients when they were not indicated, inappropriate behavior during examinations, or dual relationships (i.e., having friends, employees, or students as patients). Malmquist and Notman (2001) described cases in which psychiatrists were alleged to have made financial boundary violations by using undue influence to persuade patients to abandon previously made financial commitments.

With regard to sexual boundary violations, the AMA's Code of Medical Ethics (American Medical Association 2016c) clearly states that sexual contact that occurs during the patient–physician relationship constitutes sexual misconduct (Opinion 9.1.1). Relationships with former patients may not always be unethical, but using information obtained in a professional relationship to further develop a relationship is unethical. Similarly, the preamble to the American Psychiatric Association's (2013) *Principles of Medical Ethics With Annotations Especially Applicable to Psychiatry* states:

> A psychiatrist shall not gratify his or her own needs by exploiting the patient. The psychiatrist shall be ever vigilant about the impact that his or her conduct has upon the boundaries

of the doctor–patient relationship, and thus upon the well-being of the patient. These requirements become particularly important because of the essentially private, highly personal, and sometimes intensely emotional nature of the relationship established with the psychiatrist. (p. 3)

Data from state medical boards and federal agencies (Sansone and Sansone 2009) indicate that fewer than 2% of all practicing physicians commit sexual boundary violations, although anonymous physician surveys suggest a prevalence of such behaviors as high as 7%. The specialties of physicians most often involved in sexual violations were family medicine, psychiatry, and obstetrics/gynecology, and most physicians involved in a boundary violation were males.

Roy v. Hartogs (1976) was the first case in which a sexual boundary violation was held to be a cause of action for malpractice. Previously, recovery for damages for such claims had to be pursued through general tort law. In this case, the patient, Julie Roy, alleged that her psychiatrist committed malpractice when he prescribed sexual intercourse as part of her therapy and that her emotional distress from this contact required her to be psychiatrically hospitalized twice. She asserted a cause of action for malpractice based on failure to treat using "professionally acceptable procedures." The court found that sexual intercourse, when prescribed as a course of treatment and in violation of professional standards, was a cause of action for a malpractice suit.

In 23 states, sexual contact between a therapist and a patient is a felony offense (Morgan 2013). State licensing boards also have established standards for determining when sexual contact is a violation of medical practice, although these standards may differ from the criteria set forth in the state's criminal code. Both statutory standards and board regulations usually specify the amount of time that must pass between the end of a treatment relationship and the beginning of a sexual relationship for the physician to avoid malpractice liability or licensure sanctions. However, seven states ban sexual contact with former patients or clients regardless of the amount of time since termination of treatment.

Occasionally, a novel circumstance may arise that has not been addressed by existing statutes. When this occurs, whether a physician's duty exists or how to carry out the duty may be unclear. In this situation, only jurisdiction-specific case law can provide guidance. In the absence of case law, consultation with colleagues or a medical board can ensure that the clinician acts within the community standard of care. Additional complications may occur in situations in which a physician's duty to provide care conflicts with another obligation. In such circumstances, physicians may wish to obtain legal advice before taking action.

Within correctional environments, even minor boundary violations can pose a risk to institutional safety or could be grounds for termination of employment (Trestman et al. 2015). Requests to communicate with people outside the institution on the prisoner's behalf or to provide the dates of court appearances may appear innocuous, but a physician who provides this information may unwittingly aid in the planning of criminal activity or escape. Similarly, a prisoner who realizes that a physician is willing to bend security rules in small ways may press for even greater "favors" (Trestman et al. 2015). The most appropriate response is to "not make the first compromise of appropriate boundaries" (Gutheil 2005, p. 480).

End-of-Life Issues

Determination of Death and Withdrawal of Life-Sustaining Treatment

Although psychiatrists usually are not directly involved in the determination of death, an understanding of the clinical assessment of death is necessary to appreciate legal distinctions between the withdrawal of life-sustaining care and the provision of fatal care (i.e., physician-assisted suicide or medical euthanasia). In 2010, the American Academy of Neurology established criteria for the clinical determination of brain death (Wijdicks et al. 2010). The criteria require that the patient be in an irreversible coma, have an absence of brain stem reflexes, and be unable to breathe independently. Withdrawal of life support—specifically, mechanical ventilation—is a necessary diagnostic test for death by neurological criteria.

Thirty-six states have adopted the model legislation for death determination suggested by the Uniform Determination of Death Act (Pope 2014). This legislation allowed states to define death by either brain death criteria or the end of circulation (McCabe 1981). The assessment of brain death requires that the physician rule out reversible causes of the coma. After this, the patient is tested for the presence of oculovestibular reflexes, and a neurological examination is performed. The patient is observed and reassessed over time to confirm no change in clinical condition. Finally, ventilator support is removed to determine the presence of apnea. A patient in a persistent vegetative state is in a coma and has no response to painful stimuli but is able to breathe independently without mechan-ical support. A patient is deemed to be in a minimally conscious state if he or she shows definite but limited awareness of the environment, such as purposeful movement, spontaneous vocalization, or reaction to painful stimuli (Cranford 2002).

In the case of *Cruzan v. Director, Missouri Dept. of Mental Health* (1990), the woman at the center of the litigation, Nancy Cruzan, was in a persistent vegetative state following a motor vehicle accident. Cruzan's parents and her hospital physicians came into conflict when the parents demanded that the physicians stop Cruzan's artificial feeding and hydration. The hospital refused to stop feeding and hydration without a court order.

At a court hearing, testimony indicated that the patient had told a roommate that she would not want to live life as a "vegetable." On the basis of this testimony, the probate court ordered the feedings stopped. The Missouri Supreme Court reversed the trial court's order, holding that the medical treatment for an incompetent person could be terminated only with clear and convincing evidence of the patient's wishes when competent. The Missouri Supreme Court held that the evidence presented (e.g., the testimony of a former roommate) did not meet a clear and convincing standard. In a 5-to-4 decision, the U.S. Supreme Court upheld this clear and convincing evidence standard and further held that a competent adult had a Fourteenth Amendment liberty interest in not being forced to undergo unwanted medical procedures, such as surgery, intravenous feeding, or intravenous hydration, in the event of a persistent vegetative state. After this decision, Cruzan's parents were able to find additional evidence of her expressed wishes when competent, and the court found that this evidence met the clear and convincing standard of proof and ordered removal of feeding and hydration.

Advance Directives

The crux of the *Cruzan* case was the absence of any legal document or written expression of Cruzan's wishes for end-of-life care. To address this problem, Congress passed the Patient Self Determination Act (1990). This legislation requires hospitals, skilled nursing homes, and hospice programs to provide newly admitted patients with information about the right to create an advance directive for medical care and to appoint a health care proxy.

An *advance directive* is a legal document that an individual completes in order to give instructions regarding desired medical care at the end of life. An advance directive may include instructions regarding cardiopulmonary resuscitation, ventilator support, provision of fluids or nutrition, percutaneous endoscopic gastrostomy tube placement, treatment of infections, or surgical procedures. An advance directive also may designate a health care proxy to make decisions about additional issues not covered in the directive. The directive is made while the individual is competent but takes effect only if the patient loses decision-making capacity. An advance directive can be revoked or changed when the patient regains competency.

In the absence of an advance directive, a hospital is obligated to provide care until a proxy decision maker, usually a spouse, an adult child, or a parent, can be identified. The health care proxy must make a treatment decision based on the patient's stated interests, if known. All 50 states now have advance directive laws; however, considerable variability exists between required formats, procedures, and portability across state lines (Castillo et al. 2011).

Additional end-of-life instruments include medical orders for life-sustaining treatment and physician orders for life-sustaining treatment. These documents have the same effect as an order written by a physician within a hospital but are portable to outside facilities. A durable power of attorney for medical care functions similarly to an advance directive, although a durable power of attorney typically designates a proxy decision maker for issues not anticipated in an advance directive or living will (Hickman et al. 2015).

Psychiatric patients also use advance directives to document preferences for treatment such as choice of medication, use of electroconvulsive therapy, and use of seclusion or restraint (Miller et al. 2011). In *Hargrave v. Vermont* (2003), the Second Circuit Court of Appeals upheld the validity of such advance directives. Nancy Hargrave had been hospitalized and committed many times for the treatment of paranoid schizophrenia. She was found to be incompetent to refuse antipsychotic medication during some of her psychiatric admissions and was medicated involuntarily as a result. Finally, Ms. Hargrave wrote a durable power of attorney in which she designated a guardian for medical decisions and also refused all psychotropic medications.

At that time, Vermont's Durable Power of Attorney Act (Vermont Code 2002) allowed an individual to document treatment wishes in advance or to appoint a guardian to make decisions while the individual was incapacitated. However, the act allowed health care professionals to override a power of attorney in order to involuntarily medicate civilly committed patients or prisoners who had been judged mentally ill. The act required a court to suspend the override for 45 days to allow time to observe the patient while untreated.

Hargrave v. Vermont was certified as a class action suit on behalf of mentally ill individuals in Vermont who had durable powers of attorney. Ms. Hargrave sued the state to bar enforcement of Vermont's involuntary medication law. Ms. Hargrave claimed that Vermont's law violated Title II of the Americans With Disabilities Act (ADA) and the Rehabilitation Act of 1973 in that it discriminated against people with mental illness. Vermont justified the override by claiming that civilly committed patients fell within the imminent dangerousness exception to the ADA. That is, actions that might otherwise be deemed discriminatory are allowed if the individual poses a "significant risk to the health or safety of others" (*Hargrave v. Vermont* 2003 at 36). The state argued that a legal determination of dangerousness at the time of commitment should hold throughout the duration of commitment and therefore fell under the "direct threat" exception. The Second Circuit Court held that there was no exception in this case, because the law allowed 45 days to make a determination, and no judicial review of the patient's dangerousness after that time was conducted. Therefore, the involuntary medication override was found to violate the ADA.

Physician-Assisted Suicide

The U.S. Supreme Court has distinguished between a patient's right to end or refuse futile care and a hypothetical right to request fatal care. Futile care is treatment that cannot provide any chance of recovery because the patient has met clinical or legal criteria for death. The AMA's (American Medical Association 2016b) Code of Medical Ethics states that no physician is obligated to provide futile care (Opinion 5.5). For a patient in a persistent vegetative or minimally conscious state, the right to refuse ordinary care, such as fluid and nutrition, is based on the right

to privacy. Such a patient has a right to avoid unwanted physical intrusion and to preserve bodily integrity.

The U.S. Supreme Court has established that as a matter of law, there is no constitutional guarantee of a "right to die" (*Vacco v. Quill* 1997). In *Washington v. Glucksberg* (1997), four physicians and three terminally ill patients, joined by the organization Compassion in Dying (now known as Compassion and Choices), sought to establish a constitutional right for a mentally competent, terminally ill person to commit physician-assisted suicide and to have the Washington State ban on physician-assisted suicide declared unconstitutional on its face. The Ninth Circuit Court of Appeals had held that Washington's statutory ban on physician-assisted suicide was a violation of the Fourteenth Amendment, and the state of Washington appealed the decision. Because all three patients had died by the time of the appeal, the court had to consider whether the law was unconstitutional under all hypothetical circumstances, not merely as applied to a specific case.

Both the trial court and the Ninth Circuit Court found that individuals have a fundamental right to control the time and manner of their death and that the ban placed an undue restriction on that right. Washington State contended that the ban was necessary to prevent a broader application to voluntary or involuntary euthanasia. The Supreme Court considered amici curiae briefs filed by the American Psychiatric Association in both *Vacco* and *Washington*. The APA advised the court that

> The principle of patient autonomy... has never been understood to give patients the right to every procedure or treatment they might demand. For example, physicians need not provide futile treatment—that is, treat-

ment that has no reasonable chance of helping the patient. Similarly, physicians should not provide patients with treatments that are known to be ineffective or harmful. Such limitations are important. If a patient may demand and receive anything from a health care professional, individuals who practice the healing arts will cease being professionals. (American Psychiatric Association 1996, 11)

In a unanimous opinion, the U.S. Supreme Court stated that a rational basis existed for distinguishing between the withdrawal of life-sustaining care and assisted suicide. Chief Justice Rehnquist wrote, "Unlike the Court of Appeals, we think the distinction between assisting suicide and withdrawing life-sustaining treatment, a distinction widely recognized and endorsed in the medical profession and in our legal traditions, is both important and logical; it is certainly rational" (*Vacco v. Quill* 1997 at 2298).

The Supreme Court also noted that many state statutes barred the use of durable powers of attorney or living wills for physician-assisted suicide. The Justices expressed concern about the difficulty of defining when an illness was "terminal" and the risk of patient coercion. They noted the state's interest in preventing euthanasia. The Court found these interests to be "compelling" and sufficient to bar a constitutional right to assisted suicide. However, Justice Stevens also opined that circumstances may arise in which a state ban on assisted suicide might be unconstitutional as applied in a specific situation: "The State's legitimate interest in preventing abuse does not apply to an individual who is not victimized by abuse, who is not suffering from depression, and who makes a rational and voluntary decision to seek assistance in dying" (*Vacco v. Quill* 1997 at 2308).

Once the U.S. Supreme Court decided in *Vacco* that individuals had no constitutional right to physician-assisted suicide, the Court was able to apply a lower standard of review to the Washington State ban. This standard, known as the "reasonable relation" test, only required that the state's law have a rational basis. The Court found that

[t]hese [state] interests include prohibiting intentional killing and preserving human life; preventing the serious public-health problem of suicide, especially among the young, the elderly, and those suffering from untreated pain or from depression or other mental disorders; protecting the medical profession's integrity and ethics and maintaining physicians' role as their patients' healers; protecting the poor, the elderly, disabled persons, the terminally ill, and persons in other vulnerable groups from indifference, prejudice, and psychological and financial pressure to end their lives; and avoiding a possible slide towards voluntary and perhaps even involuntary euthanasia. (*Washington v. Glucksberg* 1997 at 2290)

The Court also noted that to support a state right to assisted suicide would require them to "reverse centuries of legal doctrine and practice, and strike down the considered policy choice of almost every State" (*Washington v. Glucksberg* 1997 at 2269).

The New Mexico Supreme Court, in considering this issue, has held that under that state's constitution, there is no right to physician-assisted suicide. The court further stated that even if the right existed, the prevention of voluntary or involuntary euthanasia would be a compelling reason to restrict the practice. The court held that "if physician aid in dying is a constitutional right, it must be made available to everyone, even when a duly appointed surrogate makes the decision, and even when the patient is unable to self-administer the life-ending medication" (*Morris v. Brandenburg* 2016 at 10).

Only five states currently have statutory laws that allow physician-assisted suicide: Oregon, Washington, Vermont, California, and Colorado. A Montana Supreme Court case, *Baxter v. Montana* (2009), essentially decriminalized the practice by allowing victim consent as a defense to homicide. All other states have criminalized assisted suicide by physicians or others through statute or case law.

For a psychiatrist working in a state institution, such as a prison or a psychiatric hospital, provision of physician-assisted suicide could carry serious implications under federal law. Under the Civil Rights of Institutionalized Persons Act (1980), state facilities have an affirmative duty to prevent suicide. A facility or individual physician participating in assisted suicide could be liable for a civil rights violation under this 1980 act or under 42 U.S.C. §1983 (Civil Action for Deprivation of Rights 1871), the federal statute that authorizes individuals to sue state agents for such violations (Department of Justice 2005).

Conclusion

Psychiatric care and the physician–patient relationship are regulated by ethical and legal standards. All practitioners should be familiar with these principles. Although issues related to informed consent and therapeutic boundaries are commonly encountered in daily practice, less common clinical circumstances require the clinician to stay abreast of current knowledge and the standard of care regarding the management of potentially dangerous patients and regarding the care of patients with terminal illness.

Key Concepts

- The physician–patient relationship is fiduciary, meaning that a physician is obliged to act solely in the patient's best interests and must be careful to avoid conflicts in duty to other individuals.

- *Informed consent* requires that the patient be advised of the nature, risks, and benefits of the proposed treatment and alternative treatments as well as the risk of refusing treatment. Informed consent usually should include any information that would be materially related to a patient's decision to accept or reject treatment.

- A *therapeutic waiver* occurs when a patient declines a risk–benefit discussion. A *therapeutic privilege* is the physician's decision to withhold information from a patient in order to avoid harm to the patient.

- In most states, clinicians have a duty to warn or protect specified third parties from actual or threatened violence by a patient.

- A *boundary violation* occurs when a physician misuses a therapeutic relationship for his or her own personal gain or for the benefit of someone other than the patient.

- An *advance directive* is executed while the individual is competent but takes effect only if the patient loses decision-making capacity. An advance directive can be revoked or changed when the patient regains competency.

- A competent patient has the right to refuse medical treatment through the use of a durable power of attorney, a medical advance directive, or a designated health care proxy. In the absence of these documents, an institution must provide care until a health care proxy can be identified or appointed.

- The U.S. Supreme Court has established that individuals have no constitutional right to physician-assisted suicide. States are free to legalize or criminalize the practice.

References

American Academy of Psychiatry and the Law: Ethics Guidelines for the Practice of Forensic Psychiatry. May 2005. Available at: http://www.aapl.org/ethics.htm. Accessed December 19, 2016.

American Medical Association: Code of Medical Ethics: Opinion 1.1.1—Patient-Physician Relationships. June 2016a. Available at: https://www.ama-assn.org/sites/default/files/media-browser/code-of-medical-ethics-chapter-1.pdf. Accessed December 29, 2016.

American Medical Association: Code of Medical Ethics: Opinion 5.5—Medically Ineffective Interventions. June 2016b. Available at: https://www.ama-assn.org/sites/default/files/media-browser/code-of-medical-ethics-chapter-5.pdf. Accessed December 29, 2016.

American Medical Association: Code of Medical Ethics: Opinion 9.1.1—Romantic or Sexual Relationships With Patients. June 2016c. Available at: https://www.ama-assn.org/sites/default/files/media-browser/code-of-medical-ethics-chapter-9.pdf. Accessed December 29, 2016.

American Psychiatric Association: Vacco v. Quill (brief). U.S. S.Ct. Briefs LEXIS 709 (1996)

American Psychiatric Association: The Principles of Medical Ethics With Annotations Especially Applicable to Psychiatry. 2013. Available at: https://www.psychiatry.org/psychiatrists/practice/ethics. Accessed December 21, 2016.

Bartlett P: Doctors as fiduciaries: equitable regulation of the doctor-patient relationship. Med Law Rev 5(2):193–224, 1997 11655266

Baxter v Montana 224 P3d 1211 (2009)

Blake V: When is a patient-physician relationship established? Virtual Mentor 14(5):403–406, 2012. Available at: http://journalofethics.ama-assn.org/2012/05/hlaw1-1205.html. Accessed December 29, 2016.

Brooks E, Gendel MH, Early SR, et al: Physician boundary violations in a physician's health program: a 19-year review. J Am Acad Psychiatry Law 40(1):59–66, 2012 22396343

Canterbury v Spence, 150 U.S. App. D.C. 263, 464 F.2d 772 (1972)

Castillo LS, Williams BA, Hooper SM, et al: Lost in translation: the unintended consequences of advance directive law on clinical care. Ann Intern Med 154(2):121–128, 2011 21242368

Civil Action for Deprivation of Rights, 42 USC §1983 (1871)

Civil Rights of Institutionalized Persons Act of 1980, 42 USC §1997 et seq. (1980)

Cranford RE: What is a minimally conscious state? West J Med 176(2):129–130, 2002 11897740

Cruzan v Director, Missouri Dept. of Mental Health, 497 U.S. 261, 110 S.Ct. 2841 (1990)

Department of Justice: Department of Justice Activities Under the Civil Rights of Institutionalized Persons Act Fiscal Year 2005. 2005. Available at: https://www.justice.gov/crt/about/spl/documents/split_cripa05.pdf. Accessed December 29, 2016.

Gutheil TG: Boundaries, blackmail, and double binds: a pattern observed in malpractice consultation. J Am Acad Psychiatry Law 33(4):476–481, 2005 16394223

Gutheil TG, Simon RI: Non-sexual boundary crossings and boundary violations: the ethical dimension. Psychiatr Clin North Am 25(3):585–592, 2002 12232972

Hargrave v Vermont, 340 F.3d 27 (2003)

Hickman SE, Keevern E, Hammes BJ: Use of the physician orders for life-sustaining treatment program in the clinical setting: a systematic review of the literature. J Am Geriatr Soc 63(2):341–350, 2015 25644280

Jablonski v U.S., 712 F.2d 391 (1983)

Johnson R, Persad G, Sisti D: The Tarasoff rule: the implications of interstate variation and gaps in professional training. J Am Acad Psychiatry Law 42(4):469–477, 2014 25492073

Kaimowitz v Michigan Dept. of Mental Health, 1 MDLR 147 (1973)

Lennon JG: Easing the medical malpractice crisis: restricting the creation of duty through an implied doctor-patient relationship. Journal of Health Care and Law Policy 7(2), 2004. Available at: http://digitalcommons.law.umaryland.edu/jhclp/vol7/iss2/6. Accessed January 14, 2016.

Lipari v Sears, 497 F.Supp. 185 (D. Neb. 1980)

Malmquist CP, Notman MT: Psychiatrist-patient boundary issues following treatment termination. Am J Psychiatry 158 (7):1010–1018, 2001 11431220

McCabe JM: The new Determination of Death Act. Am Bar Assoc J 67(11):1476–1478, 1981. Available at: http://www.jstor.org/stable/20748267. Accessed June 4, 2016.

Miller D, Hanson A, Daviss S: Shrink Rap: Three Psychiatrists Explain Their Work. Baltimore, MD, Johns Hopkins University Press, 2011, p 124

Morgan S: Criminalization of psychotherapist sexual misconduct. May 2013. Available at: http://www.naswca.org/associations/7989/files/7_13_legal_issue.pdf. Accessed February 7, 2016.

Morris v Brandenburg, 2016 N.M. LEXIS 151 (N.M. June 30, 2016)

National Conference of State Legislatures: Mental health professionals' duty to warn. September 28, 2015. Available at: http://www.ncsl.org/research/health/mental-health-professionals-duty-to-warn.aspx#1. Accessed February 15, 2016.

New York State Office of Mental Health: NY Safe Act. 2013. Available at: https://www.omh.ny.gov/omhweb/safe_act/index.html. Accessed February 15, 2016.

Patient Self Determination Act, 42 USC 1395 cc (1990)

Pope TM: Legal briefing: brain death and total brain failure. J Clin Ethics 25(3):245–257, 2014 25192349

Price M, Recupero PR, Norris DM: Mental illness and the National Instant Criminal Background Check System, in Gun Violence and Mental Illness. Edited by Gold LH, Simon RI. Washington, DC, American Psychiatric Publishing, 2015, pp 127–158

Roy v Hartogs, 381 N.Y.S. 2d 587 (1976)

Sansone RA, Sansone LA: Crossing the line: sexual boundary violations by physicians. Psychiatry (Edgmont) 6(6):45–48, 2009 19724761

Schloendorff v Society of New York Hospital, 211 N.Y. 125, 105 N.E. 92, 93 (1914)

Shultz MM: From informed consent to patient choice: a new protected interest. Yale Law J 95(2):219–299, 1985

Tarasoff v Regents of University of California, 17 Cal. 3d 425, 551 P.2d 334, 131 Cal. Rptr. 14 (1976)

Trestman RL, Appelbaum KL, Metzner JL (eds): Oxford Textbook of Correctional Psychiatry. New York, Oxford University Press, 2015, p 65

Truman v Thomas, 27 Cal. 3d 285, 611 P.2d 902, 165 Cal. Rptr. 308 (1980)

Vacco v Quill, 521 U.S. 793, 117 S.Ct. 2293 (1997)

Vars F: Illusory consent: when an incapacitated patient agrees to treatment. 87 Or. L. Rev. 353 (2008)

Vermont Code, Decedents' Estates and Fiduciary Relations, Powers of Attorney, Title 14, ch 123, §§3508, 3509 (2002)

Washington v Glucksberg, 521 U.S. 702, 117 S.Ct. 2258 (1997)

Wijdicks EFM, Varelas PN, Gronseth GS, et al; American Academy of Neurology: Evidence-based guideline update: determining brain death in adults: report of the Quality Standards Subcommittee of the American Academy of Neurology. Neurology 74(23):1911–1918, 2010 20530327

CHAPTER 9

Legal Regulation of Psychiatric Treatment

Barry W. Wall, M.D.

Stuart A. Anfang, M.D.

Landmark Cases

**Application of the President and Directors of Georgetown College,
331 F.2d 1000 (1964)**

Rouse v. Cameron, 373 F.2d 451 (1966) (AAPL only)

Wyatt v. Stickney, 344 F.Supp. 387 (1972)

O'Connor v. Donaldson, 422 U.S. 563, 95 S.Ct. 2486 (1975)

Youngberg v. Romeo, 457 U.S. 307, 102 S.Ct. 2452 (1982)

Rennie v. Klein, 720 F.2d 266 (1983)

Rogers v. Commissioner of Dept. of Mental Health,
390 Mass. 489, 458 N.E.2d 308 (1983)

Washington v. Harper, 494 U.S. 210, 110 S.Ct. 1028 (1990)

Zinermon v. Burch, 494 U.S. 113, 110 S.Ct. 975 (1990)

Hargrave v. Vermont, 340 F.3d 27 (2003)

Laws and regulations are intertwined with most elements of psychiatric treatment; becoming knowledgeable about the historical evolution of these laws and regulations assists in understanding the legal parameters governing the practice of psychiatry. For centuries, persons with mental illness have faced marginalization, treatment inequities, and stigmatization. In the nineteenth century, patients isolated in state asylums and mental hospitals had no right to association, privacy, or speech. Institutionalized patients had no input or control over the type, location, or duration of their treatment. All treatment was involuntary because no distinction between involuntary and voluntary admission existed. Well into the twentieth century, most institutionalized patients continued to lack basic human rights or the assurance that hospitalization would be humane and bear some relation to treatment and that they might again live freely in their own communities when possible.

In the civil rights era of the mid-twentieth century, legal advocates began addressing many of these inequities. Psychiatrists, other professional groups, and stakeholders began to advocate for voluntary treatment and transition to community-based treatment. In the ensuing years, a wide array of antidiscrimination laws, regulations, policies, and programs have come into effect that aim to reduce the stigma, discrimination, and disparities associated with mental health and substance use disorders and their treatment. In this chapter, we review the legal regulation of psychiatric treatment, including issues relating to mental health parity, the Patient Protection and Affordable Care Act of 2010, voluntary hospitalization, consent for hospitalization, the right to treatment, the right to refuse treatment, and proxy decision making.

Mental Health Parity and the Patient Protection and Affordable Care Act of 2010

The term *mental health parity* generally refers to the legal mandate that insurance providers offer health insurance benefits for mental health and substance use disorder services on par with covered medical and surgical benefits. Prior to 1996, health insurance policies typically covered services for mental illness or substance use disorders at far lower levels, with frequently higher deductibles, than those for medical or surgical services. These disparities prompted a movement toward mental health parity. Since 1996, several laws and regulations have been implemented with the goal of achieving mental health parity, although full parity for all plans in all states has not yet been achieved (Sarata 2011).

Three federal laws have started the process of creating federal mental health parity requirements. The Mental Health Parity Act (MHPA) of 1996 (Mental Health Parity Act 1996) requires parity in annual and aggregate lifetime limits of insurance coverage. The Mental Health Parity and Addiction Equity Act (MHPAEA) of 2008 (Mental Health Parity and Addiction Equity Act 2008b) expands parity requirements to treatment limitations, financial requirements, in-network and out-of-network covered benefits, and substance use disorders. Unfortunately, neither of these laws mandate the coverage of specific mental and substance use disorders. They require parity in benefits only when an insurer chooses to cover both mental health and medical-surgical services.

The Patient Protection and Affordable Care Act, also known as the Affordable Care Act (ACA) or "Obamacare," is the third key federal law that has helped in the movement to achieve mental health parity. President Barack Obama signed the ACA into federal law on March 23, 2010 (Patient Protection and Affordable Care Act 2010). The ACA is intended to increase the quality and affordability of health insurance, decrease the number of uninsured people by expanding coverage, and reduce health care costs.

Taken together, the MHPA, MHPAEA, and ACA achieve two goals necessary in achieving full mental health insurance coverage parity. First, these laws expand the reach of the applicability of the federal mental health parity requirements. Second, they create a mandated benefit for the coverage of certain mental health and substance use disorder services determined through rulemaking (Beronio et al. 2013).

In November 2013, the Departments of Health and Human Services (DHHS), Labor, and the Treasury issued final rules to implement the MHPAEA for private insurers (Internal Revenue Service, Department of the Treasury et al. 2013). These rules began to improve coverage levels for mental health and substance use treatment covered by commercial insurance plans. In April 2015, DHHS released another rule proposing that the implementation of the parity law should include low-income Americans insured through the government's Medicaid managed care and Children's Health Insurance Program plans (Centers for Medicare and Medicaid Services and Department of Health and Human Services 2016). The proposed regulation is similar to that released in November 2013 for private insurers.

Whether an insurance plan is subject to federal mental health parity regulations depends on the size and the kind of plan. Three types of health plans must follow federal mental health parity rules:

1. Qualified health plans as established by the ACA
2. Medicaid non–managed care benchmark and benchmark-equivalent plans
3. Plans offered through the competitive marketplace that covers individuals

Medicaid fee-for-service plans and most of Medicare do not have to comply with federal mental health parity. Currently, about one-half of all covered Americans are enrolled in large self-insured health insurance plans that are subject to federal parity. The federal parity law does not require plans to offer coverage for mental health or substance use disorders, but if they are covered, then the law requires that that coverage be equal to coverage for other health conditions (National Conference of State Legislatures 2015).

The federal parity law also applies to all plans available through state and federal health insurance marketplaces. State-regulated group health plans must continue to follow state requirements to provide coverage for specific, or all, mental health and substance use disorders. If a state has stronger parity laws than the federal laws, then health insurance plans regulated in that state must follow the state laws. For example, if state law requires plans to cover mental health conditions, then they must do so, even though federal parity makes inclusion of mental health benefits optional. Federal parity replaces state law only when the state law "prevents the application" of federal parity requirements (Final Rules Under the Paul Wellstone and Pete Domenici Mental Health Parity and Addiction Equity Act of 2008; Internal Revenue Service, Department of the Treasury et al. 2013). For example, if a state law requires some coverage for mental health conditions, then the federal requirement of equal coverage will prevail over the state law.

Unfortunately, mental health parity does not necessarily ensure good mental health coverage or adequate mental health treatment. If a health insurance plan's mental health, substance use, and medical and surgical benefits are very limited, then mental health and substance use disorder coverage will remain limited even in a plan subject to federal parity or in a state that has a strong parity law.

Additionally, health insurers use federal mental health parity clinical criteria to approve or deny mental health or substance use treatment, which may result in more limited coverage. Nevertheless, pursuant to the ACA, all health plans must release their standards for medical necessity determinations on request. The reason for denial of coverage also must be made available on request. Finally, even though benefits theoretically may be available, accessing timely services through an available provider may present a practical challenge.

Since 2014, the ACA has provided one of the largest expansions of mental health and substance use disorder coverage in a generation. However, expansions have occurred unevenly and have been heavily criticized by ACA opponents. Gaps in coverage still exist, and many people with some coverage of mental health and substance use disorders do not currently receive the benefit of federal mental health parity protections. About one-third of those who are currently covered in the individual market have no coverage for substance use disorder services, and nearly 20% have no coverage for mental health services, including outpatient therapy visits and inpatient crisis intervention and stabilization (Beronio et al. 2013).

In addition, even when individual market plans provide these benefits, the federal mental health parity law does not ensure that coverage for mental health and substance use disorder services is generally comparable to coverage for medical and surgical care. Significant confusion and concerns remain regarding insurance companies' and employers' responsibility under the law and the government's authority to impose penalties and ensure compliance under MHPAEA. Advocates claim that consumers still face barriers to obtaining recommended mental health

and substance use services. Achieving true mental health parity will take additional time and effort as well as rigorous regulation.

Patient Rights and Voluntary Psychiatric Hospitalization

Civil Rights of Institutionalized Persons Act and Protection and Advocacy for Individuals With Mental Illness Act

Since the movement away from institutionalization and toward community treatment, psychiatrists and other mental health professionals, mental health attorneys, and persons with mental illness have increasingly focused on patient rights and patient autonomy. A firm distinction now exists between voluntary and involuntary hospitalization. Voluntary hospitalization is the act of a person choosing to be admitted to a psychiatric hospital or other mental health facility. Voluntary patients are free to leave the hospital when they wish, even against medical advice. A period of notice of the wish to be discharged is usually required so that the hospital can determine whether the discharge is safe or whether involuntary commitment proceedings should be initiated.

The number of voluntary hospitalizations relative to total psychiatric admissions increased in the United States from 10% in 1949 to 45% in 1980. A 1986 survey of 1,508,302 admissions to psychiatric inpatient settings of all types showed that 71% were voluntary (Cournos et al. 1993). However, in the past several decades, the United States has experienced a dramatic decline in the number of available inpatient psychiatric beds. In 1960, the United States had 298 public psychiatric hospital beds per 100,000 persons. By 2010, that number had declined to 14 beds per 100,000 persons (Treatment Advocacy Center 2010).

The current demand for inpatient psychiatric care has far exceeded capacity, and most admissions occur in emergency situations, when a patient is deemed a danger to self or others. Many public sector systems restrict psychiatric admission to involuntary patients as a means of holding down the inpatient census and associated costs (Wall 2013). Consequently, across all facility types (public and private), 59% of all persons who received inpatient mental health services in 2010 were involuntarily admitted for care (Substance Abuse and Mental Health Services Administration 2014).

Protection and advocacy services have strengthened because of concerns among mental health advocates that widespread abuses have continued in hospitals even after deinstitutionalization. Some states began establishing protection and advocacy services for inpatients during the civil rights era. In the 1980s, the U.S. Congress also passed two important protection and advocacy acts.

The Civil Rights of Institutionalized Persons Act (CRIPA) of 1980 is a U.S. federal law that protects the rights of people in state or local correctional facilities, nursing homes, mental health facilities, and institutions for people with intellectual and developmental disabilities. The U.S. Department of Justice enforces CRIPA. CRIPA does not create new rights, but it allows the U.S. attorney general to intervene on behalf of institutionalized people whose rights may have been violated, because institutionalized persons may feel uncomfortable or be unable to report abuse in these government-run institutions.

In 1985, a U.S. Senate subcommittee investigation determined that individuals with mental illness were vulnerable to mistreatment and neglect, particularly in hospitals and institutions. In response to these hearings, Congress passed the Protection and Advocacy for Individuals With Mental Illness Act (PAIMI) of 1986. PAIMI created a federally funded, national system of patient advocacy. This legislation gives lawyers, known as *patient advocates*, the authority to investigate patient allegations of neglect, abuse, and civil rights violations. In 2000, PAIMI was amended to include individuals receiving community-based care in need of advocacy; however, protection and advocacy still must prioritize services to persons in institutional settings (Protection and Advocacy for Individuals With Mental Illness Act of 1986 2000).Currently, 57 PAIMI advocacy agencies are in operation, with 1 in each state and the District of Columbia, 5 in U.S. territories, and 1 serving several Native American tribes. PAIMI data from 1997 to 2004 indicate a slow but steady decline in cases related to abuse and neglect and a significant increase in civil rights matters such as claims of discrimination, obtaining public benefits, and issues pertaining to guardianship and informed consent. The decline in abuse and neglect cases may reflect the effect of external scrutiny by PAIMI agencies.

However, other factors influencing this decline may include the reduced number of state hospital beds (where most abuse and neglect complaints arise) and the increased adherence to the moral values of patient autonomy and providing respectful treatment. Between 1997 and 2004, the percentage of PAIMI patients residing in institutions at the time of their initial intake meeting with an advocate declined from more than 70% to 58%, as the percentage of PAIMI patients residing in community settings at intake increased from 20% to 41% (Center for Mental Health Services 2006).

Consent for Hospitalization

Early statutes regulating voluntary hospitalization specified that a patient must be legally competent to consent to hospitalization. Subsequent laws eliminated this requirement to encourage people to seek and obtain treatment when needed (Appelbaum and Gutheil 2007). In 1990, the U.S. Supreme Court ruling in *Zinermon v. Burch* addressed the requirements for voluntary consent for psychiatric hospitalization. Darnell Burch was found wandering along a Florida highway disoriented, hallucinating, and hurt. He was taken to a local private psychiatric inpatient unit, where he signed a voluntary admission form. After 3 days, Burch was transferred to Florida State Hospital, where he also signed a voluntary admission form. He was diagnosed with schizophrenia, given antipsychotic medications, and hospitalized for 5 months without a hearing.

After discharge, Burch sued in federal court alleging a violation of due process of law because he had been incompetent to consent to voluntary admission. The U.S. Supreme Court held that Burch was entitled to raise his claim in federal court. The ruling narrowly focused on whether a specific section of the federal civil rights laws was an available remedy. The Court explicitly stated that it would not rule on the issue of whether a voluntary patient must be competent to consent to admission. However, it expressed a broad range of concerns apart from the narrow decision itself, including questioning whether hospital personnel should assume that a mentally ill patient who agrees to voluntary hospitalization is making a knowing and willful decision.

The issues articulated in *Zinermon* illustrate the frequent tension between autonomy and paternalism in mental health matters. Balancing the ability to make one's own decision to be hospitalized and the possibility of being unable to do so because of active symptoms of mental illness raises legitimate concerns about when a person should autonomously decide and when the state should intervene to make decisions. It is preferable, when possible, for people to initiate their own mental health treatment, because this reflects, among other values, respect for autonomy and the provision of humane and respectful treatment.

Right to Treatment

In 1960, Morton Birnbaum, a physician and a lawyer, proposed a constitutionally protected right to treatment for persons in psychiatric hospitals on the basis of substantive due process (Birnbaum 1960). The theory was based on the quid pro quo argument that a psychiatric patient should be entitled to receive active treatment, not just confinement and basic services, in exchange for loss of freedom.

Legal advocates, mental health professionals, and persons with mental illness have used the concept of the right to treatment to improve mental health services across all settings. However, no constitutionally enshrined right to treatment has been definitively established. Court rulings on the matter have been narrow. Even though many lower courts have found a right to treatment for involuntary patients, courts have had little power to enforce full state compliance with treatment measures.

The earliest court decision regarding the right to treatment was *Rouse v. Cameron* (1966). Charles Rouse was involuntarily committed to St. Elizabeth's Hospital in Washington, D.C., in 1962 after he was adjudicated not guilty by reason of insanity on a misdemeanor offense of carrying a dangerous weapon. He challenged his detention and claimed that he received no treatment. The D.C. Circuit Court of Appeals, in its decision, recognized a right to treatment for the first time, stating, "The purpose of involuntary hospitalization is treatment, not punishment" (*Rouse v. Cameron* 1966, at 452). The Appeals Court based its decision on a Washington, D.C., statute that mandated treatment for involuntarily committed patients with mental illness: "A person hospitalized in a public hospital for a mental illness shall, during his hospitalization, be entitled to medical and psychiatric care and treatment" (Code of the District of Columbia §21-562 1978). By relying on statute, the court did not have to find a constitutional basis for the right to treatment.

The Fifth Circuit Court of Appeals also endorsed a constitutionally based right to treatment by upholding a district court ruling in *Wyatt v. Stickney* (1972). Ricky Wyatt was part of a class-action suit challenging deplorable conditions in the Alabama state hospitals. The district court held that failure to actively treat involuntary patients abridged Fourteenth Amendment rights of both due process and equal protection because treatment was the quid pro quo for involuntary loss of liberty: "To deprive any citizen of his or her liberty upon the altruistic theory that the confinement is for altruistic reasons and then fail to provide adequate treatment violates the very fundamentals of due process" (*Wyatt v. Stickney* 1972, at 785). This case, however, never went to the U.S. Supreme Court, so the constitutional right to treatment did not extend beyond the Fifth Circuit.

The Fifth Circuit Court of Appeals also upheld a constitutional right to treatment in *Donaldson v. O'Connor* (1974). Kenneth Donaldson, a nondangerous person diagnosed with schizophrenia, was held at Chattahoochee State Hospital in Florida for 14 years. He refused medications and electroconvulsive therapy because of his Christian Scientist beliefs. The hospital denied offers by friends to care for Donaldson should he be released. The Appeals Court ruled that the Fourteenth Amendment guarantees a constitutional right of a civilly committed person to receive treatment to have a reasonable opportunity to improve or cure his condition. The case was appealed to the U.S. Supreme Court in *O'Connor v. Donaldson* (1975), where the issue of a right to treatment was avoided, and the Court's holding was limited to confinement questions (see Chapter 10, "Civil Commitment").

The U.S. Supreme Court ultimately addressed the question of a right to treatment in *Youngberg v. Romeo* (1982), although the ruling was narrowly defined. Nicholas Romeo, committed to Pennhurst State Hospital in Pennsylvania, was a profoundly intellectually disabled man with an infant-level IQ. Romeo's mother became concerned by the numerous injuries he incurred while living at Pennhurst. She filed a suit on her son's behalf, alleging violation of his rights, including failing to institute appropriate measures to avoid injuries, routinely restraining him for prolonged periods, and failing to provide appropriate treatment.

The Supreme Court agreed with the Third Circuit Court of Appeals' holding that involuntary patients had constitutionally protected liberty interests under the due process clause of the Fourteenth Amendment. These included reasonably safe conditions of confinement, freedom from unreasonable body restraints, and minimally adequate training to accomplish the first two goals. By basing this right on constitutional liberty interests alone, the Supreme Court narrowly defined what elements of treatment are required, so the Court made no finding of a general right to treatment under the Constitution. Efforts to expand patients' right to treatment have continued through state laws, CRIPA, PAIMI, the ACA and its related statutes and rules, and other avenues of advocacy.

Right to Refuse Treatment

Beginning in the late 1960s, states began to move toward the "dangerousness" model of civil commitment for mental illness—that is, that individuals could be involuntarily hospitalized if they had a mental illness and potentially presented imminent risk of harm to themselves or others. As the rationale for involuntary hospitalization shifted away from treatment and more toward safety (derived from the state's "police power"), courts began to recognize the patient's right to refuse treatment, especially treatment interventions that seemed particularly intrusive, such as antipsychotic medication and electroconvulsive therapy (Appelbaum 1994).

Over the course of the 1970s and 1980s, two different approaches—the treatment-driven professional judgment model and the rights-driven model—evolved regarding the right to refuse treatment. The *treatment-driven professional judgment* approach recognizes the patient's privacy interest in objecting to involuntary treatment but allows physicians' judgment to be the ultimate determinant of whether treatment refusal can be overridden. In the professional judgment model, when a patient objects, the objection is reviewed by a medical expert or panel (sometimes including the treating physician and sometimes an independent reviewer). If the recommended treatment is considered

appropriate, then treatment is allowed. Patients can object to involuntary treatment but do not necessarily have a right to refuse appropriate treatment.

The landmark case establishing the professional judgment model to override treatment refusal is *Rennie v. Klein* (1983). John Rennie was a civilly committed involuntary patient in a New Jersey state hospital who objected to the forced administration of antipsychotic medication. The Third Circuit Court of Appeals found that the exercise of professional judgment (in this case, having a second physician review the case) to prevent the patient from endangering himself or others can override a patient's objection to treatment with antipsychotic medication.

To date, the Supreme Court has not directly ruled on a federal constitutional right to refuse treatment in civil commitment. However, two Supreme Court decisions, *Youngberg v. Romeo* (1982) and *Washington v. Harper* (1990) (see Chapters 21, "Correctional Settings and Prisoner Rights," and 22, "Psychiatric Treatment in Correctional Settings"), have supported the treatment-driven approach, endorsing the "professional judgment" model of review by a clinical decision-maker, often independent of the treating clinician.

In a *rights-driven* approach, courts require an external judicial review and more attention to formal due process rights and procedures (Appelbaum and Gutheil 2007). Contemporaneous with the *Rennie* decision, several states adopted this rights-driven model, which emphasizes individuals' rights to control what happens to their own bodies. The justification for upholding or overriding treatment refusal in these states is grounded not in the U.S. Constitution but in state constitutions, statutes, or common law arguments about autonomy. The rights-driven model goes beyond the minimum professional judgment review mandated in *Rennie* and mandates the need for more external protections and judicial oversight in order to override the patient's objection to treatment.

Because voluntary patients cannot be treated against their will unless found to lack decision-making capacity, involuntary patients similarly must be found incompetent; involuntary hospitalization due to dangerousness does not suffice to establish incompetence. Rights-driven models require a more formal evaluation of the refusing patient's competence and the appropriateness of recommended treatment. States vary in terms of procedures and oversight, but the key feature is provision for review by someone other than a physician/clinician, a move away from *Rennie's* endorsement of professional judgment.

The landmark case that established the rights-driven model of treatment refusal is *Rogers v. Commissioner of Dept. of Mental Health* (1983). In *Rogers*, a class action suit brought in a Massachusetts Federal District Court arguing for a constitutional right to refuse treatment, the class of plaintiffs was a group of involuntarily committed patients at Boston State Hospital who were refusing treatment with antipsychotic medication. Eventually, *Rogers* reached the U.S. Supreme Court, which remanded the case to the Massachusetts Supreme Judicial Court for an ultimate decision. This state court's ruling is binding only within Massachusetts, but the rights-driven approach has been adopted by some states.

The *Rogers* decision affirmed that an involuntarily committed patient is considered competent to refuse treatment until judicially found incompetent. Following a full adversarial hearing with adequate due process protections, the judge can then decide what the incompe-

tent patient would have chosen if competent. In other words, the judge makes a *substituted judgment* for the now-incompetent ward. This substituted judgment needs to take into account the following factors:

- The patient's previously expressed preferences
- The patient's religious convictions
- The probable side effects
- The prognosis with and without treatment
- The potential effect on the patient's family

Some have argued that this judicial approach is more costly in time (potential delay in treatment and longer hospitalizations) and resources (cost of attorneys, court time, potential independent experts), but rights advocates maintain that the added protections are necessary to maintain the patient's rights and autonomy (Appelbaum and Gutheil 2007). Note that both the rights-driven and the treatment-driven models allow for "emergency" interventions, which are often narrowly defined, when a physician can temporarily override a patient's (presumably incompetent) treatment refusal because serious imminent harm is likely.

Override of Treatment Refusal

As discussed in Chapter 8, "Physician–Patient Relationship in Psychiatry," the doctrine of informed consent has evolved in medicine over the past 50 years, moving from the notion of "simple consent (or assent)" to the requirement of obtaining a more complete and adequate informed consent from the patient (Berg et al. 2001). Informed consent requires that the patient have sufficient information to make the decision; that the decision be voluntary (not coerced); and that the patient be competent (have decision-making capacity) to offer consent. Evolving standards for obtaining informed consent prompt the questions of when an override of an individual's refusal of treatment is acceptable, under what circumstances, and by whose legal standing.

The state typically relies on two principles when infringing on an individual's autonomous rights: 1) the principle of police power, used to ensure the safety of the community, and 2) the parens patriae principle, whereby the state protects those unable to protect and care for themselves. Parens patriae is typically invoked in the civil setting for treatment refusal in medical cases. For example, in **Application of the President and Directors of Georgetown College** (1964), a 25-year-old woman with a 7-month-old child required an emergency blood transfusion as a result of a bleeding ulcer. She and her husband were Jehovah's Witnesses and refused consent for the transfusion. The hospital petitioned the court to override her treatment refusal.

The court, after paying a personal visit to the patient, found that the woman came to the hospital seeking help, did not want to die, was in extremis, and could not make her own decision. The court held that the state's role as parens patriae extended to both her and her 7-month-old infant. The court therefore issued an order authorizing the hospital to administer blood transfusions. Although such a case might be decided differently in 2017, given the evolution of case law and the use of advanced directives and health care proxies, **Georgetown** remains an important example of the delicate balance between the state's authority and the individual's autonomy (Appelbaum 1994).

Proxy Decision Making

The courts have established the individual's right to accept or refuse treatment via an informed consent process. As a result, courts also have had to consider the practical implications of obtaining informed consent when the person who should be the decision maker is not competent. Additional court decisions have begun to shape the contours of the circumstances and parameters when a substitute (proxy) decision maker can act and what due process protections need to be in place.

When substituted judgment is used to make this determination, a court-appointed guardian attempts to determine what the incompetent individual's wishes would have been had the individual been competent (see, e.g., *Superintendent of Belchertown State School v. Saikewicz* 1977). In some states, courts retain the authority to make the final decision, assuring judicial protection of the individual's due process rights. Other states give court-appointed guardians full authority without requiring further judicial review. Regardless, a substituted judgment is not merely what decision might be in the general "best interest" of a hypothetical patient but what a specific individual would decide if he or she were competent to make a treatment choice.

Many jurisdictions have held that certain kinds of treatment (e.g., antipsychotic medications, electroconvulsive therapy) require special authorization and special due process protections, presumably because of the more intrusive nature of the proposed treatment. The scientific basis for this "special" status might be questionable. For example, why should a guardian be able to give consent for a ward's high-risk neurosurgery but require a judge's oversight to consent to the administration of even a small dose of an antipsychotic medication? Nevertheless, legal advocates often have been successful at portraying antipsychotic medication as an "extraordinary" intervention requiring special oversight and protections (Appelbaum and Gutheil 2007).

The legal approach of holding the patient's autonomous right to decide above the state's parens patriae power and outlining very specific due process protections required to override and appoint a suitable proxy was ultimately the logic followed in *Rogers v. Commissioner of Dept. of Mental Health* (1983), as discussed earlier, and *Hargrave v. Vermont* (2003), as discussed in Chapter 8. This patient's rights–driven approach, with its full panoply of judicial involvement and due process protections, is jurisdiction specific and can vary significantly from one jurisdiction to another.

Conclusion

After centuries of marginalization, treatment inequities, and limited rights for patients with mental health disorders, in the last 50 years, we have seen a wide array of antidiscrimination laws, regulations, policies, and programs intended to reduce stigma, discrimination, and treatment disparities. These protections are grounded in federal and state statutes, federal and state case law, and administrative regulations. Clinicians and forensic psychiatric consultants need to be aware of the statutory and case law relevant to their jurisdiction.

Key Concepts

- Federal and state parity laws in the early twenty-first century have provided the largest expansions of mental health and substance use disorder coverage in a generation; however, expansions have occurred unevenly, and consumers still face significant barriers to obtaining mental health treatment.

- State and federal laws provide important protections for institutionalized persons and persons with severe mental illness. Oversight is handled at the federal or state level by designated agencies.

- The U.S. Supreme Court has not recognized a constitutionally based right to treatment; however, efforts to define those rights are found in case law decided by lower courts as well as federal and state statutes and regulations.

- The right to refuse treatment has been approached by two different models. The treatment-driven model has resulted in use of a more medical professional judgment approach; the rights-driven model has resulted in a more legal substituted judgment approach.

- The state typically relies on two principles when infringing on an individual's autonomous rights in regard to involuntary commitment and treatment: those of police power and parens patriae.

- Clinicians and forensic psychiatric consultants need to be aware of the statutory and case law relevant to their jurisdiction in assessments of treatment refusal in involuntarily committed civil patients and in advising courts and guardians of relevant issues in proceedings to override treatment refusals.

References

Appelbaum PS: Almost a Revolution: Mental Health Law and the Limits of Change. New York, Oxford University Press, 1994

Appelbaum PS, Gutheil TG: Clinical Handbook of Psychiatry and the Law, 4th Edition. Philadelphia, PA, Lippincott/Williams & Wilkins, 2007

Application of the President and Directors of Georgetown College, 331 F.2d 1000 (1964)

Berg JW, Appelbaum PS, Lidz CW, et al: Informed Consent: Legal Theory and Clinical Practice, 2nd Edition. New York, Oxford University Press, 2001

Beronio K, Po R, Skopec L, Glied S: Affordable Care Act will expand mental health and substance use disorder benefits and parity protections for 62 million Americans. February 2013. Office of the Assistant Secretary for Planning and Evaluation Research Brief, Office of Health Policy. Available at: https://aspe.hhs.gov/system/files/pdf/76591/rb_mental.pdf. Accessed December 30, 2016.

Birnbaum M: The right to treatment. Am Bar Assoc J 46:499–505, 1960

Center for Mental Health Services: Mental Health, United States, 2004 (DHHS Publ No SMA-06-4195). Edited by Manderscheid RW, Berry JT. Rockville, MD, Substance Abuse and Mental Health Services Administration, 2006

Centers for Medicare and Medicaid Services (CMS), HHS: Medicaid and Children's Health Insurance Program (CHIP) programs; Medicaid managed care, CHIP delivered in managed care, and revisions related to third party liability: final rule. Fed Regist 81(88):27497–27901, 2016

Civil Rights of Institutionalized Persons Act of 1980, 42 USC §1997 et seq. (1980)

Code of the District of Columbia §21-562. Medical and psychiatric care and treatment; records. 1978. Available at: https://beta.code.dccouncil.us/dc/council/code/sections/21-562.html. Accessed December 30, 2016.

Cournos F, Faulkner LR, Fitzgerald L, et al: Report of the task force on consent to voluntary hospitalization. Bull Am Acad Psychiatry Law 21(3):293–307, 1993 8148512

Donaldson v O'Connor, 493 F.2d 507 (1974)

Hargrave v Vermont, 340 F.3d 27 (2003)

Internal Revenue Service, Department of the Treasury; Employee Benefits Security Administration, Department of Labor; Centers for Medicare and Medicaid Services, Department of Health and Human Services: Final rules under the Paul Wellstone and Pete Domenici Mental Health Parity and Addiction Equity Act of 2008; technical amendment to external review for multi-state plan program: final rules. Fed Regist 78(219):68239–68296, 2013

Mental Health Parity Act, Pub. L. No. 104-204 (1996). Available at: https://www.congress.gov/104/plaws/publ204/PLAW-104publ204.pdf. Accessed December 30, 2016.

Mental Health Parity and Addiction Equity Act of 2008. H.R. 6983, 2008a. Available at: https://www.congress.gov/bill/110th-congress/house-bill/6983. Accessed December 30, 2016.

Mental Health Parity and Addiction Equality Act of 2008; Application of Mental Health Parity Requirements to Medicaid Managed Care Organizations, CHIP, and Alternate Benefit Plans (Crisis Management Status-2333-P). Department of Health and Human Services, Centers for Medicare and Medicaid Services, 42 CFR Parts 438, 440, 456, and 457 [CMS-2333-P] RIN 0938-AS24, 2008b. Available at: http://www.reginfo.gov/public/do/eAgendaViewRule?pubId=201504andRIN=0938-AS24. Accessed December 30, 2016.

National Conference of State Legislatures: Mental Health Benefits: State Laws Mandating or Regulating. December 30, 2015. Available at: http://www.ncsl.org/research/health/mental-health-benefits-state-mandates.aspx. Accessed December 30, 2016.

O'Connor v Donaldson, 422 U.S. 563, 95 S.Ct. 2486 (1975)

Patient Protection and Affordable Care Act, Pub. L. No. 111-148 (2010). Available at: https://www.healthcare.gov/where-can-i-read-the-affordable-care-act. Accessed December 30, 2016.

Protection and Advocacy for Individuals With Mental Illness Act of 1986, 42 USC 10801 et seq. (2000)

Rennie v Klein, 720 F.2d 266 (1983)

Rogers v Commissioner of Dept. of Mental Health, 390 Mass. 489, 458 N.E.2d 308 (1983)

Rouse v Cameron, 373 F.2d 451 (1966)

Sarata AK: Mental Health Parity and the Patient Protection and Affordable Care Act of 2010: Congressional Research Service Report 7-5700 R41249. December 28, 2011. Available at: http://www.ncsl.org/documents/health/MHparity&mandates.pdf. Accessed December 30, 2016.

Substance Abuse and Mental Health Services Administration: National Mental Health Services Survey (N-MHSS): 2010: Data on Mental Health Treatment Facilities. BHSIS Series S-69 (DHHS Publ No SMA-14-4837). Rockville, MD, Substance Abuse and Mental Health Services Administration, 2014. Available at: http://archive.samhsa.gov/data/DASIS/NMHSS2010_Web.pdf. Accessed December 30, 2016.

Superintendent of Belchertown State School v Saikewicz, 370 N.E.2d 417, 373 Mass. 728 (1977)

Treatment Advocacy Center: Trends and Consequences of Closing Public Psychiatric Hospitals, 2012: Table 2. Patients in public psychiatric hospitals per total population. 2010. Available at: http://www.treatmentadvocacycenter.org/trends-and-consequences-of-closing-public-psychiatric-hospitals-2012/tables. Accessed December 30, 2016.

Wall BW: State hospitals as "the most integrated setting according to their needs." J Am Acad Psychiatry Law 41(4):484–487, 2013 24335318

Washington v Harper, 494 U.S. 210, 110 S.Ct. 1028 (1990)

Wyatt v Stickney, 344 F.Supp. 387 (1972)

Youngberg v Romeo, 457 U.S. 307, 102 S.Ct. 2452 (1982)

Zinermon v Burch, 494 U.S. 113, 110 S.Ct. 975 (1990)

CHAPTER 10

Civil Commitment

Reena Kapoor, M.D.

Landmark Cases

Lake v. Cameron, 364 F.2d 657 (1966)

Lessard v. Schmidt, 349 F.Supp. 1078 (1972)

Wyatt v. Stickney, 344 F.Supp. 387 (1972)

O'Connor v. Donaldson, 422 U.S. 563, 95 S.Ct. 2486 (1975)

Addington v. Texas, 441 U.S. 418, 99 S.Ct. 1804 (1979)

Parham v. JR, 442 U.S. 584, 99 S.Ct. 2493 (1979)

Youngberg v. Romeo, 457 U.S. 307, 102 S.Ct. 2452 (1982)

Jones v. U.S., 463 U.S. 354, 103 S.Ct. 3043 (1983)

Kansas v. Hendricks, 521 U.S. 346, 117 S.Ct. 2072 (1997)

Olmstead v. L. C. ex rei. Zimring, 527 U.S. 581, 119 S.Ct. 2176 (1999)

Kansas v. Crane, 534 U.S. 407, 122 S.Ct. 867 (2002)

U.S. v. Comstock, 560 U.S. 126, 130 S.Ct. 1949 (2010)

Civil commitment—that is, the involuntary hospitalization of psychiatric patients—occurs within a complex clinical, legal, and regulatory framework. Modern procedures for civil commitment arose in the mid-twentieth century in response to concerns about patients with mental illness, who historically had little say in their hospitalization or treatment and who often were warehoused indefinitely in asylums. In this chapter, I review the evolution of laws and clinical practice around involuntary hospitalization, as well as the more recent development of alternative forms of civil commitment, such as mandatory outpatient treatment and commitment of sex offenders.

Historical Perspective

Courts, legislatures, families, and health care professionals have long debated how best to care for individuals with mental illness, particularly those who cannot care for themselves. In the early years of the United States, communities and families had broad latitude to make determinations regarding individuals with mental illness. These individuals were often confined in jails and alms-houses in unsanitary and brutal conditions with little legal oversight. Treatment was often nonexistent and confinement was indefinite. Many people spent their entire lives in institutions (Shorter 1997).

In the early nineteenth century, Dorothea Dix (2006) led a social reform movement aimed at treating people with mental illness more humanely. This movement resulted in moving confined individuals out of jails and into newly built psychiatric hospitals. These "asylums" promised a protected, tranquil environment in which patients could recover from mental illness. Most hospitals allowed admission based on a family member's request, and, once admitted, patients could be released only by petitioning the courts for a habeas corpus hearing. As a result, psychiatric hospital populations grew steadily, with hundreds of thousands of patients institutionalized in the United States at the turn of the twentieth century (Shorter 1997).

By the 1940s and 1950s, hospital populations swelled beyond the hospitals' capacity to provide meaningful care. In the 1960s, reform efforts began anew, this time with an emphasis on patients' civil rights. The Community Mental Health Act of 1963 marked a major change in the American approach to the treatment of mental illness, shifting the primary locus of care from large asylums to smaller community treatment centers. Additionally, the development of antipsychotic medication allowed some patients with psychotic symptoms to improve enough to live safely outside of institutions.

By the early 1970s, the emphasis on community-based treatment had firmly taken hold, and state hospital populations were reduced by half. By 2013, approximately 40,000 state hospital beds remained (Lutterman 2015), representing a 95% reduction in the psychiatric hospital population since the 1950s (Torrey et al. 2014). Deinstitutionalization has not been without unforeseen consequences, most notably the rising population of homeless and incarcerated people with mental illness (Lamb 1984). Nevertheless, models for involuntary psychiatric treatment continue to emphasize patient autonomy and community-based psychiatric care.

Rationale for Civil Commitment

Legal scholars traditionally cite two rationales for the government's authority to detain involuntarily mentally ill individuals: 1) police powers and 2) parens patriae. The concept of police powers refers to the state's authority to act as necessary to maintain societal order. When problematic social behavior in people with mental illness makes them dangerous to themselves or others, the government has the right to detain them in the interest of public safety under a police powers model. *Parens patriae* (Latin for "parent of the country") refers to the government's obligation to act in the best interest of its citizens, just as parents act in the best interest of their children. In some states, if individuals are gravely disabled or not making responsible decisions about care for their mental illness, the state may act to protect them, including ordering hospitalization or involuntary treatment.

For physicians, the rationale for involuntary hospitalization is based on principles of medical ethics dating back to the time of Hippocrates. The ethical principles of *autonomy* (respecting the patient's right to make his or her own choices) and *beneficence* (acting in the patient's best interest) both apply to civil commitment. Physicians are generally obligated to respect patients' autonomy in choosing their own course of treatment. However, severe mental illness may impair the ability to make rational choices; individuals with such mental illnesses are therefore not truly autonomous. In these circumstances, physicians may provide treatment, including hospitalization, over a patient's objection if the treatment is in the patient's best interest.

Involuntary Hospitalization

Procedures for involuntary hospitalization of psychiatric patients vary from state to state, but all follow the same general format and are based on common principles. Figure 9–1 depicts a typical civil commitment framework.

To protect patients' autonomy, physicians are given limited decision-making power in involuntary hospitalization proceedings, and strict limits are placed on the length of time that individuals can be detained without judicial review. Although some differences between jurisdictions are found, generally patients can be kept in the hospital for only a few days before a court must hold a hearing. When reviewing the appropriateness of civil commitment in each case, courts rely on principles outlined in a series of landmark decisions in the latter half of the twentieth century.

Least Restrictive Alternative

The District of Columbia (D.C.) Court of Appeals decision in *Lake v. Cameron* (1966) placed limits on civil commitment by articulating what became known as the "least restrictive alternative" doctrine for psychiatric treatment. In 1962, Catherine Lake, a 60-year-old woman, was found wandering the streets in Washington, D.C. Police officers took her to D.C. General Hospital, where she was examined by physicians and diagnosed with "chronic brain syndrome associated with aging." She was transferred to St. Elizabeths Hospital, the public psychiatric hospital of Washington, D.C., and civilly committed. Lake remained at St. Elizabeths for the next 3 years and filed several habeas corpus petitions requesting her release.

In considering Lake's appeal of her involuntary commitment, the D.C. Court of Appeals stated that courts do not have a binary choice between hospitalization and unconditional discharge. Instead, courts should consider alternative placements, such as nursing homes or community supervision, and have an obligation to permit treatment in the least restrictive setting. Although Lake did not achieve her objective of discharge from St. Elizabeths (where she remained hospitalized until her death in 1971), the principle set forth in her appellate case has endured.

Subsequent court cases have continued *Lake's* emphasis on community treatment when possible. In *Olmstead v. L. C.* (1999), the U.S. Supreme Court considered whether people with mental illness and developmental disabilities have

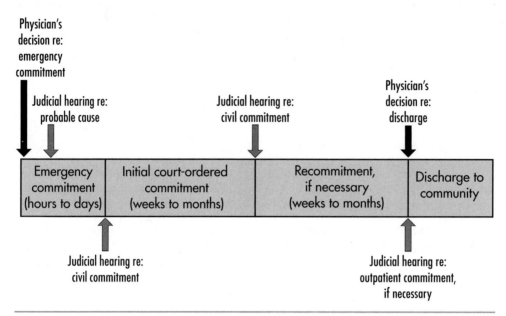

FIGURE 10–1.   Example of a civil commitment scheme.

a right to live outside institutional settings. In *Olmstead*, two patients of Georgia Regional Hospital, L.C. and E.W., petitioned the court for release from the hospital, claiming that failure to place them in the community was discriminatory under the Americans With Disabilities Act of 1990. The Court ruled that states have an obligation to provide community-based care for individuals who could safely live in such settings.

The state's mental health agency contended that the patients' delayed release was a result of cost considerations rather than discrimination, an argument that the Supreme Court found unconvincing. The Court held that "unjustified isolation" of individuals with mental illness or developmental disabilities is a form of discrimination in violation of the Americans With Disabilities Act. Disabled individuals must be placed in the community if

[a] the State's treatment professionals have determined that community placement is appropriate, [b] the transfer from institutional care to a

less restrictive setting is not opposed by the affected individual, and [c] the placement can be reasonably accommodated, taking into account the resources available to the State and the needs of others with mental disabilities. (*Olmstead v. L. C.* 1999, at 587)

Although the *Olmstead* decision was somewhat deferential to medical judgment and patient preference, *Lake* and *Olmstead* generally made clear that involuntary hospitalization is a disposition of last resort, suitable only for those patients who are too ill or dangerous to live safely in the community. The question of what constitutes "dangerousness" was not explicitly addressed by these decisions. However, other landmark court cases and state statutes have addressed this issue.

Dangerousness Standard

In the first half of the twentieth century, commitment laws were paternalistic, employing flexible criteria and giving broad discretion to physicians. Connecticut enacted a typical law, which stated that involuntary confinement required the person to be mentally ill and a "fit subject for confinement" (*Mayock v. Martin* 1968). By the 1960s, some jurisdictions, influenced by the civil rights movement, began narrowing the criteria for commitment, focusing more on patients' behavior than on their need for treatment (Anfang and Appelbaum 2006).

In 1975, the U.S. Supreme Court further altered civil commitment law with its decision in *O'Connor v. Donaldson* (1975). Kenneth Donaldson had been confined in Chattahoochee State Hospital in Florida for 15 years despite agreement among his doctors that he was not dangerous and that a reasonable discharge plan was available. Donaldson repeatedly requested release, and his legal appeals eventually reached the U.S. Supreme Court. In its decision, the Court held that "a State cannot constitutionally confine, without more, a nondangerous individual who is capable of surviving safely in freedom by himself or with the help of willing and responsible family members or friends" (*O'Connor v. Donaldson* 1975, p. 576).

Following this decision, many states amended their civil commitment statutes to replace vague criteria such as "fit subject for confinement" with a requirement to prove that the individual was either dangerous to self or others or gravely disabled. Today, most states use some version of "mentally ill and dangerous" as the requirement for civil commitment, although their exact definitions of mental illness and dangerousness vary considerably. In a few states, persons can be involuntarily hospitalized if they are gravely disabled or not making responsible decisions regarding their treatment, without a showing of dangerousness.

Definitions of Mental Disorder

All states specify that an individual must have a mental illness or mental disorder in order to be involuntarily committed. In some jurisdictions, "mental illness" for the purposes of civil commitment is limited to specific diagnoses, whereas others simply require a "substantial mental disorder." The mental disorder also must be severe enough to affect an individual's functioning in an important domain of life, such as judgment, behavior, the ability to recognize reality, or the ability to care for basic needs.

Some states are deliberately inclusive in their definitions of mental illness, specifying (as in the case of New Jersey) that mental illness for the purpose of civil commitment is "not limited to psychosis or active psychosis" (New Jersey Stat Ann. §30:4 2015). Other states exclude specific diagnoses or diagnostic categories, such as in Arizona, where individuals with substance use disorders, intellectual disability, and antisocial personality disorder are ineligible for civil commitment unless these disorders are accompanied by a "disorder of emotion, thought, cognition, or memory" (Ariz Rev Stat §36–501 2016).

Although this wide variation among state statutes makes unifying principles about mental illness difficult to discern, mental health professionals generally agree that the illness must be substantial enough to cause impairment in one or more functional areas (Pinals and Mossman 2012). Psychotic disorders almost always meet this definition, as do major mood disorders such as bipolar disorder and major depressive disorder. Although rarely specified in statute, conditions such as borderline personality disorder and anorexia nervosa also may meet the threshold in some cases.

Definitions of Dangerousness

Just as with definitions of mental illness, state statutes use different definitions of the "risk" or "dangerousness" that makes an individual eligible for civil commitment. Dangerousness can include relatively straightforward circumstances, such as recent suicide attempts or threats to harm another person, but also may include "softer" criteria, such as the inability to care for oneself or threats to property.

All states allow civil commitment based on "danger to self," and most allow it for "grave disability." Danger to self and grave disability are related concepts, because both refer to an individual's risk of self-harm rather than harm to others. Common examples of danger to self include suicide attempts, self-injurious behavior, or suicidal plans. Grave disability typically refers to an individual's inability to meet basic needs for food, shelter, or hygiene. Both of these criteria attempt to limit the group of individuals with mental illness eligible for civil commitment to those whose behavior can cause substantial self-harm, excluding those with merely odd behavior or idiosyncratic beliefs.

All states also permit civil commitment for patients who present a danger to others, although some require a recent "overt act" (e.g., violent or reckless behavior) and specify a time frame in which the behavior must have occurred (e.g., within the past month). Danger can include potential bodily harm, and a few states also permit civil commitment based on the risk of serious property damage. Common examples of danger to others include recent aggressive acts, credible threats of violence, or attempts to harm another person.

Finally, some states allow civil commitment based on a patient's need for treatment or the risk for deterioration. After the *O'Connor* decision, most states considered need for treatment alone an insufficient justification for commitment, but a few states, such as South Carolina, still allow commitment under these circumstances (S.C. Code Ann. §44–17–580 1976). Others allow commitment when need for treatment is combined with additional factors, such as the inability of a patient to provide informed consent for treatment. Need for treatment statutes are similar to those requiring grave disability; the court must find that the individual will experience serious functional impairment without involuntary treatment.

Jurisdictions that require a showing of dangerousness for civil commitment create significant limitations and challenges (Appelbaum and Gutheil 2007). First, many nondangerous patients in need of treatment, such as those who are manic or quietly delusional, may be denied beneficial care. Second, mental health clinicians are notoriously poor at assessing risk of dangerousness (see Chapter 28, "Violence Risk Assessment").

Treatment During Involuntary Hospitalization

Despite the legal system's emphasis on civil liberties and patients' rights, the courts have not articulated rigorous legal standards for providing treatment during hospitalization. For a few years in the 1970s, it appeared that the courts might do so. In *Wyatt v. Stickney* (1972), a U.S. District Court in Alabama first articulated a "right to treatment" principle, stating that hospitalized patients had a right to individualized treatment, not just custodial care, in institutions. However, subsequent U.S. Supreme Court decisions in *O'Connor v. Donaldson* (1975) and *Youngberg v. Romeo* (1982) (see Chapter 9, "Legal Regulation of Psychiatric Treatment") stopped short of defining a Constitutional right to treatment. Instead, these cases discussed a right to safety in institutions and a right to discharge for nondangerous individuals. The Court left what happened within the walls of the hospital largely to the discretion of mental health professionals.

Committed patients do not, however, automatically lose all ability to make choices about their treatment. In many states, the administration of particular treatments, such as psychotropic medication or electroconvulsive therapy, against a patient's wishes requires a separate judicial determination from the initial civil commitment proceeding (see Chapter 9). This provides an added layer of protection for patients' civil liberties and makes clear that admission to a psychiatric hospital, even involuntarily, does not necessarily equate with a lack of capacity to provide informed consent for treatment.

Due Process Requirements

Courts view civil commitment as a serious deprivation of liberty, and the due process rights afforded to individuals facing commitment reflect this perception. In *Lessard v. Schmidt* (1972), a Wisconsin federal district court ruled that due process rights in civil commitment proceedings had to mirror those of defendants in criminal proceedings. Alberta Lessard was involuntarily hospitalized after a suicide attempt. She filed suit against the state, arguing that the civil commitment procedures were unconstitutional. In reviewing Lessard's case, the federal district court noted that confinement in a psychiatric institution is similar to incarceration, because both conditions significantly restrict individuals' freedom of movement. The *Lessard* court concluded that a series of procedural protections are required in civil commitment cases, including

- Timely notice of the allegations on which the request for commitment is based
- A probable cause hearing within 48 hours of confinement
- A full hearing on the grounds for commitment within 2 weeks
- The right to representation by counsel

- Exclusion of hearsay evidence
- The right against self-incrimination

Other state court rulings have added further protections, such as the right to periodic judicial review of commitment (e.g., *Fasulo v. Arafeh* 1977).

The U.S. Supreme Court decision in ***Addington v. Texas*** (1979) addressed the necessary standard of proof in civil commitment proceedings. Frank Addington, committed to a Texas psychiatric hospital after threatening his mother, challenged his commitment on the basis that the "clear and convincing" standard of proof required by the state was insufficient. Mr. Addington argued that the state should be required to prove his dangerousness beyond a reasonable doubt. The Court reasoned that, because of the significant deprivation of liberty at stake, a standard of proof higher than a mere "preponderance of the evidence" was necessary in civil commitment proceedings. However, proof beyond a reasonable doubt would be nearly impossible to establish, given the uncertainty of psychiatric diagnosis and assessment of dangerousness. The Court held that the "clear and convincing" standard of evidence in civil commitment proceedings was sufficient to meet Constitutional requirements.

Outpatient Civil Commitment

Changes in civil commitment laws are one of the many factors that contributed to the deinstitutionalization of the 1960s and 1970s (Lutterman 2015). Today, fewer psychiatric hospital beds are available, fewer individuals with serious mental illness are hospitalized, and hospital lengths of stay are relatively short. Many clinicians have observed that individuals with serious mental illness live in a world of "revolving doors," alternating between homelessness, inpatient hospitalization, and incarceration, but rarely receiving adequate mental health treatment. In response to these concerns, states began to look for alternative solutions, including outpatient civil commitment.

Outpatient civil commitment, also known as *mandated community treatment, assisted outpatient treatment*, and *involuntary outpatient commitment*, refers to the process by which courts can order individuals to adhere to a regimen of mental health treatment while living in the community. Outpatient commitment can be used as a transition from involuntary hospitalization, an alternative to involuntary hospitalization, or a preventive intervention for those at risk for deterioration to the point of needing involuntary hospitalization. Washington, D.C., enacted the first outpatient commitment statute in the United States in 1972 (Group for the Advancement of Psychiatry 1994). Since that time, interest in outpatient commitment has grown steadily. By 2015, 45 states had adopted outpatient commitment statutes, although many did not implement or fully fund the programs (Council on Psychiatry and Law 2015).

Legal Framework

As with involuntary hospitalization, states vary widely in the criteria and procedures used in their outpatient commitment programs. New York has one of the most well-developed systems, commonly known as "Kendra's Law" or assisted outpatient treatment. Individuals are eligible for assisted outpatient treatment if they have a mental illness, are "unlikely to survive safely in the community," have a history of treatment noncompliance that has resulted in serious violent behavior or repeated hospitalizations, and are unlikely to engage voluntarily in treatment (New

York State Office of Mental Health 2006). The court must find that assisted outpatient treatment is the least restrictive alternative and that the individual is likely to benefit from the treatment.

The necessary standard of proof for outpatient commitment in New York is "clear and convincing evidence." The initial commitment period can last up to 6 months and can be extended for additional periods of up to a year at a time. If an individual does not adhere to the mandated treatment plan of outpatient commitment and the individual's mental status deteriorates, a physician can request that the police transport the individual to a hospital. The person can be held at the hospital for up to 72 hours to allow for a determination of the necessity of involuntary hospitalization.

Outpatient commitment statutes in other states follow the same basic model as New York's assisted outpatient treatment process, allowing commitment under three main circumstances: as part of a hospital discharge plan, as an alternative to hospitalization, or as a measure to prevent clinical deterioration. Patients are ordered to remain in treatment for the duration of the commitment but are not necessarily ordered to take a particular medication (or any medication at all). As with involuntary hospitalization, the commitment is subject to periodic review by the courts, with the burden on the state to prove that the patient meets commitment criteria.

The American Psychiatric Association (APA) has reviewed state outpatient commitment statutes three times, publishing reports in 1987, 1999, and 2015 (American Psychiatric Association 1987; Council on Psychiatry and Law 2015; Gerbasi et al. 2000) that supported the practice under limited circumstances. The 2015 APA Resource Document recommended that states use criteria for outpatient commitment nearly identical to those used in New York. The APA also recommended that the patient must have a detailed treatment plan and a physician who agrees to take responsibility for the treatment (Council on Psychiatry and Law 2015).

Empirical Evidence

Scientific studies have reported the efficacy of outpatient civil commitment in preventing rehospitalization and arrest for people with serious mental illness. Early studies conducted before 1990 were often critiqued on methodological grounds. More recent research, which has attempted to address these concerns by controlling for selection bias and using larger sample sizes, has shown promising results. Outpatient commitment can result in earlier detection of psychiatric deterioration, improved access to care by families (Copeland and Heilemann 2008), and decreased rates of hospitalization (Segal and Burgess 2006). Additionally, individuals under outpatient commitment orders have lower arrest rates (Hiday and Wales 2003; Link et al. 2011). Patients' and clinicians' attitudes toward outpatient commitment are generally positive when the programs are adequately implemented and limited to a subset of patients (Swartz et al. 2009).

Despite these positive studies, the APA's 2015 review of the outpatient commitment literature concluded that no clear consensus exists about the efficacy of outpatient commitment across different jurisdictions (Council on Psychiatry and Law 2015). The review concluded that the effectiveness of outpatient commitment programs depends largely on their design and implementation, the availability of intensive community-based services, and the duration of the court order. Whether the benefit of outpatient commitment results from the increased intensity of treat-

ment patients receive or from the court order itself remains unclear.

Questions about racial bias in outpatient commitment persist, because African American individuals are more likely to be committed than are Caucasian individuals. Studies investigating this issue have found that African Americans are subject to outpatient commitment at higher rates primarily because they are overrepresented in the criminal justice and involuntary hospitalization populations, which are often precursors to outpatient commitment (Swanson et al. 2009). Additional criticism includes concerns that outpatient commitment extends the trend of mental health treatment becoming more coercive, potentially distorting the therapeutic mission of the psychiatric profession (Hiday 1996).

Finally, critics of outpatient commitment have noted its practical limitations (Rowe 2013). The threat of outpatient commitment may deter some patients from seeking care. In addition, busy police officers may be reticent to bring patients who have not adhered to their mandated treatment to the hospital for evaluation, and overcrowded emergency departments may be unable to locate inpatient psychiatric beds when patients need admission. Thus, the promise of outpatient commitment, to treat patients at a lower symptom threshold and prevent clinical deterioration, remains unrealized because of the inadequate implementation of statutory provisions and lack of resources.

Special Populations

Adults with diagnoses of serious mental illness, such as schizophrenia or bipolar disorder, constitute most of the individuals subject to civil commitment proceedings. However, several special populations are also subject to commitment.

Juveniles

Children are not typically autonomous agents when making choices about their health and well-being; they rely on parents to be proxy decision makers and to act in their best interest (see Chapter 24, "Forensic Evaluations of Children and Adolescents"). Psychiatric hospitalization raises potential conflicts between children and parents, causing courts to consider whether to allow parents to admit their children without judicial oversight. In *Parham v. JR* (1979), the U.S. Supreme Court considered a case in which two children were admitted to a Georgia state hospital after repeated behavior problems at home. At the time, the hospital allowed children to be admitted "voluntarily" based on a parent's request and a physician's determination that the child was mentally ill and in need of treatment. J.R.'s attorneys argued that this process was insufficient to protect children's rights, and a judicial hearing, such as the hearings held when adults faced civil commitment, was necessary. The Supreme Court disagreed, holding that the hospital's medical fact-finding process was sufficient to meet Constitutional requirements (see also Chapter 25, "Evaluations of Juveniles in Civil Law").

Forensic Patients

Two types of forensic patients are often hospitalized for extended periods: insanity acquittees (those adjudicated not guilty by reason of insanity) and patients whose competency to stand trial cannot be restored. Most states use civil commitment proceedings with these populations. After individuals are found not guilty by reason of insanity or nonrestorable by the criminal court, they return to the hospital for evaluation of whether they meet criteria for civil commitment. The same "dangerousness" standard for civil commitment

applies, although forensic patients sometimes spend years in the hospital before successfully proving that they have been sufficiently rehabilitated to no longer pose a risk to society (Monson et al. 2001). The U.S. Supreme Court has held that insanity acquittees can be confined longer than the maximum possible term of incarceration for their offense, because hospitalization and incarceration serve different purposes (treatment vs. punishment) (*Jones v. U.S.* 1983) (see Chapter 19, "Evaluation of Criminal Responsibility").

Some states—most notably, Oregon and Connecticut—do not use civil commitment procedures for the management of insanity acquittees. Individuals found not guilty by reason of insanity by the courts in these states are committed to the jurisdiction of a psychiatric security review board, a separate regulatory body that oversees the patients' treatment in the hospital or community (Conn Gen Stat §17a-593c 2015; Ore Rev Stat §161.351 2015). The psychiatric security review board's primary mandate is to maintain public safety, so these boards can be hesitant to approve patients' progression through the treatment system. Many patients committed to a psychiatric security review board's jurisdiction will spend years, if not decades, in a high-security hospital setting before being granted conditional release. In addition, once released to the community, patients are subject to many of the same restrictions as individuals under outpatient civil commitment, including orders to comply with intensive mental health treatment.

Individuals With Substance Use Disorders

Although some states, such as Indiana and Maine, include substance use disorders in their statutory definitions of mental illness that qualify for civil commitment, many states have separate provisions that allow for commitment of individuals with severe drug or alcohol problems. The rationale for civil commitment of people with substance use disorders is similar to that of mental illness. Individuals with severe alcohol or drug abuse problems may pose a danger to themselves through major medical complications of substance use or to others by engaging in reckless or violent behavior. In severe cases of substance use disorder, the capacity to make rational choices about treatment may be impaired. In these circumstances, the court may order involuntary hospitalization for substance abuse treatment. Some states, including North Dakota and Wisconsin, permit the involuntary hospitalization of pregnant women based not on a danger to self but rather on the danger of substance use to the fetus (Pinals and Mossman 2012).

Sex Offenders

Individuals who commit sexual offenses may be subject to civil commitment under so-called sexually violent predator statutes after completion of a prison sentence (see Chapter 23, "Forensic Assessment of Sex Offenders"). Sexually violent predator commitment laws allow states to confine individuals indefinitely or at least until judged not likely to be dangerous. As of 2012, 22 states, the District of Columbia, and the federal court system had enacted sexually violent predator statutes (National District Attorneys Association 2012).

Sexually violent predator statutes differ from other civil commitment statutes in two significant ways. First, they are used only at the end of a criminal sentence, leading some to question whether their true purpose is to detain individuals whom society finds intolerable rather than providing treatment. Second, in addition to the requirement for dangerousness, the sexually violent predator statutes use the term *mental abnormality* instead of *mental illness* as a requirement for commitment. Diagnoses such as antisocial personality disorder, pedophilia, and paraphilia not otherwise specified have all satisfied the requirement for mental abnormality under sexually violent predator commitment statutes (Smith et al. 2010).

The APA has opposed sexually violent predator commitment laws, in part because of their perception that the definition of mental abnormality is overly broad. In addition, the APA noted that treatment options in most sexually violent predator commitment facilities are limited, and very few people have ever been released from the programs (American Psychiatric Association 1999). The U.S. Supreme Court has consistently disagreed with this position, ruling that sexually violent predator commitment statutes are constitutional (***Kansas v. Crane*** 2002; ***Kansas v. Hendricks*** 1997; ***U.S. v. Comstock*** 2010) (see Chapter 23). The Court's decisions in these cases has sent a strong message that civil commitment of sex offenders is permissible, despite the objections of civil rights advocates and the mental health community.

Conclusion

Civil commitment in the United States underwent significant changes in the latter half of the twentieth century, evolving from a paternalistic system of care to one in which patients' liberty interests are highly valued. Under current law, civil commitment in all jurisdictions is permissible when an individual is both mentally ill and dangerous. In some jurisdictions, persons also can be committed if gravely disabled or not capable of making responsible decisions in managing their mental illness. States use different definitions of mental illness and dangerousness in their commitment statutes, but all require proof by clear and convincing evidence and permit involuntary confinement only when an individual cannot live safely in the community.

Some have argued that current laws promote civil liberties at the expense of nondangerous patients, who are left to languish in the streets without treatment. However, courts and legislatures have continued to base civil commitment statutes on criteria requiring mental illness and dangerousness and in many states have expanded civil commitment statutes to include outpatient commitment, individuals with substance use disorders, forensic patients, and sex offenders. Each program is unique, but all civil commitment schemes are bound by a common principle: that the government can, in limited cases, authorize confinement and treatment for individuals who have mental illness and pose a risk to themselves or society.

Key Concepts

- Individuals with mental illness have a right to be treated in the least restrictive setting possible.

- Individuals facing civil commitment are afforded due process rights that mirror those in criminal proceedings, including written notice of the allegations against them, representation by counsel, an adversarial hearing, and protections against self-incrimination.

- Courts must find by clear and convincing evidence that the individual meets criteria for civil commitment.

- Civilly committed individuals retain the ability to consent to or refuse treatment.

- Outpatient civil commitment, a growing trend among states, can reduce hospitalization and arrest rates for some individuals, but its success is closely tied to proper implementation and the availability of intensive treatment services in the community.

- In addition to adults with serious mental illness, several other populations may be subject to civil commitment: juveniles, forensic patients (those involved in the criminal justice system), patients with substance use disorders, and sexually violent predators.

References

Addington v Texas, 441 U.S. 418, 99 S.Ct. 1804 (1979)

American Psychiatric Association: Involuntary Commitment to Outpatient Treatment: Report of the Task Force on Involuntary Outpatient Commitment. Washington, DC, American Psychiatric Association, 1987

American Psychiatric Association: Dangerous Sex Offenders: A Task Force Report of the American Psychiatric Association. Washington, DC, American Psychiatric Association, 1999

Americans With Disabilities Act of 1990, Pub. L. No. 101-336, 104 Stat. 328 (1990)

Anfang SA, Appelbaum PS: Civil commitment—the American experience. Isr J Psychiatry Relat Sci 43(3):209–218, 2006 17294986

Appelbaum PS, Gutheil TG: Clinical Handbook of Psychiatry and the Law, 4th Edition. Philadelphia, PA, Lippincott/ Williams & Wilkins, 2007

Ariz Rev Stat (A.R.S) §36–501 (2016)

Community Mental Health Act of 1963, 77 Stat. 282, Pub. L. No. 88-164 (1963)

Conn Gen Stat §17a-593c (2015)

Copeland DA, Heilemann MV: Getting "to the point": the experience of mothers getting assistance for their adult children who are violent and mentally ill. Nurs Res 57(3):136–143, 2008 18496098

Council on Psychiatry and Law: Resource Document on Involuntary Outpatient Commitment and Related Programs of Assisted Outpatient Treatment. Arlington, VA, American Psychiatric Association, 2015. Available at: file:///C:/ Users/Owner/Downloads/resource-2015-involuntary-outpatient-commitment.pdf. Accessed December 30, 2016.

Dix D: "I tell what I have seen"—the reports of asylum reformer Dorothea Dix. 1843. Am J Public Health 96(4):622–625, 2006 16551962

Fasulo v Arafeh, 378 A.2d 553 (1977)

Gerbasi JB, Bonnie RJ, Binder RL: Resource document on mandatory outpatient treatment. J Am Acad Psychiatry Law 28(2):127–144, 2000 10888178

Group for the Advancement of Psychiatry (GAP): Committee on Government Policy: Forced Into Treatment: The Role of Coercion in Clinical Practice, Report No 137. Washington, DC, American Psychiatric Press, 1994

Hiday VA: Outpatient commitment: official coercion in the community, in Coercion and Aggressive Community Treatment: A New Frontier in Mental Health Law. Edited by Dennis DL, Monahan J. New York, Springer Science+Business, 1996, pp 33–52

Hiday VA, Wales HW: Civil commitment and arrests. Curr Opin Psychiatry 16:575–580, 2003

Jones v U.S., 463 U.S. 354, 103 S.Ct. 3043 (1983)

Kansas v Crane, 534 U.S. 407, 122 S.Ct. 867 (2002)

Kansas v Hendricks, 521 U.S. 346, 117 S.Ct. 2072 (1997)

Lake v Cameron, 364 F.2d 657 (1966)

Lamb HR: Deinstitutionalization and the homeless mentally ill. Hosp Community Psychiatry 35(9):899–907, 1984 6479924

Lessard v Schmidt, 349 F.Supp. 1078 (1972)

Link BG, Epperson MW, Perron BE, et al: Arrest outcomes associated with outpatient commitment in New York State. Psychiatr Serv 62(5):504–508, 2011 21532076

Lutterman T: Tracking the history of state psychiatric hospital closures from 1997 to 2015. July 2015. Available at: https://media.wix.com/ugd/186708_afa348 ce61184f4d902ae55c29fcb7b7.pdf. Accessed December 30, 2016.

Mayock v Martin, 157 Conn. 56 (1968)

Monson CM, Gunnin DD, Fogel MH, et al: Stopping (or slowing) the revolving door: factors related to NGRI acquittees' maintenance of a conditional release. Law Hum Behav 25(3):257–267, 2001 11480803

National District Attorneys Association: Civil commitment of sex offenders. April 2012. Available at: http://ndaa.org/ pdf/Sex%20Offender%20Civil%20 Commitment-April%202012.pdf. Accessed December 30, 2016.

New Jersey Stat Ann. §30:4 (2015)

New York State Office of Mental Health: An explanation of Kendra's Law. May 2006. Available at: https://www.omh.ny.gov/ omhweb/Kendra_web/Ksummary.htm. Accessed December 31, 2016.

O'Connor v Donaldson, 422 U.S. 563, 95 S.Ct. 2486 (1975)

Olmstead v L. C. ex rei. Zimring, 527 U.S. 581, 119 S.Ct. 2176 (1999)

Ore Rev Stat §161.351 (2015)

Parham v JR, 442 U.S. 584, 99 S.Ct. 2493 (1979)

Pinals DA, Mossman D: Evaluation for Civil Commitment. New York, Oxford University Press, 2012

Rowe M: Alternatives to outpatient commitment. J Am Acad Psychiatry Law 41(3):332–336, 2013 24051584

S.C. Code Ann. §44–17–580 (1976)

Segal SP, Burgess PM: The utility of extended outpatient civil commitment. Int J Law Psychiatry 29(6):525–534, 2006 17070577

Shorter E: A History of Psychiatry: From the Era of the Asylum to the Age of Prozac. New York, Wiley, 1997

Smith J, Kapoor R, Baranoski MV: After commitment of sexual predators: a survey of states. Article presented at the 41st annual meeting of the American Academy of Psychiatry and the Law, Tucson, AZ, October 23, 2010

Swanson J, Swartz M, Van Dorn RA, et al: Racial disparities in involuntary outpatient commitment: are they real? Health Aff (Millwood) 28(3):816–826, 2009 19414892

Swartz MS, Swanson JW, Steadman HJ, et al. New York State Assisted Outpatient Treatment Program Evaluation. Durham, NC, Duke University School of Medicine, June 2009. Available at: http://www.omh.ny.gov/omhweb/resources/publications/aot_program_ evaluation. Accessed December 31, 2016.

Torrey E, Zdanowicz M, Kennard A, et al: The treatment of persons with mental illness in prisons and jails: a state survey. April 8, 2014. Available at: http://www.treatmentadvocacycenter.org/storage/documents/treatment-behind-bars/treatment-behind-bars.pdf. Accessed December 31, 2016.

U.S. v Comstock, 560 U.S. 126, 130 S.Ct. 1949 (2010)

Wyatt v Stickney, 344 F.Supp. 387 (1972)

Youngberg v Romeo, 457 U.S. 307, 102 S.Ct. 2452 (1982)

CHAPTER 11

Confidentiality in Psychiatric Practice

Richard Martinez, M.D., M.H.
Patrick Fox, M.D.

Landmark Cases

In re Lifschutz, 2 Cal. 3d 415; 467 P.2d 557 (1970)

***Tarasoff v. Regents of University of California*,
17 Cal. 3d 425, 551 P.2d 334, 131 Cal. Rptr. 14 (1976)**

***Doe v. Roe*, 400 N.Y.Supp. 2d 668; 93 Misc.2d 201 (1977)**

***People v. Stritzinger*, 34 Cal. 3d 505, 668 P.2d 738 (1983)**

***State v. Andring*, 342 N.W.2d 128 (Minn. 1984)**

***Jaffee v. Redmond*, 518 U.S. 1; 116 S.Ct. 1923 (1996)**

Understanding the concepts of confidentiality and privilege in the practice of psychiatry and psychotherapy requires an appreciation of our society's expectation for privacy in certain personal and professional relationships. Intimate information, whether pertaining to health, finances, or private thoughts and beliefs, would not be comfortably shared with others if not for the expectation that this information would remain confidential.

From a legal perspective, the U.S. Supreme Court has not identified a specific constitutional right to privacy, but the Court has identified a broad liberty interest that adopts a right of personal privacy in various aspects of our lives (see, e.g., *Roe v. Wade* 1973). Privacy protections usually involve two elements: first, the protection from disclosures considered personal; and second, the preservation of independence to make private decisions without state coercion. Therefore, communications and decisions related to reproduction and marriage, contraception, abortion, family relationships, and child rearing and education have all found protections in the law.

However, the protection of privacy and independent decision making is not absolute. State interests must be considered when conflicts arise between the protection of privacy and the need for state regulatory, investigative, and prosecutory activities. Criminal prosecution of offenders, protection of third parties, and the need to share information to maintain a viable health care system have been defined as legitimate state interests. Therefore, legal regulations and case law regarding confidentiality and privilege usually involve a balance between conflicting interests. In this chapter, we review the evolving legal framework regarding confidentiality issues and the psychiatrist–patient and the psychotherapist–patient relationship.

Confidentiality and Privilege

The concepts of confidentiality and privilege are often confused. Although the ethical duty of physicians to maintain confidentiality in the physician–patient relationship has been recognized as far back as the Hippocratic tradition, the legal concept of privilege has been defined and shaped only in recent years. The law has recognized that patients have a privilege to privacy and confidentiality, transforming the physician's ethical duty to maintain confidentiality into the patient's privilege to privacy in legal proceedings but with important exceptions to privi-

leged communication. Justifications for breaching confidentiality are based on professional responsibilities to protect third parties and the public at large.

The legal evolution of the patient's privilege construct begins with the case of **In re Lifschutz** (1970). Dr. Joseph Lifschutz was jailed after a judge ruled that he was in contempt of court for refusing to obey a court order instructing him to answer questions and produce records relating to communications with a former patient. This patient had filed a civil assault claim against another individual and had claimed damages for pain and suffering, resulting in the subpoena of Dr. Lifschutz's records.

Dr. Lifschutz filed a writ of habeas corpus, arguing that the court order to release his former patient's record was invalid because of Dr. Lifschutz's constitutional right to privacy, his patient's right to privacy, and infringement on Dr. Lifschutz's professional practice. Dr. Lifschutz argued that his situation was an equal protection violation because clergypersons could not be compelled to reveal confidential communications under similar circumstances. The California Supreme Court confirmed the lower court's finding that Dr. Lifschutz was in contempt, and his writ of habeas corpus was denied.

The Court acknowledged the importance of confidentiality in the practice of psychotherapy. However, the Court reasoned that the psychotherapist–patient privilege is not absolute, and under the concept of litigant-patient exception, limited disclosure would not undermine the constitutional rights of privacy claimed by Dr. Lifschutz. The Court also reasoned that Dr. Lifschutz's patient, not Dr. Lifschutz, had the privilege of privacy and that Dr. Lifschutz's patient had waived that right when the patient put his mental state at issue by claiming damages for pain and suffering.

The California Supreme Court also rejected Dr. Lifschutz's claims that compelling disclosure violated his ability to practice his profession effectively as a psychotherapist and that psychotherapy requires an absolute guarantee of confidentiality for its effectiveness and success. The Court acknowledged the uniqueness of psychotherapy and the importance of privacy protections in a profession in which a patient's private thoughts and emotions are often the foundational materials that guide professional treatment.

Nevertheless, the Court held that the psychotherapist–patient relationship is subject to reasonable disclosure under certain circumstances. Compelled disclosures involve balancing reasonable disclosures that serve governmental interests with preserving confidentiality. The Court identified "zones of privacy" legitimate to Lifschutz's claims but disagreed that the privacy claim is absolute. In some instances, physicians may assert the privilege on behalf of their patients, but when the patient has taken actions to forfeit the privilege or has failed to take action to assert the privilege, the physician cannot assert such privilege for the patient.

In *Jane Doe v. Joan Roe and Peter Poe* (1977), the Supreme Court of New York addressed the legal and ethical aspects of the physician's obligation to maintain confidentiality. Whereas **In re Lifschutz** clarified the concept of the patient's privilege of protected privacy, in *Doe v. Roe*, the Court defined the fundamental obligation of the physician to protect the patient's confidentiality and the consequences of violating this obligation. In this case, Dr. Joan Roe, a psychoanalyst, and her psychologist husband published a book that contained verbatim and extensive aspects of a patient's thoughts, feelings, emotions, fantasies, and other biographical and diagnostic information. The patient, Jane Doe, who had terminated her treatment 8 years prior to the book's publication, claimed breach of privacy and filed an injunction to stop publication of the book.

The New York Supreme Court held that Ms. Doe's information should have been kept confidential. The judge considered the relationship between patient and psychiatrist as a covenant, one that requires exceptional protection of the patient's privacy and secrets because of the requirement of "an atmosphere of unusual trust, confidence and tolerance" (*Doe v. Roe* 1977 at 675). The court rejected the defendants' claims that the scientific contribution of the book justified the disclosure and that the First Amendment protected their right to publish the book.

The Court concluded that the obligation to protect the confidences of patients is both an ethical obligation in the Hippocratic tradition and the American Medical Association's codes of ethics and a legal construct, warranting remedies through tort law. The court also considered damages and compensation for the plaintiff after clearly stating that an obligation to maintain confidentiality was owed. Punitive damages were not granted in the case because the Court did not believe that the defendant's actions were willful, malicious, and wanton but were "simply stupid" (*Doe v. Roe* 1977 at 679).

Limits of Privilege in State Prosecution in Crimes Against Persons

In *People v. Stritzinger* (1983), the California Supreme Court considered the boundaries of exceptions to the privilege of psychologist–patient confidentiality involving crimes against persons.

In *Stritzinger*, the Court supported the defendant/appellant's claim that certain rulings during his criminal trial involving charges of child molestation violated psychotherapist–patient privilege. Dr. Walker, a clinical psychologist, evaluated the defendant, Carl Stritzinger, and his stepdaughter, Sarah, in 1981, at the request of Stritzinger's wife, after she learned that her husband had been involved in various acts of sexually inappropriate behavior with her daughter.

When Sarah discussed these inappropriate behaviors with Dr. Walker, he notified the child welfare agency. The next day, a deputy from the sheriff's office contacted Dr. Walker. Dr. Walker was hesitant to disclose information about Stritzinger's treatment but agreed to talk again with the deputy after seeing Mr. Stritzinger in the next few days. After Dr. Walker expressed concerns about his patient's confidentiality, the deputy informed Dr. Walker that the circumstances fell under an exception to the psychotherapist–patient privilege. Dr. Walker proceeded to disclose to the deputy, in a conversation that Dr. Walker recorded, specific information from his session with Stritzinger.

Stritzinger was charged with crimes relating to his abuse of his stepdaughter. At trial, the Court overruled Stritzinger's claim that Dr. Walker's testimony be excluded on the basis of psychotherapist–patient privilege. Dr. Walker, over objection, was required to testify after his recorded interview with the deputy was played in court. Stritzinger was found guilty of lewd and lascivious conduct with a minor, a felony conviction, along with numerous misdemeanor charges of child molestation.

Stritzinger appealed his conviction on the grounds that his psychotherapist–patient privilege, as defined in his right to privacy and by statute in California, was violated, leading to his conviction.

The California Supreme Court agreed. Citing the previous decision in *Lifschutz* and other cases, the California Court considered the balancing of Stritzinger's privilege with the state's interests in seeking justice and truth. The majority opinion acknowledged that in certain criminal proceedings, the state may have a bona fide claim to compelling disclosure, including communications between a psychotherapist and a patient. Nevertheless, the Court concluded that Dr. Walker had discharged his duty of notification to child welfare authorities with his initial telephone report and in his initial conversation with the deputy. His second conversation with the deputy was not only unnecessary but also in violation of the psychotherapist–patient privilege. The California Court confirmed that Dr. Walker had a duty to report the alleged abuse but did not have an obligation to extend his involvement and become an agent of the investigation itself. The California Court reversed the conviction.

The decision in *State v. Andring* (1984) provided further clarification on how child abuse criminal prosecution must be balanced with a patient's privilege. David Andring was charged with criminal sexual conduct involving his 10-year-old stepdaughter and his 11-year-old niece. After Andring was released on bond, he entered a crisis intervention treatment unit. In individual and group treatment, Andring disclosed his alleged sexual conduct with his niece and stepdaughter, believing that these were confidential communications. At trial, the court granted the state's request for records from Andring's group sessions but denied the request for records from his individual sessions.

This decision underwent pretrial appeal to the Minnesota Supreme Court. The higher court was asked specifically to consider whether group therapy communications fall under the physician-patient privilege and therefore should not be admitted as evidence at trial. Although the Minnesota Supreme Court recognized that the physician–patient privilege did not preempt the child abuse reporting and investigation requirements, the Court ruled that satisfying the need for information for criminal investigation and prosecution required only that information defined in the statute. In Minnesota, this included "the identity of the child; the identity of the parent, guardian, or other person responsible for the child's care; the nature and extent of the child's injuries; and the name and address of the reporter" (*State v. Andring* 1984 at 133).

The Court reasoned that the disclosure should be balanced with the important public interest of offering rehabilitative treatment to child abusers and that an absolute override of the privilege in reporting requirements would undermine the benefits of alleged abusers seeking help. In regard to the admissibility of Andring's group therapy communications, the Minnesota Supreme Court overturned the trial court's decision, ruling that these also should be privileged, and, therefore, the trial court erred in ordering disclosure of the group therapy communications.

Tarasoff and the Duty to Protect Third Parties

The duty to protect others also constitutes a legally mandated exception to the physician's obligation to maintain confidentiality. The California Supreme Court first established a "duty to warn" third parties who are in foreseeable danger in *Tarasoff I* (*Tarasoff v. Regents of the Univ. of California* 1974). The Court modified their decision in *Tarasoff v. Regents*

of University of California (1976), also known as *Tarasoff II*, stating that therapists had a "duty to protect" a third party from a dangerous patient. This was a controversial decision at the time, but most states now have statutory or case law defining mental health professionals' duties to third parties when concerns about patients' potential violence toward others arise (Johnson et al. 2014; Kachigian and Felthous 2004).

In 1969, Prosenjit Poddar stabbed and killed Tatiana Tarasoff. Poddar had reported his intention to kill Tarasoff to his psychologist at the University of California student health clinic. Although the psychologist and clinic notified the campus police, Tarasoff was not directly warned. Tarasoff's parents sued the psychologist and the University of California. In *Tarasoff II*, the California Supreme Court ruled that although no one had a legal duty to control someone else's conduct, when a special relationship exists, a duty to protect identifiable third parties exists. In its ruling, the court stated that the "protective privilege [of confidentiality] ends where the public peril begins" (*Tarasoff v. Regents of University of California* 1976 at 442).

This decision established that once a therapist determines or should have determined that a patient poses a serious danger, the therapist has a duty to "exercise reasonable care to protect the foreseeable victim of that danger" (*Tarasoff v. Regents of University of California* 1976, at 439). Actions that might constitute the exercise of reasonable care in protecting the potential victim could include warning the potential victim, hospitalizing the patient, and contacting proper authorities, including the police. More than 35 states recognize *Tarasoff*-like duties (Fox 2010). However, states vary in how a victim is identified, what constitutes a threat, how to define imminence of a threat, which mental health professionals have this duty, and what actions are required or permissible in the breach of confidentiality (Fox 2010; Johnson et al. 2014).

Federal Psychotherapist–Patient Privilege

In *Jaffee v. Redmond* (1996), the U.S. Supreme Court considered the question of a federal psychotherapist–patient privilege. In 1991, Mary Redmond, a police officer, shot and killed Ricky Allen. Carrie Jaffee, the administrator of Mr. Allen's estate, filed a claim in federal district court alleging that Redmond violated Allen's constitutional rights by using excessive force. After the shooting, Officer Redmond had entered therapy with a social worker and had completed about 50 psychotherapy sessions. Jaffee requested access to the social worker's therapy records.

Attorneys representing Redmond argued that these records were protected from involuntary disclosure by a psychotherapist–patient privilege. Officer Redmond and her therapist refused to respond to the trial judge's order to provide records or testify. The judge advised members of the jury to presume, because Redmond refused to waive her privilege of confidentiality, that the contents of the unavailable notes would have been unfavorable. The jury awarded Allen's estate more than $500,000.

On appeal, the Seventh Circuit Court reversed the decision on the grounds that a psychotherapist–patient privilege is recognized in Rule 501 of the Federal Rules of Evidence. The court acknowledged that the privilege is not absolute and that circumstances could arise in which the disclosure of confidential information outweighs an individual's pri-

vacy interests for evidentiary and truth-seeking goals. However, the appeals court did not agree that such conditions existed in this case.

The U.S. Supreme Court, on hearing the appeal of the Seventh Circuit Court's ruling, recognized that federal jurisdictions up to this point had not uniformly recognized a patient's privilege of privacy in communications with a psychotherapist. The Court considered whether the privilege of barring disclosure of communications between a psychotherapist and a patient outweighs the need for evidence in the pursuit of the truth. The Court acknowledged that as with the spousal and attorney–client privileges, the psychotherapist–patient relationship requires trust and confidence that what is shared will remain private and protected. However, the Court also considered how this asserted privilege serves the public's interests.

The Supreme Court reasoned that just as the spousal privilege serves the institution of marriage and the attorney–client privilege supports open communication for the ends of the law and promotion of justice, the psychotherapist–patient privilege allows for the important provision of mental and emotional treatment for citizens. The provision of psychotherapy is a public good no less important than the provision of services that support physical health. In its final opinion, the Court ruled that "confidential communications between a licensed psychotherapist and her patients in the course of diagnosis or treatment are protected from compelled disclosure under Rule 501 of the Federal Rules of Evidence" (*Jaffee v. Redmond* 1996 at 1). The Court also argued for inclusion of social workers within the scope of the privilege and made clear that the notes documenting the private communications between Redmond and her therapist during the counseling sessions were privileged and protected from compelled disclosure.

Federal Privacy Regulations

Health Insurance Portability and Accountability Act (HIPAA)

Prior to 1996, no federal privacy law or standards protected how insurers, health care providers, and employers collected, stored, or transmitted sensitive health information. The Health Insurance Portability and Accountability Act of 1996 (HIPAA) established the first comprehensive federal protections for health privacy. HIPAA was enacted by Congress to ensure the continuity of insurance coverage, to protect the confidentiality of patient health information, and to ensure the security of such information. Many states have enacted stricter confidentiality and privilege laws than HIPAA. When state and federal law differ, the stricter privacy standard applies.

The Privacy Rule

HIPAA encourages development of electronic health information technologies but recognizes that easier information sharing creates security and privacy concerns. To address these privacy concerns, HIPAA provides protections for specific types of health information in the possession of certain health care entities, defined as "covered entities." Protected health information includes individually identifiable health information transmitted or maintained in any form or medium, including information about an individual's physical or mental condition, provision of health care, or payment for provision of health care (Table 11–1)

(U.S. Department of Health and Human Services, 45 CFR § 160.103, 2002).

Protected health information does not include the following:

- Deidentified information
- Employment records
- Education records covered by Family Educational Rights Privacy Act
- Student health records of certain postsecondary education clinics (20 U.S.C. § 1232g)
- Medical information for an individual deceased more than 50 years (U.S. Department of Health and Human Services, 45 CFR § 160.103, 2002)

HIPAA's definition of covered entities includes health plans, health care clearinghouses, and health care providers who transmit any health information in electronic form in connection with specific types of "standard" transactions (Table 11–2).

Covered entities do not include many organizations that hold health information, such as life insurers, workers' compensation carriers, automobile insurers, or disability insurers. Additionally, most state and local police or other law enforcement agencies, many state agencies such as child protective services, most schools and school districts, and employers are not considered HIPAA-covered entities.

Permitted uses and disclosures. The HIPAA Privacy Rule (U.S. Department of Health and Human Services, 45 CFR § 160.103, 2002, 45 CFR Part 160; Part 164, subparts A and E, 2002) was enacted in a manner to protect sensitive health information while reducing unnecessary barriers to the effective delivery of care. A covered entity *must* disclose protected health information

- To individuals when they request access to their own protected health

TABLE 11–1. **Individually identifiable health information**

Name

Address

All elements (except years) of dates related to an individual

Telephone numbers

Fax number

E-mail address

Social Security number

Medical record number

Health plan beneficiary number

Account number

Certificate or license number

Vehicle identifiers

Device identifiers (Web uniform resource locator [URL])

Internet Protocol (IP) address

Biometric identifiers, including finger or voice prints

Full-face photographic images and any comparable images

Any other unique identifying number, characteristic, or code

TABLE 11–2. **HIPAA-covered entities in connection with standard transactions (45 CFR § 162)**

Health claims and equivalent encounter information

Enrollment and disenrollment in a health plan

Eligibility for a health plan

Health care payment and remittance advice

Health plan premium payments

Health claim status

Referral certification and authorization

Coordination of benefits

First report of injury

information, a disclosure that does not require the individual's written authorization (45 CFR § 164.524).

- To the U.S. Department of Health and Human Services when the agency is conducting a compliance investigation or enforcement action.

The Privacy Rule also permits health care providers to share information for the timely and effective provision of care and for administrative operations that support the delivery of care, such as claims payment, quality assurance, and performance improvement. Except as otherwise permitted or required by the Privacy Rule (such as when individuals seek access to their own protected health information), an individual's written authorization is required for a covered entity to disclose protected health information. To be valid,

written authorizations must include the information listed in Table 11–3.

In addition to treatment, payment, and health care operations, the Privacy Rule permits a covered entity to disclose protected health information without the individual's written authorization to meet specific public interests. See Table 11–4 for a list of public interest and benefit activities as defined by HIPAA (45 CFR § 164.512).

As such circumstances permit, rather than compel the disclosure of protected health information, covered entities are advised to rely on professional judgment and ethics to determine whether a disclosure should or must be made. The Privacy Rule also permits disclosure of protected health information to an individual's employer without the individual's consent if the evaluation is necessary to meet state or federal laws for medical surveillance of the workplace, to assess for a work-related injury, and to monitor for exposure to certain substances. Employers may predicate employment on an employee's agreement to authorize disclosure of protected health information in these circumstances (Gold and Metzner 2006, p. 1879).

TABLE 11–3.	Required elements of a valid written authorization to disclose protected health information

Description of protected health information to be released

Identification of who will disclose the protected health information

Identification of who will receive the protected health information

Purpose of the disclosure

Use of expiration date or expiration event

Inclusion of required statements (revocation, no conditioning, potential for redisclosure)

Right to revoke in writing and the exceptions and instructions regarding the procedure or a reference to the Notice of Privacy Practices if this information is there

Inclusion of a statement about the covered entity's ability or inability to condition the authorization on treatment, payment, eligibility, or enrollment

Inclusion of a statement that once disclosed, the protected health information may no longer be protected by the Health Insurance Portability and Accountability Act Privacy Rule or an alternative statement if the disclosure is to another covered entity

Inclusion of a statement if use or disclosure is for marketing purposes, and the covered entity will receive remuneration

Signature of patient, with date

Uses and disclosures to law enforcement. Law enforcement officers are not HIPAA-covered entities and are not required to comply with the HIPAA Privacy Rule. A covered entity may disclose protected health information to law enforcement officials for law enforcement purposes in several circumstances (U.S. Department of Health and Human Services, 45 CFR § 160.103, 2002, 45 CFR § 164.512[f][1], 2002). Protected health information may be disclosed to law enforcement to avert a serious threat to public

TABLE 11–4.	Written authorization not required for a covered entity to release protected health information

As required by law, such as mandated reporting requirements

Public health activities

Health oversight activities

Judicial and administrative proceedings

Law enforcement functions

To facilitate cadaveric organ donation and transplants

Research

To avert a serious threat to health and safety

Workers' compensation claims as authorized by law

Specialized governmental functions

health and safety (U.S. Department of Health and Human Services, 45 CFR § 160.103, 2002, 45 CFR § 164.512[j], 2002) and as required by law, such as for the reporting of certain physical injuries (e.g., gunshot or stab wounds) or in response to an arrest warrant. Disclosure is also permissible to aid law enforcement officers in identifying or locating suspects, fugitives, missing persons, or material witnesses.

HIPAA Lawful Custody Exception

HIPAA recognizes that an individual's health information should remain protected but allows exceptions when a correctional institution or law enforcement agency has custody of an individual. Correctional institutions are not "health plans" within the strict definition of that term, because they are a government-funded program whose principal purpose is something other than providing or paying for the cost of health care (U.S. Department of Health and Human Services, 45 CFR § 160.103, 2002, 45 CFR § 160.103[2], 2002). However, if a correctional institution or contracted business associates provide health care and electronically transmit standard transactions, these institutions or associated businesses are required to comply with HIPAA.

Confidentiality of Alcohol and Drug Abuse Patient Records

The federal alcohol and drug abuse confidentiality regulations (Confidentiality of Alcohol and Drug Abuse Patient Records, 42 CFR Part 2, 1972) were created in 1972, ensuring strict confidentiality of alcohol or drug abuse treatment records. These regulations were developed to encourage individuals with an alcohol or drug abuse problem to seek treatment without fear of criminal prosecution or stigmatization. Strict confidentiality was considered necessary to foster therapeutic trust, to encourage disclosure, to promote help-seeking behavior, and to reduce stigma associated with substance use disorders (Tipping 2014).

The federal alcohol and drug abuse confidentiality regulations apply to all programs defined as "federally assisted programs" that hold themselves out as "providing, and provides, alcohol or drug abuse diagnosis, treatment or referral for treatment" (Confidentiality of Alcohol and Drug Abuse Patient Records, 42 CFR Part 2, 1972). As with HIPAA, the federal alcohol and drug abuse confidentiality regulations were not intended to prevent information sharing between entities with a legitimate need to share information for clinical purposes. Rather, these federal statutes were intended to limit the instances in which information could be shared without an individual's consent and to establish standards for how substance use disorder treatment information is to be shared.

A federally assisted program may disclose or share information about a patient's substance abuse treatment if the program has obtained the patient's written consent. The federal alcohol and drug abuse confidentiality regulations require that disclosure consents include specific elements in order to be valid (Table 11–5) (Confidentiality of Alcohol and Drug Abuse Patient Records, 42 CFR Part 2, 1972, 42 CFR §§ 2.31, 2.32, 1972). Patient-identifying information may be disclosed without the patient's consent only in special, limited circumstances (Table 11–6) (Confidentiality of Alcohol and Drug Abuse Patient Records, 42 CFR Part 2, 1972, 42 CFR § 2.12[c], 1972). Although most states have enacted stricter privacy laws than HIPAA, few states have substance use disorder confidentiality laws stricter than the federal alcohol and drug abuse confidentiality regulations.

Relevance of Federal Privacy Regulations to Forensic Evaluations

The applicability of HIPAA and the federal alcohol and drug abuse confidentiality regulations to forensic evaluations has garnered increased attention in recent years. Resolving whether the federal regulations apply to the performance of a forensic evaluation can depend on several factors, such as

- Whether the forensic evaluator is a covered entity.
- The specific type of forensic evaluation performed.
- The associated limits to confidentiality.
- Relevant state privacy law.
- By whom the evaluator is retained.

If a forensic psychiatrist qualifies as a HIPAA-covered entity, the psychiatrist

TABLE 11–5.	Required elements in all 42 CFR Part 2–compliant consent forms

Specific name or general designation of the program or person permitted to make the disclosure

Name and title of individual, or name of the organization, to which the disclosure is to be made

Name of patient

Purpose of disclosure

How much and what kind of information is to be disclosed

Signature of patient (or patient's representative)

Date on which consent is signed

Statement that consent is subject to revocation at any time (except to the extent that the consent has already been relied on)

Date, event, or condition on which the consent will expire if not revoked (patient is allowed to revoke the consent at any time)

TABLE 11–6.	Circumstances in which 42 CFR Part 2 regulations do not apply

Service-connected veterans receiving care through the Department of Veterans Affairs

Information shared within the armed forces or between the armed forces and the Department of Veterans Affairs

Information shared between a treatment facility and an entity having direct administrative control or between program personnel

Information shared through a valid Qualified Service Organization Agreement

Patient commits a crime on the premises of the treatment facility or against program personnel

Child abuse and neglect reporting as required by state law

Collection of death or other vital statistics

is under the same HIPAA confidentiality requirements as any other HIPAA-covered entity. The same privacy protections that apply to information obtained for treatment purposes apply to information obtained for nontreatment purposes, such as forensic evaluations, unless specific exceptions apply (Gold and Metzner 2006, p. 1880). For example, although the Privacy Rule allows exceptions for evaluations ordered in response to a judicial order, subpoena, or discovery request (Confidentiality of Alcohol and Drug Abuse Patient Records, 42 CFR Part 2, 1972, 45 CFR 164.512[e][i] and [ii], 1972), forensic evaluations that are not court-ordered, such as employment-related evaluations and disability determination evaluations, are subject to HIPAA's confidentiality rules.

The Privacy Rule also applies to all forensic evaluations not exempt from the HIPAA Privacy Rule, even if requested by an evaluee's attorney. In such instances, evaluators are urged to obtain written consent from the evaluee to provide the forensic report to third parties and should provide the evaluee with HIPAA's Notice of Privacy Practices (Glancy et al. 2015, p. S7). In addition, even if an evaluator is not a HIPAA-covered entity, states are increasingly adopting strict standards for confidentiality. Evaluators should refer to their state's confidentiality statutes governing the confidentiality of specific court-ordered evaluations, such as competency to stand trial, criminal responsibility, and mental condition evaluations, to determine whether such reports may be released without the consent of the evaluee.

Traditionally, forensic psychiatrists performing evaluations at the request of third parties have considered the report, which inevitably contains protected health information, to belong to the party that paid for the evaluation. Forensic psychiatrists therefore typically have not provided evaluees with copies of their reports, even when evaluees have submitted written requests to obtain copies of their evaluations. However, case law and interpretations of the provisions of HIPAA have found that such evaluations are subject to the HIPAA's requirements regarding protected health information, including an evaluee's right to access to the report if requested (Gold and Metzner 2006).

HIPAA compels a covered entity to disclose protected health information, including forensic reports, to individuals when the individuals request access to their protected health information, unless specific exceptions apply (45 CFR 164.524). Some forensic psychiatrists may not be HIPAA covered; however, as discussed earlier, state laws may exist that also require disclosure of forensic reports. In the event that state law is silent on this issue, forensic psychiatrists should bear in mind that HIPAA increasingly is becoming the national standard of care for provisions regarding confidentiality of protected health information (Gold and Metzner 2006). In the event that forensic reports are disclosed to other parties, HIPAA requires that HIPAA-covered psychiatrists keep a log of all disclosures of protected health information (Gold and Metzner 2006).

Exceptions to evaluees' rights to access their reports include information obtained for use in an administrative, civil, or criminal action or proceeding (Confidentiality of Alcohol and Drug Abuse Patient Records, 42 CFR Part 2, 1972, 45 CFR 164.524[a][1][ii], 1972). In these instances, however, evaluees retain the right to access the protected health information relied on to generate the exempted report. Forensic evaluations performed by a covered entity that do not qualify for this litigation exception must be provided to an evaluee if requested, such as evaluations requested by the evaluee's attor-

ney, disability evaluations, or fitness for duty evaluations. As in other areas of psychiatric practice, a therapeutic privilege exception to HIPAA does exist, whereby the evaluator can deny access to the protected health information if, "in the exercise of professional judgement, the access requested is reasonably likely to endanger the life or physical safety of the individual or another person" (Confidentiality of Alcohol and Drug Abuse Patient Records, 42 CFR Part 2, 1972, 45 CFR 164.524[a][3][i], 1972).

The only exception in regard to forensic evaluations is HIPAA's acknowledgment that certain types of evaluations cannot go forward without authorization of the release of information. The Privacy Rule specifies that an individual's medical treatment cannot be conditioned on the individual signing an authorization for the disclosure of information. However, the rule expressly allows independent medical evaluations by physicians to require an evaluee to sign an authorization for the release of protected health information to the third party requesting the independent medical evaluation as a condition of performing the evaluation (Confidentiality of Alcohol and Drug Abuse Patient Records, 42 CFR Part 2, 1972, 45 CFR §164.508, 1972). For example, a HIPAA-covered psychiatrist may condition the provision of a mental health evaluation paid for by an insurer or employer on the evaluee's prior authorization to disclose the results of that examination to the insurance company or employer (Gold and Metzner 2006).

HIPAA's provisions have important implications for forensic psychiatrists. First, when commencing a forensic evaluation, the evaluee should be informed as to the specific purpose of the evaluation, by which party the forensic evaluator has been retained, about any applicable limits of confidentiality, with whom information from the evaluation will be shared, about other parties who could potentially have access to the information, and whether the evaluee or his or her legal representative will have access to the completed evaluation. Forensic psychiatrists conducting third-party evaluations may refuse to conduct such evaluations unless specifically permitted by law or with a valid, written consent to release the information to the third party.

Second, forensic evaluators must be aware of the federal and their state's provisions concerning the evaluee's access to the forensic report and materials relied on by the evaluator in forming the opinion. Psychiatrists should not sign agreements with third parties, such as disability insurers or the evaluee's employer, indicating that the evaluator will not release the report to the evaluee, because HIPAA provides individuals unqualified access to their own protected health information. Even non-HIPAA-covered psychiatrists should consider releasing forensic reports directly to evaluees on receiving a written request to do so. In the event of litigation, refusal to do so may constitute a breach of a HIPAA-informed standard of care (Gold and Metzner 2006).

Conclusion

Although confidentiality is the ethical obligation of the health professional to protect the patient's privacy, privilege to prevent disclosure of health information is a legal right that belongs to the patient. State and federal case law has shaped the concepts and practices of confidentiality and privilege and has defined exceptions to the protected privilege of confidential communications and records. Communicating with other health care providers for purposes of providing care, protection of third parties, mandated reporting requirements, public health considerations, and governmental audits are some of the exceptions to this protected privilege. In our evolving digital world, federal and state regulation, guided by case law and ethical traditions in medicine, has dramatically shaped organizational practices involving confidentiality and privilege in the health professional–patient relationship.

HIPAA established federal minimum standards for the protection of health information. In states with stricter patient privacy standards, the stricter rules will apply. Although HIPAA's privacy rules apply only to covered entities, evolving standards and case law in many states are expanding the privacy requirements for treaters who are not considered HIPAA-covered entities to mirror HIPAA's privacy protections. Psychiatrists performing forensic evaluations in a state must be aware of and comply with that state's specific privacy protections pertaining to health care information. Evaluators also should be aware that for some forensic evaluations, such as disability or insurance evaluations, evaluees have a right under HIPAA to access their protected health information.

Key Concepts

- *Privilege* is a legal right of privacy owned by the patient.

- Privilege is waived by patients under certain conditions, such as in certain criminal proceedings or in civil claims in which patients have placed their mental condition at issue.

- *Confidentiality* is an ethical duty owed by physicians and health professionals to their patients.

- Confidentiality is not absolute; exceptions include meeting duties to third parties and other public safety issues.

- Reasonable steps to protect identified third parties from harm may include hospitalization of the patient, warning the potential victim, and contacting law enforcement.

- HIPAA's privacy rule sets minimum standards for protecting confidential patient information. In states with stricter rules, those state rules will govern.

- Evaluees are entitled to access forensic psychiatric reports produced by HIPAA-covered psychiatrists, conducted for disability, insurance, and other purposes, because evaluees are entitled to access their own protected health information.

References

Confidentiality of Alcohol and Drug Abuse Patient Records, Code of Federal Regulations, Title 42, Part 2. 1972. Available at: https://www.ecfr.gov/cgi-bin/text-idx?rgn=div5;node=42%3A1.0.1.1.2. Accessed January 1, 2017.

Doe v Roe, 400 N.Y.Supp. 2d 668; 93 Misc.2d 201 (1977)

Fox PK: Commentary: so the pendulum swings—making sense of the duty to protect. J Am Acad Psychiatry Law 38(4): 474–478, 2010 21156905

Glancy GD, Ash P, Bath EP, et al: AAPL practice guideline for the forensic assessment. J Am Acad Psychiatry Law 43(2)(suppl):S3–S53, 2015 26054704

Gold LH, Metzner JL: Psychiatric employment evaluations and the Health Insurance Portability and Accountability Act. Am J Psychiatry 163(11):1878–1882, 2006 17074937

Health Insurance Portability and Accountability Act of 1996, Pub. L. No. 104-191, 110 Stat. 1936 (1996)

In re Lifschutz, 2 Cal. 3d 415; 467 P.2d 557 (1970)

Jaffee v Redmond, 518 U.S. 1; 116 S.Ct. 1923 (1996)

Johnson R, Persad G, Sisti D: The Tarasoff rule: the implications of interstate variation and gaps in professional training. J Am Acad Psychiatry Law 42(4):469–477, 2014 25492073

Kachigian C, Felthous AR: Court responses to Tarasoff statutes. J Am Acad Psychiatry Law 32(3):263–273, 2004 15515914

People v Stritzinger, 34 Cal. 3d 505, 668 P.2d 738 (1983)

Roe v Wade, 410 U.S. 113, 93 S.Ct. 705 (1973)

State v Andring, 342 N.W.2d 128 (Minn. 1984)

Tarasoff v Regents of the Univ. of California, 13 Cal. 3d 177, 529 P.2d 553, 118 Cal. Rptr. 129 (1974)

Tarasoff v Regents of University of California, 17 Cal. 3d 425, 551 P.2d 334, 131 Cal. Rptr. 14 (1976)

Tipping K: Privacy issues for justice and health exchanges: separating fact from fiction. Paper presented at the Policy Academy on Cross Boundary Corrections Information Exchange hosted by the National Governors' Association, Washington, DC, June 17, 2014.

U.S. Department of Health and Human Services: The HIPAA Privacy Rule, 45 CFR Part 160; Part 164, Subparts A and E (2002)

PART III

Civil Issues and Litigation

CHAPTER 12

Professional Liability in Psychiatric Practice

Donna Vanderpool, M.B.A., J.D.

Landmark Cases

Roy v. Hartogs, 381 N.Y.S. 2d 587 (1976)

Clites v. Iowa, 322 N.W.2d 917 (Iowa Ct. App. 1982)

Psychiatry is one of the least often sued medical specialties (Jena et al. 2011; Studdert et al. 2016). Most lawsuits filed against psychiatrists do not result in payment to the plaintiff (Jena et al. 2011). In fact, most such suits are dismissed or are not pursued to trial. Legal claims can be settled at any time before, during, and after trial. In addition, courts may dismiss suits for a variety of legal reasons. Nevertheless, liability for forensic activities is possible, and psychiatrists who conduct forensic evaluations and provide testimony in the courts should understand both their liability exposure and its potential consequences.

Sources of Professional Liability

Physicians are subject to various sources of professional liability, including the following:

- *Civil liability*—tort action (citizen vs. citizen), such as malpractice, to compensate those suffering a loss caused by another
- *Criminal liability*—criminal prosecution (state vs. citizen)
- *Administrative action*—investigation (administrative agency vs. regulated

individual), such as by a state licensing board or the U.S. Department of Health and Human Services
- *Peer review*—investigation (group vs. group member), such as by a state medical association or specialty society

Many different tort actions, such as intentional infliction of emotional distress or wrongful death, can be brought against physicians. However, malpractice is the most common tort action. Table 12–1 lists the causes of action asserted against psychiatrists in malpractice claims.

Professional liability can result from the physician's acts or omissions or the acts or omissions of others. For example, a supervising psychiatrist will likely be named in complaints brought against a supervisee nurse practitioner. Physician employers also can be held vicariously liable for the actions of their employees under the legal doctrine of *respondeat superior* (i.e., an employer is responsible for the actions of employees performed within the course of their employment).

Advances in medical treatment can increase claims of professional liability: as patients' expectations increase, tolerance for adverse outcomes decreases. In addition, as the cost of care for patients who experience adverse outcomes continues to increase, legal actions to compensate for costs of care offer the possibility of awards to cover those costs. In the United States, medical malpractice actions first appeared in the mid to late 1800s due, in part, to advances in the ability to treat compound fractures (Mohr 2000). Patients began alleging that their doctors had been negligent in setting their fractured limbs, which the patients claimed resulted in a disability. Before that time, limbs with complicated traumatic injuries such as compound fractures usually were amputated, so negligent setting of fractures was not a cause for lawsuits.

Elements of Malpractice

The statutory requirements to file a medical malpractice action vary by state, but all states require the plaintiff (the patient or the patient's estate) to prove four elements to prevail in a medical malpractice action. These four elements of a medical malpractice case have been referred to as the "4 D's": duty, dereliction, damages, and direct causation.

1. *Duty*. Plaintiff has to prove that the physician had a duty to the patient to meet the standard of care. Typically, duty is created once a treatment relationship is established. However, even in the absence of a treatment relationship, such as a forensic evaluation, courts may impose duties on the physician as discussed below (see section "Liability for Forensic Activities").
2. *Dereliction (negligence)*. Plaintiff has to prove that the care delivered did not meet the standard of care or that the physician breached the duty.
3. *Damages (injury)*. Plaintiff has to prove that the patient experienced harm, which can be physical, financial, or emotional.
4. *Direct causation*. Plaintiff has to prove that the defendant physician's negligence directly caused the patient's injuries. This is typically the most difficult element to prove.

Standard of Care

Medical malpractice is defined as the act(s) or continuing conduct of a physician that does not meet the standard of care and results in injury to the patient. The standard of care owed to patients by physicians was defined in *Clites v. Iowa* (1982). Timothy Clites, a severely intellectually disabled individual, resided in a state residential treatment program for more than 10 years. During this time, he was

TABLE 12–1. **The Psychiatrists' Program® cause of loss—claims and lawsuits, 2007–2016**

Primary allegation	All ages	Adults	Minors
Incorrect treatment	37%	37%	32%
Medication issues	18%	17%	19%
Suicide/attempted suicide	15%	15%	15%
Incorrect diagnosis	6%	6%	7%
Other (e.g., inappropriate discharge, failure to monitor)	7%	8%	7%
Unnecessary commitment	4%	5%	3%
Breach of confidentiality	3%	3%	4%
Improper supervision	3%	2%	7%
Vicarious liability	2%	2%	3%
Improper discharge	1%	1%	1%
Forensic	1%	1%	1%
Duty to warn/protect	1%	1%	1%
Abandonment	1%	1%	–
Boundary violation	1%	1%	–

Note. "Primary allegation" is the main allegation by plaintiffs' attorneys of what the psychiatrist did wrong. "Incorrect treatment" will represent a high percentage of cases because plaintiffs' attorneys often use a broad, general allegation initially; this category includes all types of cases, including suicide and psychopharmacology. The category labeled "Improper supervision" refers to supervision of patients as well as of other providers.
Source. The Psychiatrists' Program. Copyright © 2016, Professional Risk Management Services, Inc. (PRMS). Used with permission.

treated with several different psychotropic medications, often used together in different combinations, and he ultimately developed tardive dyskinesia. Clites's father sued for damages based in part on a claim of negligent prescription of medication. The trial court found that the defendants had failed to provide reasonable medical treatment to Clites and that negligence was the proximate cause of his tardive dyskinesia.

The defendants appealed, claiming, among other issues, that the district court had applied an incorrect standard of care in the finding of negligence in the administration of tranquilizers. The court held that the state did not comply with the standard of care, in that a patient in Clites's circumstances and subjected to treatment with psychotropic medication must be closely monitored with regular visits by a physician, tests, and physical examinations. The court articulated the appropriate standard of care: "Doctors are held to such reasonable care and skill as is exercised by the ordinary physician of good standing under like circumstances" (p. 919).

In contrast to intentional wrongdoing, such as battery, professional negligence is considered accidental. An outcome detrimental to a patient is not necessarily evidence of negligence. The exercise of prudent professional judgment can result in an adverse clinical outcome. However, if the physician has not been negligent, even the most adverse outcome is legally not considered malpractice.

Plaintiffs suing a physician for medical malpractice generally file suit in state court. Although state court systems vary, typically physicians are sued in the county where the patient was treated. Each court has its own rules and procedures that must be followed. Medical malpractice actions are sometimes filed in the federal court system, such as when a federally employed physician is sued under the Federal Tort Claims Act or when the parties are from two different states.

Professional negligence can occur only when the standard of care is not met. Professional liability cases typically require expert testimony to elucidate the particular standard of care in any specific clinical situation. An expert witness is a person with special education, training, and experience who possesses superior knowledge in a subject about which persons having no particular training are incapable of forming an accurate opinion or deducing correct conclusions. In a medical malpractice case, the expert witness testifies about the accepted professional standard of care, gives an opinion about whether the defendant met the standard of care, and concludes whether the alleged breach of the standard of care (negligence) was the proximate cause of any alleged injuries.

An expert witness's opinions and testimony about the standard of care rely on a combination of factors including, but not limited to, the following:

- Federal and state statutes, such as laws promulgated by federal and state legislatures (e.g., the federal Controlled Substances Act)
- Federal and state agency regulations, such as state licensing boards and the federal Drug Enforcement Agency (DEA)
- Federal and state case law, including legal opinions previously decided by state and federal courts
- Other materials from regulatory bodies, such as rules, guidelines, and policy statements from state and federal regulatory agencies, including U.S. Food and Drug Administration–approved drug label information
- Authoritative clinical guidelines, such as treatment guidelines from reputable professional organizations (but not health plans' utilization review guidelines)
- Policies and guidelines from professional organizations, such as ethics statements and resource documents from the American Medical Association (AMA), the American Psychiatric Association (APA), and the American Academy of Psychiatry and the Law (AAPL)
- Professional literature, such as authoritative treatises or clinical textbooks and journal articles
- Regulatory and institutional accreditation standards, facility policies, and procedures

Clinical guidelines by themselves do not set the standard of care. Rather, guidelines are just one piece of evidence that the judge and jury will use to determine the applicable standard of care in a given case. Physicians who provide treatment that deviates from widely accepted guidelines may not have been negligent in their treatment, but the reasoning behind such deviations should be adequately documented and supported by current practice and professional literature. For example, off-label use of certain medications is a common and accepted practice, but physicians prescribing a medication for an off-label use should document their rationale and be able to cite professional literature supporting the off-label use.

Expert Witness Testimony in Medical Malpractice Cases

Table 12–2 presents a summary of the litigation process in a medical malpractice case.

TABLE 12–2. Civil litigation process in a medical malpractice case

Summons and complaint	Documents filed with the court by plaintiff initiating a lawsuit; lists initial allegations against defendant
Answer	Document filed with the court by defendant; responds to all allegations in summons and complaint
Discovery	Both sides obtain facts and information about the case from each other; may include depositions, interrogatories, production of documents, and other sources of information
Pretrial motions	Requests to the court for an order or ruling on some aspect of the case
Jury selection	Potential jurors are questioned by the judge and attorneys (known as *voir dire*) for both sides to determine whether a juror's background, opinions, or life experiences may affect his or her impartiality to decide the case
Opening statements	Both sides' attorneys outline their version of the case and what they intend to prove
Testimony of plaintiff, plaintiff's expert, defendant, and defendant's expert	May include redirect and re–cross-examination of plaintiff, defendant, and witnesses
Closing statements	Both sides' attorneys summarize the evidence that has been presented and the relation of the evidence to the issues in the case
Jury deliberations and verdict	Jurors provide an opinion on liability and, if the verdict is for plaintiff, damages the jury believes should be awarded to plaintiff
Judgment	Case resolution entered by the court; may or may not be the same as the verdict
Postjudgment motions	Several motions are possible, including a motion for the court not to accept an unsupported verdict and enter a "judgment notwithstanding the verdict"
Appeal	The nonprevailing party asks an appellate court to review whether the trial court committed an error that adversely affected the outcome of the case

In professional liability cases, experts must hold their opinions with "reasonable medical certainty" or "reasonable medical probability"; that is, the expert must believe that the opinion is more likely than not accurate. For example, if experts are asked, based on reasonable medical certainty, whether the injuries were the result of the defendant psychiatrist's actions, experts may answer yes if they believe that those actions were "more likely than not" the cause of the injury.

Expert witnesses are generally deposed during the discovery phase of a malprac-tice claim. A *deposition* is a formal question and answer session in which one party to the lawsuit asks witnesses oral questions under oath. Depositions enable a party to discover information that may be used at trial. In addition, testimony obtained during a deposition creates a record that preserves the testimony for use at trial. Although depositions are usually conducted in an attorney's office and are less formal than courtroom proceedings, they are considered testimony that may be admitted or brought up at trial.

Deposition questions and testimony differ from courtroom testimony in several respects. One of the most significant is relevance. Attorneys at a deposition may ask broad-ranging questions, because the purpose of the deposition is to discover evidence that may be relevant at trial. The attorney for the opposing party in the lawsuit questions the deponent, and the deponent's attorney may object to inappropriate or irrelevant lines of questioning. However, the deponent typically has to answer the questions. At trial, this testimony may in fact be deemed inadmissible, but this cannot and does not prevent attorneys at the deposition from asking questions that the deponent must answer under oath.

The deposition of an expert witness is intended to allow the opposing party an opportunity to fully elucidate the expert's opinions and the bases of those opinions. Expert witnesses also should expect to be questioned about their education, training, experience, and prior testimony in other cases, because the opposing party may use this information to argue that the court should not recognize the proffered clinician as an expert. Motions to exclude the expert witness can be made before trial through a motion *in limine* or during trial when the proffered expert is questioned through a *voir dire* examination.

The trial court judge determines if a witness is qualified to testify as an expert. Once the court has decided that a witness may testify as an expert, the jury must decide, after listening to the expert's testimony, what weight should be given to the expert's opinion. Expert witnesses should be prepared to testify about all their opinions in the case at hand, even if a report has been provided. In many jurisdictions, although experts may rely heavily on their reports, only the expert's testimony and not the report will be admitted as evidence.

Boundary Violations

Boundary issues can range from accepting small gifts as a token of a patient's appreciation to financial exploitation (Chapter 8, "Physician–Patient Relationship in Psychiatry"). Typically, boundary violations become the subject of a complaint or litigation when they involve sexual misconduct, either alone or together with other inappropriate or exploitative behavior.

Lawsuits involving allegations of psychiatrists having sexual relations with their patients can be brought as a malpractice action. In *Roy v. Hartogs* (1976), Julie Roy sued her psychiatrist, Dr. Hartogs, for emotional and mental injuries. Dr. Hartogs claimed that he engaged in sexual intercourse with the plaintiff as part of her therapy. Ms. Roy claimed psychological injuries as a result of this treatment. Dr. Hartogs was found liable, and Ms. Roy was awarded both compensatory and punitive damages. The court, in considering this matter as a malpractice case, found that "sex under cloak of treatment is an acceptable and established ground for disciplinary measures taken against physicians either by licensing authorities or professional organizations" (p. 591).

States vary in how they address the issue of psychiatrists and other mental health professionals who engage in sexual contact with patients. In some states, sexual relations with patients has long been considered a criminal act, typically a felony punishable by imprisonment and fines. In California, sexual contact with a patient is considered unprofessional conduct and is also punishable by imprisonment and fine (Cal. Bus. and Prof. Code § 729, 2013). Recently, states without such an explicit prohibition have been enacting laws to criminalize sexual contact with patients.

Notably, the defendant psychiatrist in *Roy v. Hartogs*, after being found liable for malpractice, sued his malpractice insurer to recover his costs and expenses. In *Hartogs v. Employers Insurance* (1977), the court found that because the psychiatrist's sexual conduct toward the plaintiff did not constitute treatment, the conduct was not medical malpractice and therefore was not covered by the physician's professional liability policy. Most of the appellate courts also have held that sexual misconduct does not constitute professional services for which a malpractice insurer is liable to pay damages. Professional liability insurance companies may explicitly exclude coverage for sexual misconduct. Alternatively, coverage (typically for defense only) could be expressly capped as a policy sublimit, for a mixed maximum amount such as $25,000.

In order to exclude coverage for a claim or lawsuit, the insurer must advise the insured of the exclusion from coverage, usually by a "Reservation of Rights" letter. Typically, a Reservation of Rights letter informs the insured that the insurer is handling the action, for example, by providing an attorney to defend the insured but "reserves the right" not to pay for certain losses not covered under the policy, such as sexual misconduct. In the absence of such an exclusion, the insurer would be required to cover any settlement or judgment.

Malpractice Insurance

Professional malpractice insurance is a contract between an insurer and an insured individual or group that provides coverage for professional liability claims. This coverage is for the policy period—that is, the time between the effective date (the date coverage first took effect) and the expiration of the policy. Issues related to insurance policies are analyzed under a strict contractual review (see, e.g., *Mazza v. Medical Mutual Insurance Co. of North Carolina* 1984). Courts are clear that any coverage limitations must be specifically ex-

pressed in the policy. Any ambiguities in an insurance policy are to be construed in favor of the insured to uphold coverage.

The two main types of medical malpractice insurance policies are referred to as *occurrence* and *claims-made*. With an occurrence policy, coverage is provided for an incident giving rise to a claim or lawsuit that occurs while the policy is in effect, regardless of when the claim is reported to the insurance company and even if the claim is reported after the policy has expired. Policy holders are given a new set of policy limits each year that an occurrence policy is renewed. Previous years' limits remain available for claims that may arise from incidents occurring during those previous years.

In claims-made policies, coverage is provided only for claims that both occur and are reported while the policy is in effect. If the incident giving rise to the claim occurred while the insured had coverage, but is reported after the policy has expired, the insurer does not provide coverage unless extended reporting coverage ("tail" coverage) has been purchased. When this type of policy is renewed, policy holders are given a new set of policy limits but do not keep the prior years' limits. Tail coverage does not extend the policy period but rather extends the time during which coverage will be provided for claims that may be reported.

Regardless of which type of policy is purchased, psychiatric malpractice policies have two sets of provisions limiting the amount of money available to pay claims, settlements, and judgments in any given year. The first is a per-incident limit (i.e., the amount of coverage for each individual claim during a policy period). The second is an aggregate limit (i.e., the amount of coverage for all combined claims during a policy period).

Malpractice policies cover certain types of expenses associated with defending a malpractice claim. They obligate the insurer to pay indemnity costs, which are the amount paid to resolve the claim or lawsuit, whether by settlement or judgment. They also obligate the insurer to pay defense costs, the amount paid for legal expenses to defend the case, such as attorneys' fees and expert witness fees. Defense costs can be significant. Malpractice insurance policies address the payment of defense costs either "inside" or "outside" of policy limits. If the policy pays defense costs inside the limit, the amount of money available to pay indemnity costs (settlements or judgments) is reduced by the amount of defense costs. On the contrary, if the policy pays defense costs outside of the policy limits, the indemnity amount is not reduced by defense costs.

Punitive damages, intended to punish the defendant and deter inappropriate behavior, may or may not be covered by insurance policies. Some courts believe that wrongdoers, not their insurers, should be punished (see, e.g., *Aetna v. McCabe* 1983), and therefore public policy interests indicate that insurers should not cover punitive damages. However, insurance companies may have to cover punitive damages if their policies do not explicitly exclude punitive damages (see, e.g., *Mazza v. Medical Mutual Insurance Co. of North Carolina* 1984).

Other significant elements in a malpractice insurance policy include the following:

- *What exactly is covered.* The definition of *professional services, practice of medicine,* or comparable terms. Additional coverage may be required for forensic activities and administrative activities, such as a position as a medical director.
- *Endorsements.* A written amendment, addition, or modification that takes precedence over the original policy provisions. These may be used to expand coverage (e.g., by adding defense coverage for administrative actions) or to restrict coverage.
- *Exclusions.* A list of activities such as criminal acts, the liability for which will be excluded from coverage.
- *"Consent to settle" provisions.* The language and types of consent provisions include

  1. *Unlimited consent.* The insured alone decides whether a case can be settled. No settlement can be made without the insured's express consent.
  2. *No consent.* The insurer alone decides when a case will be settled, and the insured has no say.
  3. *Limited with a hammer clause.* The insured is allowed to accept or reject settlement. However, the insured then would be personally responsible for any judgment or settlement in excess of the previously rejected settlement amount.
  4. *Limited with arbitration.* In the event that the insured and the insurer do not agree on settling the claim, both agree to arbitration to come to a decision.

Professional Liability: Other Venues

Licensing Board Complaints

All physicians are required to have a license granted by a state licensing board to practice medicine in that state, and all states have a state licensing board. Physicians do not have a right to a state license; a license to practice medicine is a privilege granted by the state, and the state licensing board controls the status of a physician's license to practice. Board hearings are less formal than civil court procedures, and physicians are not protected by rights available in civil courts, such as due process, but they may be represented by legal counsel. A complaint made to a state board may result in suspension or limitation of a physician's license. The physician may be required to undergo treatment or to be supervised by another physician who will report to the board in order to regain full licensure status.

Filing a board complaint rather than a civil complaint can be an appealing option, particularly to forensic evaluees and other third parties such as companies or law firms that retain forensic psychiatrists. Unlike civil litigation, in which a complaining party must have legal standing to proceed with a lawsuit, licensing board complaints can be filed by anyone, including evaluees, patients, patients' friends and families, and government representatives, such as state attorneys general and Medicaid program representatives. Board complaints do not require that the complainant have an injury, as is the case with malpractice lawsuits. Also, unlike litigation, board complaints may not be precluded by statutes of limitations. Finally, licensing boards generally investigate all complaints, even if complaints appear to lack merit.

Although state medical licensing board practices may vary somewhat, typically complaints are initially screened to determine whether immediate investigation is needed (as in the case of allegations of sexual behavior with patients), whether more information is needed (such as medical records), and whether the complaint is within the board's jurisdiction. Minor violations may result in an administrative citation or a fine rather than formal discipline. For example, failure to provide patients access to their records is typically considered a minor violation and is easily rectified. In this type of case, the state board might advise the licensee

of the violation, advise him or her to come into compliance, and impose a fine.

If the initial review indicates that a more significant violation may have occurred, the licensing boards will investigate, and depending on the result of the investigation, the case may be closed, referred for enforcement, or referred for other action, such as criminal prosecution. A board investigation into major violations such as sexual contact with a patient may result in formal charges and a hearing. The charges may be accepted by the licensee, similar to a settlement agreement in litigation. Penalties can include fees, supervision, and license revocation. If the physician contests the charges and the accompanying discipline imposed by the board, typically licensees have the ability to appeal. Depending on the jurisdiction, appeals from disciplinary actions may be heard by administrative law judges or by state trial courts.

As previously mentioned, professional liability insurance policies may cover the defense of administrative actions such as those brought by a licensing board. If such coverage is provided, psychiatrists are advised to contact their insurer immediately on notice of a board complaint or investigation so that an attorney can be appointed to assist in responding to the board.

Peer Review Actions

Physicians are subject to peer review by the various professional organizations to which they belong. Most professional organizations, including specialty societies and state medical associations, have a mechanism through which complaints about members can be investigated, and sanctions can be imposed. For example, AAPL uses the APA's process for investigation of ethical complaints received about its members. Peer review actions, although not limited to investigations of forensic activities, are addressed later in this chapter (see "Liability for Forensic Activities" section) specifically in regard to liability for forensic activities.

National Practitioner Data Bank

Congress established the National Practitioner Data Bank (NPDB) as an information clearinghouse for information about a health care practitioner's qualifications to practice medicine. The NPDB is primarily a flagging system serving to alert users that a more comprehensive review of the qualifications and background of a health care practitioner or provider may be prudent. The NPDB's requirements, established and governed by provisions found in several laws, are administered by the U.S. Department of Health and Human Services (2015).

State licensing boards, hospitals, and professional societies such as the AMA and the APA must report adverse actions affecting the licensure, membership, and clinical privileges of a health care practitioner. Malpractice insurers are required to report any medical malpractice insurance payment made on the physician's behalf to the NPDB, regardless of the amount. This report is submitted online and consists of demographic information about the physician and the patient, information about the alleged malpractice and injury, and payment information. Once the insurer submits the report, the physician will receive a copy and be given an opportunity to add his or her own comments.

NPDB information is not available to the general public. The information is confidential, and only eligible entities, as defined by the law, are entitled to access it (U.S. Department of Health and Human Services 2015). NPDB records are available to state licensing boards, hospitals, other health care entities, professional societies, and certain federal agencies. In the case of a medical malpractice action and under certain limited circumstances, a plaintiff's attorney or a pro se plaintiff may query the NPDB. Practitioners are entitled to self-query at any time (U.S. Department of Health and Human Services 2015).

Liability for Forensic Activities

Historically, psychiatrists did not face professional liability exposure for forensic activities because forensic evaluators have no treatment relationship with a forensic evaluee. Without a treatment relationship, no duty is owed to the evaluee. In recent years, however, courts have begun to depart from this traditional rule. The current judicial trend is to impose malpractice liability even absent the traditional physician–patient relationship (Appelbaum 2001; Gold and Davidson 2007). Courts also may expect nonmembers to follow a professional organization's ethics code, such as that of the AAPL (*Sugarman v. Board of Registration in Medicine* 1996). In addition, state medical boards and professional associations have become much more active in reviewing forensic activities.

Professional Liability and Independent Medical Evaluations

In some states, performing independent medical evaluations (IMEs) can be considered the practice of medicine, creating two issues for forensic practitioners: oversight and licensure. If IMEs are considered the practice of medicine, physicians may be subject to oversight by the licensing board in the jurisdiction where the IME is performed (Gold and Davidson 2007; Simon and Shuman 1999). Therefore, before agreeing to perform an IME in a state in which the psychiatrist is not licensed, a forensic psychiatrist should determine whether medical licensure is required. Forensic clinicians may be able to find preliminary state licensure requirements for expert witnesses in the Federation of State Medical Boards (2016) Web site publication, "Expert Witness Qualifications: Board-by-Board Overview." Psychiatrists also should consider checking with the medical board in the state in which the IME will be conducted.

Courts have defined four possible duties owed by nontreating physicians such as forensic psychiatrists to evaluees (Vanderpool 2011). First is the possible duty not to injure the evaluee. Most courts that have considered these claims have found that the duty not to injure an evaluee is almost always required. This duty is recognized in case law and may include emotional injury. Notably, courts generally have found that adverse outcomes from IME reports are not an adequate basis for a lawsuit based on this duty.

The second possible duty, although currently the view held in only a minority of courts, is the duty to properly diagnose the evaluee. The third possible duty, the view held by a majority of courts, is the duty to inform the evaluee about a potentially serious medical condition, such as imminent risk of suicide. This duty may be required by state regulation, is recognized in case law, and is required by AMA Code of Medical Ethics Opinion 1.2.6 (American Medical Association 2016). Courts have found that the duty to inform cannot be delegated to others. Accordingly, psychiatrists should ensure that all IME contracts allow the evaluating psychiatrist to notify the evaluee directly of any serious medical conditions.

The final possible duty is the duty to maintain confidentiality. That this duty exists is also the view of most courts that have heard such cases and is recognized in case law. Maintaining confidentiality in evaluations conducted for purposes other than treatment is required by state and federal statutes and regulations, such as Standards for Privacy of Individually Identifiable Health Information (2000) (Standards for Privacy of Individually Identifiable Health Information (2000) [HIPAA] Privacy Rule) and Confidentiality of Alcohol and Drug Abuse Patient Records (1987), and is required by professional organizations such as the AAPL, APA, and AMA (Gold and Davidson 2007; Vanderpool 2011).

The duty to maintain confidentiality includes the obligation to disclose only relevant information to third parties. For example, AAPL's "Practice Guideline for the Forensic Evaluation of Psychiatric Disability" (Gold et al. 2008) states: "information that is not relevant to the disability evaluation should be considered confidential. Consent to release information in disability evaluations does not give a psychiatrist *carte blanche* to reveal all information obtained during the evaluation by anyone who is interested in it" (Gold et al. 2008, p. S10). In addition, the Genetic Information Nondiscrimination Act of 2008 (29 CFR § 1635.8[a]) prohibits disclosure of genetic information (defined to include family history) to employers.

Another confidentiality issue involves dangerous evaluees. Courts have found the duty to warn extends beyond treating providers to those performing IMEs (*Gavin v. Hilton Worldwide, Inc.* 2013). Finally, in terms of attorneys' requests for an expert's IME reports from other, unrelated cases, at least one court has prohibited the disclosure of unrelated confidential information (*Graham v. Dacheikh* 2008).

For psychiatrists who are covered providers under HIPAA, the Privacy Rule's requirements apply to all disclosures of protected health information, regardless of the purpose for which the protected health information was created (Gold and Metzner 2006). Once a provider meets the regulatory definition of a health care provider subject to HIPAA's regulations, then that provider must comply with the Privacy Rule's requirements for all uses and disclosures of protected health information. To assist covered providers in fulfilling this legal obligation, the Privacy Rule has an exception at 45 CFR § 164.508(b)(4)(ii) that expressly allows physicians conducting IMEs to require the evaluee to sign an authorization for the release of protected health information to the third party requesting the IME as a condition of performing the IME. This provision stands in contrast to the general rule that the provision of health services cannot be conditioned on the individual signing an authorization for the disclosure of information.

In terms of the evaluee's access to records, HIPAA's Privacy Rule is clear that an evaluee has a right, with only limited exceptions, to his or her own protected health information, regardless of the fact that a third party paid for the evaluation and that the evaluating physician is not a treatment provider. This also may be true under state law. For example, New Hampshire's Board of Medicine has specified that IME evaluees are entitled to a copy of IME records (Taylor 2002). Psychiatrists conducting IMEs, disability evaluations, and evaluations for nontreatment purposes should ensure that contracts with third parties do not prohibit the disclosure of information to the evaluee.

Other administrative actions initiated by IME evaluees are also possible. As discussed earlier, evaluees can always file a complaint with the evaluator's licensing board or a professional organization or institution to which the evaluating psychiatrist belongs. Psychiatrists should be certain that their professional liability insurance covers all their forensic services as well as all venues in which complaints may be brought.

Professional Liability for Providing Expert Witness Testimony

Professional liability for psychiatric expert witness activities (Binder 2002) typically falls into one of three categories:

1. Malpractice lawsuits
2. Licensing board investigations and discipline
3. Professional organization peer review and discipline

Criminal liability for testimony, such as perjury, is also possible, but such actions are rare because medical opinions are based on professional judgment.

Malpractice Lawsuits

Litigation against experts is possible, although two types of immunity from professional liability are relevant for physicians performing civil forensic activities: quasi-judicial immunity and witness immunity. Quasi-judicial immunity is generally available only when the physician is retained by and reports directly to the court. Witness immunity generally protects the physician's actual testimony, whether at trial or at deposition, as well as any statements, opinions, or findings that are set forth in any report.

Physicians should be aware that these immunities are only immunity from suit, not immunity from investigation by a licensing board or professional association or from criminal prosecution for perjury. Physicians providing expert testimony are most likely immune from a civil lawsuit based on expert testimony. Because of the availability of immunity from civil suits, licensing boards in recent years have become more active in policing expert witness activities.

Courts generally have found that witness immunity precludes claims brought by one party in civil litigation against the expert testifying for the other party. In terms of a party suing its own expert, a few cases have arisen, mostly involving financial or math errors by the expert, such as an error in the expert's calculation of lost profits. However, lawsuits may be brought for other issues.

For example, in *Pace v. Swerdlow* (2008), the plaintiff's physician expert, without consulting the retaining attorney, drafted an "addendum" to his deposition testimony close to the time of trial changing his opinion. The addendum directly opposed the plaintiff's claims and supported the opposing side's arguments. After the trial court granted the defendant's motion for summary judgment, the plaintiff filed suit against the expert, alleging, among other claims, malpractice and fraud. The expert filed a motion to dismiss, claiming witness immunity. The trial court granted the expert's motion to dismiss; the plaintiff appealed. The appellate court agreed with the plaintiff that the expert's change of opinion so close to trial damaged the plaintiff's case and held that the expert may have proximately caused the plaintiff's case to be dismissed prematurely.

Licensing Board Investigations and Discipline

As is the case when performing IMEs, providing expert witness testimony can constitute the practice of medicine in some jurisdictions, even in the absence of treatment (Gold and Davidson 2007; Simon and Shuman 1999; Vanderpool 2011). Accordingly, the expert's activities in these jurisdictions are subject to state regulation and oversight. Even in states where providing expert testimony is not considered the practice of medicine, states still may have the ability to regulate experts. As pointed out by the California attorney general, "the Board may discipline a physician for unprofessional conduct even though the actual misconduct does not constitute the practice of medicine or cause harm" (Office of the Attorney General, State of California 2004, p. 7).

Licensing boards mainly regulate three areas of expert activities: disciplining for unprofessional conduct, controlling when a state license is required, and creating standards for expert testimony. When licensing boards promulgate regulations related to the provision of expert testimony, the regulations may apply to all experts testifying in that state, regardless of whether they are licensed to practice in the state. For example, under Mississippi law,

> Any physician who performs medical expert activities [in Mississippi], whether or not licensed to practice medicine in Mississippi, may be disciplined or otherwise held professionally accountable by the [Mississippi] Board, upon a finding by the Board that the physician is unqualified as evidenced by behavior including, but not limited to, incompetent professional practice, unprofessional conduct, or any other dishonorable or unethical conduct likely to deceive, defraud, or harm the public. (Miss. Admin. Code 30-17-2635:8.6, 1972)

Professional Organization Peer Review and Discipline

The ability of a professional society to sanction a member for giving improper testimony was validated in *Austin v. American Association of Neurological Surgeons*

(2001). Accordingly, professional societies have increased their investigations and sanctions of expert witness testimony, resulting in more lawsuits against the societies and against expert witnesses alleging defamation. State medical associations may have programs to review complaints about expert testimony by their members and also may refer cases to the state licensing board for review.

Peer review sanctions can have serious consequences. In addition to compromising hospital or organizational privileges, suspension or expulsion from professional organizations is reportable to the NPDB.

Conclusion

Psychiatrists often assume that because no physician–patient relationship exists in forensic examinations, such examinations and related activities such as writing reports and providing testimony do not create liability exposure. Court decisions and state regulations in recent years have indicated that forensic evaluators in fact owe certain duties to evaluees. Psychiatrists should understand their legal and ethical duties and the potential consequences that may arise from breach of these duties.

Key Concepts

- Although psychiatry is one of the least often sued medical specialties, psychiatrists are exposed to several types of professional liability for forensic activities, including civil lawsuits, criminal prosecution, administrative actions, and peer review actions.

- Courts increasingly are imposing liability on psychiatrists performing forensic activities, such as independent medical evaluations, even in the absence of a treatment relationship.

- To prevail in a malpractice action, the plaintiff must prove that the psychiatrist had a duty, the duty was breached, and the psychiatrist's breach directly caused harm to the patient.

- Malpractice insurers are required to report any malpractice payment made on the insured's behalf to the National Practitioner Data Bank.

- The four possible duties an independent medical evaluation provider may owe to the evaluee are to not injure; to diagnose properly; to inform the evaluee of a serious medical condition; and to maintain confidentiality.

- Psychiatrists providing forensic services are subject to peer review and discipline by the various professional organizations to which they belong.

- Physicians providing forensic services should not assume that their insurance policy covers forensic services and should confirm coverage for those activities with their insurer.

References

Aetna v McCabe, 556 F.Supp. 1342 (1983)

American Medical Association: AMA Code of Medical Ethics: Opinion 1.2.6—Work-Related and Independent Medical Examinations. 2016. Available at: http://www.ama-assn.org/ama/pub/physician-resources/medical-ethics/code-medical-ethics.page. Accessed January 2, 2017.

Appelbaum PS: Law and psychiatry: liability for forensic evaluations: a word of caution. Psychiatr Serv 52(7):885–886, 2001 11433104

Austin v American Association of Neurological Surgeons, 253 F.3d 967 (7th Cir 2001)

Binder RL: Liability for the psychiatrist expert witness. Am J Psychiatry 159(11):1819–1825, 2002 12411212

Cal. Bus. and Prof. Code § 729 (2013)

Clites v Iowa, 322 N.W.2d 917 (Iowa Ct. App. 1982)

Confidentiality of Alcohol and Drug Abuse Patient Records, 42 CFR Part 2 (1987)

Federation of State Medical Boards: Expert witness qualifications: board-by-board overview. 2016. Available at: https://www.fsmb.org/Media/Default/PDF/FSMB/Advocacy/GRPOL_ExpertWitness.pdf. Accessed January 2, 2017.

Gavin v Hilton Worldwide, Inc., 2013 WL 1402350 (N.D. Cal. 2013)

Genetic Information Nondiscrimination Act, 29 CFR § 1635 (2008)

Gold LH, Davidson JE: Do you understand your risk? Liability and third-party evaluations in civil litigation. J Am Acad Psychiatry Law 35(2):200–210, 2007 17592166

Gold LH, Metzner JL: Psychiatric employment evaluations and the Health Insurance Portability and Accountability Act. Am J Psychiatry 163(11):1878–1882, 2006 17074937

Gold LH, Anfang SA, Drukteinis AM, et al: AAPL practice guideline for the forensic evaluation of psychiatric disability. J Am Acad Psychiatry Law 36(4 suppl):S3–S50, 2008 19092058

Graham v Dacheikh, 991 So.2d 932 (Fla. App. 2 Dist. 2008)

Hartogs v Employers Insurance, 89 Misc.2d 468 (1977)

Jena AB, Seabury S, Lakdawalla D, et al: Malpractice risk according to physician specialty. N Engl J Med 365(7):629–636, 2011 21848463

Mazza v Medical Mutual Insurance Co. of North Carolina, 319 S.E.2d 217 (1984)

Miss. Admin. Code 30-17-2635:8.6 (1972)

Mohr JC: American medical malpractice litigation in historical perspective. JAMA 283(13):1731–1737, 2000 10755500

Office of the Attorney General, State of California. Opinion of Bill Lockyer, Attorney General, and Gregory L. Gonot, Deputy Attorney General (03-1201). Available at: http://ag.ca.gov/opinions/pdfs/03-1201.pdf. Updated April 28, 2004. Accessed January 2, 2017.

Pace v Swerdlow, 519 F.3d 1067 (10th Cir. 2008)

Roy v Hartogs, 381 N.Y.S. 2d 587 (1976)

Simon RI, Shuman DW: Conducting forensic examinations on the road: are you practicing your profession without a license? J Am Acad Psychiatry Law 27(1):75–82, 1999 10212028

Standards for Privacy of Individually Identifiable Health Information [Health Insurance Portability and Accountability Act of 1996 Privacy Rule], 45 CFR § 164 (2000)

Studdert DM, Bismark MM, Mello MM, et al: Prevalence and characteristics of physicians prone to malpractice claims. N Engl J Med 374(4):354–362, 2016 26816012

Sugarman v Board of Registration in Medicine, 662 N.E.2d 1020 (Mass. 1996)

Taylor P (ed): New Hampshire Board of Medicine Newsletter. July 2002. Available at: https://www.oplc.nh.gov/medicine/documents/newsletter-november-2001.pdf. Accessed January 2, 2017.

U.S. Department of Health and Human Services, Health Resources and Services Administration: NPDB Guidebook. Rockville, MD, U.S. Department of Health and Human Services, 2015. Available at: http://www.npdb.hrsa.gov/resources/aboutGuidebooks.jsp. Accessed December 31, 2016.

Vanderpool DL: Risk of harm to the forensic expert: the legal perspective, in Ethical Issues in Forensic Psychiatry. Edited by Sadoff RL. New York, Wiley-Blackwell, 2011, pp 197–211

CHAPTER 13

Competencies in Civil Law

Susan Hatters Friedman, M.D.

Ryan C.W. Hall, M.D.

Landmark Case

State v. Hurd, 86 N.J. 525, 432 A.2d 86 (1981)

Capacity (in clinical terms) or *competence* (in legal terms) refers to whether a person has the necessary abilities to adequately make a specific decision (such as to refuse psychiatric treatment) or complete a specific task (such as writing a will). Individuals are not incompetent simply because they have a mental illness. In clinical evaluations and as a matter of law, adults are presumed to be competent until adjudicated otherwise.

The evaluation of capacity or competency is task-specific rather than global. An individual may be competent to complete one task but not another. Evaluators should consider the specific task in question when conducting a competency or capacity evaluation. Competency reports and testimony should explain how specific symptoms functionally impact specific capacities.

In this chapter, we discuss general principles of psychiatric civil competency evaluations. However, legal statutes governing civil competencies vary among jurisdictions. Therefore, evaluators should review relevant local legal standards. Factors often critical in evaluations include the factual understanding of the situation or problems in question and the likely consequences of an action or a decision, the ability to rationally manipulate information and perform tasks, and the communication of choice (Glancy et al. 2015). Cognitive impairments, psychotic symptoms, mood symptoms, or extreme anxiety may affect any or all of these elements of capacity.

Guardianship

A guardian has the legal authority and duty to care for another person and that person's property. The need for a guardian may arise because of a legal status, such as being a minor, or when a person becomes incapacitated or disabled. Most jurisdictions use behavioral functioning, cognitive functioning, or necessity for determining the need for a guardian (American Bar Association Commission on Law and Aging and American Psychological Association 2005). A guardianship is a fiduciary relationship (i.e., another party's interests are placed above the guardian's interests) when making decisions about the ward's person or property (American Bar Association Commission on Law and Aging and American Psychological Association 2005; Soliman and Hall 2015).

The legal theories under which the court can initiate a guardianship are the concepts of *parens patriae* (i.e., the state as a parent) and individual and public welfare. States often limit guardians' authority regarding "extraordinary" treatment such as electroconvulsive therapy, amputations, psychiatric medications, and withdrawal of life-sustaining treatments (American Bar Association Commission on Law and Aging and American Psychological Association 2005; Soliman and Hall 2015). Since a guardianship involves an incapacitated person, the process of establishing a guardianship is almost always involuntary.

Several instruments, such as power of attorney, advance directives, living wills, and pre-need guardianships (legal documents submitted to a court specifying that a guardian is to be appointed if needed), allow individuals to express their wishes while competent. However, these executed documents are not necessarily dispositive and may be revoked or challenged. An allegation of undue influence or lack of free will when the document was executed could be the basis of a legal challenge (American Bar Association Commission on Law and Aging and American Psychological Association

2005; Hall et al. 2005; Soliman and Hall 2015).

Evaluations for purposes of appointing a guardian are more encompassing than other types of capacity evaluations, and multiple types of guardianship exist. *Full guardianship* (also known as *general guardianship*, *plenary guardianship*, or *chancery guardianship*) requires the guardian to make all significant decisions affecting a ward's well-being including physical custody, education, health, activities, and general welfare (American Bar Association Commission on Law and Aging and American Psychological Association 2005). In general, the legal system attempts to limit infringement on people's autonomy. For this reason, least restrictive alternatives to guardianships are often sought, or a guardian may be appointed only for specific or limited tasks, such as

- *Medical treatment or health decisions:* actions necessary to provide medical care, food, shelter, clothing, personal hygiene, or care without which serious and imminent physical injury or illness is likely to occur
- *Financial decisions:* actions necessary to obtain, administer, and dispose of real and personal property, intangible property, business property, benefits, and income

Psychiatrists providing guardianship evaluations should understand the specific type of guardianship being sought.

- *Guardian of estate only (conservator):* makes decisions about money and property.
- *Guardian of person:* makes medical decisions and decisions about placement (e.g., nursing home, hospitalization, rehabilitation).
- *Emergency temporary guardian:* often appointed with a finding by the court

of imminent need such as concerns about safety, physical or mental health dangers, or property being misappropriated.

- *Guardian ad litem, law guardian, or special advocate:* usually a lawyer appointed by the court who appears in a lawsuit or during an emergency court issue on behalf of an incompetent person (or minor) but does not have authority outside of the legal case.

When performing a guardianship evaluation, psychiatrists need to identify the retaining party (e.g., the court, the attorney representing the subject of the evaluation, or the attorney representing the party challenging competency). They also should understand that their role is usually one of independent evaluator and not treatment provider. Most important, psychiatrists should understand why one party believes that the subject needs a guardian, or what medical or psychiatric incapacity is giving rise to the claim of a need for a guardian (American Bar Association Commission on Law and Aging and American Psychological Association 2005). Identification of the reason a guardianship is being pursued helps the expert in obtaining appropriate collateral information, including sworn statements from others involved, medical records, and past legal documents or contracts.

A guardianship report often contains the individual's history, collateral information, mental status examination, diagnosis, prognosis, and potential treatment options (American Bar Association Commission on Law and Aging and American Psychological Association 2005; Glancy et al. 2015). Although treating physicians, including psychiatrists, may provide information regarding need for a guardianship, avoiding dual agency

roles is generally ethically advisable. Ideally, evaluators in guardianship hearings should not be the evaluee's treatment provider (Reid 2008; Strasburger et al. 1997).

Understanding the context in which the question of guardianship arises may help the evaluator assess potential conflicts of interest in others, such as motives for pursuing guardianship or sources of bias in individuals providing collateral information (Hall et al. 2005). The context also will guide the psychiatric evaluator in asking appropriate questions in the evaluation.

For example, an evaluator conducting a financial guardianship evaluation should review financial documents, ask questions related to sources of income and property, and examine how the evaluee makes financial decisions. Extensive questioning about medical information or medical decision making might not be necessary. Financial capacity, that is, the ability to manage financial affairs in one's own interest, requires performance skills such as balancing a checkbook and judgment skills (American Bar Association Commission on Law and Aging and American Psychological Association 2005). Questions might be included about saving for retirement, investments, donations, financial advisers, as well as the thought process involved in making these decisions.

Although an evaluee's psychiatric diagnosis (if any) must be considered and reported, diagnosis alone does not determine whether a guardian is needed. Guardianship evaluations focus on abilities such as executive function, memory, concentration, language, and their effect on daily or specific functioning. Cognitive screening instruments such as the Mini-Mental State Examination, the Montreal Cognitive Assessment, and the Clock Drawing Test are often used to help identify potential deficits (American Bar Association Commission on Law and Aging and American Psychological Association 2005; Hall 2015). Depending on the history and degree of impairment, more in-depth psychometric testing may be warranted (American Bar Association Commission on Law and Aging and American Psychological Association 2005).

A guardianship by its very nature limits an individual's rights. Therefore, courts have developed a system of checks and balances to ensure that a potential ward's rights are not violated. These actions can take the form of reviewing the need for a guardian at regular and specified intervals, such as each year, or at special request; appointing an independent monitor who may investigate, seek information, examine documents, or interview the ward and report findings to the court; or periodically asserting the continued need for guardianship by a health care provider.

The process by which a guardianship is established often begins with a petition to determine incapacity. The petition usually identifies the person bringing the action and the facts explaining why the person filing the petition believes the subject of the petition lacks competency. The finding of incompetency is often determined in a formal court hearing. The legal standard of proof for a finding of incompetency is usually "clear and convincing evidence," and the petitioner bears the burden of proof. Jurisdictions may use the lower standard of "preponderance of the evidence" to terminate a guardianship because maintaining a guardianship violates fundamental rights if it is more likely than not that the subject has regained capacity.

Many jurisdictions have mechanisms for emergency guardianship hearings. However, situations arise in which temporary substitute decision makers need to be identified in time-critical or emergency situations prior to court hearings, especially when health care decisions must be made (Soliman and Hall 2015). Many jurisdictions first will consider previously executed documents such as powers of attorney, advanced directives, or living wills, reflecting an individual's wishes designating a specific decision maker if the person becomes incapacitated. If these documents do not exist, statutes often define a family hierarchical approach, such as spouse, then parents or adult children, then siblings, and so on, for health emergency situations (Shand and Hall 2015; Soliman and Hall 2015). In these situations, surrogates are expected to use either "substituted judgment" to make decisions that the incapacitated person would have wanted or a "best interest" standard if the individual's wishes are unknown or unclear.

Competency to Make Medical Decisions

Competence to make medical decisions is considered in four parts: communication of a choice, ability to understand relevant information, ability to appreciate one's illness and its likely consequences, and rational manipulation of information (Appelbaum and Grisso 1988). The ability to express a choice is impaired if a person cannot clearly communicate. This component is also lacking if a person vacillates about a decision or is unable to maintain a choice long enough for that decision to be implemented. Competence to consent to or refuse treatment involves the ability to provide informed consent (see Chapter 8, "Physician–Patient Relationship in Psychiatry," for further discussion), including understanding the risks of, benefits of, adverse effects of, and alternatives to treatment (American Bar Association Commission on Law and Aging and American Psychological Association 2005; Glancy et al. 2015).

The meaning of *understanding* differs from the meaning of *appreciating* (Saks and Jeste 2006). *Understanding* may be conceptualized as comprehending the meaning of the issues involved in the treatment. *Appreciating* the issue may be understood as grasping how the information about the treatment applies to oneself. To determine either understanding or appreciation, evaluees may be asked to paraphrase the information provided (Appelbaum and Grisso 1988). Delusions, lack of insight, and pathological distortion may affect both understanding and appreciation (Appelbaum 2007). Appreciation also may be affected by psychosis, with lack of insight into the person's own mental or physical illness.

In considering the ability to reason, the evaluator may ask how the subject arrived at the choice, a process that includes consequential thinking, comparative judgments about risk of treatment versus treatment refusal, and probability judgments about the likelihood of outcomes (Saks and Jeste 2006). The evaluee's ability to repeat the information the evaluator has provided is not sufficient. Evaluees should be asked to explain the basis for their decision(s) and the risks and benefits associated with the decision(s) in their own words. Evaluees may express personal considerations in their decision-making process, such as wishes to avoid dependency or pain (American Bar Association Commission on Law and Aging/American Psychological Association Assessment of Capacity in Older Adults Project Working Group 2008).

Rational manipulation of information in this context includes use of logical thinking in comparing risks and benefits

of treatments (Mossman and Shoemaker 2010). Psychosis, dementia, extreme anxiety, or depression may affect these cognitive abilities (Appelbaum and Grisso 1988). The process of decision making, rather than the outcome, is most important. If evaluees can show intact cognitive abilities, they have a right to accept or reject treatments.

Evaluators have to make a judgment regarding the evaluee's level of understanding, appreciation, and reasoning required to make a medical decision (Saks and Jeste 2006). These judgments may differ, depending on the severity of the medical problem and the risks of the procedure. Arguments for a "sliding scale" have been made, with a higher standard applied when considering a more serious medical procedure than that required for a low-risk intervention (American Bar Association Commission on Law and Aging/American Psychological Association Assessment of Capacity in Older Adults Project Working Group 2008).

An evaluee must understand enough to make a reasonable decision but need not understand information at the level of a physician. Similarly, the evaluator must consider how far an evaluee's beliefs or reasoning deviate from social norms before the evaluee may be thought to lack capacity to appreciate the issue in question (Saks and Jeste 2006). Even mentally intact people may make decisions that are not fully rational or that do not follow purely logical decision-making processes. This may be a result of misunderstanding probabilities, fantasies about a physician's unlimited or exceptional skill, or overvaluing the experiences of close friends (Saks and Jeste 2006).

Normal aging, without dementia, leads to changes in cognitive functioning (Gatz 2006). Usually, normal aging most affects short-term memory, as well as learning and retaining new information (Gatz 2006). Memory lapses, such as forgetting someone's name, difficulty multitasking, and slower information processing, also have been noted (Gatz 2006). Thus, considering competency to make a medical decision in an older individual who does not have dementia requires consideration of the cognitive changes associated with normal aging.

Mental illness does not in itself indicate that a person lacks the capacity to make medical decisions (Saks and Jeste 2006). For example, an evaluee may hold a long-standing delusion about being the president of the United States, but this delusion may not impair the understanding of risks of, benefits of, and alternatives to surgery. In addition, although an individual's diagnosis may be stable over time, symptoms can wax and wane, resulting in changes in capacity. In such cases, capacity may best be considered a *state* rather than a *trait* (Saks and Jeste 2006). For example, as dementia progresses, decision-making capacity is often impaired (Mossman and Shoemaker 2010). Minor impairments in comprehension and memory that initially did not limit the person's decision-making capacities may become limiting as impairments worsen.

Evaluating and documenting decision-making capacity should go beyond recording a diagnosis and should include documenting the abilities to understand, appreciate, reason, and communicate choices while recording the evaluee's preferences and values (McSwiggan et al. 2016). The use of psychometric tests or structured judgment instruments should be considered when relevant or appropriate. Unfortunately, studies have found that few capacity evaluations explain the cognitive, functional, and mental health issues that may affect evaluators' conclusions (McSwiggan et al. 2016).

Except in urgent situations, if the cause of incompetency is potentially remediable, then efforts should be made to restore competency (Appelbaum 2007). If such efforts are unsuccessful and the evaluee continues to lack capacity, a substitute decision maker is sought.

In recent years, consideration of capacity has been shifting from an all or none model to one that preserves and promotes autonomy and least restrictive practices. For example, courts and evaluators may be asked to determine what kind of support individuals with "decision-making disabilities" require in order to be most autonomous in their decision making (Peisah et al. 2013). Autonomy is promoted by seeking assent (agreement) rather than consent in minors and adults adjudicated to be incompetent. Shared and collaborative decision making have been suggested, promoting both autonomy and evaluee involvement despite varying abilities. Collaborative decision making focuses on the evaluee's wishes and values, influences how the evaluee makes decisions, and helps promote identity and self-esteem (Peisah et al. 2013).

In the United States, the age of consent for medical procedures varies by jurisdiction (Coleman and Rosoff 2013). In the case of abortions, in most states pregnant minors can bypass parental consent requirements by obtaining judicial authorization (Friedman et al. 2015). Forensic psychiatrists may be asked to evaluate whether the minor is sufficiently mature and well enough informed to decide intelligently whether to have an abortion (Friedman et al. 2015). Alternatively, courts may grant a waiver of parental consent for abortion when parental notification is not in the minor's "best interest." This usually arises in cases in which the minor has been abused, circumstances that evaluators should document in their reports.

Informed consent and decision-making capacity in pregnancy create additional considerations in situations that seemingly place the interests of a pregnant woman and her fetus at odds (Hall et al. 2015). However, treatment issues can be reframed as attempts to find the best option for the mother–fetus dyad. Thus, disclosures should include the potential risks to both mother and fetus of treatment as well as untreated mental illness. This allows the pregnant woman to make her own best decision, with balanced information, after considering the relative risks of potential outcomes (Friedman 2015).

All states allow a competent person to designate a proxy decision maker for medical decisions should the individual become incapacitated, and the capacity to appoint a proxy decision maker may be retained despite a person being found otherwise incompetent in other areas of functioning (Kim and Appelbaum 2006). The capacity required to appoint a proxy decision maker is the cognitive ability to make a meaningful choice about who this decision maker should be (Kim and Appelbaum 2006). Otherwise, the medical decisions made by family members approached for consent may not reflect the views that the individual held when previously competent, for example, before the progression of dementia.

Evaluators should not assume that a person has received all the necessary information because he or she has signed a consent form. Similarly, capacity to consent to research needs to be considered before evaluees sign informed consent forms. Treatment in a research protocol is primarily in the interest of science (and future others) rather than in the interest of the individual research participant (Kim and Appelbaum 2006). The standard to consent to an experimental treatment research project therefore is likely higher than the standard to consent to routine treatment (Saks and Jeste 2006).

Testamentary Capacity

Testamentary capacity is the ability to write a valid will or to execute a valid codicil or addendum to an existing will. Testamentary capacity requires that the testator or testatrix understands what a will is and knows the extent of his or her financial holdings, his or her natural (familial) heirs, the will's effect on others, and the general plan for distribution of the estate (Sageman 2003). The individual must have testamentary capacity at the time the will is executed, not consistently over time, for the will to be valid (American Bar Association Commission on Law and Aging and American Psychological Association 2005).

Many of the elements for assessing testamentary capacity are derived from a judicial opinion in a famous 1870 case, *Banks v. Goodfellow* (Hall et al. 2009; Shulman et al. 2015). Individuals have testamentary capacity if they

- Understand the nature of the act in which they are engaged.
- Appreciate the effect of the act.
- Understand the extent of their property.
- Know their natural heirs.
- Are not influenced by delusions in making the provisions of the will.

Elements of knowledge and understanding need not be exact. For example, individuals executing wills do not need to know the exact dollar value of their stock holdings. However, they do need to show a general understanding of their assets and their approximate current value (Hall et al. 2009).

Some have suggested that when long-held beliefs are abandoned in changing a will, an additional factor to consider is the concept of *stability of beliefs* (e.g., family values, financial beliefs, guiding principles, nature of relationships) or at least whether the individual has a clear rationale for the change (American Bar Association Commission on Law and Aging and American Psychological Association 2005; Hall et al. 2009; Merikangas 2015; Rodgers and Baird 2015; Shulman et al. 2015). This concept has become more important because as average life expectancy increases, the prevalence of dementia is expected to increase (Prince et al. 2013).

Although some argue for a notion of stability in cognition when it comes to making testamentary decisions, other jurisdictions and case law recognize the concept of a *lucid interval* (American Bar Association Commission on Law and Aging and American Psychological Association 2005). This implies that a will is valid even if the evaluee has a waxing and waning illness, as long as the will was executed during a period of functionality (American Bar Association Commission on Law and Aging and American Psychological Association 2005). To preserve a record indicating testamentary capacity, video recordings may be made, especially when beneficiaries anticipate that a will is likely to be contested. However, recordings may not prove testamentary capacity definitively, especially when they have been made under apparent duress. Alternatively, a family member or involved other may make a recording but ask leading questions or questions that do not validate concepts such as appreciation of value or extent of the property. Recordings also may be found to be unreliable when they are placed in the context of additional collateral information (Hall et al. 2009).

Most jurisdictions do not allow for a will to be directly challenged while the testator is living (Hall et al. 2009), so typically testamentary capacity evaluations are conducted postmortem. Therefore, these assessments often rely on review of

- Medical records.
- Collateral information such as written statements, interviews, and depositions of people close to the testator.
- Legal records, including past wills and other contracts that are entered into around the time the will was made.
- Financial records.
- Recordings (in some cases).

In postmortem cases, physicians often comment on how physical illness or medication could have affected the cognitive abilities of the testator, how illnesses typically progress, cognitive abilities in question, and how changes in cognitive abilities could affect relationships and the ability to make decisions.

In some cases, a testamentary assessment will be conducted and documented just before a will is executed as a preventive measure to reduce the likelihood that the will may be overturned later. In these cases, evaluators should review medical, legal, and financial records prior to and concurrent with the capacity evaluation to ensure accuracy of the responses. Although no single question may prove or disprove testamentary capacity in all situations, contemporaneous testamentary capacity evaluations should include questions such as

- Why change your will now?
- Do you understand that the new will invalidates the previous will?
- What are the differences between the old will and the new will?
- What are the important relationships in your life?
- Who did you consider including or not including in the will and why?

TABLE 13–1. **Warning signs for the potential presence of undue influence**

Changes in financial management enrich the new beneficiary.

The testator makes changes to professional services (e.g., new bankers, stockbrokers, attorneys, physicians).

The testator is socially isolated from family, friends, and other stable relationships but not the new beneficiary.

New professional and personal relationships with the testator are formed that involve only individuals approved by the person suspected of undue influence.

New gifts are made to community institutions, such as some portions of funds going to a religious group, charity, or community/government endowment, to encourage support in the community for a relationship involving undue influence.

The person suspected of undue influence moves into the testator's home or controls the testator's schedule.

The testator suddenly develops a mistrust of family members, particularly about financial affairs.

The person suspected of undue influence accompanies the testator to most important transactions, not leaving the testator alone during transactions to speak for himself or herself.

The testator expresses feelings of helplessness or dependency that only the person suspected of undue influence can address (e.g., "He alone prevents me from going to a nursing home").

- What are your important or major assets?
- Why divide the estate in this way?
- How will people feel about this division?
- What are the economic implications to yourself and others (e.g., tax concerns, ease of access to funds)?

Challenges to wills often include the allegation that a beneficiary had *undue influence* over a testator. Therefore, testamentary capacity evaluations often must consider whether a beneficiary has misused or abused a position of trust or power in his or her relationship with the testator such that he or she has deprived the testator of free will (American Bar Association Commission on Law and Aging/American Psychological Association Assessment of Capacity in Older Adults Project Working Group 2008; Hall et al. 2005). Table 13–1 reviews warning signs of undue influence.

In considering the issue of undue influence, in addition to actions directly taken by another, an evaluator may need to consider factors such as

- Physical limitations that place a testator at risk for becoming isolated.
- Sensory loss, such as vision or hearing impairment, that makes it harder for the testator to communicate or obtain information.
- Effects of medications that may cloud cognition or be used to manipulate a testator, such as pain or anxiety medications being withheld or given as a way to punish or reward behavior.
- Manipulation of testator by controlling access to addicting substances such as alcohol or cigarettes (e.g., "Do as I say, or you will not be able to smoke").

Capacity to Contract

A contract is a legally binding agreement voluntarily made between two parties. A higher level of capacity is required to enter into a contract than is required to make a will because a contract involves a competing interest. In a will, a testator is distributing his or her own assets; in a business contract, the person is contracting with another entity that has different interests. Questions about capacity to contract might be raised after an unusual contract is made by someone who was in the throes of mania, psychosis, intoxication, or dementia.

Competency to enter into a contract requires meaningful understanding of the nature, terms, and effects of the contract (Mossman and Shoemaker 2010; Sageman 2003). If the business transaction in a contract is complicated, a higher level of understanding may be needed. The most important test for this capacity therefore focuses primarily on cognition.

In an evaluation of capacity to enter a contract, questions should be posed about the meaning of the contract, its terms, and its permanency. Do evaluees understand what they are losing or gaining? Do they understand that the contract is permanent rather than temporary? For example, how do evaluees explain selling their property at a lower-than-market value price, and are the reasons given rational or irrational? What do the evaluees believe will happen if the contract does not go through? Was the contract influenced or motivated by delusional thinking?

Competency to enter into a marriage contract might be raised as an issue by the family of a person with an intellectual disability, severe mental illness, or dementia (Sageman 2003). To be competent to marry, evaluees should understand the nature of marriage and the obligations and duties it entails.

Competence to divorce may gain importance over time because of an aging population susceptible to dementia and the increased social acceptability and frequency of divorce (Mossman and Shoemaker 2010). Symptoms of mental illness may cause persons seeking divorce to make judgments not in their own best interests during the litigation or may not recognize the potential significant negative outcomes of a divorce. Capacity to divorce is similar to capacity to contract. Evaluators should assess whether the evaluee has the capacity to understand the meaning of divorce, can express a clear and consistent desire for divorce for reality-based reasons, and can understand and participate in divorce proceedings (Mossman and Shoemaker 2010). Evaluators could ask how divorce was decided on, how the person believes divorce will affect him or her, and what the person believes will happen should he or she not obtain a divorce (Mossman and Shoemaker 2010). The presence of delusional reasons for seeking a divorce also should be explored.

Testimonial Capacity

Testimonial capacity is the ability, when testifying in court, to remember and report what has been observed and understanding the importance of doing so accurately. Testimonial capacity involves cognitive, memory, and communication skills. It requires the ability to recall information about the subject at issue and the ability to understand the legal duty to testify truthfully. In simpler terms, testimonial capacity requires a cognitive ability to distinguish between the truth and a lie, a moral understanding that lying is bad, and a practical understanding that lying in court could result in punishment.

Adult witnesses are presumed to be competent, unless shown to be incompetent, under Rule 601 of the Federal Rules of Evidence (2017a). Three requirements for any witness to be competent to testify include 1) the person's cognitive and moral abilities being of a sufficient level (Myers 1993), 2) personal knowledge of the relevant facts (under Rule 602 of the Federal Rules of Evidence [2017b]), and 3) the understanding of the religious oath or secular affirmation to testify truthfully (under Rule 603 of the Federal Rules of Evidence [2017c]).

Concerns have been raised for centuries regarding children's ability to testify (Friedman and Howie 2013). Children as young as 3 years may be competent to testify (Myers 1993). Children by age 3 or 4 years can tell the difference between the truth and a lie, or real from pretend. They also know that they could be punished for lying. Young children may be asked obvious true-or-false questions to ascertain their knowledge and ability to tell the truth, such as "I am a woman. Is that true or not true?" Obviously, questions posed to young children should use simple language.

In testimonial capacity evaluations of individuals with mental illness, opinions should explain why specific symptoms impair a witness's relevant functional capacities and recommend approaches that may optimize the witness's function. For example, in the case of a young child or someone with intellectual disability, evaluators might recommend that simply worded questions be used in court.

A psychiatric evaluation of competence to testify is not commonly required if an adult witness or older child witness has intelligence levels that fall within normal ranges. However, psychiatrists may be asked to evaluate younger children. A psychiatrist also might be asked to evaluate the ability to form memories, communicate appropriately, and appreciate the meaning of the oath in witnesses with intellectual disability, dementia, or a substance use disorder.

Less commonly, testimonial capacity may be questioned in persons with psychotic disorders because of impaired reality testing and judgment (Melamed 2008). Symptoms of posttraumatic stress disorder in a child, including intrusive thoughts about the defendant and avoid-

ant behavior, also can interfere with testimonial capacity (Quinn 1986). Psychiatrists may be called to educate the jury about child development and recall and recognition memory.

Five cognitive capacities are required to be able to testify (Myers 1993). These include the ability to

1. Observe.
2. Demonstrate memory.
3. Communicate (when developmentally appropriate questions are posed).
4. Distinguish the truth from a lie.
5. Understand the obligation to tell the truth in testimony.

When evaluating testimonial capacity, psychiatrists should avoid suggesting or creating new memories. They should begin by obtaining a free narrative through open-ended questions and avoid leading questions. Psychiatrists should consider the following issues:

- Does the evaluee appreciate the meaning of the oath and the meaning of truth and lies and what can happen if he or she lies in court?
- How does the evaluee understand the event? Does this comport with collateral data?
- Does the evaluee have the capacity to lay down new memories and to retrieve them?
- Is the evaluee especially suggestible? (Young children may be more suggestible to authority figures.)

Additionally, evaluation of testimonial capacity should take place in a single examination, because repeated interviews lead to the risk of introducing material to those who are suggestible.

Evaluators should use caution in differentiating evaluations of credibility or truthfulness from issues of testimonial competency (Quinn 1986). Credibility of testimony is the purview of the fact finder, and expert testimony on credibility is not admissible. Assessment of lying is not outside the ken of the layperson or within the special knowledge of psychiatry. Rather, as noted earlier in this chapter, the evaluator should assess whether the evaluee understands the difference between the truth and a lie and the risk of perjury.

A witness's suggestibility also may require some comment. Suggestibility is a type of memory distortion related to repetitive or misleading questions and a desire to please (Bala et al. 2010). This occurs more commonly among children, especially under circumstances when children might be repetitively questioned by a parent. Young children in particular may feel that they need to provide some answer to questions, even when they actually do not know the answer (Bala et al. 2010) or if questioned by an authority figure.

Hypnotically refreshed testimony can be excluded in a person who otherwise has testimonial capacity. The state bears the burden of proof of the acceptability of the victim's hypnotically enhanced testimony with a "clear and convincing evidence" standard. Psychiatrists may be called to testify about hypnosis and its reliability. *State v. Hurd* (1981) considered the admissibility of a victim's testimony that was hypnotically enhanced to refresh memory about a crime. Concerns about the reliability of hypnosis-enhanced witness memory led to the court's adoption of six procedural safeguards, often referred to as the Orne criteria (so-called after their developer, Dr. Martin Orne), to decrease the risk of biased testimony:

1. The hypnotist should be a psychiatrist or psychologist trained in hypnosis.
2. The hypnotist should be an independent professional.
3. Information given to the examiner about the case should be written rather than verbal.
4. Victims should be examined before the hypnosis to determine what facts they recall.
5. The hypnosis should be video recorded.
6. Only the victim and hypnotist should be present in the session.

The hypnotist should have no preconceptions about the perpetrator in order to avoid the risk that the victim may confabulate to please the hypnotist.

Firearms Capacity

Federal law prohibits individuals who have been adjudicated as mentally ill (meaning primarily individuals who have been civilly committed) from owning firearms (American Psychiatric Association 2014; Fisher et al. 2015; Hall and Friedman 2013; Price et al. 2016). Many states have passed additional restrictions that make it easier for people with suspected mental illness to be placed in firearm-prohibited categories. For example, in 2014, Florida passed a law allowing admitting physicians to submit paperwork to the courts indicating that individuals involuntarily brought to the hospital for evaluation would have been involuntarily committed if they had not voluntarily agreed to psychiatric admission (Florida Statute 790.065(2)(I)4, 2014). A magistrate of the court then reviews the paperwork and can adjudicate the person as unfit to own a firearm.

The National Instant Criminal Background Check System Improvement Amendments Act of 2007 encouraged states to establish procedures for restoration of firearm rights to those who were barred because of mental health adjudications (Gold and Vanderpool 2016; Price et al. 2016). Jurisdictions approach removal from the list in different ways, such as legislating time limits before a due process claim to restore the right to own firearms can be sought (e.g., 5 years) or allowing that a person may reach a level of stability or that the person is no longer "disabled" (Gold and Vanderpool 2016; Simpson 2007). Some states do not require medical or psychiatric opinions in the restoration process (Fisher et al. 2015). However, increasing numbers of individuals prohibited for mental health reasons are seeking to have their firearm rights restored, resulting in the need for psychiatric opinions regarding the ability to safely own firearms (Gold and Vanderpool 2016; Simpson 2007).

Firearm capacity involves assessment of both current and future risk. People with mental illness who are compliant with treatment may be no greater risk to the general population than are other members of a community (Monahan et al. 2001). A history of civil commitment has not been shown to be the best long-term marker for gun violence or lack of firearm capacity (Gold and Vanderpool 2016). For example, someone involuntarily committed for severe depression may go years or a lifetime without a recurrence. However, there is no guarantee that an individual will remain compliant with treatment or that individuals who are currently psychiatrically stable will remain so.

Gun restoration evaluations, also known as *relief from disability evaluations*, are a relatively new and unique type of capacity evaluation. These evaluations combine traditional capacity questions that address current state abilities with risk assessment evaluations based on probabilities for the future and the need for treatment. Other risk assessment evaluations may serve as an initial framework

for the evaluation (e.g., police officer returning to duty) but may not fully meet the needs for general firearm capacity involving a broad population (Anfang et al., in press; Gold and Vanderpool 2016). In addition, other capacity evaluations result in documents or actions that can be revisited if capacity changes in the future (such as establishing an irrevocable trust), whereas firearm capacity fluctuations can result in very real future danger.

Evaluators providing firearm capacity evaluations, especially if not indemnified by state law, may increase their liability exposure if they find that someone has current capacity only to have an event occur at some unknown time in the future. Liability issues may become a significant concern, given that risk assessment accuracy generally decreases over time, and most states do not identify or require the evaluator to comment on likelihood for deterioration of capacity. Moreover, although laws appear to be written to prevent mass shootings, a far more likely outcome is self-harm (American Psychiatric Association 2014; Gold 2013; Hall and Friedman 2013).

Evaluators therefore should clearly define the limitations of their opinions and the evidence base on which they rely when providing firearm capacity evaluations. For example, caution may be needed in how the violence risk assessment portion of the evaluation is presented, because instruments such as the Historical Clinical Risk Management 20, Classification of Violence Risk, and Violence Risk Assessment Guide may not be normed specifically for this population (see Chapter 28, "Violence Risk Assessment"). For example, tools normed on mentally ill offenders may not adequately address self-harm risk for the general population with mental illness (Fisher et al. 2015; Friedman et al. 2013; Gold and Vanderpool 2016).

As in other capacity evaluations, the evaluator should obtain appropriate collateral information, including medical records relevant to the initial loss of gun rights, records pertaining to past violence, military records, current treatment records, and potential criminal records. In addition, evaluations should address diagnosis, violence history and risk, self-harm risk, and insight into the need to continue treatment (Fisher et al. 2015). Prognosis and stability with and without treatment also may be more important because gun ownership may take future risk into account.

As in other types of forensic evaluations, optimally, evaluators should not be the evaluee's treatment provider. This helps maintain the objectivity of the evaluation and reduces the risk that the evaluation will interfere with the physician–patient relationship. In addition, evaluators conducting assessments of their own patients may increase their potential liability if a negative outcome occurs (Gold and Vanderpool 2016).

Conclusion

Competency is specific to a particular issue. Evaluations should consider not only the diagnosis but also the symptoms that specifically impair the capacity to perform the task or act in question. The capacity to perform one act is not necessarily the same as the capacity to perform a different act. These abilities, and thus the person's capacity, may change over the course of time, such as with disease progression or treatment.

Key Concepts

- Adults are considered competent unless adjudicated otherwise.

- Competency is task-specific or act-specific. Evaluators should consider the effect of specific symptoms on the specific act at issue.

- In cases of capacity to make medical decisions, the person must be able to understand and appreciate the information about the treatment, its risks, and the risks of not treating; manipulate information rationally; and communicate a decision.

- A person may be competent to make a will (distributing assets) and at the same time not be competent to enter into a contract because of the requirement to consider competing interests.

- Testamentary capacity requires that at the time of execution of a will, the testator knew the nature and extent of his or her financial holdings, the persons who would naturally inherit, and the cogent reasons for his or her disposition choices.

- Testimonial capacity requires the ability to recall facts about the issue and the understanding of the duty to testify truthfully, a separate issue from credibility.

- Firearm restoration evaluations are a unique type of capacity evaluation in which risk of danger to self and others also must be considered.

References

American Bar Association Commission on Law and Aging and American Psychological Association: Assessment of Older Adults With Diminished Capacity: A Handbook for Lawyers. Washington, DC, American Bar Association and American Psychological Association, 2005. Available at: http://www.apa.org/pi/aging/resources/guides/diminished-capacity.pdf. Accessed January 2, 2017.

American Bar Association Commission on Law and Aging/American Psychological Association Assessment of Capacity in Older Adults Project Working Group: Assessment of Older Adults With Diminished Capacity: A Handbook for Psychologists. Washington, DC, American Bar Association and American Psychological Association, 2008. Available at: https://www.apa.org/pi/aging/programs/assessment/capacity-psychologist-handbook.pdf. Accessed January 2, 2017.

American Psychiatric Association: Position statement on firearm access, acts of violence and the relationship to mental illness and mental health services. Approved by the Board of Trustees, December 2014. Approved by the Assembly, November 2014. Available at: https://www.psychiatry.org/file%20library/about-apa/organization-documents-policies/policies/position-2014-firearm-access.pdf. Accessed January 2, 2017.

Anfang SA, Gold LH, Meyer DJ: Guideline for the forensic assessment of disability. J Am Acad Psychiatry Law (in press)

Appelbaum PS: Clinical practice: assessment of patients' competence to consent to treatment. N Engl J Med 357(18):1834–1840, 2007 17978292

Appelbaum PS, Grisso T: Assessing patients' capacities to consent to treatment. N Engl J Med 319(25):1635–1638, 1988 3200278

Bala N, Evans A, Bala E: Hearing the voices of children in Canada's criminal justice system: recognising capacity and facilitating testimony. Child Family Law Quarterly 22:21–45, 2010

Banks v Goodfellow, LR 5 Q.b. 549 (1870)

Coleman DL, Rosoff PM: The legal authority of mature minors to consent to general medical treatment. Pediatrics 131(4):786–793, 2013 23530175

Federal Rules of Evidence: Rule 601: competency to testify in general, in Federal Rules of Evidence, 2017 Edition. 2017a. Available at: https://www.rulesofevidence.org/article-vi/rule-601. Accessed January 2, 2017.

Federal Rules of Evidence: Rule 602: need for personal knowledge, in Federal Rules of Evidence, 2017 Edition. 2017b. Available at: https://www.rulesofevidence.org/article-vi/rule-602. Accessed January 2, 2017.

Federal Rules of Evidence: Rule 603: oath or affirmation to testify truthfully, in Federal Rules of Evidence, 2017 Edition. 2017c. Available at: https://www.rulesofevidence.org/article-vi/rule-603. Accessed January 2, 2017.

Fisher CE, Cohen ZE, Hoge SK, et al: Restoration of firearm rights in New York. Behav Sci Law 33(2–3):334–345, 2015 25711715

Florida Statute §790.065(2)(I)4 (2014)

Friedman SH: The ethics of treating depression in pregnancy. J Prim Health Care 7(1):81–83, 2015 25770721

Friedman SH, Howie A: Salem witchcraft and lessons for contemporary forensic psychiatry. J Am Acad Psychiatry Law 41(2):294–299, 2013 23771943

Friedman SH, Hall RCW, Sorrentino RM: Commentary: women, violence, and insanity. J Am Acad Psychiatry Law 41(4): 523–528, 2013 24335325

Friedman SH, Hendrix T, Haberman J, et al: Judicial bypass of parental consent for abortion: characteristics of pregnant minor "Jane Doe's." J Nerv Ment Dis 203(6):401–405, 2015 26034870

Gatz M: Cognitive capacities of older adults who are asked to consent to medical treatment or to clinical research. Behav Sci Law 24(4):465–468, 2006 16883616

Glancy GD, Ash P, Bath EP, et al: AAPL practice guideline for the forensic assessment. J Am Acad Psychiatry Law 43(2 suppl): S3–S53, 2015 26054704

Gold LH: Gun violence: psychiatry, risk assessment, and social policy. J Am Acad Psychiatry Law 41(3):337–343, 2013 24051585

Gold LH, Vanderpool D: Relief from disabilities, in Gun Violence and Mental Illness. Edited by Gold LH, Simon RI. Arlington, VA, American Psychiatric Association Publishing, 2016, pp 339–380

Hall RCW: Mental status: examination, in Wiley Encyclopedia of Forensic Science, 2015, pp 1–8. Available at: http://onlinelibrary.wiley.com/doi/10.1002/9780470061589.fsa287.pub2/full. Accessed January 2, 2017.

Hall RCW, Friedman SH: Guns, schools, and mental illness: potential concerns for physicians and mental health professionals. Mayo Clin Proc 88(11):1272–1283, 2013 24138962

Hall RCW, Hall RCW, Chapman MJ: Exploitation of the elderly: undue influence as a form of elder abuse. Clin Geriatr 13:28–36, 2005

Hall RCW, Hall RCW, Myers W, et al: Testamentary capacity: history, physicians' role, requirements, and why wills are challenged. Clin Geriatr 17:18–24, 2009

Hall RCW, Friedman SH, Jain A: Pregnant women and the use of corrections restraints and substance use commitment. J Am Acad Psychiatry Law 43(3):359–368, 2015 26438814

Kim SYH, Appelbaum PS: The capacity to appoint a proxy and the possibility of concurrent proxy directives. Behav Sci Law 24(4):469–478, 2006 16883617

McSwiggan S, Meares S, Porter M: Decision-making capacity evaluation in adult guardianship: a systematic review. Int Psychogeriatr 28(3):373–384, 2016 26412394

Melamed Y: Testimony by mentally ill individuals. J Am Acad Psychiatry Law 36(3):393–397, 2008 18802190

Merikangas JR: Commentary: Contested wills and will contests. J Am Acad Psychiatry Law 43(3):293–297, 2015 26438806

Monahan J, Steadman HJ, Silver E, et al: Rethinking Risk Assessment: The MacArthur Study of Mental Disorder and Violence. New York, Oxford University Press, 2001

Mossman D, Shoemaker AN: Incompetence to maintain a divorce action: when breaking up is odd to do. St Johns Law Rev 84:117–197, 2010

Myers JEB: The competence of young children to testify in legal proceedings. Behav Sci Law 11:121–133, 1993

Peisah C, Sorinmade OA, Mitchell L, et al: Decisional capacity: toward an inclusionary approach. Int Psychogeriatr 25(10):1571–1579, 2013 23809025

Price M, Recupero PR, Norris DM: Mental illness and the National Instant Criminal Background Check System, in Gun Violence and Mental Illness. Edited by Gold LH, Simon RI. Arlington, VA, American Psychiatric Association Publishing, 2016, pp 127–158

Prince M, Bryce R, Albanese E, et al: The global prevalence of dementia: a systematic review and metaanalysis. Alzheimers Dement 9(1):63–75.e2, 2013 23305823

Quinn KM: Competency to be a witness: a major child forensic issue. Bull Am Acad Psychiatry Law 14(4):311–321, 1986 3801683

Reid WH: The treatment-forensic interface. J Psychiatr Pract 14(2):122–125, 2008 18360199

Rodgers C, Baird JA: Commentary: The lucid interval: coping with unscientific terminology. J Am Acad Psychiatry Law 43(3):298–299, 2015 26438807

Sageman M: Three types of skills for effective forensic psychological assessments. Assessment 10(4):321–328, 2003 14682478

Saks ER, Jeste DV: Capacity to consent to or refuse treatment and/or research: theoretical considerations. Behav Sci Law 24(4):411–429, 2006 16883609

Shand JP, Hall RCW: Consent in psychiatric emergencies: what clinicians need to know. Psychiatr Times 32:17–20, 2015

Shulman KI, Hull IM, DeKoven S, et al: Cognitive fluctuations and the lucid interval in dementia: implications for testamentary capacity. J Am Acad Psychiatry Law 43(3):287–292, 2015 26438805

Simpson JR: Bad risk? An overview of laws prohibiting possession of firearms by individuals with a history of treatment for mental illness. J Am Acad Psychiatry Law 35(3):330–338, 2007 17872555

Soliman S, Hall RCW: Forensic issues in medical evaluation: competency and end-of-life issues. Adv Psychosom Med 34:36–48, 2015 25832512

State v Hurd, 86 N.J. 525, 432 A.2d 86 (1981)

Strasburger LH, Gutheil TG, Brodsky A: On wearing two hats: role conflict in serving as both psychotherapist and expert witness. Am J Psychiatry 154(4):448–456, 1997 9090330

CHAPTER 14

Personal Injury

Kenneth J. Weiss, M.D.

Clarence Watson, J.D., M.D.

Landmark Cases

Dillon v. Legg, 68 Cal. 2d 728, 441 P.2d 912 (1968)

Ibn-Tamas v. U.S., 407 A.2d 626 (D.C. 1979)

Whereas the aim of criminal law is intended, in part, to maintain social control, civil law is concerned with settling disputes between parties, whether individuals, groups, corporate entities, or governments. The essential format is that one party, the plaintiff, alleges having been wronged by the other party, the defendant, and seeks monetary damages. Thus, through a bit of legal logic, compensation would make the plaintiff "whole." Alternatively, the defendant could be found blameless.

Unlike criminal justice, with rights in favor of the defendant, civil lawsuits, in theory, begin with a level playing field. Besides medical malpractice, civil litigation most relevant to psychiatrists is the resolution of personal injury claims. Be-

cause civil cases are about money rather than freedom, expert witnesses may be under great pressure from retaining attorneys, whose clients have much to gain or lose.

Mental health professionals often evaluate claims of emotional distress or psychiatric injury brought about by a defendant's actions or inaction. Personal injury may be claimed as a result of negligence, intentional or unintentional, or violation of law, such as discrimination or harassment. Forensic psychiatrists are asked to determine whether the plaintiff was injured and, if so, to assess causality (if applicable), degree of impairment, and prognosis. Such assessments are among the most complex and ethically challenging tasks within forensic psychiatry.

Legal Principles

The notion that a person who has been intentionally or negligently injured by another should be financially compensated for those injuries is a fundamental tenet of civil law. We live in a litigious society in which private wrongs, whether legitimate or frivolous, are brought before the civil court system in pursuit of legal remedies. Although such avenues for compensation are likely to be taken for granted now, ancient legal systems offered no such remedies (Wigmore 1894).

Personal injury law, or *tort law*, allows an injured party to be financially made "whole" by the person causing the injury. Unlike criminal law, in which the government prosecutes defendants for unlawful acts against citizens or society in general, civil tort lawsuits involve a plaintiff suing a defendant to rectify the private wrongs or injuries experienced by the plaintiff. If successful in proving a defendant's liability for those injuries, usually by a standard of preponderance of the evidence, a plaintiff may recover a judgment of monetary damages meant to compensate the plaintiff for those injuries.

Contemporary tort law in the United States evolved from ancient Anglo-Saxon customs in which laws were limited to crimes against the social group, and private wrongs received little to no legal cure. At that time, private injuries were resolved within the context of a clan system, in which blood feuds or private wars were used to exact vengeance for such injuries (Stone 1950). Gradually, in an effort to reduce claim-based violence between clans, the introduction of monetary payments in lieu of feud became an option in settling private claims. Under that system, the injuring party could choose to feud or to provide money to the injured party. Eventually, the amount of money, or the "bot," awarded to the injured party was set by public decree and depended on the type of injury suffered (Nordstrom 1966).

Law of Torts

Tort law can be divided into three categories, depending on the nature of the defendant's conduct: strict liability, intentional torts, and negligent tort. *Strict liability* involves a defendant's liability for a plaintiff's injuries even when the defendant did not intend to harm the plaintiff and otherwise acted with care. In other words, a defendant may be deemed liable without evidence of fault. The plaintiff's claim simply must show that the defendant marketed, manufactured, or sold a defective product (e.g., seat belt or airbag) that caused harm to the plaintiff during the intended use of the product.

Intentional torts involve a defendant acting in a specific manner to produce a particular result. Intentional torts include assault, battery, and infliction of mental or emotional distress. Assault involves an individual intentionally causing apprehension of harmful or offensive contact in another. Battery, by contrast, is the intentional infliction of actual harmful or offensive contact. A claim of intentional infliction of emotional distress may be substantiated when a plaintiff can prove that a defendant wanted to cause the plaintiff emotional distress, knew (or should have known) with substantial certainty that the plaintiff would experience emotional distress, and recklessly disregarded the high probability that the plaintiff would experience emotional distress.

In claims of intentional infliction of emotional distress, the plaintiff must prove what was in the mind of the defendant—that the defendant intended to cause harm. The plaintiff also must show that the defendant's intentional behavior was extreme and outrageous and that the plaintiff suffered actual severe emotional distress. Typically, the measure of severe distress is based on whether a reasonable person in the plaintiff's position would have experienced that distress. However, when a defendant has knowledge that a plaintiff is particularly sensitive or emotionally vulnerable, those particular characteristics of the plaintiff are taken into account, and the reasonable person standard may be set aside.

Negligent torts involve a defendant's careless conduct that places the plaintiff at unreasonable risk of harm, and injury occurs. In order to establish that a defendant's conduct was negligent, plaintiffs must prove several elements. First, they must prove that the defendant had a legal duty to behave in a certain manner. For example, a licensed driver has a legal duty to operate his or her vehicle in a manner that avoids unreasonable risk of harm to fellow motorists and pedestrians. Second, plaintiffs must prove that the defendant breached that legal duty and created an unreasonable risk of harm. Third, plaintiffs must establish that the defendant's conduct was the proximate cause of the harm suffered. Lastly, plaintiffs must show that they experienced actual damages.

Damages

In intentional tort lawsuits, plaintiffs are not required to experience or prove actual physical harm in order to recover financial damages awards. In those cases, nominal damages may be awarded to a plaintiff even if no physical harm has occurred. For example, a plaintiff who becomes frightened by a defendant's intentional and outrageous conduct may be awarded a nominal amount that recognizes the plaintiff's claim. Compensatory damages may be awarded in cases in which physical injury occurs, including

pain and suffering, medical expenses, and other economic losses. In addition to nominal and compensatory damages, a plaintiff in an intentional tort case may be awarded punitive damages when the defendant's conduct is considered outrageous or malicious. Such awards are intended to penalize defendants financially for their conduct and typically involve large monetary sums.

Generally, a plaintiff filing a negligence claim must prove that an actual physical injury was caused by a defendant's conduct in order to recover damages. Accordingly, nominal damages are not awarded in negligence lawsuits. Once a plaintiff proves that actual physical harm was inflicted, the plaintiff may be awarded damages for economic loss, pain and suffering, mental distress associated with the injury, and "hedonic" damages related to plaintiff's loss of ability to enjoy previous life activities. Punitive damages usually are not awarded unless the defendant's negligent behavior is deemed particularly reckless or "willful and wanton."

Zone of Danger

Although physical injuries are generally expected to form the basis of a negligence lawsuit, in certain circumstances, a plaintiff may recover damages for mental distress alone. A defendant may be liable for the mental suffering of plaintiffs who fall "within the zone of danger" of the defendant's negligence. For example, if a defendant causes an accident and a plaintiff is close enough to be in danger of immediate bodily injury but escapes physical harm, the defendant may be liable for the plaintiff's resulting emotional distress. Severe emotional distress in these cases may involve the plaintiff having various psychiatric disorders including anxiety, depression, and posttraumatic stress disorder (PTSD).

Defendants also may be found liable for negligent infliction of emotional distress in situations in which a plaintiff is not within the zone of danger but is instead a bystander. In **Dillon v. Legg** (1968), the plaintiff, Margery Dillon, was crossing a street with her two daughters. The defendant, Mr. Legg, while driving his car, struck and killed one of the children. Dillon filed suit against Legg, seeking damages for her deceased daughter, her surviving daughter, and herself. The trial court granted Legg's motion for summary judgment, based on the argument that Dillon was not "within the zone of danger." On appeal, the California Supreme Court reversed the trial court's decision, stating that the zone of danger for emotional injury was broader than that for physical danger and that no distinction could be drawn between physical and emotional injury.

Thus, a plaintiff who witnesses a close relative endure sudden and serious bodily injury caused by a defendant's negligence may recover damages for mental suffering without being in the physical zone of danger. Typically, these cases require that the close relative be a child, spouse, parent, or sibling of the plaintiff. Circumstances that may increase or decrease the mental distress include whether the plaintiff was close enough to the scene to witness the accident directly or whether the plaintiff's shock arose from hearing about it after the accident. Both circumstances are compatible with the DSM-5 diagnostic criteria for PTSD (American Psychiatric Association 2013).

Eggshell Plaintiff Doctrine: Relevance of Predisposing Factors

Under common law, a defendant may not escape liability for a plaintiff's inju-

ries simply because the plaintiff has a preexisting condition, including a psychiatric disorder that creates susceptibility to experiencing harm that the defendant could not foresee (*Vosburg v. Putney* 1891). Accordingly, a plaintiff's preexisting condition, which contributes to a more serious injury than would have been expected, will not negate damages owed by the defendant. Therefore, the defendant takes the plaintiff as he or she finds him or her and is responsible for all causally related damages, even though the plaintiff was more susceptible to injury because of a preexisting condition.

Assessing the Personal Injury Plaintiff

The general method and format for the examination of the plaintiff follows the outline described in the American Academy of Psychiatry and the Law (AAPL) Guideline for Forensic Assessment (Glancy et al. 2015) and elsewhere in this volume. The following annotations apply to personal injury evaluations.

From the Top Down

Whether retained by plaintiff or defense counsel, the essential elements of a psychiatric evaluation include agency, purpose, scope, one or more legal questions to be illuminated, the review of documents, the examination itself, and collateral sources. If a report is requested, these elements should be addressed in the written work product.

Agency

The expert witness's client is either plaintiff or defense counsel. The retaining attorney typically will vet the expert for qualifications, experience, publications relevant to the matter at hand, and testimony in prior cases. Testifying uniformly across cases is not essential; however, disparities in an expert's prior testimony will be exploited during deposition or trial. Generally, experts are required or asked to produce a list of prior cases in which they provided testimony so that both parties can determine whether the expert typically testifies for plaintiffs or defendants. If the balance is highly skewed, then attorneys may make claims of bias.

In regard to the business aspects of forensic psychiatric practice, most expert witnesses issue retaining agreements specifying terms: hourly rates versus flat rates, compensation for time blocked out for depositions and testimony, cancellation fees, and so forth. Experts should receive a retainer fee, when possible, before commencing work, with the expectation of further billing and full compensation at the time a report is issued. Compensation should come directly from the attorney's office or firm. Retaining attorneys also should understand that an expert's opinions are independent and may or may not be useful in supporting or refuting a claim. When experts are retained by defense attorneys, experts' opinions can range anywhere from total rebuttal of the plaintiff's expert to complete agreement.

Purpose and Scope

The underlying legal question should be straightforward: Does the individual have a mental disorder or suffering as a result of the alleged incident? If so, what is the disorder, how long will it last, what constitutes appropriate treatment, and how much will treatment cost? Often, the psychiatric expert will offer opinions exclusively on the "damages" side of the litigation (e.g., the medical conditions payable to the plaintiff) and not at all on the "liability" side (e.g., fault in accidents,

problems with products, whether discrimination or harassment occurred). The expert's opinions should respond to the questions asked and not stray into the domain of the fact finder.

In cases in which traumatic brain injury (TBI) is alleged, the forensic psychiatrist may request that a formal neuropsychological assessment and/or neuroimaging be conducted by respective professionals, while retaining overall assessment of mental health (see Chapter 5, "Psychological Testing in Forensic Psychiatry," and Chapter 7, "Neuroimaging and Forensic Psychiatry"). Psychiatrists should be aware that performing psychometric tests without adequate training, applicable certification, or experience can spell disaster for the admissibility, weight, or credibility of their opinions. Similarly, although the literature on TBI and mild TBI and concussion is helpful, such disorders are typically beyond the scope of the general psychiatrist (Katz et al. 2015). However, relying on the findings of other professionals (e.g., psychologists, neurologists, neuroradiologists) is acceptable practice; other professionals' findings inform psychiatric opinions and give them additional dimension.

Materials

Expert witnesses are entitled to use a variety of materials. The range of records that might be available for review is summarized in Table 14–1 (Ciccone and Jones 2010). Although psychiatric history may not detract from the current claim of injury, evaluating psychiatrists need to develop an understanding of the plaintiff's lifetime functioning, both before and after the event in question. Thus, while the eggshell plaintiff rule prevails, the expert witness's role is to attribute the contribution of the event to the plaintiff's subsequent functioning and provide a determination of its net effect.

TABLE 14–1.   Personal injury evaluations: relevant records

Medical records	Nonmedical records
Medical and psychiatric treatment records, including laboratory and imaging reports	Police records, including witness statements
Hospitalization records	Workplace accident reports
Substance use disorder treatment records	Legal records, including other expert reports
Psychological test results and reports	Employment records
Pharmacy records	Military records
Emergency department records, including records from prior to the event	Financial records
Ambulance, first-responder reports	Academic records

Source.   Adapted from Ciccone and Jones 2010.

Assessing Causation: Independent Medical Examination

Although attributing causation may seem straightforward when the sequence of events suggests it, causation in forensic psychiatric evaluations requires careful attention. Plaintiff's attorneys often claim that the event in question caused all the subsequent problems in a plaintiff's life, not just psychiatric problems. Defense counsel typically seeks to attribute a plaintiff's psychiatric symptoms to causes other than the defendant's behavior.

Causality: Physical-Mental or Mental-Mental?

Personal injury claims include nonpsychiatric damage to the body (*physical*) and traumatic experiences that leave psychiatric sequelae (*mental-mental*). Pain and disability contributing to mental disorders (*physical-mental*) further complicate forensic evaluation. Physical damage to the brain may require both neuropsychological and neuropsychiatric evaluations (see Chapters 5 and 7 for further discussion). The psychiatric expert witness in physical-mental cases may not have to opine on the original causation; rather, opinions may be requested regarding whether a direct link exists between the physical injuries and the resultant mental state.

In mental-mental cases, a statement of causality typically is requested, although the form of causation opinions may vary by jurisdiction. In some jurisdictions, causation is not a required expert opinion or is a determination made by the trier-of-fact (i.e., judge or jury). The plaintiff must prove that "but for" the defendant's negligence, harm would not have occurred. Generally, experts use language such as "the mental disorder was a direct result of the accident" or "the accident was a substantial factor in bringing about the mental condition." The legal term *proximate cause* expresses the same concept, underscoring that the behavior of the defendant and not some intervening act brought about damage to the plaintiff. If a preexisting mental disorder was exacerbated, the language can be modified accordingly.

Reports must reflect the language requirements of the jurisdiction, in terms of both causality and degree of scientific certainty. The expert witness may need to carefully parse out the causal nexus and what is or is not attributable to the event, remembering that the defendant may be liable for the plaintiff's episode of psychiatric illness indexed to the event. In reports focusing on psychiatric damages and not on liability, the language should steer clear of statements about the defendant's negligence. For example, a psychiatric expert witness would not be addressing negligence of a surgeon, no matter how obvious, only the physical-mental connection. In all cases, expert opinions must be expressed explicitly in locally appropriate language reflecting "reasonable scientific [or medical or psychiatric] certainty." This standard is the 50.01% or more likely than not rule. Anything less will be viewed as inadmissible speculation.

Avoiding Bias

Unless solicited by a neutral mediator, psychiatric examinations of personal injury litigants are not strictly "independent"; rather, they represent partisan work products. In some jurisdictions, the use of the term *independent medical examination* is banned from any documents related to workers' compensation claims or in cases in which the evaluating physician is paid by an insurance company (e.g., Delaware Code Online 1999). The goal of making injured persons "whole" through financial damage awards is achieved through an adversarial process that creates pressures on expert witnesses. For example, plaintiffs' attorneys may portray their clients as having PTSD, a favored plaintiff's diagnosis (see "Posttraumatic Stress Disorder" section later in this chapter). Similarly, defense attorneys often urge evaluators to seek alternative causes for the plaintiff's distress—specifically, causes for which the defendant could not be liable. Of course, a plaintiff may have both an alternative cause of

stress or a preexisting vulnerability and a new injury or an exacerbation of a preexisting injury for which the defendant may be liable.

Forensic psychiatrists should always be mindful of these expectations to avoid bias in their evaluations, opinions, and reports. The forensic psychiatrist's task is to elucidate mental health issues as objectively as possible (American Academy of Psychiatry and the Law 2005). The expert's findings may not be entirely congruent with the attorney's expectations but should not be subject to revision by or negotiation with retaining counsel. Attorneys are free to retain other experts to render opinions should they be dissatisfied with one expert's conclusions.

Assessing Damages

Expert witnesses do not directly quantify monetary awards but aid in the calculation by prognosticating recovery (or permanence) and treatment needs. The evaluation often is complicated by the presence of physical injury, and the psychiatrist's opinion therefore may rely on a prognostication of conditions outside general psychiatric knowledge. In these cases, psychiatrists should be certain to use all expert reports, including those of other health professionals, vocational specialists, and forensic economists.

Damages Due to Pain

Chronic pain conditions present particularly complex issues. If the underlying physical condition is deemed permanent, the psychiatric expert can suggest a treatment plan based on the patient's resilience and capacity to adjust to pain or loss of function. However, the medical determination of degrees and permanence of pain itself relies on the patient's subjective reports. Objective measures for assessing pain are still lacking (Greely 2015). Although the forensic expert's experience may provide a guideline for matching congruence of pain with the nature and extent of injuries, such experience is not necessarily adequate. Experts should consider and respect variability in pain thresholds and tolerance and should not simply conclude that an evaluee is magnifying discomfort.

Hedonic Damages

Over time, the jurisprudence of personal injury claims has permitted inclusion of nonphysical injuries for the fact finder's consideration. The pain and suffering associated with physical injury may be self-evident and not require dedicated expert testimony, but some plaintiff attorneys will want a more detailed analysis of the relation between the alleged harm and the quality of life. These matters are often referred to as *hedonic* injuries because they encompass the capacity to derive pleasure from life. Forensic evaluators therefore need to understand the effect of the alleged injury on the plaintiff's social and interpersonal functioning and relationships (Weiss 2011). These types of damages include diminished interest in social and leisure activities, feelings of detachment or distance in important relationships, and anhedonia. Irrespective of whether hedonic damages are separately compensable, the forensic evaluator should document the evaluee's experiences in this regard.

Posttraumatic Stress Disorder

PTSD was first included in DSM-III (American Psychiatric Association 1980). Attorneys quickly realized that PTSD, by

definition, indicates causality and provided a gateway to damages (Smith 2011). Documented vehicle accidents, natural disasters, victimizations, and similar subjectively traumatic events obviate, in many cases, the need for expert testimony on causality. Other issues, such as the severity of the condition, its duration, related impairments, and recommended treatment, still require assessment.

DSM-5 (American Psychiatric Association 2013) has provided more support for claims of trauma, especially under the new category, "Trauma- and Stressor-Related Disorders," which permits a dimensional approach to trauma-related diagnoses, from adjustment disorders through PTSD (Levin et al. 2014). From a lawyer's perspective, a PTSD diagnosis or another diagnosis from DSM-5's "Trauma- and Stressor-Related Disorders" amounts to "diagnosing liability" (Smith 2011). The trauma criterion for PTSD has been expanded in DSM-5 and now includes learning about a traumatic event occurring to a close family member or friend, without directly experiencing or witnessing it. However, evaluators still must determine whether the event in question constitutes a traumatic event, distinguishing it from an ordinary stressor that elicits either a pathological reaction (adjustment disorder) or a normative response (no psychiatric diagnosis).

A clinical presentation must include significant distress or functional impairment to be classified as a mental disorder. In the adversarial justice system, expert witnesses may feel pressure to diagnose PTSD or a less causally certain condition, such as major depressive disorder. Unlike the clinical treatment situation, in which the patient's narrative is accepted as true, no such attitude can prevail in the forensic setting. Forensic professionals are faced with the task of assessing the traumatic event and the proportionality of the reported subjective symptoms (Simon 2008). The detection of functional impairment may be aided by collateral interviewing of family members or others, when feasible.

According to DSM-5, a traumatic event must be personal, potent, and unusual. Plaintiff and defendant may agree on exposure to a traumatic stressor, such as a witnessed accident, or contest traumatic exposure, such as in unwitnessed harassment. Regardless, forensic psychiatrists should bear in mind that the quality and intensity of a person's reported symptoms do not validate the factual basis of a traumatic event. The error of assuming that because an individual has a diagnosis of PTSD, the individual must have experienced the traumatic exposure as claimed is not uncommon. However, neither the factual basis of the alleged trauma nor the reported symptoms can be accepted at face value in the setting of litigation. In addition, courts are not likely to admit opinions that use syndromes not recognized as psychiatric diagnoses in DSM-5, such as battered-spouse syndrome, to imply verification of an alleged traumatic stressor (see, e.g., *Ibn-Tamas v. U.S.* 1979).

Clinical Guidance

Forensic professionals should be vigilant for feigned, rote, or rehearsed responses designed to establish a diagnosis of PTSD. Not everyone exposed to a traumatic stressor develops PTSD. The reasons for the variability undoubtedly involve combinations of personal experience, genetic and epigenetic factors, and unknown constitutional vulnerabilities or protections. Many persons' stress responses resolve over time, whereas others' are chronic and unremitting. Given the eggshell plaintiff doctrine, defense experts using research into vulnerability and genomics may have little traction

(Sharma et al. 2016; Skelton et al. 2012). Neuroplasticity and psychological resilience also may play a role in healing from trauma but currently cannot be measured for prognostication (Kays et al. 2012). For example, reduced hippocampal volume may be associated with PTSD, but whether this is the result of psychic trauma or a preexisting risk factor for the development of PTSD is not clear (Kays et al. 2012).

Objective Testing

The validation and quantification of PTSD symptoms in litigation are similar to that in clinical practice. No single test constitutes a gold standard for the psychometric assessment of PTSD in the personal injury context, especially in regard to assessing malingered PTSD (Guriel and Fremouw 2003). Some clinicians prefer to administer broad-spectrum inventories, such as the Minnesota Multiphasic Personality Inventory–2 or the Millon Clinical Multiaxial Inventory—4th Edition. These tests are used to obtain evidence of inconsistencies and feigning and to explore differential diagnostic possibilities. Several other instruments have been designed to assess specifically for malingering in presentations of PTSD symptoms (see Chapter 6, "Evaluation of Malingering"). However, forensic psychiatrists without appropriate training who administer such inventories and simply append the database-generated report run the risk of undermining the credibility of their opinions. A psychologist trained in the interpretation of the instrument would be in a better position to explain the findings and defend the methodology.

Clinical rating instruments that focus on specific dimensions of PTSD may have utility. However, forensic psychiatrists are well advised to be able to show evidence of training and experience in their use. The best known is the Clinician-Administered

PTSD Scale for DSM-5 (CAPS-5; Weathers et al. 2013). This instrument can aid clinicians in establishing current PTSD and changes in an individual's PTSD over time, which can track treatment response. The CAPS-5 requires an index trauma and is susceptible to confirmation bias. Accordingly, clinicians using assessments such as CAPS-5 should be mindful of the litigation context and of the reliability of the subjective responses of the evaluee. Neither the CAPS-5 nor another instrument replaces the clinical examination, but its validity and reliability add weight to interview findings.

The Report

Forensic experts should not issue a report until the retaining attorney requests that they do so. Evaluators should first discuss the findings with the attorney. Whereas a written report is "discoverable," discussions with the attorney constitute work product and are not discoverable. Attorneys may not wish to use the expert's findings, and they may not want documentation of findings or opinions that are not supportive of their client's case. Reports should be fair and comprehensive, showing an understanding of the case and the evaluee (Norko and Buchanan 2011), and in keeping with the American Academy of Psychiatry and the Law's (2005) ethical admonition of striving for objectivity.

Reviewing a report with attorneys can be helpful in identifying errors such as mistaken dates or typos. Many experts bristle when asked to make changes. Given the fact that the expert's findings represent one piece of evidence in a complex matter, such requests should be taken seriously and changes made that do not alter the essential findings. On the other hand, the expert's opinions, if conscientious and honest responses to the legal questions posed, should not be altered. For example, requests to change a diagnosis from adjustment disorder to PTSD or to revise an opinion about prognosis to appear better or worse invade the expert's autonomy and should be politely declined.

Conclusion

The assessment of personal injuries contains a microcosm of principles within the practice of forensic psychiatry. Evaluations tax many core skills of evaluators: interviewing, data interpretation, differential diagnosis, appreciation of the multiple forces acting on persons, ability to convey a person's narrative in writing, cause-and-effect reasoning, and mindfulness of the ethical principles that underlie the work. The complexity of these evaluations renders adherence to ethical principles of striving for objectivity all the more imperative.

Key Concepts

- Claims of personal injury can be made on the basis of emotional damage (e.g., posttraumatic stress disorder) or physical injury producing emotional damage (e.g., chronic pain and disability) or both.

- The expert witness should review available objective and corroborating evidence, because the plaintiff's claims of emotional distress are often based largely on self-report.

- Forensic clinicians consulting in lawsuits should be vigilant for pressure from attorneys and to remain objective.

- The diagnosis of posttraumatic stress disorder should be supported by clinical data, not simply checklists, and will be scrutinized for conformity to DSM-5 criteria.

- Psychometric testing, when applicable, should be conducted by a clinician trained in the use of the instrument and who can support its validity and reliability in an evidentiary hearing.

- Malingering of psychiatric symptoms always should be considered in a personal injury claim.

- The forensic report should "connect the dots" between the event in question and the clinical condition of the plaintiff, specifically stating causality in the language of the jurisdiction.

References

American Academy of Psychiatry and the Law: Ethics Guidelines for the Practice of Forensic Psychiatry. May 2005. Available at: http://www.aapl.org/ethics.htm. Accessed June 12, 2017.

American Psychiatric Association: Diagnostic and Statistical Manual of Mental Disorders, 3rd Edition. Washington, DC, American Psychiatric Association, 1980

American Psychiatric Association: Diagnostic and Statistical Manual of Mental Disorders, 5th Edition. Arlington, VA, American Psychiatric Association, 2013

Ciccone JR, Jones JCW: Personal injury litigation and forensic psychiatric assessment, in The American Psychiatric Publishing Textbook of Forensic Psychiatry, 2nd Edition. Edited by Simon RI, Gold LH. Arlington, VA, American Psychiatric Publishing, 2010, pp 261–282

Delaware Code Online: Chapter 206: Formerly Senate Bill No. 150: An Act to Amend Title 19 of the Delaware Code Relating to Worker's Compensation. July 20, 1999. Available at: http://delcode.delaware.gov/sessionlaws/ga140/chp206.shtml#TopOfPage. Accessed January 2, 2017.

Dillon v Legg, 68 Cal. 2d 728, 441 P.2d 912 (1968)

Glancy GD, Ash P, Bath EP, et al: AAPL practice guideline for the forensic assessment. J Am Acad Psychiatry Law 43 (2 suppl): S3–S53, 2015 26054704

Greely HT: Neuroscience, mindreading and the courts: the example of pain. J Health Care Law Policy 18:171–206, 2015

Guriel J, Fremouw W: Assessing malingered posttraumatic stress disorder: a critical review. Clin Psychol Rev 23(7):881–904, 2003 14624820

Ibn-Tamas v U.S., 407 A.2d 626 (D.C. 1979)

Katz DI, Cohen SI, Alexander MP: Mild traumatic brain injury, in Handbook of Clinical Neurology, Vol 127 (3rd Series), Traumatic Brain Injury, Part I. Edited by Grafman J, Salazar AM. Amsterdam, The Netherlands, Elsevier BV, 2015, pp 131–155

Kays JL, Hurley RA, Taber KH: The dynamic brain: neuroplasticity and mental health. J Neuropsychiatry Clin Neurosci 24(2): 118–124, 2012 22772660

Levin AP, Kleinman SB, Adler JS: DSM-5 and posttraumatic stress disorder. J Am Acad Psychiatry Law 42(2):146–158, 2014 24986341

Nordstrom RJ: Toward a law of damages. Case West Reserve Law Rev 18(1):86–102, 1966

Norko MA, Buchanan A: Introduction, in The Psychiatric Report: Principles and Practice of Forensic Writing. Edited by Buchanan A, Norko MA. Cambridge, UK, Cambridge University Press, 2011, pp 1–9

Sharma S, Powers A, Bradley B, et al: Gene x environment determinants of stress- and anxiety-related disorders. Annu Rev Psychol 67:239–261, 2016 26442668

Simon RI: Forensic psychiatric assessment of PTSD claimants, in Posttraumatic Stress Disorder in Litigation, 2nd Edition. Edited by Simon RI. Washington, DC, American Psychiatric Publishing, 2008, pp 41–90

Skelton K, Ressler KJ, Norrholm SD, et al: PTSD and gene variants: new pathways and new thinking. Neuropharmacology 62(2):628–637, 2012 21356219

Smith DM: Diagnosing liability: the legal history of posttraumatic stress disorder. Temple Law Rev 84:1–69, 2011

Stone FF: Touchstones of tort liability. Stanford Law Rev 2:259–284, 1950

Vosburg v Putney, 80 Wis. 523, 50 N.W. 403 (Wis. 1891)

Weathers FW, Blake DD, Schnurr PP, et al: The Clinician-Administered PTSD Scale for DSM-5 (CAPS-5). 2013. Available at: https://www.ptsd.va.gov/professional/assessment/adult-int/caps.asp. Accessed January 2, 2017.

Weiss KJ: Forensic musings: the metaphysics of "hedonic loss." Am J Forensic Psychiatry 32:5–16, 2011

Wigmore JH: Responsibility for tortious acts: its history. Harv Law Rev 7:315–337, 1894

CHAPTER 15

Psychiatric Evaluation in Discrimination and Harassment Claims

Liza H. Gold, M.D.

Landmark Cases

Meritor Savings Bank v. Vinson, 477 U.S. 57, 106 S.Ct. 2399 (1986)

Harris v. Forklift Systems, Inc., 510 U.S. 17, 114 S.Ct. 367 (1993)

Oncale v. Sundowner Offshore Services, Inc., 523 U.S. 75, 118 S.Ct. 998 (1998)

Bragdon v. Abbott, 524 U.S. 624, 118 S.Ct. 1952 (1998)

Olmstead v. L.C. ex rei. Zimring, 527 U.S. 581, 119 S.Ct. 2176 (1999)

United States v. Georgia, 546 U.S. 151, 126 S.Ct. 877 (2006)

Psychiatric evaluations can become central in the resolution of workplace conflict or litigation involving disability claims, need for accommodations, causation, damages, and other issues. Mental and emotional injuries constitute the bulk of exposure in much federal and civil employment litigation (McDonald and Kulick 2001). Psychiatrists can best assist attorneys, employers, insurers, or finders of fact by providing opinions regarding relevant psychiatric issues based on careful evaluation of the totality of circumstances in each case.

This chapter reviews the salient psychiatric issues in the evaluation of the employment discrimination and harassment claims. Legal claims of harassment, discrimination, and/or retaliation may be brought under the 1964 Civil Rights Act (CRA) or state civil rights anti-discrimination statutes, the Age Discrimination in

Employment Act (1967), the Americans with Disabilities Act (ADA) (1990), or through the U.S. Equal Employment Opportunity Commission (EEOC) or its state equivalents. Many employment claims are filed jointly, often with personal injury claims such as wrongful termination or intentional infliction of emotional distress, with multiple complaints arising from the same incident(s).

Identifying the Legal and Psychiatric Issues in Employment Claims

Workplace complaints of discrimination and harassment are common. In fiscal year 2015, the EEOC received almost 90,000 complaints of discrimination, resulting in 356.6 million dollars of monetary benefits to claimaints (Equal Employment Opportunity Commission [EEOC] 2016a). Almost 64,000 of these were discrimination claims under Title VII of the CRA: about 28,000 were harassment charges; about 31,000 were claims of racial discrimination; and about 40,000 were claims of retaliation. About 27,000 were claims of disability discrimination in violation of the ADA (EEOC 2016a).

Psychiatric issues in employment related harassment and discrimination claims, including personal injury claims, typically involve at least one of the following three areas of assessment (Gold et al. 2016):

- Whether the employee has a psychiatric diagnosis, and if so, its duration, symptoms, and prognosis.
- Whether the disorder has resulted in a work-related impairment.
- The etiology or causation of the disorder and, specifically, its relationship to the evaluee's work.

Table 15–1 identifies which combination(s) of these three categories are relevant in specific types of employment litigation.

Anti-Discrimination Laws

Anti-discrimination laws have been enacted to address and prevent disparate treatment of specific classes of individuals in the workplace. Title VII of the 1964 Civil Rights Act (CRA) and parallel state statutes prohibit discrimination on the basis of sex, gender, race, color, religion, age, or national origin. The CRA was amended in 1978 to include discrimination on the basis of pregnancy (EEOC 1978). Notably, federal law does not protect individuals from private sector employment discrimination on the basis of sexual orientation, although this may be changing (see EEOC 2016b). However, federal government employees are protected from this type of discrimination, and about half of all states also have laws prohibiting discrimination on the basis of sexual orientation (Ritter 2016).

The CRA and additional federal and state statutes have created a variety of avenues in addition to those provided by tort litigation through which individuals who believe they have been unfairly treated in the workplace can seek legal redress. The CRA also established the EEOC to enforce federal anti-discrimination statutes; many states and smaller jurisdictions have similar enforcement agencies.

Workplace discrimination against women and racial minorities, although often more subtle than in the past, is the most common type of discrimination claim. However, employment discrimination is not limited to these groups (Stockdale et al. 2015). Disparate treatment of a

TABLE 15–1.   **Summary of salient issues in employment evaluations**

Type of claim or evaluation	Legal or statutory definition of psychiatric disability/ impairment	Degree of impairment or injury relevant	Prognosis relevant	Causation relevant	Liability relevant
Discrimination/ retaliation Civil rights	No	Yes	Yes	Yes	Yes
ADA	Yes	Yes	Possibly	No	No
Personal Injury	No	Yes	Yes	Yes	Yes

ADA=Americans with Disabilities Act of 1990.

protected group may include harassment, discrimination, or unequal treatment on the basis of sex, gender, religion, national origin, pregnancy, or age (and in some cases, sexual orientation); disparities in pay or employment patterns; and limited occupational choices for men or women or for members of racial or religious groups.

As more federal and state statutes against workplace harassment and discrimination have been enacted over past years, employment litigation has increased (see EEOC 2016a). Virtually every federal employment discrimination lawsuit contains an allegation that the plaintiff suffered mental and emotional distress at the hands of the defendant employer (McDonald and Kulick 2001); many are filed jointly with tort claims such as negligent or intentional infliction of emotional distress. Thus, forensic psychiatrists are frequently asked to provide evaluations and testimony regarding psychiatric injury, causation, diagnosis, and prognosis.

Discrimination Law and Sexual Harassment

A review of the evolution of sexual harassment law, a unique type of employment discrimination, demonstrates the dynamic nature of employment discrimination law in the past decades. The EEOC first defined sexual harassment in 1980 as "unwelcome sexual advances, requests for sexual favors, and other verbal or physical conduct of a sexual nature." The EEOC (1980) stated this conduct constitutes illegal sexual harassment when

1. Submission to such conduct is made either explicitly or implicitly a term or condition of an individual's employment.
2. Submission to or rejection of such conduct by an individual is used as the basis for employment decisions affecting such individual.
3. Such conduct has the purpose or effect of unreasonably interfering with an individual's work performance or creating an intimidating, hostile, or offensive working environment.

The essential component of sexual harassment is "unwelcome conduct" (i.e., conduct lacking the elements of choice and mutuality) based on sex or gender and increasingly, sexual orientation. Sexual harassment is the only form of discrimination in which conduct must be demonstrated to be unwelcome. Overt or covert coercion in sexual harassment or discrimination typically relies on the power of the perpetrator to affect a target's economic status. Thus, sexual harassment and gender discrimination are not necessarily motivated by sexual interest or attraction.

The EEOC has defined two types of sexual harassment: *quid pro quo* and hostile work environment. *Quid pro quo* harassment refers to situations in which work conditions or job benefits are explicitly or implicitly contingent upon or involve the exchange of sexual favors. *Quid pro quo* sexual harassment was established as a form of illegal sexual discrimination under Title VII in 1976 (see *Williams v. Saxbe* 1976). *Hostile work environment* sexual harassment refers to continuous, frequent, or repetitive patterns of offensive and unwelcome behavior that adversely affect the terms or conditions of employment. This category encompasses discrimination on the basis of gender alone, and can include behaviors such as sexually oriented joking or teasing, unwelcome displaying of sexual images or objects, unwelcome touching or propositions, or hostile treatment based solely on gender (EEOC 1980).

The U.S. Supreme Court established that hostile environment sexual harassment was also a violation of Title VII in *Meritor Savings Bank v. Vinson* (1986). In *Meritor*, the Court held that to prevail in a hostile environment claim, the unwelcome or offensive behaviors must be so pervasive, repetitive, or severe that they alter the conditions of employment and create an abusive working environment. The Court also ruled that a plaintiff's voluntary participation in the alleged behavior did not legally establish that the defendant's actions were welcome.

In *Meritor*, Michelle Vinson was terminated after a 4-year sexual relationship with her supervisor, Sidney Taylor. Ms. Vinson claimed that she had participated in the relationship because she feared losing her job. A federal district court held that Ms. Vinson was not the victim of sexual harassment because the sexual relationship was voluntary. However, the Supreme Court held that the proper inquiry regarding a sexual harassment claim was not whether a plaintiff's participation was voluntary, but whether the behavior was unwelcome.

In *Harris v. Forklift Systems, Inc.* (1993), the Supreme Court unanimously held that a plaintiff is not required to suffer psychological harm or prove that she was psychologically injured in order to prevail in a sexual harassment claim. Teresa Harris alleged that the president of Forklift Systems, Inc., Charles Hardy, created a hostile work environment through his abusive, vulgar, and offensive sexual comments and actions. His reported conduct included calling Ms. Harris "a dumb ass woman" and requesting that Ms. Harris and other female employees retrieve coins from the front pockets of his pants. Ms. Harris quit and filed a sexual discrimination suit under Title VII.

The court stated that the presence of psychological harm is relevant to determining whether the plaintiff found the environment abusive, but is not necessary to establish illegal discrimination. While acknowledging the lack of a precise test to determine whether an environment is hostile or abusive, the Court stated that all circumstances should be evaluated. These include the frequency of the conduct, its severity, whether the conduct was physically threatening or humiliating or was merely an offensive comment, and whether it unreasonably interfered with an employee's work performance. The Court also stated that both objective and subjective perspectives must be considered in determining the validity of the claim.

In *Oncale v. Sundowner Offshore Services, Inc.* (1998), the Supreme Court ruled that same-sex harassment could constitute an illegal form of sex discrimination under Title VII. Joseph Oncale worked on an oil platform with seven other men for Sundowner Offshore Services, Inc. Coworkers labeled Mr. Oncale a "homosexual" and subjected him to offensive and humiliating behaviors, including threatening him with rape and sodomizing him with a bar of soap. Mr. Oncale complained to supervisors, who took no action. Mr. Oncale filed a complaint, stating he was being subjected to discrimination because of his gender. The Supreme Court unanimously held that Title VII protection in the workplace applies to same-sex harassment and other types of sexual harassment not motivated by "sexual desire." The Court concluded that regardless of the gender of the victim or perpetrator, any type of discrimination based on sex may be actionable if it objectively disadvantages the victim in the workplace.

Thus, illegal "sex-based" discrimination encompasses behaviors based on biological sex and on social and cultural gender constructs, such as targeting individual men or women due to failure to conform to gender stereotypes (see *EEOC v. Boh Brothers Construction Co.* 2013; *Price Waterhouse v. Hopkins* 1989). Notably, the percentage of men filing sexual and gender-based harassment claims has steadily increased in the wake of these and other decisions, from 9.1% in 1992 to 17.1% in 2015 (EEOC 2016a).

Filing a Harassment or Discrimination Claim

The EEOC enforces federal statutes that prohibit harassment, discrimination, and retaliation against individuals who have filed good faith complaints or participated in investigatory proceedings. The facts of a case may support a variety of legal claims, alone or in conjunction with a Title VII action. However, Title VII requires that plaintiffs must exhaust EEOC administrative remedies for claims of discrimination and retaliation before jurisdiction in federal district court can be granted. Filing a claim under state antidiscrimination laws may be a more desirable option for plaintiffs wishing to expedite proceedings, since state laws do not require exhausting EEOC remedies before litigating.

Psychiatric Issues in Title VII Claims

Psychiatrists retained in harassment and discrimination cases may be asked to address causation of emotional injury, psychological symptoms and/or diagnoses, related functional impairment, and issues relating to treatment, treatment costs, and prognosis (Gold 2004). These evaluations require the identification of psychiatric disorders, present and past level of functioning, and likelihood of recovery. Questions regarding prognosis, with and without treatment, which require assessment of the plaintiff's motivation for recovery, are relevant to legal damage assessments.

The psychiatric outcome of workplace experiences such as harassment and discrimination depends on multiple factors and circumstances (Gold 2004; Vasquez et al. 2003). Psychiatric factors that may affect claims of causation and damages should also be considered, such as possible alternate causation of claimed emotional distress and pre-existing mental health disorders or problems. Nonpsychiatric factors, such as adverse employment actions (e.g., being laid off due to a reduction in force or being placed on a

TABLE 15–2.   Relevant factors in harassment and discrimination evaluations

Characteristics of the harassment or discrimination: frequency, duration, magnitude

Plaintiff's emotional, psychological, and workplace responses to the harassment

If the plaintiff complained, the employer's responses to the complaints and/or harassment

Availability of support for the plaintiff inside and outside the workplace

Plaintiff's resources, strengths, vulnerabilities

Plaintiff's past psychiatric history

Plaintiff's employment history

Potential psychological symptoms or effects of underlying medical conditions or medications

Previous or concurrent trauma, sources of stress, or distress

Plaintiff's present or past substance use history

Effects of adverse employment actions or workplace conflict

Effects of litigation (see, e.g., Strasburger 1999)

Emotional effects of retaliation, if clinically distinct from the effects of the claimed harassment

performance improvement plan) and workplace conflict (with coworkers or supervisors) should also be examined. Table 15–2 provides a review of issues that should be assessed.

The issues of functional impairment, prognosis, and potential recovery are integral to damage assessments. Current level of impairment is assessed through evaluation of the claimant's history, behavior, and examination findings. The claimant's pre- and post-incident(s) functional capacities should be compared. Prognostic opinions should be based on an assessment of functioning, the effects of preexisting and current psychiatric status, the natural history of the specific disorder, and the actual or potential effects of treatment. Comparison of the plaintiff's personality, behavior, employment history and functioning before and after the alleged harassment or discrimination is crucial in assessments of changes in functioning and in the determination of motivation for recovery and willingness to enter treatment (Gold 2004).

Motivation to obtain treatment can be particularly problematic in the context of litigation. Plaintiffs are legally obligated to minimize their damages. Nevertheless, plaintiffs may focus on legal issues rather than on accessing treatment, which often prevents resolution of psychiatric symptoms. Even when plaintiffs obtain treatment, the stress of litigation typically exacerbates symptoms, particularly when litigation becomes more active, for example, before a deposition or trial (Lawson and Fitzgerald 2016; Strasburger 1999).

A review of all relevant documents and a thorough psychiatric evaluation can provide information relevant to many of the psychiatric and legal issues in harassment and discrimination cases. Clinicians should conduct a clinical interview, record review, and, when possible, collateral interviews with third parties. They should obtain as extensive a history as possible, including review of past and current sources of trauma and distress, and review of the claimant's litigation history, employment history, and history of interpersonal relationships. Record review should include medical, legal, psychiatric, pharmacy, EEOC, investigative, and employment records. In cases in which civil charges are filed in conjunction with or after the filing of criminal charges such as assault, battery, or rape, police records may be available.

Attorneys may exert pressure on experts to provide opinions beyond the boundaries of the expert's psychiatric training and experience, and sometimes past the boundaries of the field of psychiatry. Evaluators should decline to provide opinions outside their areas of expertise or opinions properly decided by the finder of fact. Psychiatrists should avoid providing opinions for which a scientific basis is lacking or which are essentially legal arguments or determinations and not psychiatric conditions, such as the credibility of the plaintiff or the plaintiff's allegations or, in sexual harassment claims, whether the alleged behavior was unwelcome.

Each case must be assessed based on its own merits and the totality of related circumstances. Relevant social science can be used to support opinions, but research findings cannot provide data about individual cases. Forensic clinicians should base their opinions on the case's specific facts and data and should be prepared to defend those opinions on that same basis. Besides the fact that a command of relevant data is an essential component of competent forensic practice, familiarity with the specific facts of the case will help overcome legal arguments that an expert's testimony is not relevant and therefore should not be admitted (Gold 2004; Goodman-Delahunty and Foote 2013).

Psychiatric Diagnoses in Employment Litigation

Systematic psychiatric assessment should integrate legal concepts of causation with the nature and extent of any injury, whether discrimination was the likely proximate cause, and effects on functioning (Goodman-Delahunty and Foote 2013). Harassment or discrimination may be, and often is, adversely correlated with job-related, psychological, and physical outcomes but the severity of the harassment is usually the primary predictor of psychological outcome (Bergman et al. 2012; Foote and Goodman-Delahunty 2005; Gold 2004). More severe outcomes in response to less severe harassing behaviors raise issues of preexisting psychiatric vulnerability, alternative causation, or malingering. Psychological testing can be helpful in diagnostic assessment and in discriminating malingered symptoms (see Chapters 5, "Psychological Testing in Forensic Psychiatry," and 6, "Evaluation of Malingering").

Posttraumatic Stress Disorder

Posttraumatic stress disorder (PTSD) is a commonly claimed and preferred plaintiff's diagnosis in civil litigation, including harassment and discrimination cases. More than any other diagnosis, PTSD implies single and external causation and focuses attention on the alleged event(s) rather than on the plaintiff (Kilpatrick and McFarlane 2014; Simon 2002). Plaintiffs in employment-related litigation often claim that workplace events such as job loss or verbal outbursts by a supervisor have caused PTSD. Likewise, treating mental health clinicians will frequently and mistakenly diagnose any stress-related response or symptom related to an adverse work experience as PTSD, particularly in the context of litigation (Rosen 1995).

The question of whether harassment and discrimination, particularly sexual harassment, can be a form of trauma that may cause PTSD is a matter of continuing debate (see, e.g., Fitzgerald et al. 2013). However, most people exposed to traumatic stressors do not develop PTSD (Breslau 2009; Kessler et al. 1995). Exposure to interpersonal conflict or unwanted job loss, whether discriminatory or not, or the more common and less severe behaviors associated with harassment and discrimination, can be distressing and stressful. However, such adverse experiences are not traumatic stressors and are unlikely to result in the development of PTSD absent a preexisting vulnerability or additional traumatic circumstances (Breslau 2009; Raabe and Spengler 2013). For example, as explicitly noted in the *Diagnostic and Statistical Manual of Mental Disorders,* 5th Edition (DSM-5), being fired does not constitute a traumatic stress that meets Criterion A, the gatekeeper criterion, for a diagnosis of PTSD (see American Psychiatric Association 2013, p. 279).

An individual who claims or demonstrates symptoms consistent with PTSD as a result of exposure to less severe, infrequent, or low magnitude forms of harassment and discrimination should be carefully assessed for the possibility of malingering, individual susceptibility to psychiatric morbidity, preexisting psychiatric disorders, or concurrent or prior traumatic exposure (Gold 2004; Lawson et al. 2013). A thorough assessment should consider possible alternative causes of trauma and non-work-related stress or distress.

Personality Disorders

Just as PTSD is a preferred plaintiff's diagnosis in employment litigation, Cluster B personality disorders, particularly borderline personality disorder (BPD), is a preferred defense diagnosis. Plaintiffs diagnosed with personality disorders provide opportunities for defendants to support legal arguments that

- A "reasonable person" would not have found the alleged behaviors unwelcome or discriminatory;
- A plaintiff misinterpreted or misperceived the alleged behaviors; and/or
- The plaintiff was "hypersensitive" or had an overly exaggerated reaction

to objectively mild or non-offensive behavior.

In addition, a personality disorder usually becomes recognizable during adolescence or early adult life and so, by definition, is a preexisting condition. Psychiatric evaluation in harassment and discrimination cases should include consideration of behavioral patterns or cognitive processes that might affect interpersonal relationships or cause perceptual distortion. Determination of an individual's tendency to invite, misinterpret, distort, or overreact to the behaviors of others is a critical part of a harassment or discrimination assessment, whether due to BPD or any other psychological process, such as an underlying psychosis or paranoid thought disorder.

However, forensic evaluators should be cautious about making a personality disorder diagnosis based solely on the events in the case and especially in the absence of an adequate longitudinal history that supports a personality disorder diagnosis (Gold 2004; Goodman-Delahunty and Foote 2013). A diagnosis of a personality disorder should be based on lifelong, pervasive, and inflexible patterns of dysfunction and maladaptive coping (see American Psychiatric Association 2013). Individuals with personality disorders typically have histories of chaotic lives, dysfunction, and problematic relationships across all spheres of functioning. Evidence of such patterns and dysfunction requires review of previous employment history and records, prior and current interpersonal functioning in other areas of life, and even prior litigation history.

The Americans with Disabilities Act (1990)

The ADA was enacted to protect the civil rights of individuals with any type of disability, including mental health disorders, in a variety of public and social circumstances, including the workplace. The ADA provides its own unique definition of disability as either "a *physical or mental impairment* that *substantially limits* one or more of the *major life activities* of such individual; a record of such an impairment; or being regarded as having such an impairment" (italics added) (42 U.S.C. §12101).

Supreme Court and lower court rulings significantly limited the class of persons entitled to protection under the ADA and narrowed the definitions of key terms such as "substantially limits" and "major life activities" (see *Murphy v. United Parcel Service, Inc.* 1999; *Sutton v. United Air Lines, Inc.* 1999; *Toyota v. Williams* 2002). Congress enacted the Americans with Disabilities Act Amendments Act (ADAAA) (2008) with the explicit intent of restoring the ADA's original intention to provide broad civil rights coverage to individuals with disabilities (Hickox 2011; Recupero and Harms 2013). The ADAAA and associated EEOC regulations (EEOC 29 C.F.R. §1630 [Appendix], 2011) expanded the interpretation of key terms in the definition of disability (Dielman et al. 2009), included less restrictive interpretations of the terms "substantially limits" and "major life activities," and explicitly mentioned major psychiatric disorders as disabilities (Recupero and Harms 2013).

Scope of the ADA: Landmark Cases

The ADA has been applied in a broad range of circumstances and in a variety of claims to change the way American society perceives and addresses the needs of individuals with disabilities. Individuals who satisfy the ADA's definition of disabilty obtain protection under all sections of the ADA, including protection against discrimination in restaurants, stores, private schools, and professional offices, as well as employment. The following landmark cases demonstrate the wide-ranging scope of this civil rights legislation.

In *Bragdon v. Abbott* (1998), the U.S. Supreme Court ruled that disparate treatment of disabled individuals without objective evidence of the need for such treatment constituted discrimination on the basis of a disability. In this case, a dentist refused to treat an HIV-positive patient in his office and would only treat her in a hospital setting, at extra cost to the patient. He claimed he required such "extra precautions" because her HIV-positive status posed a "direct threat" to his health and safety, a circumstance that allows exception to ADA regulations, but he provided no objective evidence to support this policy. The Court held that although no one is required to provide treatment or accommodation if that treatment presents a direct threat to safety, the risk assessment must be based on medical or other objective evidence. Additionally, HIV qualifies as a disability under the ADA because it affects a major life activity, reproduction.

In *United States v. Georgia* (2006), the Supreme Court held that state prison facilities were not exempt from the provisions of the ADA protecting the civil rights of individuals with disabilities. Tony Goodman, a paraplegic held in a Georgia state prison, sued Georgia in federal court for violating his rights under the ADA. Mr. Goodman claimed that prison conditions such as lack of handicapped accessible facilities resulted, among other things, in denial of medical treatment as well as privileges granted to nondisabled prison inmates. The Court unanimously agreed with Mr. Goodman, denying Georgia's argument that state prisons were immune from suit for damages under the ADA.

The Supreme Court has also made clear that the ADA applies to individuals with mental illness and used the ADA to open the door for people with disabilities and their families to demand a full range of community services as alternatives to services provided only in institutional settings. In *Olmstead v. L.C. ex rei. Zimring* (1999), two Georgia women with diagnoses of mental health disorders and intellectual disabilities were repeatedly admitted to and discharged from a Georgia state hospital but were not provided with community-based services. Their treating physicians agreed the women could live in the community with appropriate support. The Georgia Department of Human Resources argued that financial constraints prevented the provision of community services. The women brought suit against the Georgia Department of Human Resources, claiming the state's refusal to provide community-based services was a violation of their rights under the ADA.

The Court agreed, ruling that "[u]njustified isolation [in a psychiatric hospital] is properly regarded as discrimination based on disability" (*Olmstead v. L.C. ex rei. Zimring* 1999 at 597). The Court affirmed that states are required to place persons with mental disabilities in integrated community settings rather than in institutions when the state's treatment professionals have determined that community placement is appropriate and if the affected individual does not oppose transfer from institutional care to a less restrictive setting.

The ADA in Employment Litigation

Title I of the ADA is intended to allow individuals with mental or physical disabilities, or a history of disabilities, or individuals regarded as having disabilities, to continue working despite disabilities. This legislation requires employers to make "reasonable accommodations" for "disabled" but qualified individuals to enable those individuals to perform "essential job functions," unless the accommodation would impose an "undue hardship" on the employer (Gold and Shuman 2009; Recupero and Harms 2013).

To access the protection of the ADA, employees have to identify themselves as having a medical or psychiatric diagnosis. Employers are then legally required to engage in an "interactive process" with the employee through which employers and employees clarify the disabled individual's needs and identify the appropriate reasonable accommodation(s) as quickly as possible. Any unnecessary delay in addressing requests for accommodations may lead to employer liability. Employees with an identified diagnosis or disability may request accommodations, but even if they do not, employers notified of a possible disability may be required to explore the need for accommodations with the employee.

Employees who are totally disabled and unable to work are not eligible for accommodation under the ADA. The ADA does not override health and safety requirements established under other Federal laws, such as those of the U.S. Occupational Safety and Health Administration, even if a standard adversely affects the employment of an individual with a disability. The ADA also does not supersede state or local laws that provide greater or equal protection for persons with disabilities, although it does preempt laws that provide less protection (Gold and Shuman 2009; Recupero and Harms 2013).

Employees claiming protection for a psychiatric disability under the ADA must provide mental health documentation to their employers. In most ADA cases, documentation is completed by treating mental health providers and does not require forensic psychiatric evaluation. If employees and employers cannot resolve disagreements over application of the ADA, such as what constitutes a reasonable accommodation or whether the employee can perform the essential functions of a job, the dispute may go to court for a final determination.

That being said, the vast majority of ADA issues, such as requests for accommodations or arguments regarding whether an individual has a disability, do not proceed to litigation. In these cases, if a dispute cannot be resolved through information provided by treating physicians, forensic psychiatric assessments may be dispositive for both employers and employees and are often requested before disputes have escalated to litigation (Gold and Shuman 2009).

Complex circumstances may also prompt a referral for a forensic ADA evaluation. For example, employers may find it difficult to determine whether an employee's behavior or performance difficulties are due to a psychiatric illness that may require accommodation or to poor work and interpersonal skills that require disciplinary action. Forensic psychiatrists can provide opinions as to whether an employee's psychiatric impairment (if any) affects occupational functioning, whether the employee poses a direct threat in the workplace (which disqualifies the employee from ADA protections), and whether reasonable accommodations may enable the employee to overcome functional impairments in performing job duties.

The ADA and Psychiatric Evaluations

Litigation or settlement of ADA claims, whether in civil courts or through the EEOC's regulatory process, do not statutorily require the provision of expert testimony. However, many ADA claims have been dismissed because of a lack of reliable professional testimony, especially when impairments, like psychiatric impairments, are "less obvious" (Hickox 2011). The determination that an individual has a psychiatric disability under the ADA statutorily requires that the individual have a diagnosable mental impairment. "Impairment" under the ADA is defined broadly, such that most "disorders" are recognized as "impairments" but not necessarily as "disabilities" (Fram 2008).

Whether an impairment rises to the level of a disability is an individualized, case-specific inquiry. The EEOC states, "An impairment is a disability…if it substantially limits the ability of an individual to perform a major life activity as compared to most people in the general population" (EEOC 2011, p. 17000). The EEOC regulations list intellectual disability, autism, major depressive disorder, bipolar disorder, PTSD, obsessive-compulsive disorder (OCD), and schizophrenia (among other diagnoses) as examples of impairments that should easily be recognized to represent a disability and to substantially limit a major life activity (EEOC 2011).

As mentioned above, ADA protections do not apply if the employee presents a direct threat in the workplace. The ADA defines "direct threat" to be "a significant risk to the health and safety of others that cannot be eliminated by reasonable accommodations" (ADA 42 USC §12111[3], 1990). The mere perception by another employee or supervisor that an individual is dangerous often is insufficient to satisfy statutory requirements. Recent violent behaviors or a plan to commit violence is an example of objective evidence of direct threat under the

ADA (Gold and Shuman 2009; Recupero and Harms 2013). Psychiatric ADA evaluations addressing "direct threat" require assessment of risk factors for violence (Schouten 2013; also see Chapter 28, "Violence Risk Assessment").

The ADA specifically excludes certain conditions and behaviors as grounds for disability (Table 15–3). For example, substance use disorders caused by current use of illegal drugs are excluded from ADA protection. However, individuals with a history of substance use but who are not current users are protected under the ADA. Bisexual and homosexual orientations, neither of which is a DSM diagnosis, also cannot be used as qualifying diagnoses leading to determinations of disability under the ADA.

The second requirement for psychiatric disability under the ADA is that the identified mental condition must "substantially limit one or more of the major life activities." The EEOC's list of potential major life activities includes, but is not limited to, "caring for oneself, performing manual tasks, seeing, hearing, eating, sleeping, walking, standing, lifting, bending, speaking, breathing, learning, reading, concentrating, thinking, communicating, and working" (Title 42, Chapter 126, Sec. 1202[2][A]). Psychiatrists should focus on the clinical aspects of an evaluee's limitations and describe the "condition, manner, or duration" of each affected activity (EEOC 2011).

Importantly, an individual with an impairment that limits a major life activity is still covered by the ADA when that impairment is in remission. Similarly, the determination of whether an impairment substantially limits a major life activity will be made without consideration of the efficacy of mitigating measures, such as medication. Employers cannot require employees to use a mitigating measure, but failure to do so might

disqualify employees from the ADA's protection. For example, failure to mitigate might render an employee unqualified for a position or may support an employer's contention that an employee presents "a direct threat" (EEOC 2011; Recupero and Harms 2013).

Functional Evaluation and Essential Job Functions

Individuals disabled under the ADA are entitled to continue to work at their job positions only if they can perform the essential job functions with or without accommodation. "Essential functions" are statutorily defined as the fundamental job duties of the employment position. A job function may be considered essential for any of several reasons, including, but not limited to, the following (29 CFR §1630.2[n][2] 2011):

1. The position exists to perform that specific function.
2. A limited number of employees are available among whom the performance of that job function can be distributed.
3. The function may be highly specialized so that incumbents in the position are hired for their expertise or ability to perform the particular function.

Psychiatric evaluators therefore need to determine whether the disabled individual can perform essential job functions (Anfang et al., in press; Recupero and Harms 2013). Evaluators should not assume they understand which job functions are essential, and should bear in mind that not all written job descriptions contain every significant or essential aspect of functioning the employee needs to be able to perform. To gain an understanding of an evaluee's essential job func-

TABLE 15–3. **Diagnoses and conditions statutorily excluded from Americans with Disabilities Act protection (42 U.S.C. §12211)**

Compulsive gambling	Pedophilia
Kleptomania	Exhibitionism
Pyromania	Voyeurism
Sexual orientation (i.e., bisexuality and homosexuality)	Other sexual behavior disorders
Gender identity disorders (not resulting from physical impairments)	Substance use disorders with current use of illegal drugs
Transvestitism	All DSM-5 "V" codes
Transexualism	

tions, evaluators should obtain a written or verbal job description from the employer as well as information from the evaluee.

Evaluating psychiatrists should then determine if the evaluee can carry out the essential functions of the job whether the evaluee has a psychiatric illness or not, and with or without accommodation. Information regarding this assessment should be obtained from both the employer and the evaluee. For example, if the evaluee is a post office letter handler, sorting mail might be an essential job function; working an occasional overnight shift might not be an essential job function. The psychiatrist then would determine if the letter handler could perform the essential function of sorting mail if no psychiatric illness existed, independent of the non-essential night-shift job function.

This assessment is critical in cases of employees who have misrepresented their training or are having problems with job performance. Such employees may have a poor work performance predating their claim of psychiatric disability, though they may assert that their poor performance is caused by their psychiatric illness. Individuals unable to perform essential job functions, with or without accommodation, cannot retain that specific job even when considered disabled under the ADA.

Reasonable Accommodations

Psychiatrists performing ADA evaluations are often asked to identify accommodations that would permit a disabled evaluee to perform essential job functions. The ADA regulations define reasonable accommodations as "modifications or adjustments to the work environment, or to the manner or circumstances under which the position held or desired is customarily performed, that enable an individual with a disability who is qualified to perform the essential functions of that position;" or "that enable [an] employee with a disability to enjoy equal benefits and privileges of employment as are enjoyed by its other similarly situated employees without disabilities" (29 CFR §1630.2[o][1] 2011).

Identifying potential accommodations requires knowledge of the essential functions of the job. It may also involve a more detailed understanding of workplace surroundings, structure, and scheduling. Many of the accommodations needed by employees with disabilities can be arranged through simple, inexpensive, and straightforward interventions (Gold and Shuman 2009; Recupero and Harms 2013) that involve increased communication, schedule changes, or changes in surroundings or the physical

TABLE 15–4.   **Possible reasonable accommodations for employees with psychiatric illness**

1. Structured time off, for example, time to attend treatment appointments during business hours

2. Altered break and work schedules (e.g., scheduling work around medical appointments)

3. Physical changes in workplace (e.g., moving location to larger or smaller spaces, access to windows)

4. Access to equipment that supports functioning (e.g., use of noise cancelling headphones to decrease external stimulation)

5. Changes in supervisory methods (e.g., providing written instructions, breaking tasks into smaller parts, more frequent meetings with supervisors)

6. Eliminating a non-essential or marginal job function that someone cannot perform because of a disability

7. Telework

8. Possible reassignment to a vacant position that the employee can perform

Source.   EEOC 1997, 2016c.

environment. The EEOC has provided examples of reasonable accommodations for persons with mental disabilities (EEOC 1997), some of which are listed in Table 15–4.

Although employers are required to provide reasonable accommodations, employees are not entitled to accommodations that cause employers "undue hardship," that is, expensive, difficult, or disruptive accommodations (29 CFR §1630.2[p] 2011). Differences of opinion between employee and employer on whether specific accommodations are reasonable, like other disputed elements of ADA claims, may become the subject of litigation. Psychiatrists may be asked to offer opinions about potential accommodations, but they do not make determinations regarding whether a specific accommodation would be considered reasonable or an undue hardship for an employer.

Suggestions for accommodations should take into account the EEOC's guidance, clinical judgment regarding the symptoms and severity of the evaluee's disorder, and an understanding of the individual's work situation. Psychiatrists recommending specific accommodations should bear in mind that employers are more likely to implement suggestions for non-complex, inexpensive accommodations.

Conclusion

A complex array of laws, agencies, regulations, and contracts governs the workplace (Gold and Shuman 2009). The complexity of employment regulations, the passions invested in employment and careers, and basic concepts of fairness in the workplace can result in conflict and litigation. Psychiatrists may be involved at various stages of discrimination, harassment, and ADA claims. Psychiatric opinions, based on professional expertise, guided by forensic and clinical psychiatric ethics and methodology, and informed by relevant social science, are of value to all parties in employment-related cases. Regardless of the legal basis of a plaintiff's claim, each case should be evaluated based on the totality of its specific circumstances.

Key Concepts

- The Equal Employment Opportunity Commission (EEOC) has defined two types of sexual harassment: *quid pro quo* and hostile work environment.

- The degree of psychiatric injury incurred, if any, should be proportional to the magnitude, frequency, and intensity of workplace experiences. Lack of proportionality exists preexisting psychological vulnerability, alternate causation, or malingering.

- Psychiatric evaluations in harassment or discrimination cases should include characteristics of the harassment, premorbid functioning of the plaintiff, prior work history, the effects of retaliation, the effects of litigation, as well as other factors.

- Psychiatric diagnoses and prognostic opinions in employment litigation should be supported by the facts of the case and the evaluee's longitudinal psychiatric and employment history.

- Psychiatrists should be familiar with the American with Disabilities Act's statutorily defined terms of "impairment," "substantial limitations," "major life activities," and "essential job functions."

- Psychiatrists should assess whether evaluees have signs and symptoms that meet criteria for a psychiatric disorder, whether they demonstrate substantial impairment of major life activities related to the disorder, and whether functional capacities related to essential and nonessential job functions are impaired.

- Psychiatrists should assess whether evaluees can perform essential job functions with or without accommodations.

- Psychiatrists should suggest accommodations that may enable individuals to perform essential job functions for which they are qualified.

References

Age Discrimination in Employment Act: 29 U.S.C. §§ 621–634. 1967. Available at: https://www.eeoc.gov/laws/statutes/adea.cfm. Accessed January 2, 2017.

Americans with Disabilities Act, Pub. Law No. 101–336, 104 Stat. 327 (1990), 42 U.S.C. §12101 et seq.

Americans with Disabilities Act Amendments Act, Pub. Law No. 110–325, 122 Stat. 3553 (2008), 42 U.S.C. §12101 et seq.

American Psychiatric Association: Diagnostic and Statistical Manual of Mental Disorders, 5th Edition. Arlington, VA, American Psychiatric Association, 2013

Anfang SA, Gold LH, Meyer DJ: Guideline for the forensic assessment of disability. J Am Acad Psychiatry Law (in press)

Bergman ME, Palmieri PA, Drasgow F, et al: Racial/ethnic harassment and discrimination, its antecedents, and its effect on job-related outcomes. J Occup Health Psychol 17(1):65–78, 2012 22409391

Bragdon v Abbott, 524 U.S. 624, 118 S.Ct. 1952 (1998)

Breslau N: The epidemiology of trauma, PTSD, and other posttrauma disorders. Trauma Violence Abuse 10(3):198–210, 2009 19406860

Civil Rights Act of 1964, Title VII, 42 U.S.C. § 2000e–2(a)(1) (1964)

Dielman SK, Morgan MA, Winkelman CL: Labor and employment law. Texas Bar J 72:27–28, 2009

EEOC v Boh Brothers Construction Co., LLC, No. 11–30770 (5th Cir. 2013)

Equal Employment Opportunity Commission: Guidelines on discrimination because of sex. 29 C.F.R. §1604.11(a), 1980. Available at: http://lor.gvtc.org/uploads/SEC622/EEOCGuidelines.pdf. Accessed January 2, 2017.

Equal Employment Opportunity Commission: The Pregnancy Discrimination Act. 1978. Available at: https://www.eeoc.gov/laws/statutes/pregnancy.cfm. Accessed January 2, 2017.

Equal Employment Opportunity Commission: EEOC enforcement guidance: the Americans with Disabilities Act and psychiatric disabilities. EEOC Notice No. 915.002, 1997. Available at: https://www.eeoc.gov/policy/docs/psych.html. Accessed January 2, 2017.

Equal Employment Opportunity Commission: Regulations to implement the equal employment provisions of the Americans with Disabilities Act. 29 C.F.R. Part 1630. Fed Regist 76(58):16978–17017, 2011

Equal Employment Opportunity Commission: Enforcement and litigation statistics. 2016a. Available at: https://www.eeoc.gov/eeoc/statistics/enforcement/index.cfm. Accessed January 2, 2017.

Equal Employment Opportunity Commission: EEOC wins key ruling in sexual orientation case. 2016b. Available at: https://content.govdelivery.com/accounts/USEEOC/bulletins/170dca2. Accessed January 2, 2017.

Equal Employment Opportunity Commission: The mental health provider's role in a client's request for a reasonable accommodation at work. 2016c. Available at: https://www.eeoc.gov/eeoc/publications/ada_mental_health_provider.cfm. Accessed January 2, 2017.

Fitzgerald LF, Collinsworth LL, Lawson AK: Sexual harassment, PTSD, and Criterion A: if it walks like a duck…. Psychol Inj Law 6:81–91, 2013

Foote WE, Goodman-Delahunty J: Evaluating Sexual Harassment: Psychological, Social, and Legal Considerations in Forensic Examinations. Washington, DC, American Psychological Association, 2005

Fram DK: Practitioners' note: the ADA Amendments Act: dramatic changes in coverage. Hofstra Labor and Employment Law Journal 26:193–221, 2008

Gold LH: Sexual Harassment: Psychiatric Assessment in Employment Litigation. Washington, DC, American Psychiatric Publishing, 2004

Gold LH: Sexual harassment, in Principles and Practice of Forensic Psychiatry, 3rd Edition. Edited by Rosner R, Scott CL. Boca Raton, FL, Taylor & Francis, 2016, pp 327–336

Gold LH, Shuman DW: Evaluating Mental Health Disability in the Workplace: Model, Process, and Analysis. New York, Springer, 2009

Gold LH, Metzner JL, Buck JB: Psychiatrtic disability evaluations, workers' compensation, fitness-for-duty evaluations, and personal injury litigation, in Principles and Practice of Forensic Psychiatry, 3rd Edition. Edited by Rosner R, Scott CL. Boca Raton, FL, Taylor & Francis, 2016, pp 307–318

Goodman-Delahunty J, Foote WE: Using a five-stage model to evaluate workplace discrimination injuries. Psychol Inj Law 6:92–98, 2013

Harris v Forklift Systems, Inc., 510 U.S. 17, 114 S.Ct. 367 (1993)

Hickox SA: The underwhelming impact of the Americans with Disabilities Act Amendments Act. Baltimore Law Review 40:417–492, 2011

Kessler RC, Sonnega A, Bromet E, et al: Posttraumatic stress disorder in the National Comorbidity Survey. Arch Gen Psychiatry 52(12):1048–1060, 1995 7492257

Kilpatrick DG, McFarlane AC: Posttraumatic stress disorder and the law: forensic considerations, in Handbook of PTSD: Science and Practice, 2nd Edition. Edited by Friedman MJ, Keane TM, Resick PA. New York, Guilford, 2014, pp 540–554

Lawson AK, Fitzgerald LF: Sexual harassment litigation: a road to re-victimization or recovery? Psychol Inj Law 9:216–229, 2016

Lawson AK, Wright CV, Fitzgerald LF: The evaluation of sexual harassment litigants: reducing discrepancies in the diagnosis of posttraumatic stress disorder. Law Hum Behav 37(5):337–347, 2013 23544390

McDonald JJ, Kulick FP: The rise of the psychological injury claim, in Mental and Emotional Injuries in Employment Litigation, 2nd Edition. Edited by McDonald JJ, Kulick FP. Washington, DC, Bureau of National Affairs, 2001, pp xiv–xxxvi

Meritor Savings Bank v Vinson, 477 U.S. 57, 106 S.Ct. 2399 (1986)

Murphy v United Parcel Service, Inc., 527 U.S. 471 (1999)

Olmstead v L.C. ex rei. Zimring, 527 U.S. 581, 119 S.Ct. 2176 (1999)

Oncale v Sundowner Offshore Services, Inc., 523 U.S. 75, 118 S.Ct. 998 (1998)

Price Waterhouse v Hopkins, 490 U.S. 228 (1989)

Raabe FJ, Spengler D: Epigenetic risk factors in PTSD and depression. Front Psychiatry 4:80, 2013 23966957

Recupero PR, Harms SE: The Americans with Disabilities Act (ADA) and the Americans with Disabilities Act Amendments Act in disability evaluations, in Clinical Guide to Mental Disability Evaluations. Edited by Gold LH, Vanderpool DL. New York, Springer, 2013, pp 259–289

Ritter L: Sexual orientation and gender identity: protected categories under Title VII? Journal of Legislation Online Supplement, Paper 1, September 6, 2016. Available at http://scholarship.law.nd.edu/jleg_blog/1/. Accessed January 2, 2017.

Rosen GM: The Aleutian Enterprise sinking and posttraumatic stress disorder: misdiagnosis in clinical and forensic settings. Prof Psychol Res Pr 26:82–87, 1995

Schouten R: Workplace violence evaluations and the ADA, in Clinical Guide to Mental Disability Evaluations. Edited by Gold LH, Vanderpool DL. New York, Springer, 2013, pp 291–308

Simon RI (ed): Posttraumatic Stress Disorder in Litigation: Guidelines for Forensic Assessment, 2nd Edition. Washington, DC, American Psychiatric Publishing, 2002

Stockdale MS, Sliter KA, Ashburn-Nardo L: Employment discrimination, in American Psychological Association Handbook of Forensic Psychology: Vol 1. Individual and Situational Influences in Criminal and Civil Contexts. Edited by Cutler BL, Zapf PA. Washington, DC, American Psychological Association, 2015, pp 511–532

Strasburger LH: The litigant-patient: mental health consequences of civil litigation. J Am Acad Psychiatry Law 27(2):203–211, 1999 10400429

Sutton v United Air Lines, Inc., 527 U.S. 471, 119 S. Ct. 2139 (1999)

Toyota Motor Manufacturing, Kentucky, Inc. v Williams, 534 U.S. 184, 122 S. Ct. 681 (2002)

United States v Georgia, 546 U.S. 151, 126 S.Ct. 877 (2006)

Vasquez MJT, Baker NL, Shullman SL: Assessing employment discrimination and harassment, in Handbook of Psychology, Volume 11: Forensic Psychology. Edited by Goldstein AM, Weiner IB. New York, Wiley, 2003, pp 259–277

Williams v Saxbe, 413 F.Supp. 654, D.D.C. (1976)

CHAPTER 16

Fitness for Duty, Impaired Professionals, and Public Safety

Marilyn Price, M.D.

Debra A. Pinals, M.D.

Fitness-for-duty (FFD) evaluations (FFDEs) have been defined as "comprehensive evaluations designed to determine if an employee is capable of performing the essential functions of his or her job" (Schouten 2012, p. 903). Although any employer may request an FFDE, these assessments commonly involve professionals whose work performance can affect public safety or the employer's liability (Wettstein 2013), such as physicians (see, e.g., Price and Meyer 2013) and law enforcement officers (see, e.g., Pinals and Price 2013). FFDE evaluees can also include other health care professionals, emergency response personnel, and public transportation professionals.

Multiple statutes and substantial case law justify ordering an FFDE in cases where public safety is an issue (Pinals and Price 2013). FFDEs are triggered by behavior that may be related to a medical condition, mental illness, or substance abuse and interferes with workplace performance or raises concerns about workplace safety (Anfang et al., in press). An employer also may request an FFD certification for an employee seeking to return to work after a period of medical leave.

Fitness-for-Duty Evaluations: General Considerations

The purpose of an FFDE is to assess whether employees whose psychological status is perceived as potentially unstable or threatening are able to safely perform their jobs. A psychiatric FFDE is intended to answer very specific questions:

- Is the employee able to perform all or some of the duties of the job, and perform them safely, without danger to self or others, including the general public?

- Does psychiatric illness impair job performance or increase the risk of danger in the performance of the job?

An examination for either inability to perform essential job functions or possible dangerousness should be tailored to seek only that information necessary to determine whether employees can perform their jobs or whether they present a direct threat unless otherwise indicated. Continued employment may be conditioned on the employee's full cooperation (Gold and Shuman 2009).

Evaluators should be aware that FFDEs can give rise to litigation if conflict regarding the employee's ability to function in the workplace cannot be resolved. Referrals for an FFDE typically arise in the context of a substantial disagreement between the employee and employer about the employee's abilities to perform job duties adequately or safely. Regardless of whether a safety or performance issue is in question, in most referrals, the employee believes he or she is able to work, while the employer believes that the employee is not able to work or not able to work safely.

Referral Process

In many cases, the need for an FFDE, particularly if a threat of violence is involved, may appear to employers to be acute. Employment decisions, such as placing an employee on administrative leave or seeking sensitive information from the employee, made in the heat of the moment by employers, can compound a sense of crisis. Consequently, referral sources often ask evaluators to complete FFD assessments quickly, on an urgent or even emergent basis.

Psychiatrists should approach requests for expedited FFDEs cautiously. Conducting these examinations under a pressured timeframe and volatile circumstances is inadvisable. In addition, the timing of a referral for an FFDE can substantially affect its findings and should also be considered upon request for provision of an FFDE examination. Evaluating an employee in the acute phase of an illness that may remit either partially or totally with treatment creates an incomplete picture of FFD. In these cases, the employee should be stabilized before an FFDE is undertaken (Gold and Shuman 2009). If it becomes evident during the initial discussion with the referring source that the evaluee needs a clinical evaluation and treatment rather than a forensic evaluation, psychiatrists should provide this opinion to the referral source at the time of the referral, rather than agree to proceed with the FFDE (Anfang et al., in press).

The referral process for an FFDE differs depending on the source of the referral (Anfang and Wall 2006). In cases involving physicians and other healthcare professionals, referrals may come from "a hospital or state physician health committee, a hospital peer review committee, a medical licensing board, or an array of health care agencies of which the health care provider is a member" (Price and Meyer 2013, p. 337). Often, the process for initiating a physician's FFDE originates with a patient or staff member complaint or problems in work performance. The law in many states requires physicians to report colleagues whom they believe to be impaired (Price and Meyer 2013), and such reporting has also been described as an "ethical obligation" for physicians (American Medical Association 2016, Opinion 9.031).

Referrals may also be prompted by sexual misconduct, other boundary violations, or other unethical behavior

(Anfang et al. 2005; Janofsky 2011). Disruptive behavior in a physician is a common reason for a psychiatric FFDE referral (Anfang and Wall 2006; Meyer and Price 2006). Generally, disruptive behavior refers to "[p]ersonal conduct, whether verbal or physical, that negatively affects or that potentially may negatively affect patient care" (American Medical Association 2016, Opinion 9.045).

For law enforcement personnel, referrals may be prompted by concerns raised by supervisors, fellow officers, or members of the public (Pinals and Price 2013). An officer will generally be placed on administrative leave until the FFDE is completed because of public safety concerns. An officer may have been referred for outpatient or inpatient treatment prior to the scheduling of an FFDE in some circumstances (Anfang et al., in press). A more detailed review of law enforcement FFDEs can be found in Chapter 30 ("Forensic Psychiatry and Law Enforcement").

For some professions, requests for an FFDE may come directly from an employer or even from an employee seeking to return to work after taking leave under the Family and Medical Leave Act of 1993 (2009) (FMLA) or through an employer-sponsored disability benefit program. Employers may require medical certification of employees' ability to work safely prior to resuming their former work responsibilities. Often, the employee's treating physician submits such certification, but referral for an evaluation by a forensic psychiatrist may be indicated in some cases.

Before accepting an FFDE referral, psychiatrists should discuss the objectives and case factors with the party requesting the evaluation to determine if they are qualified to perform the assessment (American Academy of Psychiatry and the Law 2005; Glancy et al. 2015). A psychiatrist with minimal training and

experience in geriatric medicine, for example, may not be the best forensic specialist to evaluate a bus driver with suspected cognitive impairment. When the referral for an FFDE is prompted by concerns about the employee's potential for violent behavior, the forensic psychiatrist should have training and expertise in violence risk appraisal (Schouten 2013; Wettstein 2013; see also Chapter 28, "Violence Risk Assessment").

Documentation

Referral questions and related records should be reviewed carefully before conducting the evaluee's mental health FFD interview. Evaluators should request a written description of the behavior that led to the request for the FFDE before scheduling the examination, including documentation about the incident and the evaluee's current job status. The referral source should furnish a job description and indices of past performance. The referral source should also provide a list of questions to guide the evaluation.

Availability of information and documentation will vary on a case-by-case basis. In addition, the Americans with Disabilities Act (ADA) or FMLA may restrict the employer's access to certain types of information. Evaluees may be responsible for supplying relevant medical/psychiatric records, as employers are often restricted from accessing this information. Evaluators should consider the source of the information and whether that source has intentionally or unintentionally provided incomplete records. Reports therefore should also clearly identify sources of information, for example, documentation provided by the evaluee as opposed to that provided by the employer, and whether that documentation appears complete or incomplete.

Additional documentation that may be relevant includes the evaluee's current job status (i.e., whether the evaluee is on medical or administrative leave, suspended, or working with or without restrictions) and the names and contact information of workplace supervisors, witnesses, and complainants, if any, who may provide collateral information. If reliable or relevant opinions cannot be offered without additional or restricted information, psychiatrists should state that the opinions offered are limited by lack of access to these records and that a final determination cannot be made without their review.

Structure of the FFDE

Relevant Laws

Employers are required through a variety of obligations to make prudent efforts to assure safety in the workplace as well as public safety (Gold and Shuman 2009). They are statutorily authorized by the ADA to require an FFDE when they have a reasonable basis for concern. Nevertheless, employers also have obligations to their employees that must be taken into consideration when the question of fitness-for-duty arises. Many laws protecting the rights of employees with health-related impairments against unfair discrimination are relevant to FFDEs, including the ADA, collective bargaining agreements, the FMLA, the Occupational Safety and Health Act of 1970 (OSHA), and state occupational health regulations. Individuals wrongly suspected or accused of threats or violent acts may bring suit against their employers for violations of these rights (Schouten 2012).

For medical professionals, Medical Practice Acts and the federal Health Care Quality Improvement Act (HCQIA) of 1986 are especially pertinent (Janofsky 2011; Price and Meyer 2013; Walker 2004). Each state has a Medical Practice Act that grants authority to a medical board in the state to investigate or discipline physicians in that jurisdiction (Grant and Alfred 2007; Law and Hansen 2010; Walker 2004). The primary responsibility of each state's medical board is to protect public safety, not to serve the interests of physicians (Meyer and Price 2012). The HCQIA formalized the process of peer review of physicians and established the National Practitioner Data Bank (2017) (NPDB), which houses records of a doctor's past malpractice judgments, disciplinary sanctions and medical license suspension, adverse clinical privilege actions from hospitals, and adverse professional society membership actions, among others.

Other laws may be pertinent, depending on individual case factors, including the Department of Transportation (DOT) regulations for Commercial Driving License (CDL) holders, the Uniformed Services Employment and Reemployment Rights Act (USERRA), workers' compensation regulations, the Genetic Information Nondiscrimination Act (GINA), the Health Insurance Portability and Accountability Act (HIPAA), and state or local employment laws (Fischler et al. 2011; International Association of the Chiefs of Police 2013; Pinals and Price 2013; Schouten 2012), among others. When unfamiliar with a particular law relevant to the forensic evaluation, psychiatrists should not hesitate to ask the retaining party for more information about the law and how it pertains to the case.

Confidentiality

FFDE reports are appropriately limited to responses and information relevant to specific referral questions. These reports typically do not need to contain certain information that might normally be included in a standard clinical or disability evaluation. For example, FFDE reports do not necessarily need to describe an evaluee's family or social history except to the extent that such information is directly related to the specific referral questions. Sensitive personal data irrelevant to the purpose of an evaluation should be omitted or summarized in the interests of privacy, especially as employers or their agents will have access to the report. Statutorily mandated requirements about the confidentiality of protected health care information (PHI) apply to FFDEs (Gold and Metzner 2006). The evaluating psychiatrist, the referral source, and the evaluee all need notice and understanding of the limitations of confidentiality and the nature of the anticipated disclosures.

Informed Consent

Informed consent is needed both to conduct an FFDE and to release the information obtained (Wettstein 2013). The psychiatrist's role, the purpose of the examination, and its potential consequences should be made clear to the evaluee. Evaluees should be made aware of all parties to whom the psychiatrist will release the information and the potential negative outcomes and consequences that may arise from the FFDE (Wall 2005). Consent should be obtained both verbally and in written form signed by the evaluee before starting the evaluation. If an evaluee refuses to provide consent both for the evaluation and the release of information, the psychiatrist should not proceed with the evaluation.

For example, physicians undergoing FFDEs may be unaware of the potential "domino effect" of unfavorable findings (Price and Meyer 2013, p. 342). Physicians who are found unfit to practice may lose their licenses or have to report disciplinary action to supervisory administrators, who may then terminate their employment (Price and Meyer 2013).

Even when a physician is found fit for duty, risks to the physician's privacy may arise as a consequence of state laws granting public access to information generated by investigatory or disciplinary proceedings (American Psychiatric Association 2004).

Similarly, police officers and military personnel declared unfit for duty for psychiatric reasons may struggle with internalized shame, loss of social support, and financial hardship. These can result from the stigma surrounding mental illness and the cultural ideals of strength and self-sufficiency often taught to young recruits and rookies (Mahoney 2013).

Dissimulation

In FFDEs and right-to-work assessments, psychiatrists will be more likely to encounter dissimulation than malingering (Wettstein 2013). *Dissimulation* involves "the concealment of genuine symptoms of mental illness in an effort to portray psychological health" (Glancy et al. 2015, p. S45). Unconscious minimization may arise from denial, lack of insight, or even represent a manifestation of illness (Rosman 2001). Conscious dissimulation, like frank malingering, is a form of intentional deception. Evaluees may conceal problems to avoid negative consequences or sanctions for their behavior (Reynolds 2002).

Evaluees who acknowledge the existence of a mental health disorder or a substance use disorder in partial remission may also attempt to minimize or downplay the severity of their current symptoms or relapse risk in order to return to work more quickly. Physicians, in particular, are often exceptionally skilled in concealing the extent of their impairment from colleagues and in attributing blame to other factors (Wettstein 2005). During the review of collateral information and the psychiatric interview, examining the evaluee's potential incentives for dissimulation, such as financial difficulties or fear of lost career opportunities, will be helpful in making determinations regarding minimization or dissimulation of symptoms.

Conducting the Evaluation

The process and specifics for conducting an FFDE of a professional whose job affects public safety will depend on the profession and employer in question. Some types of FFDEs carry additional or specialized inquiries. FFDEs of law enforcement officers, for example, require psychiatrists to offer an opinion as to whether the evaluee can safely operate a firearm, especially in high-stress, chaotic situations, an essential job function (Pinals and Price 2013; see also Chapter 30). Regardless of the type of job involved, in most cases the evaluation should include a review of collateral information; a detailed psychiatric interview, including a mental status examination; an assessment of impairment and the relationship to specific job functions; an assessment of risks associated with that job to the employee and to the safety and welfare of the general public; and the presentation of the psychiatrist's opinions and recommendations. In some cases, a formal violence risk assessment may be required (see Chapter 28).

Collateral Information

In FFDEs, the need to review extensive collateral information is essential (Table 16–1).

In FFDEs of physicians, collateral information might also include past judgments for or against the physician or

disciplinary actions (such as previous license suspension) by a state medical board, credentialing agency, peer-review committee, or other entity. In examinations of police officers, employers might also provide information that includes "work performance, conduct, commendations, citizen letters of appreciation or complaint, disciplinary and civil claims history, remediation efforts, internal affairs investigations, involvement in critical incidents and use of force incidents, incident reports of any triggering events, earlier periods of disability, previous referral to EAP, and available treatment records" (Pinals and Price 2013, p. 378; see also Chapter 30).

Reviewing collateral information *before* performing the psychiatric interview allows evaluators to identify relevant questions beforehand. However, examiners should be sensitive to the potential for bias that may arise from reviewing materials provided by a party with an interest in the case outcome (Glancy et al. 2015). As noted above, the source of collateral information should be clearly identified in the report.

In FFDEs, conducting interviews with third parties in order to collect additional collateral information may be helpful. These third parties may include members of the evaluee's family, coworkers (subordinates, supervisors, and peers), and treatment providers, among others (Wettstein 2013). The evaluee's written consent (i.e., release of information) enabling these third parties to speak with the forensic psychiatrist is often necessary (Anfang et al., in press; American Psychiatric Association 2004). Even where the law does not require the evaluee's consent to these third-party contacts, obtaining consent honors the ethical principle of respect for persons (Buchanan and Norko 2013).

Psychiatrists may find it necessary to request or recommend the collection of

TABLE 16–1. **Collateral information in fitness-for-duty evaluations (FFDEs)**

Medical and psychiatric treatment records

A written job description from the employer

Copies of past job performance evaluations or disciplinary actions

Copies of written reports or complaints that relate to the reason for the FFDE referral

Legal documents related to previous workers' compensation cases or periods of occupational disability

Results of psychological testing, including pre-employment testing

Educational history, such as academic transcripts and the evaluee's curriculum vitae

Documents relating to criminal history, such as arrest records

Military history documents, including discharge type

Legal history, including previous civil litigation

Electronic communications, such as emails, blog posts, Twitter feeds, and other social media activity

additional data, such as pharmacy records, neuropsychological evaluation (see Chapter 5, "Psychological Testing in Forensic Psychiatry"), laboratory tests, or neuroimaging (see Chapter 7, "Neuroimaging and Forensic Psychiatry"). Toxicology screens may be helpful because alcohol or substance abuse can often contribute to problematic workplace behavior. Recommendations or requests for additional data should be tailored to specific questions. For example, if dementia is a consideration, formal neuropsychological testing and focused diagnostic testing to identify the suspected cognitive impairments and their cause may be indicated (Glancy et al. 2015).

Psychiatric Interview

At the initial meeting, examinees should be encouraged to review the events leading to the FFDE from their perspective, and to include opposing points of view, even if they believe those opposing points of view are invalid. After reviewing the employee's version of events, the evaluator should be prepared to ask specific questions in order to explore in detail any discrepancies between the evaluee's description of events as compared to the versions of collateral sources.

The psychiatric interview should include a full history and mental status examination. While gathering a family history may be part of a routine general psychiatric evaluation, obtaining genetic information, including family history, may be prohibited by GINA for certain professionals (see Chapter 12, "Professional Liability in Psychiatric Practice"). The evaluee's educational and occupational histories are especially relevant in FFDEs (Glancy et al. 2015; Pinals and Price 2013). Questioning should specifically address work-related capacities (Anfang et al., in press). If the evaluee has a history of disciplinary actions, eliciting further detail about these incidents and their resolution will be helpful (Anfang and Wall 2006).

Determining the approximate onset of occupational difficulties is important. The sudden appearance of performance or behavior problems in an older professional who previously enjoyed an exemplary work record and successful career, for example, should lead the evaluator to consider a neurocognitive disorder in the differential diagnosis (Peisah and Wilhelm 2007). Similarly, "neurological disorders, such as seizures, the sequelae of traumatic brain injury, and certain endocrine disorders, should always be considered when formulating cases involving impulsivity, violence, or sexually anomalous behavior" (Glancy et al. 2015, p. S17).

Psychiatrists should consider the impact that investigatory and disciplinary proceedings may be having on the professional in question. For physicians, the experience of being investigated can be profoundly demoralizing, even if complaints are spurious and the physician is found not to be impaired (Meyer and Price 2012; Verhoef et al. 2015). Evaluees undergoing FFDEs often experience significant emotional distress over having their professional competence questioned, being investigated or disciplined, and fearing they may lose professional status, career opportunities, or even their livelihood. For law enforcement officers, being found unfit for duty may also result in a loss of significant psychosocial supports, particularly peer socialization among police officers (Anfang and Wall 2006).

Finally, acute and long-term risk assessment and risk mitigation are an important part of all FFDEs when evaluees have been referred for disruptive, threatening, or dangerous behavior, or for concerns regarding public safety. Evaluators should be certain they understand safety or danger concerns relevant to the specific FFDE, and address them directly with the evaluee. Static and dynamic factors that indicate heightened risk of violence, if present, should be reviewed and discussed.

Assessment of Impairment

As with disability evaluations, psychiatrists conducting FFDEs may be required to provide an estimate of the evaluee's current level of impairment and expected level of impairment in the future, with or without treatment. An evaluee's fitness for duty or work impairment will depend on the specific responsibilities of the job in question and any potential interaction between the evaluee's job and their psychiatric condition. For example, "a physician with bipolar disorder might be restricted from working excessive irregular work hours. This might be impairing for a solo practitioner obstetrician, but might not present a significant problem for an office-based allergist" (Anfang and Wall 2006, p. 678).

The psychiatrist assessing impairment should also consider the potential impact of treatment. For example, medication side effects such as a slowed reaction time or drowsiness could have significant FFD implications for someone who carries a firearm, operates public transport, or operates machinery. A finding that an evaluee is unfit for a particular job is not synonymous with a finding of disability in other contexts. Nevertheless, some referring sources may request a specified level of impairment that could be relevant to future determinations of eligibility for disability benefits. If this information is requested, the American Medical Association's *Guides to the Evaluation of Permanent Impairment* (American Medical Association 2008) may be helpful (Glancy et al. 2015).

Scope of the Evaluation and Report, and Evaluee's Privacy

FFD report formats will vary depending on case specifics, but general guidelines are available to help evaluators who are unsure as to FFD report standards or expectations (see, e.g., Granacher 2011; Janofsky 2011; Wettstein 2010, 2013). When deciding what information to present in the forensic report, the examiner should remain cognizant of the applicable laws and the specific questions requested by the referring party. For example, an FFD certification in the context of an employee returning after FMLA leave need not be as exhaustive as a report involving a physician's FFD (American Psychiatric Association 2004; Falls and Nellermoe 2014). FFD reports for state licensing authorities (e.g., medical boards, bar examiners) often must be more detailed. Similarly, the interests of public safety typically outweigh the evaluee's privacy interests in the context of FFDEs of law enforcement professionals (International Association of the Chiefs of Police 2013).

In some cases, the examining psychiatrist may not have sufficient information to formulate a definitive opinion. Such limitations should be disclosed in the forensic report (American Academy of Psychiatry and the Law 2005; Buchanan and Norko 2013). For example, the scope of FFD reports for law enforcement personnel and other professionals may be limited by union contracts (Anfang and Wall 2006). Alternatively, a physician's FFD may also depend on questions of medical skill that cannot be assessed through a psychiatric interview (American Psychiatric Association 2004). If evaluators suspect shortcomings in a medical professional's clinical skills or knowledge base, they should recommend referral for additional skills evaluation (Anfang et al. 2005; Price and Meyer 2013).

Psychiatrists often must limit the information in the written report to data that relate specifically to the question being asked by the employer (e.g., "Is it safe for this person to return to work?"). Not only do many employees prefer to limit the amount of personal information disclosed to their employer, many employers themselves prefer to receive the minimum information necessary to lessen the risk of a future ADA lawsuit (Schouten 2012). Sharing more clinical information than is necessary with an employer may subject the examining psychiatrist to liability for breach of confidentiality (Schouten 2012; see also Chapter 12). Although FFDEs of physicians for state boards of medical licensure often require comprehensive reports, "[s]ensitive personal information may be spared or summarized in the report if it is not directly related to the fitness questions" (American Psychiatric Association 2004, p. 1). Finally, when preparing the FFDE report, psychiatrists covered under HIPAA should take into consideration the evaluee's right to access the report (see Chapter 11, "Confidentiality in Psychiatric Practice").

Presenting Opinions and Making Recommendations

Psychiatrists should offer opinions about the presence of a psychiatric illness and the extent, if any, to which the illness has interfered with the evaluee's ability to function effectively and safely in the specific work setting. However, the diagnosis of a psychiatric disorder may or may not be relevant to an evaluee's fitness for duty. The terms *illness* and *impairment* are not synonymous (Federation of State Medical Boards of the United States 2011; Glancy et al. 2015). An evaluee may have significant impairment in terms of occupational functioning without meeting criteria for a DSM psychiatric illness. For example, a judge who routinely berates and insults defendants and verbally abuses attorneys may have maladaptive personality traits and coping strategies rather than mental illness. Conversely, many persons who *do* have symptoms that meet criteria for a serious DSM-5 mental illness are nonetheless highly skilled and minimally impaired in occupational functioning, particularly if the condition is in remission or well controlled by treatment.

The evaluator should provide a description of how a psychiatric illness or impairments affects job-related capacities and thus FFD. These opinions should all be accompanied by descriptions of specific areas of impairments, including insight and judgment, and should be well supported by data and the foundation for opinions should be discussed in detail in the report. Referral sources will also expect reports to address the evaluee's work status by offering one of the following opinions:

1. The employee is fit for duty and able to return to work without restriction, with or without treatment.
2. The employee is fit for duty with certain restrictions, with or without treatment.
3. The employee is temporarily unfit for duty, but the likelihood that impairments may resolve with treatment is high. Return to work should be based on the condition that the evaluee receive treatment.
4. The employee is unfit for duty and is likely remain so permanently
5. The employee is unfit for duty and it is too early or there is not enough information to determine whether the employee may be able to return to work in the future.

Evaluators may conclude that evaluees have no impairment and may return to the workplace and include the data that supports this opinion. Reports should not simply conclude that there is no problem and that, therefore, the examinee is fit for duty (Anfang et al. 2005; Anfang and Wall 2006).

In many cases, the question "Is the evaluee fit for duty?" does not have a simple yes-or-no answer (Glancy et al. 2015). Evaluees may be able to perform some, but not all, of their duties. Similarly, evaluees might be unfit currently but might be expected to improve significantly with treatment (Glancy et al. 2015). Conversely, evaluees with minor impairments may be able to perform their jobs safely at present but may need to plan for future retirement if a progressive disorder is discovered.

The evaluator should explain what restrictions or limitations might apply. "Restrictions are most easily understood as what an individual *should not* do, whereas limitations can be described as what the individual *cannot* do because of the severity of psychiatric symptoms" (Anfang and Wall 2006, p. 678). In FFDEs, the evaluator is often asked to provide recommendations as to whether workplace monitoring, monitoring of treatment compliance, or some other type of monitoring is necessary to ensure the employee's continued fitness for work (Glancy et al. 2015; Price and Meyer 2013). The forensic psychiatrist could also recommend education, skill-building, and other activities that may help restore the evaluee's fitness for duty (Wall 2005).

If the psychiatrist opines that the evaluee is currently unfit for duty but that treatment may restore an acceptable level of functioning, the employer may request an estimate of the amount of time reasonably expected for completion of successful treatment (Glancy et al. 2015). Recommendations for workplace monitoring contracts may also be offered (Anfang et al., in press).

The psychiatrist is frequently expected to make recommendations for treatment of the evaluee's condition (American Psychiatric Association 2004; Wettstein 2013). In the case of physicians and other healthcare professionals, treatment and monitoring of an impaired professional is often coordinated and overseen by a Physician Health Program (PHP). PHPs are "program[s] of prevention, detection, intervention, rehabilitation and monitoring of licensees with potentially impairing illnesses, approved and/or recognized by the state medical board" (Federation of State Medical Boards of the United States 2011).

When no patient harm has occurred, a physician may be monitored by the PHP, through a *voluntary track,* which has enhanced protection of the physician's confidentiality and privacy (Federation of State Medical Boards of the United States 2011). When a patient has been harmed, or when a licensee is referred to a PHP by a medical licensing board, typically that physician is followed through the PHP's *mandated track,* which involves the provision of periodic progress reports to the medical board (Federation of State Medical Boards of the United States 2011). The Federation of State Physician Health Programs (FSPHP) states that "[r]ehabilitation of physicians with potentially impairing health conditions is the primary function of PHPs" (Federation of State Physician Health Programs 2005, p. 4).

Finally, the psychiatrist may also offer opinions regarding the evaluee's long-term prognosis (Gold and Shuman 2009). Opinions about prognosis should be based on careful consideration of multiple factors outlined in Table 16–2.

For example, peer-reviewed literature supports a strong likelihood of successful recovery from substance abuse and mental illness among physicians who are actively engaged in treatment (Price and Meyer 2013; Wettstein 2005). Conversely, a history of multiple "second chances" and continuing performance problems or recidivism in spite of treatment or attempts at accommodations do not bode well for the evaluee's fitness for duty, at least in his or her most recent occupation (Price and Meyer 2013; Regenbogen and Recupero 2012).

Ethical Considerations

Appropriateness of the Fitness-for-Duty Evaluation

Evaluators should be alert to misuse of the FFDE process. The employer may maintain that the FFDE is needed because the employee has exhibited mental impairment affecting performance or has posed a threat in the workplace. However, in some cases, employers attempt to use psychiatric FFDEs for inappropriate reasons, such as to resolve managerial problems or as retaliation against a whistleblower or an employee who has filed a complaint of sexual harassment, racial, or age discrimination (Schouten 2012).

Examining psychiatrists should give evaluees an opportunity to explain their side of any work-related conflicts that preceded the referral for an FFD assessment (Meyer and Price 2006). Employees may assert that the FFDE was retaliatory and will be used to discredit them or to justify their termination. The evaluator's role is to provide a response to the referral questions and avoid becoming an advocate for either employer or employee (Anfang et al., in press). The psychiatric report should clearly indicate if an evaluee does not demonstrate a psychiatric disorder or symptom as the basis for problematic workplace behavior or for workplace conflict.

Honesty and Objectivity: Bias in FFDEs

Bias is a potential difficulty in FFDEs just as it can be in most forensic psychiat-

---

TABLE 16–2. Factors impacting prognosis in fitness-for-duty evaluations

Natural course of any diagnosed psychiatric or other illness

Side effects or expected benefits of treatment

Expected treatment compliance

Personality factors unique to the evaluee

Interactions between the evaluee's symptoms and job functions

---

ric evaluations. An evaluee or third party (such as the evaluee's attorney or the referring agency) may exert pressure on the psychiatrist to offer an opinion that the evaluee is fit for duty. However, prematurely declaring a professional fit for duty is contrary to the interests of public safety. In addition, such opinions are potentially detrimental to the evaluee, who may face additional discipline or potential job loss due to poor performance (Schouten 2012).

In some cases, such as FMLA return-to-work scenarios, the FFD certification may be requested from the treating physician, which can raise ethics issues related to dual-role conflict (i.e., serving as both the treating clinician and the forensic evaluator) (Strasburger et al. 1997). In FFDEs, assessments of fellow physicians and other colleagues can pose special problems with respect to transference issues (Anfang and Wall 2006). The American Psychiatric Association states that "[t]he evaluating psychiatrist should not have any current or past treatment or employment relationship with the physician being examined" (American Psychiatric Association 2004, p. 2).

Prioritizing Safety

The forensic psychiatrist must consider the safety and well-being of the evaluee as well as those whose safety may be affected by an impaired professional. The examiner should perform a thorough assessment of the risk for harm to the eval-uee or others, including inquiries about suicidal or homicidal ideation (see Chapters 27, "Suicide Risk Assessment," and 28). Such assessments are particularly critical for members of professions at statistically increased risk, such as anesthesiologists (Price and Meyer 2013) and police officers (Pinals and Price 2013). Psychiatrists should also consider occupational factors that may increase risk, such as access to firearms in the case of military, police officers, and security guards, and industrial chemicals or gases in manufacturing plant workers and laboratory technicians.

In some cases, as discussed earlier, the performance of a psychiatric FFDE may need to be deferred to arrange emergency treatment (Wettstein 2013). If the examinee makes a credible threat to harm someone during the course of the psychiatric interview, such disclosure may trigger a *Tarasoff* duty for the forensic psychiatrist to warn or protect endangered third parties even though the evaluee is not a patient (Gutheil and Brodsky 2010; *Tarasoff v. Regents of the University of California* 1976). Additional considerations are necessary when determining if a firearm can be safely returned to a law enforcement officer who had been placed on restricted duty (Pinals and Price 2013). While the examiner may understandably develop feelings of empathy toward the evaluee, FFD assessments of professionals place a stronger obligation on protecting the safety of the public.

Conclusion

Forensic psychiatrists can expect to receive more requests for FFDEs and right-to-work assessments in the years to come, not only for physicians and law enforcement professionals, but also for workers in diverse professions that may affect the safety of the public or the viability of the employer's economic activity. For psychiatric FFDEs, psychiatrists must clarify the precise referral question(s) and tailor the assessment to the needs of the retaining party, the specifics of the job in question, factors related to conditions (and their treatment) that the evaluee may have, and applicable laws. Careful consideration of the common ethical issues in FFDEs will help the forensic psychiatrist to balance the rights and dignity of the evaluee with the critical need to protect public safety.

Key Concepts

- Referrals for fitness-for-duty evaluations (FFDEs) are usually made by employers who have become concerned about whether the referred employee can continue to function safely in the workplace.

- Occupations that can have a significant impact on public safety, such as medical professionals and law enforcement officers, are typically the subjects of FFDEs.

- Psychiatrists should be certain to understand the reason for the referral, and have access to adequate collateral information, including why concerns arose.

- Psychiatrists should correlate impairments with specific job functions; an individual may have a psychiatric illness and not be occupationally impaired.

- FFDEs should include assessment of risks of safety for the evaluee and the public.

- FFDE reports should contain only that information relevant to the FFD evaluation; psychiatrists are required to maintain confidentiality of nonrelevant information gathered during the course of the evaluation.

References

American Academy of Psychiatry and the Law: Ethics guidelines for the practice of forensic psychiatry. May 2005. Available at: http://www.aapl.org/ethics.htm. Accessed December 19, 2016.

American Medical Association: Guides to the Evaluation of Permanent Impairment, 6th Edition. Edited by Andersson GBJ, Cocchiarella L. Chicago, IL, American Medical Association, 2008

American Medical Association: Code of medical ethics. 2016. Available at: http://www.ama-assn.org/ama/pub/physician-resources/medical-ethics/code-medical-ethics.page? Accessed January 3, 2017.

American Psychiatric Association: Resource document—guidelines for psychiatric "fitness for duty" evaluations of physicians. 2004. Available at: https://www.psychiatry.org/psychiatrists/search-directories-databases/library-and-archive/resource-documents. Accessed January 3, 2017.

Anfang SA, Wall BW: Psychiatric fitness-for-duty evaluations. Psychiatr Clin North Am 29(3):675–693, 2006 16904505

Anfang SA, Faulkner LR, Fromson JA, et al: The American Psychiatric Association's resource document on guidelines for psychiatric fitness-for-duty evaluations of physicians. J Am Acad Psychiatry Law 33(1):85–88, 2005 15809244

Anfang SA, Gold LH, Meyer DJ: Practice guideline for the forensic evaluation of psychiatric disability. J Am Acad Psychiatry Law (in press)

Buchanan A, Norko M: The forensic evaluation and report: an agenda for research. J Am Acad Psychiatry Law 41(3):359–365, 2013 24051588

Falls JS, Nellermoe EM: Navigating the FMLA minefield: seven common mistakes employers make. South Carolina Lawyer 25:44–49, 2014

Family and Medical Leave Act of 1993, 29 C.F.R. § 825.300 (2009)

Federation of State Medical Boards of the United States: Policy on Physician Impairment. Euless, TX: Federation of State Medical Boards, 2011

Federation of State Physician Health Programs: Physician Health Program Guidelines, December 2005 Edition. 2005. Available at: http://www.fsphp.org/resources/guidelines. Accessed January 3, 2017.

Fischler GL, McElroy HK, Miller L, et al: The role of psychological fitness-for-duty evaluations in law enforcement. Police Chief 78:72–78, 2011

Glancy GD, Ash P, Bath EP, et al: AAPL practice guideline for the forensic assessment. J Am Acad Psychiatry Law 43(2)(Suppl):S3–S53, 2015 26054704

Gold LH, Metzner JL: Psychiatric employment evaluations and the Health Insurance Portability and Accountability Act. Am J Psychiatry 163(11):1878–1882, 2006 17074937

Gold LH, Shuman DW: Evaluating Mental Health Disability in the Workplace: Process, Model, and Analysis. New York, Springer, 2009

Granacher RP: Employment: disability and fitness, in The Psychiatric Report: Principles and Practice of Forensic Writing. Edited by Buchanan A, Norko MA. New York, Cambridge University Press, 2011, pp 172–186

Grant D, Alfred KC: Sanctions and recidivism: an evaluation of physician discipline by state medical boards. J Health Polit Policy Law 32(5):867–885, 2007 17855720

Gutheil TG, Brodsky A: Commentary: Tarasoff duties arising from a forensic independent medical examination. J Am Acad Psychiatry Law 38(1):57–60, 2010 20305076

Health Care Quality Improvement Act (HCQIA), 1986, 42 U.S.C. 11101 et seq.

International Association of the Chiefs of Police: IACP Police Psychological Services Section: psychological fitness-for-duty evaluation guidelines. 2013. Available at: http://www.theiacp.org/portals/0/documents/pdfs/PsychFitnessforDutyEvaluation.pdf. Accessed January 3, 2017.

Janofsky JS: Competency to practice and licensing, in The Psychiatric Report: Principles and Practice of Forensic Writing. Edited by Buchanan A, Norko MA. New York, Cambridge University Press, 2011, pp 145–157

Law MT, Hansen ZK: Medical licensing board characteristics and physician discipline: an empirical analysis. J Health Polit Policy Law 35(1):63–93, 2010 20159847

Mahoney K: Whose choice? Psychotropic medication and the armed forces. South Calif Rev Law Soc Justice 22:201–232, 2013

Meyer DJ, Price M: Forensic psychiatric assessments of behaviorally disruptive physicians. J Am Acad Psychiatry Law 34(1):72–81, 2006 16585237

Meyer DJ, Price M: Peer review committees and state licensing boards: responding to allegations of physician misconduct. J Am Acad Psychiatry Law 40(2):193–201, 2012 22635290

National Practitioner Data Bank: Reporting requirements and query access. 2017. Available at: https://www.npdb.hrsa.gov/resources/tables/reportingQueryAccess.jsp. Accessed January 3, 2017.

Occupational Safety and Health Act, Pub. L. No. 91–596, 84 Stat. 1590, 1970

Peisah C, Wilhelm K: Physician don't heal thyself: a descriptive study of impaired older doctors. Int Psychogeriatr 19(5):974–984, 2007 17506910

Pinals DA, Price M: Fitness-for-duty of law enforcement officers, in Clinical Guide to Mental Disability Evaluations. Edited by Gold LH, Vanderpool DL. New York, Springer, 2013, pp 369–392

Price M, Meyer DJ: Fitness-for-duty evaluations of physicians and health care professionals: treating providers and protecting the public, in Clinical Guide to Mental Disability Evaluations. Edited by Gold LH, Vanderpool DL. New York, Springer, 2013, pp 337–367

Regenbogen A, Recupero PR: The implications of the ADA Amendments Act of 2008 for residency training program administration. J Am Acad Psychiatry Law 40(4):553–561, 2012 23233478

Reynolds NT: A model comprehensive psychiatric fitness-for-duty evaluation. Occup Med 17(1):105–118, v, 2002 11726340

Rosman JP: Malingering: distortion and deception in employment litigation, in Mental and Emotional Injuries in Employment Litigation, 2nd Edition. Edited by McDonald JJ, Kulick FB. Washington, DC, The Bureau of National Affairs, 2001, pp 409–453

Schouten R: Psychiatric consultation in problem employee situations. Psychiatr Clin North Am 35(4):901–913, 2012 23107569

Schouten R: Workplace violence evaluations and the ADA, in Clinical Guide to Mental Disability Evaluations. Edited by Gold LH, Vanderpool DL. New York, Springer, 2013, pp 291–308

Strasburger LH, Gutheil TG, Brodsky A: On wearing two hats: role conflict in serving as both psychotherapist and expert witness. Am J Psychiatry 154(4):448–456, 1997 9090330

Tarasoff v Regents of the University of California, 551 P.2d 334 (Cal. 1976)

Verhoef LM, Weenink JW, Winters S, et al: The disciplined healthcare professional: a qualitative interview study on the impact of the disciplinary process and imposed measures in the Netherlands. BMJ Open 5(11):e009275, 2015 26608639

Walker YN: Protecting the public. The impact of the Americans with Disabilities Act on licensure considerations involving mentally impaired medical and legal professionals. J Leg Med 25(4):441–468, 2004 15764506

Wall BW: Commentary: The clinical implications of doctors' evaluating doctors. J Am Acad Psychiatry Law 33(1):89–91, 2005 15809245

Wettstein RM: Commentary: Quality improvement and psychiatric fitness-for-duty evaluations of physicians. J Am Acad Psychiatry Law 33(1):92–94, 2005 15809246

Wettstein RM: The forensic psychiatric examination and report, in The American Psychiatric Publishing Textbook of Forensic Psychiatry, 2nd Edition. Edited by Simon RI, Gold LH. Washington, DC, American Psychiatric Publishing, 2010, pp 175–203

Wettstein RM: Fitness-for-duty evaluations, in Clinical Guide to Mental Disability Evaluations. Edited by Gold LH, Vanderpool DL. New York, Springer, 2013, pp 309–336

CHAPTER 17

Psychiatric Disability

Albert M. Drukteinis, M.D., J.D.

Determinations of psychiatric disability are regularly included in conjunction with claims of mental injury and damages. In fact, the evaluation of psychiatric disability is one of the most common requests made of general and forensic psychiatrists and nonpsychiatric clinicians. Mental disorders do not automatically equate to disability; therefore, psychiatric disability determinations involve nonmedical and vocational considerations. This chapter addresses various categories of functional impairments that can result in disability and discusses how to probe those categories and corroborate functional limitations in the context of a person's history. The chapter also discusses the difference in scope in the assessment of disability between a treating psychiatrist and forensic psychiatrist and provides a basic guideline to assess a patient's disability objectively.

General Issues in Disability Assessments

Scope of Psychiatric Disability

Psychiatric disability claims are frequent and not likely to decrease. Most individuals with mental disorders, even many of those with serious psychiatric disorders, are employed, at least at some time in their lives (Erickson and Lee 2008). However, claims of disability for mental disorders have increased 168% between 2000 and 2013, representing nearly 30% of all Social Security Disability Insurance (SSDI) adult beneficiaries, with a cost in 2013 alone of over 30 billion dollars (Social Security Administration 2000, 2013).

In addition to Social Security disability claims, psychiatrists are often asked to provide opinions on short-term and long-term disability for private insurance, workers' compensation, personal injury claims, military veterans' benefits, state and federal employees' disability retirement programs, accommodations under the Americans with Disabilities Act, fitness-for-duty evaluations, and incapacity under the Family and Medical Leave Act. These claims are often accompanied by additional issues of causation, work-relatedness, service connection, or specific occupational impairment. However, work capacity remains the central determinant of functional impairment for which disability claims are brought and the issue upon which psychiatrists are asked to opine.

Therefore, psychiatrists can expect to confront disability issues as a routine part of their practice and should be familiar with how to provide objective opinions and avoid common pitfalls. In forensic psychiatry, the issue of objectivity is so central that the *Ethics Guidelines for the Practice of Forensic Psychiatry* of the American Academy of Psychiatry and the Law (AAPL) recommends that psychiatrists avoid serving as both treating clinician and forensic evaluator (American Academy of Psychiatry and the Law 2005). Practically, however, disability issues arise so frequently in the course of treatment that psychiatrists would find it impossible to recommend an independent forensic evaluation in every instance, despite recognizing that providing disability evaluations may raise questions about their objectivity. However, there should be recognition of a difference in the capabilities of treating psychiatrists and those forensically trained, even among otherwise qualified clinicians (Christopher et al. 2011; Gold 2011).

Defining Disability

An individual with a mental disorder is not automatically disabled because of that mental disorder. As elementary as that sounds, misconception about this principle is the main source of errors in disability evaluations. The American Medical Association (AMA) *Guides to the Evaluation of Permanent Impairment*, 6th Edition (American Medical Association 2008), makes a distinction between impairment and disability. *Impairment* is defined as "a significant deviation, loss, or loss of use of any body structure or body function, in an individual with a health condition, disorder, or disease" (p. 5). Such alteration of an individual's health status is assessed by medical means. In contrast, *disability* is defined as "activity limitations and/or participation restrictions in an individual with a health condition,

disorder or disease" (p. 5). Disability is assessed by medical and nonmedical means. Therefore, a mental disorder may or may not result in impairment, and impairment may or may not result in a disability.

Despite the distinction between the terms, *impairment* and *disability* are often used interchangeably. Although a fact-finder (e.g., the court, a governmental agency, an insurance company panel) makes the final determination of disability, medical opinions on disability may be appropriate. Medical opinions are routinely requested and offered on disability, including both its degree and expected duration (Drukteinis 2003). Opinions regarding disability require more than a medical consideration of symptoms and health status. How and why the capacity to meet an occupational demand has been altered must be identified.

Measuring Disability

Medical and surgical specialties widely utilize the AMA *Guides* (American Medical Association 2008) to evaluate disability, particularly for workers' compensation claims. The *Guides* provides criteria for assigning a percentage value to functional disability. The chapter titled "Mental and Behavioral Disorders" discusses three types of psychiatric disorders for which percentage impairment ratings can be calculated (American Medical Association 2008, p. 349):

- *Mood* disorders, including major depressive disorder and bipolar affective disorder
- *Anxiety* disorders, including generalized anxiety disorder, panic disorder, phobias, posttraumatic stress disorder, and obsessive-compulsive disorder[1]
- *Psychotic* disorders, including schizophrenia

The premise underlying the *Guides* selection of these diagnoses is that in serious mental illnesses, occupational impairment is obvious, whereas disability is more difficult to assess, especially in more subtle conditions in which litigation or personality factors may coexist. However, when the *Guides* is used in the evaluation of psychiatric disability, no other psychiatric diagnoses, such as substance use disorders or somatoform disorders, are ratable by a percentage impairment. The actual method of arriving at a psychiatric impairment rating in the AMA *Guides*, 6th Edition, is based on a median, or middle, value of percentages derived from the Brief Psychiatric Rating Scale (Hedlund and Viewig 1980; Overall and Gorham 1988); the Global Assessment of Functioning Scale (GAF) from the *Diagnostic and Statistical Manual of Mental Disorders*, 4th Edition, Text Revision (DSM-IV-TR) (American Psychiatric Association 2000, pp. 32–34); and the Psychiatric Impairment Rating Scale (American Medical Association 2008, pp. 356–360). Where psychiatrists are required to provide a percentage of psychiatric impairment, careful reading and study of the AMA *Guides*, 6th Edition, is highly recommended (American Medical Association 2008).

Notably, even though limited to three diagnostic categories, the *Guides* rating method has no evidence supporting its reliability or validity in the assessment of psychiatric disability. The *Diagnostic and Statistical Manual of Mental Disorders*, 5th Edition (DSM-5), has eliminated its previously recommended use of the Global Assessment of Functioning (GAF) Scale (along with the multiaxial system for diagnosis) because of the lack of conceptual clarity and questionable psychometrics in routine practice (American Psychiatric Association 2013, p. 16). This may create confusion in the long term for the use of the AMA *Guides* in mental disorders. DSM-5 recommends that psychiatrists consider a new tool for assessment of global functioning and impairment, the World Health Organization Disability Assessment Schedule 2.0 (WHODAS 2.0) (American Psychiatric Association 2013, pp. 745–748). WHODAS 2.0 is a patient self-report assessment tool in which the assessment of impairment and disability is separate from diagnostic considerations; can reflect any medical illness, psychiatric illness, or comorbid condition; and does not imply the etiology of impairments (Üstün et al. 2010). However, as a self-report instrument lacking internal indices of validity, WHODAS 2.0 creates difficulties for forensic psychiatrists, since an individual's assessment of his or her degree of impaired functioning may not accord with the appraisal of professional experts under the best of circumstances (Gold 2014).

Psychiatrists should not assume that in the jurisdiction where they practice, percentage ratings for mental disorders are allowed or that the AMA *Guides*, 6th Edition, is recognized as the means to arrive at a rating. Psychiatrists should also be careful not to blur physical and psychiatric impairment in an attempt to demonstrate the patient's overall functional limitations. Physical impairment ratings should be assessed separately by medical specialists. A percentage rating for psychiatric impairment may also not be required or acceptable either for Social Security disability benefits or under a pri-

---

[1] Although posttraumatic stress disorder and obsessive-compulsive disorder are no longer classified as anxiety disorders in DSM-5, the AMA *Guides* have yet to be revised to reflect this fact.

vate disability insurance policy, both of which have their own categories of impairment and may rely on descriptive language rather than percentages (see discussion in the next section of this chapter). Similarly, in workers' compensation claims, some jurisdictions will limit "stress" or psychiatric claims to those that include a physical component; also, they may or may not recognize percentage ratings for mental injury.

Types of Disability Evaluations

Social Security Disability

Disability determinations for the U.S. Social Security Administration (SSA) are based on their own set of definitions and rules. The SSA, the largest supplier of disability benefits in the country, offers benefits through Social Security Disability Insurance (SSDI), supported by funds obtained from an individual's prior work (Federal Insurance Contributions Act [FICA]), and through Supplemental Security Income (SSI), supported by revenued funds of the U.S. Treasury to individuals who have limited or no prior work history.

For SSA purposes, a disabling psychiatric condition is one with "documentation of a medically determinable impairment(s), consideration of the degree of limitation such impairment(s) may impose on (one's) ability to work, and consideration of whether these limitations have lasted or are expected to last for a continuous period of at least 12 months" (Social Security Administration 2015a). This means that the individual cannot work at all or, if 55 years of age or older, is unable to perform past relevant work (Social Security Administration 2015c).

The SSA lists nine diagnostic categories that may qualify for Social Security benefits, including personality disorders and substance use disorders.

With regard to the mental impairment that may flow from those conditions, each diagnostic category is assessed by a specific set of medical findings (Paragraph A criteria), as well as evidence of impairment-related functional limitations (Paragraph B criteria), two of which are required for disability to be deemed present (Social Security Administration 2015b). These include:

- Marked restriction in activities of daily living.
- Marked difficulties in maintaining social functioning.
- Marked difficulties in maintaining concentration, persistence, or pace.
- Repeated episodes of decompensation, each of extended duration.

Several diagnostic categories include additional functional criteria (Paragraph C criteria) that add to the severity of impairment or provide an alternative analysis if the Paragraph B criteria threshold is not met. For example, one such category is schizophrenia spectrum and other psychotic disorders, in which a residual disease process results in such marginal adjustment that decompensation is predicted with minimal demands (Social Security Administration 2015b).

Although psychiatrists may provide opinions on these impairments, the ultimate determination of disability is based increasingly on vocational considerations—that is, nonmedical factors—rather than on the nature and level of impairment. In SSDI determinations, the psychiatrist is asked or expected to determine not whether the patient is disabled but only to report on the mental disorder and level of impairment. Typically, SSDI claims rely on information provided by treating psychiatrists who are believed to be in the best position to provide the relevant information in regard to their patients' diagnoses and functional impairments.

Workers' Compensation

Workers' compensation systems provide limited disability benefits for injuries or illnesses that arise out of and in the course of employment. Benefits are intended to replace lost wages and pay for medical expenses related to the injury. Liability on the part of the employer does not have to be shown.

Psychiatric claims generally fall under one of three categories: 1) physical-mental (i.e., a physical event or injury causing a mental injury), 2) mental-physical (i.e., a psychological event such as a sudden shock, causing a physical injury, such as a cardiac arrest), and 3) mental-mental (i.e., a psychological event causing a psychological injury) (Gold et al. 2008). Historically, mental-mental claims were regarded as lacking an objective basis and therefore not recognized. Gradually, more jurisdictions have recognized mental and emotional disability claims and the psychological pressures that lead to them (see, e.g., *Carter v. General Motors* 1960).

In some jurisdictions, mental impairment is assessed using the AMA *Guides*, 6th Edition, including a percentage of impairment rating. In other jurisdictions, percentages are not used or required and variable categories of impairment are addressed (Gold et al. 2008). In addition, unlike SSDI claims, which require total inability to work for at least 12 months, workers' compensation claims are also broken down according to their degree and their likely duration (Gold et al. 2008, pp. S28–S31):

- Temporary partial disability
- Temporary total disability
- Permanent partial disability
- Permanent total disability

Depending on the type of mental disorder, a temporary disability may be understandable, but a permanent one would not be expected. Similarly, a given mental disorder may cause an individual to be disabled from one type of work but not another or prevented from working full-time but not part-time. (One of the most common opinions provided by psychiatrists is that the patient can only work part-time.) Such opinions may be reasonable, but only if formed from a complete understanding of the specific nature of the individual's work duties. In workers' compensation claims, as in all disability claims, determination of whether the disorder leads to work-related problems, or work-related problems lead to the disorder, is challenging.

Every workplace has its own unique environment, and the jobs within that environment may require unique skills. Therefore, generalized categories of impairment do not always provide sufficient guidance in assessing work impairment. Psychiatrists should consider obtaining the claimant's job description that may explicitly or implicitly identify the mental functioning requirements.

It may also be helpful to consider mental impairment in terms of four broad intersecting domains in which a larger number of potential functional requirements unique to the job could fall: physical, cognitive, affective, and social (Gold and Shuman 2009). For example, the *physical* domain could include maintaining endurance, stamina, and work pace; the *cognitive* domain could include the ability to understand and follow directions, or problem solve; the *affective* domain could include stress tolerance and mood consistency; and the *social* domain could include the ability to work with a team and to accept supervision (Gold and Shuman 2009, pp. 102–103). Unless specific categories of impairment need to be addressed, domains of function may allow cataloging a wide range of functional requirements into an organized scheme.

Private Disability Insurance

Private disability insurers offer an individually paid option of a safety net for those who can afford it or whose employer includes it as a benefit. Private disability insurance is essentially a private contract, subject to agreed terms and conditions. Although insurance policies are subject to the state's regulatory system, private disability insurance payments are typically much higher than those for Social Security disability and workers' compensation. Insurance carriers, therefore, will often contest disability claims and will investigate social, personal, and employment circumstances relevant to the claim (see Gold and Shuman, 2009, pp. 192–208).

Psychiatrists may be asked by the insurance carrier to supply mental health information to validate the claim of disability. Initially such claims are for *short-term disability* (typically 6 months only), and then *long-term disability*, which may or may not have a time limit for mental disorders (e.g., 2 years). Regardless of the information and opinions provided by the psychiatrist, the insurance carrier may require an independent or forensic examiner to evaluate the patient. That examiner may also contact the psychiatrist to seek additional information or to pose questions that remain unanswered about the claim. Treating psychiatrists may wish to limit their opinions to that information that is routinely gathered in the treatment relationship (e.g., diagno-

sis, treatment, prognosis, observed functional limitations). Expected time for recovery may also be provided if possible. However, psychiatrists should be aware of the issues that might be raised and litigated even if their own opinions are more circumscribed.

Many private disability insurance policies require that the insured claimant be disabled from any occupation or work in order to receive disability benefits. Others define disability narrowly as an inability to perform the functions of the claimant's own occupation, that is, the job the insured person was actually doing when the disability was incurred. This type of policy was popular in an era when professionals, such as physicians and attorneys, often purchased private disability insurance and seldom claimed psychiatric disability. For example, a vascular surgeon might be disabled even if he or she can no longer perform surgery but can still practice in other areas of medicine. Regardless, whether the person is partially or totally disabled requires a comprehensive and objective assessment.

Another commonly contested issue in private disability claims arises when a change in employment circumstances, such as a demotion or the loss of a job, triggers or accompanies a disability claim. Normally, such a situation would not qualify for private disability insurance benefits. However, distinctions in such cases may not be clear. For example, workers may claim that if not for their mental disorder, they would not have been demoted or terminated. If psychiatrists do not have sufficient information about the employment circumstances, they should not assume that a mental disorder led to the change in employment circumstances. Forensic psychiatrists should seek additional information from the employer. A proper assessment will require careful investigation and corroboration along a timeline of when the change in employment circumstances occurred and if objective impairment was evident at that time.

The Disability Assessment

The Pitfalls of Self-Report

Generally, psychiatrists make an assessment of disability based on the diagnosis of a sufficiently severe mental disorder and on their intuition about the credibility of the patient's self-report. This method is not particularly objective and typically relies on scanty information provided by patients regarding their functioning and vocational abilities. Self-reports of impairment may not be reliable or complete because of the subjective nature of mental disorders and the investment of the patient in gaining disability status. Without following individuals through the course of a typical day and monitoring their activities, a thorough understanding of their actual functioning is not possible. In that sense, all assessments of disability are only an approximation.

Nevertheless, this approximation can be made more reliable by probing categories of function in detail, seeking clear examples of impairment, obtaining reliable corroboration, understanding the nature of the patient's work, using relevant assessment instruments, and eliminating alternative explanations for disability claims. These steps may require more time and effort than a treating psychiatrist can provide, but they are necessary for a forensic psychiatrist or for a psychiatrist assuming a forensic role in the assessment of disability.

Psychiatrists conducting a disability evaluation should expand their assessment after making a diagnosis to address whether there is impairment, since a diagnosis alone does not provide specific information about impairment. Conclusory statements such as "I can't take the stress of work anymore" or "I can't seem to function" should not be accepted at face value. The circumstances, degree, frequency, and context of those claims must be ascertained. Using the categories of functioning outlined in the AMA *Guides* or by the SSA is a reasonable starting point. Psychiatrists should dissect each category in detail, seeking specific examples. If patients are unable to give reliable examples of impairment, are evasive, or can only discuss impairment in vague generalities, then they have not sufficiently demonstrated an impairment or disability. In contrast, concrete examples of impaired function can be compelling and are less likely to be contrived.

Corroboration of a disability can be either internal (i.e., directly heard or observed by the evaluator) or external (i.e., from outside sources such as reports of family, friends, or employers, or other witnesses' observations). The forensic psychiatrist conducting a comprehensive psychiatric evaluation of disability should also seek corroboration from medical and psychiatric records, employment files, and tax returns, all of which could help chronicle a person's functioning over time. Treating psychiatrists may not have access to all this information, and should be aware that their opinions on disability have only a limited foundation.

Even with corroboration of the evaluee's claims, the reliability of all sources of information must also be taken into account. For example, family members may be as invested in a disability claim as the patient and may distort the patient's mental symptoms in support of the claim. In adversarial situations such as personal injury litigation or workers' compensation, an employer or other party may also be biased against a claim of disability and provide misleading information. The inherent bias of all informants as well as the consistency of reported information should be scrutinized.

One method of obtaining internal corroboration from the patient is to survey a typical day in the patient's life. Tracing the day, hour by hour, can sometimes reveal areas of preserved functioning that demonstrate the potential for work or rehabilitation. Questioning a person in detail about a typical day makes it more difficult for the person to rely on generalized descriptions of impairment. The person's hobbies, recreation, and social interactions can be a rich source of information. A full schedule of personal activities can demonstrate a lack of credible impediment to work. The absence of activity may reveal someone who is passively accepting an invalid role.

Psychiatrists who are trying to determine whether a patient is able to work should have an adequate understanding of the nature of the job. Often, assumptions about a patient's job are poorly founded or based on stereotypes. Patients may also misrepresent their work duties or overemphasize those duties that are particularly strenuous. Speaking to the employer, with the patient's permission, can reveal a more balanced description of specific work requirements. It may also lead to an awareness of possible accommodations for the patient's mental disorder or opportunities for modified work duties. A formal job description may be helpful to review so that actual employment duties can be addressed.

Assessment tools traditionally used by psychiatrists can also help objectify impairment so that an opinion is not based solely on a patient's self-report. A carefully performed mental status examination or a battery of psychological tests may reveal cognitive impairment, severity of clinical complaints, vulnerability to fragmentation under stress, exaggeration, and other useful impairment parameters. A dramatic or histrionic presentation, or one that is inconsistent with the history of complaints, can raise doubt about the severity of the mental disorder. An angry, belligerent presentation could lead a psychiatrist to conclude that the patient is very symptomatic, when such a presentation actually represents a defensive posture to avoid scrutiny. A patient's ease during the psychiatric interview and in conversation, as well as more formal testing of mental processes, may suggest adequate cognitive functioning despite claims to the contrary.

Finally, the psychiatrist should consider alternative explanations for the patient's disability claim. The most common alternative explanation for claims that are poorly supported is that the individual is choosing not to work rather than being unable to work. Because of the subjective nature of mental disorders, this distinction is challenging for psychiatrists or forensic evaluators. Choosing not to work as opposed to being unable to work due to impairment lie on opposite sides of a continuum in which both circumstances may be operative. Evaluating psychiatrists are tasked with assessing which factor is more substantial. The best tool for this critical element of the evaluation is an accurate and reliable longitudinal history tracing the evolution of the claimed impairment in relationship to the individual's working life. The narrative that a longitudinal history reveals may be as important in the determination of disability as the science regarding the mental disorder (Drukteinis 2014).

Confounding Factors

The thorniest confounding factor facing treating psychiatrists in performing disability assessments for their own patients is the potentially damaging effect on the therapeutic alliance. The effects of providing an objective opinion on disability that disagrees with the patient's conviction that disability exists can disrupt the treatment alliance. In addition, because of the therapeutic alliance, most psychiatrists are prone to give their patients the benefit of the doubt. At the same time, a variety of psychiatric attitudes and countertransference dynamics may also enter into the decision-making process (Mischoulen 2002). Among these are judgments about the patient's character and work ethic, identification with the patient, and rescue fantasies.

If the psychiatrist's opinion on disability is favorable to the patient, at least in the short run, the therapeutic alliance may be strengthened. On the other hand, even if the opinion on disability is unfavorable, communicating this to the patient can become part of the therapeutic process (Mischoulen 2002). Psychiatrists should address the underlying psychological issues leading to the patient's misperception of disability in a nonjudgmental manner, recognizing that the patients may genuinely perceive that they are disabled. Additionally, an opinion in favor of disability may be considered by some patients to be unfavorable, given that they may not want to see themselves disabled and will insist on continuing to work even when a mental disorder creates significant impairment.

Alternatively, treating psychiatrists can limit the consequences of providing an unfavorable opinion on disability by limiting their reporting to the diagnosis and claimed symptomatology, forgoing any conclusions about work impairment or disability. The administrative fact-finder then makes the determination. This is the same process the SSA requires of treating clinicians. However, in claims other than those involving SSDI, this stance often falls short of the inquiring party's needs. Without the psychiatrist's support, this approach may leave the patient administratively stranded.

In addition to the psychiatrist's concern for the therapeutic alliance, malingering, symptom exaggeration, and secondary gain are also potential confounding factors in a disability claim and should be considered in the assessment. External incentives for malingering, such as avoiding work and financial compensation from disability benefits, are common in disability claims. Malingering and symptom exaggeration have been estimated to occur in up to 30% of disability claimants (Aronoff et al. 2007; Chafetz and Underhill 2013; Mittenberg et al. 2002).

Malingering is difficult to detect solely through unstructured interviews, so psychiatrists should consider using instruments specifically designed to assess for malingering (see Chapter 6, "Evaluation of Malingering"). Factors that suggest malingering are poor motivation, circumstances for disability other than illness, atypical or exaggerated symptoms, inconsistencies in the presentation or narrative, and activity or behavior that is incongruent with the claim. The reasonable certainty that someone is malingering almost requires an admission of faking or an observation of flagrant contradiction to claims of impairment (Hurst 1940). These occur rarely, and making the diagnosis of malingering inevitably has a pejorative effect. On the other hand, symptom exaggeration and magnification are common and may be completely, mostly, or at least partially unintentional.

DSM-5 indicates that among factors that could lead to the suspicion of malingering is the presence of antisocial personality disorder (American Psychiatric Association 2013). However, it is more likely that sociopathic effects on disability claims are on a continuum and parallel to symptom exaggeration and malingering (Drukteinis 2008), so that the actual diagnosis of antisocial personality disorder may be less relevant. The more relevant assessment is determining the degree to which symptoms are genuine versus exaggerated, whether impairment from symptoms is substantial versus minimal, and how much can be attributed to being unable to work versus choosing not to work. Without evidence to the contrary, psychiatrists should explain to patients that their symptoms are inconsistent or without adequate objective basis rather than to call them malingerers or, in effect, liars.

Because disability benefits influence the reporting and perhaps the experiencing of symptoms (Gold et al. 2008; Kwan and Friel 2002; Rogers and Payne 2006), the potential for secondary gain should always be considered. *Secondary gain* refers to environmental responses to being sick that reinforce symptoms. Examples include financial reimbursement, attention from the family, or avoidance of less-than-satisfactory work conditions. The absence of rehabilitation efforts that might demonstrate the patient's motivation toward recovery and the decision to claim long-term disability before receiving treatment are both indicators of potential for symptom exaggeration or secondary gain.

Iatrogenic factors can lead to a mutually reinforcing concept of invalidism between patient and psychiatrist and block a patient's recovery. Such factors can be introduced by over-pathologizing someone's condition. They can also arise if the psychiatrist prematurely supports a disability claim or extends it to the point that the patient cannot recover the initiative or energy to reenter the workforce. In addition, medication side effects can create impairments and should be regularly reevaluated for their potential role in maintaining impairment. There is little justification for side effects of medication to be the primary cause of work impairment. In long-term treatment, perpetual focus on illness and impairment becomes a self-fulfilling prophecy (Seligman 2002).

Disability and Specific Mental Disorders

Although some patients with very severe mental disorders can work in a limited capacity or in a sheltered setting, certain disorders clearly are more likely to result in work impairment. Psychotic conditions such as schizophrenia or severe bipolar disorders routinely lead to major impairment in social and occupational functioning. Similarly, certain chronic anxiety and depressive disorders that are unresponsive to treatment can be disabling, if not for all work, then perhaps for the type of work that the patient was formerly capable of doing. Posttraumatic stress disorder, which is the subject of much litigation involving disability claims, may be quite disabling for certain types of work, particularly if the trauma occurred in a similar work setting. However, few objective data support chronic total disability from posttraumatic stress disorder (Drukteinis 2003).

Somatic symptom and related disorders (previously called "somatoform disorders") present a unique conundrum in disability claims in that the impairment is due to physical symptoms, but prominent psychological factors and emotional distress are involved (American Psychiatric Association 2013, pp. 309–327). In some of these cases, such as chronic pain disorders, the disability is said to be caused by physical symptoms and therefore is not technically a mental health issue. However, a secondary psychological reaction is asserted as an independent impairment (Drukteinis 2000, 2009). For example, patients may claim disability due to back pain, but medical evidence shows that a sedentary work capacity is still present. Patients may then claim that depression caused by inability to work at their former job or chronic pain itself has resulted in total disability. This scenario arises in situations where percentage ratings are sought for physical and mental impairment as part of settlement negotiations.

Even more controversial are disability claims for addictive and personality disorders (Frisman and Rosenheck 2002; Grant et al. 2005). Should disability be granted for an individual's maladaptive behavior? Are these conditions over which an individual has no control? Political, philosophical, public policy, and social science considerations are involved in this controversy. Practically, however, if a period of temporary disability can be used to help with psychological growth and recovery, even for these conditions, disability benefits may be justified. Permanent disability for such claims, on the other hand, should be more carefully examined.

In general, disability determinations should take into account the natural course of a mental disorder, the expected effects of adequate treatment, and a realistic prognosis. Work, by and large, is healthy and restorative for most people, even those with mental disorders, and should be encouraged. Disability can have an eroding effect on the individual. Therefore, opinions about disability, particularly permanent disability, should be cautiously considered.

Conclusion

Disability determinations are a challenging area of forensic and clinical psychiatry that cannot be avoided. Psychiatrists should refer to accepted categories of potential impairment in addition to reporting symptoms and making a diagnosis. Assessing whether impairment exists according to these categories can be accomplished through a careful and detailed review coupled with reliable corroboration. The therapeutic alliance with the patient and its accompanying bias are challenging but not insurmountable. If disability status can be seen as both a benefit and potential harm to the patient, then a more objective judgment will be easier to make and communicate to the patient as part of the therapeutic process. Referral to a forensic psychiatrist in complex cases is encouraged, or when damage to the therapeutic alliance is foreseeable. More detailed guidelines for evaluation are available in the AAPL *Practice Guideline for the Forensic Evaluation of Psychiatric Disability* (Gold et al. 2008).

Key Concepts

- A mental disorder does not automatically equate to a disability.

- Disability determinations must involve nonmedical and vocational considerations.

- Disability must be demonstrated, not presumed.

- All disability determinations are an approximation, since it is impossible to completely know a person's functioning.

- Therapeutic alliance and countertransference issues can create an inherent bias for the psychiatrist when evaluating patients for disability.

- Disability benefits can be an important safety net for a patient with a mental disorder, but they can also have an eroding effect that is unhealthy.

References

American Academy of Psychiatry and the Law: Ethics guidelines for the practice of forensic psychiatry. May 2005. Available at: http://www.aapl.org/ethics.htm. Accessed December 19, 2016.

American Medical Association: Guides to the Evaluation of Permanent Impairment, 6th Edition. Edited by Andersson GBJ, Cocchiarella L. Chicago, IL, American Medical Association, 2008

American Psychiatric Association: Diagnostic and Statistical Manual of Mental Disorders, 4th Edition, Text Revision. Washington, DC, American Psychiatric Association, 2000

American Psychiatric Association: Diagnostic and Statistical Manual of Mental Disorders, 5th Edition. Arlington, VA, American Psychiatric Association, 2013

Aronoff GM, Mandel S, Genovese E, et al: Evaluating malingering in contested injury or illness. Pain Pract 7(2):178–204, 2007 17559488

Carter v General Motors, 361 Mich 577, 106 NW2d 105 (1960)

Chafetz M, Underhill J: Estimated costs of malingered disability. Arch Clin Neuropsychol 28(7):633–639, 2013 23800432

Christopher PP, Arikan R, Pinals DA, et al: Evaluating psychiatric disability: differences by forensic expertise. J Am Acad Psychiatry Law 39(2):183–188, 2011 21653261

Drukteinis AM: Overlapping somatoform syndromes in personal injury litigation. Am J Forensic Psychiatry 21:37–66, 2000

Drukteinis AM: Disability determination in PTSD litigation, in Posttraumatic Stress Disorder in Litigation: Guidelines for Forensic Assessment, 2nd Edition. Edited by Simon RI. Washington, DC, American Psychiatric Publishing, 2003, pp 141–161

Drukteinis AM: Disability and sociopathy, in International Handbook of Psychopathic Disorders and the Law. Edited by Felthous A, Sass H. Chichester, UK, Wiley, 2008, pp 137–154

Drukteinis AM: Pain disorders in litigation: psychiatric update and evaluation guide. Am J Forensic Psychiatry 30:5–105, 2009

Drukteinis AM: Forensic historiography: narratives and science. J Am Acad Psychiatry Law 42(4):427–436, 2014 25492068

Erickson W, Lee C: 2007 Disability Status Report: United States. Ithaca, NY, Cornell University Rehabilitation Research and Training Center on Disability Demographics and Statistics, 2008

Frisman LK, Rosenheck R: The impact of disability payments on persons with addictive disorders. Psychiatr Ann 32:303–307, 2002

Gold LH: Commentary: Challenges in providing psychiatric disability evaluations. J Am Acad Psychiatry Law 39(2):189–193, 2011 21653262

Gold LH: DSM-5 and the assessment of functioning: the World Health Organization Disability Assessment Schedule 2.0 (WHODAS 2.0). J Am Acad Psychiatry Law 42(2):173–181, 2014 24986344

Gold LH, Shuman DW: Evaluating Mental Health Disability in the Workplace: Model, Process, and Analysis. New York, Springer, 2009

Gold LH, Anfang SA, Drukteinis AM, et al: AAPL practice guideline for the forensic evaluation of psychiatric disability. J Am Acad Psychiatry Law 36(4)(suppl):S3–S50, 2008 19092058

Grant BF, Hasin DS, Stinson FS, et al: Co-occurrence of 12-month mood and anxiety disorders and personality disorders in the US: results from the national epidemiologic survey on alcohol and related conditions. J Psychiatr Res 39(1):1–9, 2005 15504418

Hedlund JL, Viewig BW: Brief Psychiatric Rating Scale: a comprehensive review. J Oper Psychiatr 11:48–65, 1980

Hurst AF: Medical Diseases of War. London, Arnold, 1940

Kwan O, Friel J: Clinical relevance of the sick role and secondary gain in the treatment of disability syndromes. Med Hypotheses 59(2):129–134, 2002 12208197

Mischoulen D: Potential pitfalls to the therapeutic relationship arising from disability claims. Psychiatr Ann 32:299–307, 2002

Mittenberg W, Patton C, Canyock EM, et al: Base rates of malingering and symptom exaggeration. J Clin Exp Neuropsychol 24(8):1094–1102, 2002 12650234

Overall JE, Gorham DR: Brief Psychiatric Rating Scale: recent developments in ascertainment and scaling. Psychopharmacol Bull 24:97–99, 1988

Rogers R, Payne JW: Damages and rewards: assessment of malingered disorders in compensation cases. Behav Sci Law 24(5):645–658, 2006 17016811

Seligman MEP: Authentic Happiness. New York, Free Press, 2002

Social Security Administration: Annual statistical report on the Social Security Disability Insurance Program. 2000. Available at: https://www.socialsecurity.gov/policy/docs/statcomps/di_asr/2000/index.html. Accessed June 13, 2017.

Social Security Administration: Annual statistical report on the Social Security Disability Insurance Program. 2013. Available at: https://www.socialsecurity.gov/policy/docs/statcomps/ di_asr/2013/index.html. Accessed June 13, 2017.

Social Security Administration: Disability evaluation under social security: 12.00 Mental Disorders—Adult. 2015a. Available at: https://www.ssa.gov/disability/professionals/bluebook/12.00-Mental Disorders-Adult.htm. Accessed June 6, 2017.

Social Security Administration: Disability evaluation under social security: 12.01 Category of Impairments, Mental Disorders. 2015b. Available at: https://www.ssa.gov/disability/professionals/bluebook/12.00-MentalDisorders-Adult.htm#12_01. Accessed June 6, 2017.

Social Security Administration: Disability Planner: How we decide if you are disabled, Steps 4 and 5. 2015c. Available at: https://www.ssa.gov/planners/disability/dqualify5.html. Accessed June 6, 2017.

Üstün TB, Kostanjsek N, Chatterji S, et al: Measuring Health and Disability: Manual for WHO Disability Assessment Schedule (WHODAS 2.0). Geneva, World Health Organization, 2010

PART IV

Criminal Justice

CHAPTER 18

Evaluation of Competencies in the Criminal Justice System

Charles L. Scott, M.D.

Landmark Cases

Dusky v. United States, 362 U.S. 402, 80 S.Ct. 788 (1960)

Wilson v. United States, 129 U.S. App. D.C. 107, 391 F.2d 460 (1968)

North Carolina v. Alford, 400 U.S. 25, 91 S.Ct. 160 (1970)

Jackson v. Indiana, 406 U.S. 715, 738, 92 S.Ct. 1845 (1972)

Colorado v. Connelly, 479 U.S. 157, 107 S.Ct. 515 (1986)

Rock v. Arkansas, 483 U.S. 44, 107 S.Ct. 2704 (1987)

Riggins v. Nevada, 504 U.S. 127, 112 S.Ct. 1810 (1992)

Godinez v. Moran, 509 U.S. 389, 113 S.Ct. 2680 (1993)

Cooper v. Oklahoma, 517 U.S. 348, 116 S.Ct. 1373 (1996)

Sell v. United States, 539 U.S. 166, 123 S.Ct. 2174 (2003)

Indiana v. Edwards, 554 U.S. 164, 128 S.Ct. 2379 (2008)

From the moment individuals are approached by police officers as possible criminal suspects until their involvement with the complex criminal justice system is finished, they may have to navigate a variety of legal tasks, consult with a range of court officials, and make decisions that can often impact the rest of their lives. Because these activities range in complexity, individuals may need different abilities to tackle the various legal scenarios facing them. The concept of *competency* refers to a person's capacity relevant to a specific task or issue. The various individual competencies are both task specific and moment specific. This chapter reviews how examiners can assess a range of competencies that defendants must muster as they meander through the maze of the criminal justice system.

Competency to Stand Trial

Legal Overview

Competency to stand trial (CST), sometimes referred to as "adjudicative competence," represents the legal construct that defendants should have the ability to participate in their own trial process. CST evaluation requests are the most common referrals for criminal forensic examination (Rogers et al. 2001). Surveys indicate that public defenders have concerns regarding CST for approximately 10%–15% of their clients (Melton et al. 2007). Conservative estimates suggest that 60,000 competency evaluations are requested per year. When the number of actively psychotic and mentally disordered inmates is taken into account, the potential number of competency evaluations could easily be twice this estimate (Rogers and Johansson-Love 2009).

Defendants are presumed competent to stand trial. However, various courtroom participants (e.g., defense attorney, judge, prosecuting attorney) can request an evaluation of a defendant's competency at any point before or during the trial process. A judge, or in some jurisdictions a jury, determines whether a defendant is competent.

The U.S. Supreme Court addressed the level of proof required to prove that a defendant is incompetent in *Cooper v. Oklahoma* (1996). In this case, Byron Keith Cooper was charged with murdering an 86-year-old man during a burglary. During his trial, Mr. Cooper exhibited bizarre behavior, such as talking to himself and to "spirits." He also reported fears that his attorney wanted to kill him. The trial court utilized the Oklahoma statute that required Mr. Cooper to prove trial incompetency by *clear and convincing evidence* (an approximate 75% level of certainty). This clear and convincing standard of proof is substantially higher than the *preponderance of evidence* standard, which requires a level of proof referenced as "more likely than not" (i.e., greater than 50%).

The trial court found that Mr. Cooper had not met the higher clear and convincing standard for proving trial incompetency. He was subsequently tried, found guilty, and sentenced to death. On appeal, the U.S. Supreme Court held that the Oklahoma statute violated due process because it allowed a defendant who was "more likely than not" incompetent to be found competent to stand trial under the clear and convincing standard and to be sentenced to death. The Supreme Court stated that a defendant should bear the burden of proving incompetence to stand trial by the preponderance of evidence standard.

The U.S. Supreme Court first established the constitutional standard for CST in *Dusky v. United States* (1960). Milton Dusky was a 33-year-old man charged with assisting in the kidnapping and rape of an underage female. A pretrial psychiatric evaluation determined that Mr. Dusky suffered from a "schizophrenic reaction, chronic undifferentiated type." The trial court noted that Mr. Dusky was oriented and could recall events, and these observations served as the court's basis for finding him competent to stand trial. After being found guilty of rape, he appealed the lower court's finding that he was competent to stand trial. The U.S. Supreme Court enunciated the following as a minimum constitutional standard for trial competency: "[W]hether he [had] sufficient present ability to consult with his lawyer with a reasonable degree of rational understanding—and whether he [had] a rational as well as factual understanding of the proceedings against him" (***Dusky v. United States*** 1960).

Melton et al. (2007) outlined the important components embedded within the ***Dusky*** CST standard:

1. The CST standard involves two prongs:
   - The ability of the defendant to understand the criminal process
   - The ability of the defendant to assist his or her attorney in the defendant's own defense
2. CST evaluations focus on a defendant's *present* ability; that is, the evaluation is needed to determine the defendant's current mental state, in contrast to sanity evaluations (discussed in Chapter 19, "Evaluation of Criminal Responsibility"), which retrospectively analyze the defendant's mental state at the time of the alleged crime.
3. The CST evaluation examines a defendant's capacity to stand trial as opposed to his or her willingness to stand trial.
4. The CST standard requires only that the defendant have a reasonable degree of rational understanding, not an absolute or perfect capacity in this regard.

5. The presence of a mental illness alone does not automatically equate with a finding of trial incompetency. The evaluator has to demonstrate the relationship, if any, of the mental disorder to trial competency deficits.

Conducting the Evaluation

Although the federal *Dusky* standard does not specifically state that a mental disease or defect is necessary to find a person incompetent to stand trial, the vast majority of state statutes require some type of mental disorder as the predicate basis for such a finding. Because state statutes have slight variations in their CST standards, examiners should be familiar with the precise language that defines trial competency in their jurisdictions.

Prior to conducting the evaluation, an examiner needs to become familiar with the charges the defendant is facing as well as the police report and witness statements regarding the alleged offense. This information is important to help assess the defendant's understanding of his or her legal situation and the relationship, if any, of the individual's mental state to a finding of trial incompetency. Additional documents that may be helpful include jail treatment records, prior psychiatric records, medical records, educational records, and prior criminal record (also known as a National Crime Information Center report). In addition to reviewing relevant records, an evaluator should understand what difficulties, if any, the defendant's defense attorney has noted in the client's ability to assist the attorney.

Diagnostic Considerations

Psychotic disorders, severe mood disorders, and cognitive impairments represent the most common diagnoses associated with findings of trial incompetency. Although less severe diagnoses could potentially render a defendant incompetent, examiners must understand that many defendants may feel sad or anxious about their legal situation. Such adjustment reactions are not usually of the type or severity that impairs a defendant's ability to participate in the legal process.

Likewise, personality disorders alone are not typically considered to be a diagnosis responsible for rendering a defendant trial incompetent. For example, a defendant with antisocial personality disorder who threatens his or her attorney may have difficulties working with counsel, but such antisocial behaviors are generally not accepted as sufficient support for a finding of trial incompetency. In other words, a defendant who chooses not to work with counsel is competent, unlike a defendant who lacks the capacity to work with counsel. Some personality disorders, however, such as a schizoid or paranoid personality disorder, may impact a defendant's psycholegal abilities, and trial courts have allowed consideration of such disorders when determining trial competency (*State v. Stock* 1971; *United States v. Veatch* 1993).

Claims of amnesia are common in the criminal justice system. According to Cima et al. (2004), 23% of male forensic inpatients charged with serious crimes claimed either partial or total amnesia for their alleged crimes. Amnesia for a criminal act is not necessarily a bar to a finding of trial competency.

The District of Columbia (D.C.) Circuit Court of Appeals addressed this issue in **Wilson v. United States** (1968). Robert Wilson and a codefendant robbed a pharmacy store and were subsequently pursued in a high-speed police chase that ultimately resulted in the getaway car crashing into a tree. Mr. Wilson suffered a significant head injury, and his partner

in crime died. Mr. Wilson could not recall anything that happened on the afternoon of the robberies, although his mental status was otherwise normal.

Despite Mr. Wilson's amnesia for the crime, he was deemed competent to stand trial and subsequently convicted. Mr. Wilson appealed, claiming that his amnesia prevented him from testifying on his own behalf (in violation of the Fifth Amendment) and effectively assisting his attorney (in violation of the Sixth Amendment). The D.C. Court of Appeals held that amnesia was not an automatic bar to a defendant being found incompetent and remanded the case back to the trial court to carefully review whether Mr. Wilson's amnesia had negatively impacted his trial competency.

The D.C. Court of Appeals outlined a two-stage process when considering an amnestic defendant. First, the trial court must predict whether the defendant's reported amnesia would render him or her competent or incompetent. If the defendant is found competent, the court must then conduct a posttrial inquiry, involving a review of six factors (Table 18–1) to evaluate whether the defendant's amnesia actually impaired his or her capacity to participate during the trial process.

Forensic Evaluation Specific to CST

After establishing a baseline regarding a defendant's general abilities and functioning, evaluators usually ask questions specifically related to trial competency. Such questions typically require the defendant to demonstrate an understanding of the following (Resnick and Noffsinger 2004):

- *Legal charges.* The defendant should be asked to describe the legal charges, his or her understanding of the seri-

TABLE 18–1. ***Wilson* factors to evaluate amnesia impact on competency to stand trial**

1. The effect of the amnesia on the defendant's ability to consult with and assist his or her lawyer

2. The effect of the amnesia on the defendant's ability to testify

3. How well the evidence could be extrinsically reconstructed, including evidence relating to the alleged offense and any plausible alibi

4. The extent to which the government assisted the defense in this reconstruction

5. The strength of the prosecution's case, including the possibility that the accused could, but for the amnesia, establish an alibi or other defense

6. Any other facts and circumstances that would indicate whether or not the defendant had a fair trial

Source. ***Wilson v. United States*** 1968.

ousness of the charges, and the potential sentence for each charge. If the defendant is unable to name the precise penal code term for the charge, the examiner should assess whether the defendant possesses an appropriate understanding of the elements of the charge. For example, if a defendant does not state precisely that he or she is charged with first-degree homicide but tells the examiner that he or she is charged with premeditated murder, the defendant has demonstrated a basic understanding of this charge.

- *Roles and responsibilities of courtroom participants.* The defendant can be asked to explain the roles of the defense attorney, prosecuting attorney, judge, witness, and jury, as well as the defendant. In addition to understanding the defendant's rational knowledge of the courtroom participants, the examiner should also evaluate whether the defendant has any irrational beliefs associated with these individuals that negatively impact the defendant's trial competency.
- *Available pleas.* The examiner should inquire into the defendant's knowledge of these various pleas: guilty, not guilty, not guilty by reason of insanity, guilty but mentally ill (if available in the governing jurisdiction), and no contest. In addition, the defendant should understand the concept of plea bargaining, which generally involves a reduced sentence in exchange for a guilty or no contest plea. If a defendant refuses to consider a plea bargain, the forensic psychiatrist should evaluate whether this refusal results from irrational thinking due to a mental disorder.

In some situations, a defendant may provide inadequate answers about the legal process due to a lack of knowledge about the justice system as opposed to an impaired ability to understand this information. A lack of knowledge alone does not equate with trial incompetency. In such a situation, the evaluator should educate the defendant and later ascertain whether the defendant had the capacity to learn and retain the information.

In addition to assessing the trial-related areas as described above, the examiner should gather information regarding the defendant's ability to assist in his or her defense. Important areas to evaluate in making this determination are reviewed in Table 18–2.

Asking a defendant to explain his or her understanding of the allegations and

TABLE 18–2.   **Abilities needed for defendants to assist in their defense**

1. To work with defense counsel
2. To appreciate their legal situation as a criminal defendant
3. To rationally consider a mental illness defense
4. To appraise evidence and estimate likely outcome of a trial
5. To have sufficient memory and concentration to understand trial events
6. To maintain appropriate courtroom behavior
7. To provide a consistent and organized account of the offense (although reported amnesia of offense does not necessarily prevent a finding of competency)
8. To formulate a basic plan of defense

Source.   Resnick and Noffsinger 2004.

evidence may assist in evaluating the defendant's understanding of the charges, potential witnesses who might testify for or against the defendant, the presence of incriminating or exculpatory evidence, the defendant's ability to communicate key information to counsel, and an understanding of available pleas based on the offense circumstances (to include a plea of insanity).

When defendants refuse to discuss the criminal allegations, experts should ask the defendants to explain why they wish to withhold this information. Some defendants refuse to provide this information based on their attorneys' instructions not to discuss their offense with anyone but legal counsel. The defendant in this situation may be demonstrating a rational ability to follow legal guidance, an important aspect of CST. In contrast, another defendant may refuse to discuss the allegations based on paranoia about the examiner or the trial process, indicating an irrational belief system and possible incompetence (Mossman et al. 2007).

Although the defendant's account of the crime is relevant in evaluating trial competency, some jurisdictions prohibit evaluators from this type of questioning. Potential concerns about taking a defendant's crime account as part of a trial competency evaluation include the possibility that this information will be used against the defendant at a later stage of the trial or may expose future legal strategies to the prosecution. To minimize this risk, an expert should consider including only a general statement in the competency reports, to the effect that the defendant was able to discuss his or her whereabouts at the time of the crime and his or her version of events surrounding the alleged offense. If the expert is later asked to testify about specific information relating to the crime provided by the defendant during the CST evaluation, the expert can seek guidance from the court about whether discussion of any potentially incriminating information is allowed before answering this question (Mossman et al. 2007).

Hypnosis and the Criminal Defendant

Hypnosis has been used by defense attorneys to help refresh defendants' memories of their roles in alleged offenses. However, memories recovered under hypnosis may be inherently unreliable. Despite these concerns, in *Rock v. Arkansas* (1987), the U.S. Supreme Court held that courts cannot automatically bar all hypnotically refreshed defendant testimony. The Court noted that to do so would violate defendants' Fifth Amendment right to testify in their own defense, Sixth Amendment right to have witnesses testify on their behalf, and Fourteenth Amendment right to due process of law that allows the presentation of evidence in court. The Court emphasized that states could establish guidelines for the court on admissibility of hypnotically refreshed memories, but could not blindly exclude such testimony.

Psychological Testing and Structured Evaluation Instruments

Several structured instruments designed to evaluate a defendant's CST have been developed and can serve as a useful guide for the evaluator. A summary of the most common structured evaluation instruments and their strengths and weaknesses is provided in Table 18–3.

For defendants who may have a developmental or intellectual disability, intelligence testing is often used to assess the degree, if any, of cognitive impairment (see Chapter 5, "Psychological Testing in Forensic Psychiatry"). The usefulness of other types of psychological tests that are commonly used in clinical evaluations, such as the Rorschach test or Draw a Person test, may be limited: "the routine administration of conventional psychological tests is unlikely to be a cost-efficient means of gathering information in most competency cases. Because the nature of the cognitive deficits in such cases is relatively specific, generalized measures of intelligence or personality are unlikely to be very helpful" (Melton et al. 2007, p. 161). The American Academy of Psychiatry and the Law (AAPL) Practice Guideline for Trial Competency also supports this position: "Psychiatrists can usually ascertain the crucial psychological data relevant to functioning as a competent criminal defendant directly from interviewing defendants and evaluating information provided by collateral sources" (Mossman et al. 2007, p. S36).

Evaluating Malingering in CST Evaluations

The forensic evaluator should also consider the possibility that the defendant may malinger psychiatric symptoms or knowledge deficits to appear incompetent to stand trial to avoid or delay prosecution. In evaluating a defendant's potential malingering of trial incompetency, the examiner should consider standard approaches to the assessment of malingered psychiatric symptoms, as outlined in Chapter 6, "Evaluation of Malingering." Factors that increase the likelihood of malingering incompetency to stand trial are reviewed in Table 18–4.

Psychological tests designed to assess malingering, such as the Structured Interview of Reported Symptoms (SIRS; Rogers 1992), Structured Inventory of Malingered Symptomatology (SIMS; Widows and Smith 2005), Miller Forensic Assessment of Symptoms Test (M-FAST; Miller 2001), Test of Memory Malingering (TOMM; Tombaugh 2009), and Minnesota Multiphasic Personality Inventory–2 (MMPI-2; Butcher et al. 1989), may be particularly helpful in determining whether the defendant is feigning or exaggerating symptoms of psychiatric illness. Three psychological tests that specifically assess malingering in the context of CST evaluations have been developed. These instruments are summarized in Table 18–5.

Assessment of Defendants Who Refuse a CST Evaluation

Evaluators may encounter a defendant who refuses to participate in the competency assessment. An evaluation refusal alone does not indicate trial incompetency; otherwise, all defendants could simply maintain their silence during an

TABLE 18–3.   Structured evaluation instruments to assess competency to stand trial

Instrument and description	Pros	Cons
Competence Assessment for Standing Trial for Defendants with Mental Retardation (Everington 1990) Contains 50 items in three sections Sections I and II use multiple-choice questions at fourth-grade reading level to evaluate understanding of legal terms and ability to assist defense. Section III includes oral questioning to elicit narrative answers.	Scoring guidelines provided Satisfactory psychometric properties	Competence assessment is limited to defendant's "understanding" abilities Multiple-choice recognition format does not allow an in-depth evaluation of defendant's understanding of legal issues
Competency Assessment Instrument (U.S. Department of Health 1973) Nonstandardized, semi-structured interview Uses 5-point Likert ratings to evaluate 13 court-related abilities	Provides organized format to focus interview with numerous sample questions High face validity	Neither administration nor scoring is standardized
Georgia Court Competency Test (Nicolson and Kugler 1991) Screening instrument Includes picture of courtroom layout Asks questions about roles of courtroom participants and defendant's relationship with counsel	Explicit scoring system Quick and easy to administer	May not adequately evaluate understanding and participation in legal process to include ability to assist counsel
MacArthur Competency Assessment Tool—Criminal Adjudication (Hoge et al. 1997) Semi-structured interview format with 22 items Utilizes a hypothetical vignette to assess a defendant's psycholegal abilities Yields information on understanding, appreciation, and reasoning competency–related abilities	Provides explicit scoring criteria Unique format allows assessment of defendant's ability to process and understand relevant information Component measures are closely related to *Dusky* criteria	Hypothetical vignette used to assess understanding and reasoning abilities does not pertain to defendant's own case

TABLE 18–3. Structured evaluation instruments to assess competency to stand trial *(continued)*

Instrument and description	Pros	Cons
Evaluation of Competency to Stand Trial—Revised (Rogers et al. 2004)	Component measures closely related to *Dusky* criteria	Limited range of potential psychopathologies to evaluate and rate
Semi-structured interview format	Includes a brief measure to screen for possible feigning	Gradations of psychopathology do not clearly translate to affect on CST
Contains three scales: Consult with Counsel, Factual Understanding of Courtroom Proceedings, and Rational Understanding of Courtroom Proceedings	Excellent psychometric properties	Internal validity issues regarding item ratings and scale interpretations
Scale scores can be converted to T-scores used to assess degree of functional capacity impairment with comparison norms from offender samples		

Source. Melton et al. 2007.

TABLE 18–4. **Factors suggesting malingered incompetency to stand trial**

Atypical presentation of psychiatric symptoms

Malingering indicated on psychological testing

Malingered responses on structured CST evaluation instruments

Mental disorder symptoms appearing only during a CST evaluation

Decline in defendant's level of functioning only during CST evaluation

Markedly impaired cognitive ability only when CST questions are asked

Excellent abilities to work on other legal cases (such as a civil lawsuit)

Performance on competency assessment not consistent with educational level or life achievement

Note. CST=competency to stand trial.

evaluation, thereby preventing their cases from moving forward. These situations require a careful approach.

First, examiners should remember that they are attempting to determine whether a defendant has a mental disorder that actually interferes with his or her *capacity* to stand trial. In particular, the examiner should consider highly organized capacities that may be relevant in assessing trial competency, even if a defendant refuses to answer questions. For example, is the individual able to learn new material, to demonstrate sustained concentration on various assigned tasks, and to advocate for his or her rights or for the rights of other patients? These capacities are important in—and relevant to—working with an attorney and facing trial.

Second, examiners should collect objective evidence to determine whether an evaluation refusal is due to a mental disorder or is more consistent with voluntary noncooperation. A defendant could refuse an examination due to severe paranoia regarding examiners and their role in the legal system. However, observations in settings outside the forensic evaluation can often clarify whether the paranoia is pervasive or only appears suddenly during testing.

CST Evaluation Outcomes

Once an evaluator has rendered his or her CST opinion, a court hearing is usually held to make a legal determination of the defendant's CST. In some cases, the attorneys stipulate to a finding without a formal hearing. A defendant found incompetent to stand trial is usually committed involuntarily to an inpatient psychiatric facility for competency restoration and treatment of the underlying mental disorder. In some jurisdictions, if the defendant is deemed not restorable and remains incompetent (e.g., due to treatment-resistant psychosis), the defendant may be involuntarily committed under the state's statutory civil commitment scheme for persons deemed nonrestorable. Inpatient competency restoration typically involves a combination of treatment for the defendant's underlying mental illness and education regarding the legal system (Noffsinger 2001).

Defendants cannot be involuntarily hospitalized indefinitely for competency restoration purposes, as indicated by the U.S. Supreme Court ruling in *Jackson v. Indiana* (1972). This case involved 27-year-old Theon Jackson, who was deaf and mute and had a severe intellectual

TABLE 18–5. Malingered trial incompetency assessment instruments

Test	Description	Malingering assessment strategy
Evaluation of Competency to Stand Trial— Revised (Rogers et al. 2004)	Semi-structured interview format	Contains 28 atypical presentation items
	Three scales that measure factual understanding, rational understanding, and ability to consult with counsel	Five scales designed to assess feigned incompetence
Inventory of Legal Knowledge (Musick and Otto 2010)	Consists of 61 true-false items about the legal system	Measures response style toward evaluation of trial competency
	Does not directly measure trial competency	Symptom validity testing approach using forced-choice paradigm
		Provides cutoff scores for likely feigning
		Scores less than chance are particularly suspicious for feigned trial incompetency
Test of Malingered Incompetence (Colwell et al. 2008)	Evaluates cognitive malingering of trial incompetency	Symptom validity testing approach using forced-choice paradigm
	Two scales with 25 items each: General Knowledge and Legal Knowledge	Provides cutoff score to identify honest *vs.* dishonest responder
	Not designed to test trial competency	

disability. He was charged with stealing money from two purses, yielding a grand total of $9.00. As a result of his severe disabilities, he was found incompetent to stand trial and involuntarily committed to a psychiatric facility until such time that he became competent.

Mr. Jackson's attorney appealed to the U.S. Supreme Court, arguing that the hospital would never be able to restore Mr. Jackson to trial competency, which would result in his effectively being involuntarily committed for the duration of his life. The Court held that an incompetent defendant cannot be held more than the reasonable period of time necessary to determine whether the defendant will regain competence in the foreseeable future. The Court famously articulated, "Due Process requires that the nature and duration of confinement bear some reasonable relation to the purpose for which the individual is committed" (*Jackson v. Indiana* 1972). Since this ruling, states have varied widely in what they consider a "reasonable" length of time of commitment for competency restoration purposes. As of 2007, nearly 30% of states specify 1 year or less, 20% specify 1–10 years, 22% link the limit to the criminal penalty for the charged offense (up to life), and 30% set no limit (Kaufman et al. 2012).

In some cases, defendants may refuse to take psychiatric medication(s) prescribed to treat the underlying mental disorder, thereby delaying or preventing competency restoration. Two important U.S. Supreme Court cases—*Sell v. United States* (2003) and *Riggins v. Nevada* (1992)—have specifically addressed the involuntary medication of pretrial defendants.

Most jurisdictions have procedures to involuntary medicate patients who are a danger to themselves or others or who are gravely disabled (see Chapter 9, "Le-

gal Regulation of Psychiatric Treatment"). In *Sell v. United States* (2003), the U.S. Supreme Court outlined the conditions under which an incompetent defendant may be involuntarily medicated when the defendant's mental condition does not result in an acute emergency, a grave disability, or a likelihood of serious harm to self or others. Charles Sell was a St. Louis dentist who had a long-standing history of delusional disorder. He was charged with multiple counts of Medicaid fraud and one count of money laundering. Dr. Sell was found incompetent to stand trial and was involuntarily committed to a hospital for competency restoration. He refused to take the antipsychotic medication prescribed for his delusional disorder. Dr. Sell challenged the involuntary medication administration, and the case was appealed to the U.S. Supreme Court.

The issue before the Court was whether the U.S. Constitution permits the government to involuntarily administer antipsychotic drugs to a nondangerous, mentally ill criminal defendant for the sole purpose of rendering the individual competent to stand trial. The U.S. Supreme Court ruled that such defendants can be given medication involuntarily but only under certain conditions. The Court specified the conditions that must be met prior to the involuntary administration of medication. These are sometimes referred to as the "*Sell* criteria" and are outlined in Table 18–6.

Once defendants are restored to competency, however, they may refuse continued forcible medications during the trial in some situations. In the case of *Riggins v. Nevada* (1992), David Riggins was charged with the stabbing death of Paul Wade in his Las Vegas apartment. Shortly after his arrest, he complained of hearing voices and was subsequently treated with thioridazine. After Mr. Rig-

TABLE 18–6. *Sell* **criteria for involuntarily medicating a defendant found incompetent to stand trial**

1. The court must find an important government interest is at stake. Both person and property crimes can be viewed as serious offenses that justify the government's interest in adjudicating criminality.

2. The court must find that the medication significantly furthers the state's interests. For example, the medication should be likely to render the defendant competent to stand trial and not have such severe side effects that it would interfere with trial competency.

3. The medication must be the most appropriate method of restoring trial competency, which cannot be achieved with less intrusive treatments.

4. The medication must be medically appropriate, taking into consideration the efficacy of the medication as well as its side effects.

Source. ***Sell v. United States*** 2003.

gins was adjudicated competent to stand trial, his attorney requested that the defendant's medication be stopped because it prejudicially affected his attitude, demeanor, and appearance at trial and interfered with his ability to assist counsel. The trial court continued the involuntary medication, and Mr. Riggins was found guilty and sentenced to death. On appeal, his attorney alleged that this involuntary medication violated his client's Fourteenth Amendment due process rights because it negatively interfered with his mental state. The attorney argued that the medication prevented the jury from seeing Mr. Riggins's true mental condition, which was particularly relevant considering that he was pleading insanity.

The U.S. Supreme Court reversed Mr. Riggins's conviction, holding that the involuntary administration of antipsychotic drugs violated his Sixth Amendment rights (ability to assist his attorney) and his Fourteenth Amendment due process rights. The Court noted that prior to involuntarily medicating a defendant at trial, the state must first demonstrate that the medication was medically appropriate, that no less restrictive alternatives were used, and that the medication was necessary for the defendant's safety or the safety of others. The Court

stated that involuntary medication might have been justified by showing that an adjudication of guilt or innocence could not be obtained using less intrusive means.

Competency to Waive Rights

Competency to Waive Miranda Rights and to Confess

The U.S. Supreme Court case of *Miranda v. Arizona* (1966) established the initial "right" that a person involved in the criminal justice system is granted the "right to remain silent." The Court held that due to the coercive nature of police interrogation in a custodial setting, the police must advise formally detained individuals that they have a right to remain silent, guaranteed by the Fifth Amendment, and a right to an attorney, guaranteed by the Sixth Amendment. Advising a suspect of these "rights" is now referred to as the "*Miranda* warning." Police are required to inform suspects that they will be provided an attorney if they cannot afford one, and that any statements they make may be used against them in court. The

Court also specified that waiving these rights must be done knowingly, intelligently, and voluntarily.

Evaluating whether a suspect *knowingly* waived his or her rights generally involves a consideration of the totality of the circumstances surrounding that individual. Factors to consider in this regard include the manner in which the warnings were given, the suspect's capacity to understand his or her rights, and whether an attorney or other third party assisted the suspect in understanding these rights.

In assessing whether a person *intelligently* waived his or her *Miranda* rights, evaluators should assess the person's ability to grasp what a "right" means and ability to understand that these rights are absolute in this circumstance. Grisso (1998) developed the Instruments for Assessing Understanding and Appreciation of Miranda Rights (IAU), a structured instrument designed to assess adolescents' and adults' ability to waive *Miranda* rights. This instrument examines the following four components relevant to evaluating a *Miranda* rights waiver:

1. Comprehension of Miranda Rights (CMR)
2. Comprehension of Miranda Rights—Recognition (CMR-R)
3. Comprehension of Miranda Vocabulary (CMV)
4. Function of Rights in Interrogation (FRI)

The Miranda Rights Comprehension Instruments (Goldstein et al. 2014) revised the IAU by rewording some of the Miranda warnings, adding a fifth warning regarding the ability to invoke the right to an attorney and to silence at any time, and providing additional juvenile normative data. The four basic test categories from the IAU remain the same with the revisions as described above.

Evaluating whether a suspect *voluntarily* waived his or her rights requires a determination that the individual chose to confess of his or her own free will and did not confess due to police coercion. In the case of **Colorado v. Connelly** (1986), the U.S. Supreme Court examined the voluntariness of a psychotic defendant's confession. In this case, Frances Connelly approached a Denver police officer. After spontaneously confessing to a murder, the officer immediately read Mr. Connelly his *Miranda* rights. At a subsequent hearing, a psychiatrist testified that Mr. Connelly had been experiencing command hallucinations to confess, which prevented him from exercising a free and rational choice to admit his crimes.

Both the trial court and the Colorado Supreme Court suppressed the confession because it was not voluntary and therefore violated Mr. Connelly's Fourteenth Amendment due process rights. On appeal, the U.S. Supreme Court reversed the lower courts' decisions and held that a confession is voluntary unless evidence indicates that the police coerced the individual's statements. Because no evidence of police coercion, intimidation, or deception was produced, Mr. Connelly's confession was considered voluntary, even though driven by his command auditory hallucinations.

Competency to Plea Bargain

Approximately 90% of criminal cases end with a plea bargain (Melton et al. 2007). Therefore, a defendant's understanding of the concept and consequences of plea bargaining is an important focus of a CST evaluation. When accepting a plea bargain, the defendant forfeits several rights, including the right to a jury trial, the right to testify on one's own behalf, the right to confront witnesses, and the right to avoid self-incrimination. Even an innocent defendant may decide to accept a plea bargain to avoid a harsh sentence. However, defendants should understand that once they plead guilty, even if they insist on their innocence outside of court, they are considered guilty of the offense as a matter of law.

In the U.S. Supreme Court case of **North Carolina v. Alford** (1970), Henry Alford was indicted for first-degree murder and faced the death penalty. The evidence against him was strong. This evidence included a police officer's testimony that shortly before the murder Mr. Alford took the gun from his home and stated he intended to kill the victim, and upon returning home Mr. Alford declared he had killed his intended target.

Mr. Alford accepted a plea bargain to second-degree murder, which removed the possibility of facing the death penalty. During the proceeding in which he pled guilty, he continued to protest his innocence. After Mr. Alford received a sentence of 30 years, he appealed, claiming that he pled guilty only because he feared the death penalty and therefore his guilty plea was involuntary. The U.S. Supreme Court held that a defendant may plead guilty while protesting his innocence. When a defendant's competency to accept a plea bargain is raised, the evaluator should determine whether the defendant voluntarily, knowingly, and understandably consented to the imposition of the prison sentence, even if refusing to admit his or her role in the crime.

Competency to Represent Oneself

Although the Sixth Amendment to the U.S. Constitution guarantees a criminal defendant the right to assistance of counsel, defendants may wish to represent themselves. Conducting one's own defense is also called a *pro se* defense; *pro se* is a Latin phrase that means "for oneself." Two U.S. Supreme Court cases have upheld a defendant's right to self-representation. In the case of *Faretta v. California* (1975), the U.S. Supreme Court held that a court cannot automatically force an attorney upon an unwilling defendant.

In the subsequent case of **Godinez v. Moran** (1993), the U.S. Supreme Court continued to uphold the right of a defendant to waive assistance by counsel. Richard Allan Moran was charged with three counts of first-degree murder after he walked into the Red Pearl Saloon and shot the bartender and a customer prior to robbing the cash register. Nine days later, he shot and killed his ex-wife and then attempted suicide by shooting himself and slitting his wrists. He survived and later confessed to the killings but pleaded not guilty to his charges.

Although two court-ordered psychiatrists noted that Mr. Moran was depressed, he was found competent to stand trial. He subsequently informed the court that he wanted to change his plea to guilty and discharge his attorneys. After being found guilty and sentenced to death, Mr. Moran appealed, claiming he was mentally incompetent to represent himself. The trial court dismissed Mr. Moran's petition, and he appealed this decision to the U.S. Supreme Court, which ruled that the competency standard to waive the right to counsel and plead guilty is the same as the standard for determining CST. The Court also noted that whether or not the defendant could represent himself adequately was irrelevant to his decision to forgo legal counsel.

The *Godinez* ruling does not necessarily prohibit a state from adopting a higher

standard of competency for self-representation than the competency to stand trial
standard. In the U.S. Supreme Court case
of *Indiana v. Edwards* (2008), Ahmed Edwards attempted to steal a pair of shoes
from an Indiana department store. When
discovered by a department store security officer, Edwards fired three shots, one
of which wounded a bystander. He was
charged with attempted murder, battery
with a deadly weapon, criminal reckless-
ness, and theft.

Mr. Edwards was found incompetent
to stand trial and committed to a state
hospital for competency restoration. After 5 years, he was adjudicated competent, and he asked to serve as his own attorney. The court refused his request and
appointed an attorney who acted on Mr.
Edwards's behalf. The jury deadlocked on
some of the charges, and at his retrial, Mr.
Edwards again asked to represent himself. The trial judge ruled that although
Mr. Edwards was competent to stand trial,
he was not competent to represent himself. Mr. Edwards was tried and convicted
of battery and attempted murder.

Mr. Edwards ultimately appealed the
case to the U.S. Supreme Court, alleging that his rights had been violated because he had not been allowed to represent himself, even though he had been
found competent to stand trial. The U.S.
Supreme Court held that a court may
deny a mentally ill defendant found competent to stand trial the right to self-
representation. However, the Court did
not articulate any standard to determine
defendants' competency to act as their
own legal counsel, nor did they overrule
the prior *Faretta* holding that addressed
a non–mentally ill defendant's right to
self-representation (*Indiana v. Edwards*
2008).

Conclusion

Competency to stand trial is the most
common type of forensic evaluation in the
criminal justice system. With the trend of
increasing criminalization of people with
mental illness, requests for CST evaluations are likely to increase. States will be
faced with several challenges to address
the increasing number of competency
evaluation requests, including the availability of qualified examiners, the availability of inpatient psychiatric beds, and
the financial burden to the state and local
counties in housing inmates with mental
illness who have been found incompetent
to stand trial. To meet this challenge, key
stakeholders should explore creating a
range of settings appropriate for competency restoration, develop rapid assessment screens to help triage and match
diagnostic and treatment services for defendants found trial incompetent, and implement evidence-based treatments in a
timely manner to prevent delays in treatment and costly use of hospital beds.

Key Concepts

- Competency-to-stand-trial evaluations focus on the defendants' *present ability* to assist their legal counsel and their understanding of the legal process.

- The presence of a mental disorder does not automatically equate with a finding of incompetency to stand trial.

- There are various trial-specific competencies, and the evaluator should evaluate
  the relationship, if any, of a mental disorder to each specific competency task.

- Even if a defendant's mental illnesses influence his or her decision to confess, the U.S. Supreme Court has held that the issue to examine in regard to voluntariness of the confession is the presence of police coercion.

- Although individuals without mental illness have a constitutional right for self-representation, the court can determine whether mental illness prevents defendants from conducting their own defense (i.e., *pro se* defense).

References

Butcher J, Dalstrom W, Graham J, et al: Manual for Administering and Scoring the MMPI-2. Minneapolis, University of Minnesota Press, 1989

Cima M, Nimjan H, Merckelbach H, et al: Claims of crime-related amnesia in forensic patients. In J Law Psychiatry 27(3):215–221, 2004 15177990

Colorado v Connelly, 479 U.S. 157, 107 S.Ct. 515 (1986)

Colwell K, Colwell JH, Perry AT, et al: The Test of Malingered Incompetence (TOMI): a forced-choice instrument for assessing cognitive malingering in competence to stand trial evaluations. Am J Forensic Psychol 26:17–41, 2008

Cooper v Oklahoma, 517 U.S. 348, 116 S.Ct. 1373 (1996)

Dusky v United States, 362 U.S. 402, 80 S.Ct. 788 (1960)

Everington C: The Competency Assessment for Standing Trial for Defendants with Mental Retardation (CAST-MR): a validation study. Criminal Justice and Behavior 17:147–168, 1990

Faretta v California, 422 U.S. 806, 95 S.Ct. 2525 (1975)

Godinez v Moran, 509 U.S. 389, 113 S.Ct. 2680 (1993)

Goldstein NES, Zelle H, Grisso T: Miranda Rights Comprehension Instruments (MRCI) Manual for Juvenile and Adult Evaluations. Sarasota, FL, Professional Resource Press, 2014

Grisso T: Instruments for Assessing, Understanding, and Appreciation of Miranda Rights. Sarasota, FL, Professional Resource Press, 1998

Hoge SK, Bonnie RJ, Poythress N, et al: The MacArthur Adjudicative Competence Study: development and validation of a research instrument. Law and Human Behavior 21:141–182, 1997

Indiana v Edwards, 554 U.S. 164, 128 S.Ct. 2379 (2008)

Jackson v Indiana, 406 U.S. 715, 92 S.Ct. 1845 (1972)

Kaufman AR, Way BB, Suardi E: Forty years after Jackson v. Indiana: states' compliance with "reasonable period of time" ruling. J Am Acad Psychiatry Law 40(2):261–265, 2012 22635300

Melton GB, Petrila J, Poythress NG, et al: Competency to stand trial, in Psychological Evaluations for the Courts: A Handbook for Mental Health Professionals and Lawyers, 3rd Edition. Edited by Melton GB, Petrila J, Poythress NG, et al. New York, Guilford, 2007, pp 125–200

Miller HA: The Miller Forensic Assessment of Symptoms Test (M-FAST) Professional Manual. Odessa, FL, Psychological Assessment Resources, 2001

Miranda v Arizona, 384 U.S. 436, 86 S.Ct. 1602 (1966)

Mossman D, Noffsinger SG, Ash P, et al; American Academy of Psychiatry and the Law: AAPL Practice Guideline for the forensic psychiatric evaluation of competence to stand trial. J Am Acad Psychiatry Law 35(4)(Suppl):S3–S72, 2007 18083992

Musick JE, Otto RK: Inventory of Legal Knowledge. Lutz, FL, Psychological Assessment Resources, 2010

Nicholson RA, Kugler KE: Competent and incompetent criminal defendants: a quantitative review of comparative research. Psychol Bull 109:355–370, 1991

Noffsinger SG: Restoration to competency practice guidelines. Int J Offender Ther Comp Criminol 45:356–362, 2001

North Carolina v Alford, 400 U.S. 25, 91 S.Ct. 160 (1970)

Resnick PJ, Noffsinger S: Competency to stand trial and the insanity defense, in The American Psychiatric Publishing Textbook of Forensic Psychiatry. Edited by Simon RI, Gold LH. Washington, DC, American Psychiatric Publishing, 2004, pp 329–347

Riggins v Nevada, 504 U.S. 127, 112 S.Ct. 1810 (1992)

Rock v Arkansas, 483 U.S. 44, 107 S.Ct. 2704 (1987)

Rogers R: Structured Interview of Reported Symptoms. Odessa, FL, Psychological Assessment Resources, 1992

Rogers R, Johansson-Love J: Evaluating competency to stand trial with evidence-based practice. J Am Acad Psychiatry Law 37(4):450–460, 2009 20018994

Rogers R, Grandjean N, Tillbrook CE, et al: Recent interview-based measures of competency to stand trial: a critical review augmented with research data. Behav Sci Law 19(4):503–518, 2001 11568958

Rogers R, Tillbrook CE, Sewell KW: Evaluation of Competency to Stand Trial, Revised (ECST-R). Odessa, FL, Psychological Assessment Resources, 2004

Sell v United States, 539 U.S. 166, 123 S.Ct. 2174 (2003)

State v Stock, 463 S.W.2d 889 (Mo. 1971)

Tombaugh TN: Test of Memory Malingering. Princeton, NJ, Pearson Education, 2009

United States v Veatch, 842 F. Supp. 480 (W.D. Okla. 1993)

U.S. Department of Health, Laboratory of Community Psychiatry: Competency to Stand Trial and Mental Illness. Publ No (AMD) 77-103. Rockville, MD, U.S. Department of Health, 1973

Widows MR, Smith GP: Structured Inventory of Malingered Symptomatology Professional Manual. Odessa, FL: Psychological Assessment Resources, 2005

Wilson v United States, 129 U.S. App. D.C. 107, 391 F.2d 460 (1968)

CHAPTER 19

Evaluation of Criminal Responsibility

Charles L. Scott, M.D.

Landmark Cases

R. v. McNaughten (Daniel M'Naghten's Case), 8 E.R. 718 (1843)

Durham v. United States, 94 U.S. App. D.C. 228, 214 F.2d 862 (1954)

Robinson v. California, 370 U.S. 660, 82 S.Ct. 1417 (1962)

Washington v. United States, 129 U.S. App. D.C. 29, 390 F.2d 862 (1967)

Powell v. Texas, 392 U.S. 514, 88 S.Ct. 2145 (1968)

Frendak v. United States, 408 A.2d 364 (1979)

Ibn-Tamas v. United States, 407 A.2d 626 (D.C. 1979)

Jones v. United States, 463 U.S. 354, 103 S.Ct. 3043 (1983)

Foucha v. Louisiana, 504 U.S. 71,112 S.Ct. 1780 (1992)

Montana v. Egelhoff, 518 U.S. 37,116 S.Ct. 2013 (1996)

Clark v. Arizona, 548 U.S. 735, 126 S.Ct. 2709 (2006)

The recognition that individuals with mental illness may not be responsible for their behavior is a concept dating back to the 1772 B.C. Code of Hammurabi. During the Roman Empire, laws existed acknowledging that some individuals with mental illness had little control of their behavior and were therefore *non compos mentis,* Latin for "of unsound mind" (Taylor 2015). The concept of insanity under English law can be traced to 1324 when the *Statute de Prerogativa Regis* ("the king's prerogative") was passed, allowing the king to seize the lands of "idiots" and "lunatics." *Lunatics* referred to persons who became insane during their life or experienced insanity interspersed with lucid intervals. English law increasingly recognized that an "insane" person should not be punished in the same way as a person who did not suffer from insanity (Crotty 1924).

Under common law, to be held criminally responsible, a person must have both an *actus reus* (Latin for "guilty act") and a *mens rea* (Latin for "guilty mind"). *Actus reus* refers to the specific voluntary criminal act, whereas *mens rea* refers to the level of intent necessary to commit the criminal act. Jurisdictions vary significantly as to how a defendant's *mens rea* at the time of the crime may be considered for evaluating the degree, if any, of personal culpability. This chapter reviews psychiatric evaluations specific to assessing mental state at the time of the offense and possible consequences when the court determines that a person's criminal acts were influenced by mental illness.

Legal Tests of Insanity

Insanity is a legal rather than a psychiatric term. The definition of *insanity* varies widely according to the jurisdiction where the alleged crime is committed. In the United States, a defendant has no constitutional right to an insanity defense. In fact, four states (Idaho, Kansas, Montana, and Utah) do not allow a defendant to plead not guilty by reason of insanity (American Academy of Psychiatry and the Law [AAPL] Practice Guideline 2014).

The most common test of insanity used in the United States is known as the *M'Naghten* standard, developed in 1843

following the trial of Daniel M'Naghten. Mr. M'Naghten was found not guilty by reason of insanity after he attempted to assassinate the prime minister of Britain and instead shot his secretary Edward Drummond. Queen Victoria, angered by the legal outcome in this case, ordered her 15 law lords to draft a new standard of criminal responsibility. The new standard read as follows: "To establish a defence on the ground of insanity, it must be clearly proved that at the time of the committing of the act, the party accused was labouring under such a defect of reason, from the disease of the mind, as not to know the nature and quality of the act he was doing, or if he did know it, that he did not know he was doing what was wrong" (*R. v. McNaughten* 1843).

This test is often referred to as the *right/wrong* test or *cognitive* test because of its emphasis on the defendant's ability to know, understand, or appreciate the nature and quality of his or her criminal behavior or the wrongfulness of his or her actions at the time of the crime. Some version of this test of insanity is used in the majority of U.S. jurisdictions (Table 19–1) (AAPL 2014).

A second insanity test is the American Law Institute's (ALI's) *Model Penal Code* (American Law Institute 1955). In essence, this test asks the evaluator to determine whether the defendant's mental disorder rendered him or her unable to appreciate the criminality of his or her conduct (i.e., distinguish right from wrong, known as the *cognitive prong*) or unable to conform his or her behavior to the requirements of the law (i.e., having an irresistible impulse, known as the *volitional prong*). Under the ALI test, mental illnesses manifested by repeated criminal or antisocial conduct are barred from being used as the basis for an insanity defense. A major criticism of this test has been the difficulty in distinguish-

TABLE 19–1. U.S. jurisdictions using *M'Naghten* or modified *M'Naghten* standard

Alabama	Minnesota	Oklahoma
Alaska	Mississippi	Pennsylvania
Arizona	Missouri	South Carolina
California	Nebraska	South Dakota
Colorado	Nevada	Tennessee
Florida	New Jersey	Texas
Georgia	New Mexico	Virginia
Iowa	North Carolina	Washington
Louisiana	Ohio	U.S. Military

ing between those individuals who could not conform their behavior and those individuals who chose not to conform their behavior. Despite this difficulty, this test is the legal standard used in 20 states (Table 19–2) (AAPL 2014).

A third test, known as the *Durham* rule or *product* test, derived from the case of *Durham v. United States* (1954). Monte Durham had a long history of imprisonment and psychiatric hospitalizations. Two months after his release from a psychiatric hospital in Washington, D.C., Mr. Durham was arrested for housebreaking. After being hospitalized for restoration of competency to stand trial, he was returned to court with a discharge diagnosis of "without mental disorder, psychopathic personality." At the time of his trial, the District of Columbia's test for insanity was whether the defendant did not know the difference between right or wrong or suffered from an irresistible impulse. The trial court rejected Mr. Durham's insanity defense, and he appealed his conviction.

On appeal, Judge David Bazelon took the opportunity to change the District of Columbia's insanity standard. He rejected the "right-wrong" test because it did not "take sufficient account of psychic realities," and he rejected the "irresistible impulse test" because it "gives no recognition to mental illness characterized by

brooding and reflection." Judge Bazelon announced a new test that allowed a finding of insanity if the defendant's unlawful act was a "product of a mental disease or defect." Under this standard, known as the product test or *Durham* rule, psychiatrists were at liberty to provide their own definitions of mental disease or defect. As a result, once an expert proposed that the defendant had a qualifying mental illness (however defined), the conclusion that a defendant's criminal behavior was a product of the mental illness was relatively easy to establish.

In a subsequent case of *Washington v. United States* (1967), Judge Bazelon expressed his frustration with mental health experts' increasing encroachment on the jury's role in determining criminal responsibility. In writing the court's opinion, he noted "that testimony in terms of 'mental disease or defect' seems to leave the psychiatrist too free to testify according to his judgment about the defendant's criminal responsibility." The Bazelon court held that psychiatrists were permitted to explain how a defendant's mental disease or defect related to the alleged offense, but psychiatrists should not speak directly to whether or not a defendant's conduct was a product or result of mental illness. The D.C. Court of Appeals eventually rejected the *Durham* test altogether in the case of *United States v. Brawner* (1972). In its place,

TABLE 19–2.   **U.S. jurisdictions using the American Law Institute (ALI) or modified ALI Model Penal Code**

Arkansas	Kentucky	Oregon
Connecticut	Maine	Rhode Island
Delaware	Maryland	Vermont
District of Columbia	Massachusetts	West Virginia
Hawaii	Michigan	Wisconsin
Illinois	New York	Wyoming
Indiana	North Dakota	

the D.C. Circuit adopted the insanity test developed in 1955 by the ALI under the Model Penal Code. The product test is currently the insanity standard used in New Hampshire.

The ALI Model Penal Code was the insanity standard in place in the District of Columbia on March 30, 1981, the day that John Hinckley attempted to assassinate President Ronald Reagan. Mr. Hinckley was diagnosed with schizophrenia and found legally insane under the ALI standard because the jury decided that at the time of the offense he could not conform his conduct to the requirements of the law. A public outcry in response to the verdict resulted in a tightening of insanity standards in both the state and federal justice systems. Four states abolished the insanity defense altogether, and 36 states reformed laws related to criminal responsibility (AAPL 2014).

In 1984, in response to the *Hinckley* verdict, Congress passed the Insanity Defense Reform Act 1984. Under this new law, Congress changed the standard of legal insanity in federal trials to more closely align with the *M'Naghten* cognitive standard. In this revised federal insanity defense test, a defendant was not responsible for criminal conduct if "as a result of a severe mental disease or defect, [he] was unable to appreciate the nature and quality or the criminality or wrongfulness of his acts" (Insanity Defense Reform Act 1984).

In addition to removing the volitional arm of the previous insanity test, the Insanity Defense Reform Act altered requirements regarding which party should bear the burden of proof. Under the previous standard, the prosecution was required to prove the defendant sane beyond a reasonable doubt. With the passage of this law, the burden of proof shifted to the defendant, who had to prove his or her insanity at the time of the offense by clear and convincing evidence. This insanity standard is the same standard required in military trials under the Uniform Code of Military Justice (AAPL 2014) (see Chapter 31, "Military Forensic Psychiatry").

Mental Disorders and the Insanity Defense

Qualifying Mental Disorders

Definitions of *mental disease* and *mental defect* that qualify for an insanity defense are usually found in case law and/or statutes. Most insanity defenses involve defendants who have a psychotic disorder or intellectual disability (AAPL 2014). Examiners should carefully review whether any disorders in their jurisdictions are prohibited from consideration for the insanity defense. Diagnoses that are commonly excluded by statute or the insanity standard include personality disorders, seizure disorders, adjustment disorders, paraphilic disorders, kleptomania, and pyromania.

Substance Use

The U.S. Supreme Court has addressed the relationship of a defendant's substance use to criminal responsibility in two landmark cases. First, in *Robinson v. California* (1962), the U.S. Supreme Court was asked to review a California statute that criminalized being under the influence of or addicted to narcotics. Lawrence Robinson was picked up by police officers, who observed that he had "tracks" on his arms consistent with intravenous heroin use. Although not under the influence of heroin at the time of his arrest, Mr. Robinson was convicted of being *addicted* to the use of narcotics. On appeal, the U.S. Supreme Court recognized that drug addiction was a disease. The majority concluded that punishing a person for the status of having a disease violated the Eighth Amendment. Justice Potter Stewart famously wrote that even "one day in prison for the 'crime' of having the common cold" would represent cruel and unusual punishment.

In the subsequent case of *Powell v. Texas* (1968), the U.S. Supreme Court again considered whether substance use should qualify as a mental disease or defect absolving a defendant from criminal blame. Leroy Powell was well known in Travis County, Texas, because he had nearly 100 convictions for public intoxication. In December 1966, he was again arrested for being under the influence of alcohol. His defense argued that in light of the *Robinson* ruling, Mr. Powell should not be arrested for having the "disease" of alcoholism. At his trial, the judge rejected the claim that Mr. Powell was not criminally responsible due to his alcoholism. He was convicted, and his case was appealed to the U.S. Supreme Court.

The U.S. Supreme Court distinguished Mr. Powell's case from their prior holding in *Robinson*. The Court noted that Mr. Powell was not convicted for having the disease of alcoholism but for the disruptive public behavior resulting from his alcohol use. The Court refused to equate alcoholism as a mental disease that would excuse a person from criminal responsibility. In fact, Justice Marshall emphasized, "Nothing could be less fruitful than for this Court to be impelled into defining some sort of insanity test in constitutional terms" (*Powell v. Texas* 1968 at 536).

All jurisdictions in the United States exclude voluntary intoxication as the *sole* mental condition permitted to justify an insanity defense (AAPL 2014). Some jurisdictions allow consideration of substance use disorders as a qualifying mental disorder for insanity in the following three circumstances:

1. *Idiosyncratic intoxication:* when a person has an unexpected and adverse mental reaction to his or her first use of alcohol. Drugs such as cocaine and methamphetamine have well-known and long-established risks and therefore do not generally qualify for idiosyncratic intoxication.
2. *Involuntary intoxication:* when a person is unaware that he or she has consumed alcohol or a substance and is therefore not responsible for any adverse resulting mental states.
3. *Permanent mental illness or cognitive impairment caused by substance use:* when a person has sustained psychiatric symptoms or cognitive impairment that extends beyond the intoxication period and substance use (e.g., alcohol-induced major neurocognitive disorder).

In some jurisdictions, these mental states are referred to as "settled insanity" or "settled psychosis," although the definitions of these terms vary widely.

Syndromes Qualifying as Mental Disorders

The "AAPL Practice Guideline for Forensic Psychiatric Evaluation of Defendants Raising the Insanity Defense" (AAPL 2014) recommends that psychiatric diagnoses used to support an insanity defense should follow the current *Diagnostic and Statistical Manual of Mental Disorders* (DSM) or *International Statistical Classification of Diseases and Related Health Problems* (ICD). When a non-DSM or non-ICD diagnosis is provided, the evaluator should cite the relevant literature to support its use.

Various "syndromes" have been proposed as qualifying for the underlying mental disease or defect component of the insanity defense. Many of these syndromes have little, if any, empirical support and are not included in accepted diagnostic classifications. Syndromes proposed for purposes of evaluating a defendant's criminal responsibility have included sexual addiction, homosexual panic, black rage, road rage, premenstrual dysphoric disorder (now an accepted DSM-5 diagnosis), paraphilic coercive disorder (rejected as a DSM-5 diagnosis), codependency, neonaticide/infanticide syndrome, and battered woman syndrome (Hunsley et al. 2012).

Of all the syndromes proposed as the basis for an insanity defense, *battered woman syndrome* (BWS) has perhaps received the most attention. The term arises from research conducted by Dr. Lenore Walker with more than 100 women in the late 1970s. This research resulted in a description of a pattern of violence that consisted of an initial courtship period followed by three phases that repeated themselves in a cyclical pattern. The first was described as the *tension-building phase*, in which the woman would attempt to please or appease her batterer out of fear. The second was the *acute battering incident*, in which the woman was at highest risk for physical or sexual injury. The third phase was the *loving-contrition* or *honeymoon phase*, during which the batterer would apologize for his behavior and exhibit temporary contrition (Walker 2006).

Although BWS is rarely used as the sole basis for an insanity defense, a woman's history of being battered has been used to explain why a woman may have believed she was acting in self-defense when charged with certain crimes. In the case of *Ibn-Tamas v. United States* (1979), Dr. Walker was asked to provide expert witness testimony about BWS to help explain why Beverly Ibn-Tamas shot her husband Yusef Ibn-Tamas to death in 1976. The defense asked Dr. Walker to describe the pattern of "wife battering" and to give her opinion regarding the similarities of Ms. Ibn-Tamas's personality and behavior to those of battered women Dr. Walker had studied.

The defense claimed that Dr. Walker's testimony was relevant and would help the jury evaluate the credibility of the defendant's claim that she shot her husband in self-defense because she believed she was in imminent danger. The trial judge excluded Dr. Walker's testimony because of concerns that her testimony would include discussion of prior violent acts of the deceased husband, invade the province of the jury in evaluating Ms. Ibn-Tamas's credibility, and clearly suggest that the deceased husband was a batterer. Ms. Ibn-Tamas was convicted of second-degree murder and appealed, claiming that the trial court erred in excluding Dr. Walker's testimony.

The D.C. Court of Appeals applied a threefold test to evaluate the admissibility of Dr. Walker's testimony. First, the subject matter must be "beyond the ken of the average laymen" and distinctly related to some science or profession. Second, the witness must have sufficient knowledge, skills, or experience to aid the trier of fact. Third, the state of the scientific knowledge must be sufficiently established to allow a reasonable opinion by the expert. The appellate court ruled that the trial court erred in finding Dr. Walker's testimony inadmissible on the ground that it would invade the province of the jury. The court also could not find justification to exclude Dr. Walker's testimony on the two other criteria, which were not even addressed by the trial court. Following this ruling, numerous courts have allowed testimony on BWS to justify self-defense behaviors even when the defendant does meet criteria for legal insanity (AAPL 2014).

Preparing for the Sanity Evaluation

When preparing to evaluate a defendant's criminal responsibility, a forensic expert should first clarify whether the expert is court appointed or retained by the defense or prosecution. Although the examiner, regardless of the retaining party, should always strive for honesty and objectivity, opinions rendered by a psychiatrist hired by the defense are not always disclosed to other parties.

Before the examiner conducts the evaluation, the defense attorney should be notified of the impending interview. The defense attorney may request to be present during the assessment and may obtain a court order allowing defense counsel to be present. In this situation, the evaluator should request that defense counsel not interrupt the examination or instruct the defendant how to respond to questions. Before the evaluation, the evaluator

should request the exact language of the jurisdiction's insanity statute and any relevant case law. Also, the examiner should review collateral records that may assist in evaluating the mental state of the defendant at the time of the offense. If the defendant refuses to sign a release for records, the expert can request that the court order the release of needed records. Collateral records that may assist in the sanity evaluation are reviewed in Table 19–3.

The forensic expert should pay particular attention to those records that describe the defendant's mental state close to the time of the crime. The following are specific areas to review in the collateral records:

- Defendant's exact statements before and after the offense
- Defendant's offense accounts to police officers and others
- Presence of any mental health symptoms near the time of the offense, particularly psychotic symptoms such as paranoia, delusions, and/or hallucinations
- Presence or absence of substance use prior to the offense
- Presence of antisocial personality traits or disorder
- Presence of a rational alternative motive rather than a psychotic motive
- History of a similar offense indicating a possible pattern of criminal behavior
- History of malingering psychiatric symptoms before or after the offense

In addition to collateral records, other evaluators' opinions may help in assessing the consistency of the defendant's presentation and account of the crime. However, examiners should first determine whether any prior psychiatric or psychological examinations are prohibited from their review. Finally, the exam-

TABLE 19–3.   Collateral records to consider in sanity evaluations

Defendant's account of crime to police or other witnesses

Audio- or videotaped statements from defendant

Witness and victim statements

911 calls (if available)

Videotape of crime or crime scene (if available)

Jail booking and treatment records following the defendant's arrest

Prior psychiatric, alcohol, and drug treatment, and medical records

Prior psychological testing

Any writings from defendant that may reflect his or her mental state or motive

Computer hard drive and communications, where appropriate

Records of prior arrests/convictions

Prior prison records

Prior educational records

Prior work records

iner may find it helpful to take a detailed social background history from family members and individuals who know the defendant, paying particular attention to the defendant's mental state in the days and hours prior to the crime.

Sanity Evaluation of the Defendant

The forensic expert should attempt to evaluate the defendant as soon as possible after the crime to assess the defendant's mental state close to the time of the crime and to minimize the risk that the defendant will learn how to malinger mental illness (Resnick and Noffsinger 2004). The forensic evaluator should explain to the defendant the nature and purpose of the interview, the limitations of confidentiality, who hired the examiner, and the fact that the examiner could testify at trial.

After providing the initial informed consent, the evaluator usually conducts a biopsychosocial psychiatric interview. Key areas to review include the defendant's past psychiatric history and prior

hospitalizations, family psychiatric history, educational history, history of learning disabilities or intellectual disabilities, and social and relationship history, particularly as related to the crime victims.

The examiner should obtain the defendant's account of the crime in an open-ended manner. For example, the evaluator might ask, "What happened on the day of the offense? Tell me everything that you remember, starting with the day before this happened." The evaluator should ask the defendant to describe his or her thoughts, feelings, and exact behaviors before, during, and after the alleged crime. After obtaining the defendant's initial account, the evaluator may need to ask more detailed specific questions to evaluate the defendant's sanity. In addition, the examiner should clarify with the defendant any inconsistent accounts of the offense provided either during the interview or to other individuals (Resnick and Noffsinger 2004). Questions that an evaluator should consider asking to help obtain the defendant's account of the crime are listed in Table 19–4.

TABLE 19–4. **Sample questions to help evaluate mental state at time of offense**

What was your relationship to the victim [if the crime involved a victim]?

When did you first have the thought to commit your offense?

Did you prepare for this? If so, how?

Had you ever tried to do this before? If so, what stopped you or why did it not work out?

What did you do immediately following this offense? Why?

Prior to committing this crime, did you know that this was against the law?

At the time that you committed this crime, did you know it was against the law?

Would you have done this if a police officer was near or at the scene? If yes, why? If no, why not?

Would you have done this if someone unexpected arrived at the scene? If yes, why? If no, why not?

Is there anything that made you think what you did was a right thing to do? If so, what?

When was the last drink of alcohol or use of any other drugs you took prior to this crime?

Were you experiencing mental illness symptom(s) at the time of the crime? If so, what? When did these symptoms start? When did these symptoms end? [The examiner may need to ask specific questions regarding the presence of hallucinations, delusions, paranoia, or other mental health symptoms.]

The evaluator should also consider the possibility that the defendant may malinger psychiatric symptoms in an attempt to be found legally insane. The examiner should be particularly familiar with characteristics of feigned hallucinations or delusions (Resnick 1999). Psychological tests designed to assess malingered psychiatric symptoms may also be useful (see Chapter 6, "Evaluation of Malingering"); however, the evaluator should keep in mind that these tests do not specifically evaluate the defendant's mental status at the time of the crime. Therefore, a finding on a psychological test that the defendant is not currently malingering symptoms does not necessarily mean that the defendant is not feigning symptoms about his or her mental state in the past.

The evaluator may encounter a defendant who refuses an insanity defense, even when strong evidence indicates that the defendant would likely meet the jurisdiction's definition of insanity. In events leading to the case of *Frendak v. United States* (1979), Paula Frendak shot a coworker in Washington, D.C., and then fled the scene. She was eventually arrested in Abu Dhabi, United Arab Emirates. After extradition, Ms. Frendak was charged with first-degree murder and carrying a pistol without a license.

During her competency to stand trial proceedings, evidence of insanity was introduced. However, Ms. Frendak refused to raise the insanity defense at trial. At the time of her trial, the *Whalen* rule, which allowed a trial judge the discretion to impose an unwanted defense on a defendant (*Whalen v. United States* 1980), was in effect. The trial judge, who found that the psychiatric evidence raised sufficient questions about Ms. Frendak's criminal responsibility at the time of the crime, opined that under the *Whalen* rule, he was required to raise the insanity defense against the defendant's objection. Ms. Frendak was found not guilty by reason of insanity and appealed, challenging the validity of the *Whalen* rule.

The D.C. Circuit Court of Appeals held that a trial judge may not force an insanity defense on a defendant found competent to stand trial if the defendant intelligently and voluntarily decides to forgo that defense. The court also noted that a finding of trial competency was not sufficient to show that the defendant was capable of rejecting an insanity defense. Furthermore, the court identified the following five reasons a defendant could rationally choose to forgo an insanity defense:

1. A person found not guilty by reason of insanity could spend more time in a psychiatric hospital than in prison.
2. A person found not guilty by reason of insanity might receive better mental health treatment in a prison than in a mental hospital, and a hospital's restrictions and routines may differ from those in prison.
3. A person might wish to avoid the stigma associated with being labeled "insane."
4. A person could lose certain rights, such as the right to own a firearm or vote, as a result of hospital commitment.
5. A person might have committed the crime as a political or religious act, and pleading insanity would diminish the importance of his or her cause.

When a defendant with mental illness refuses an insanity defense, the evaluator should carefully determine whether this decision represents a rational refusal or is instead an irrational decision arising from mental illness.

The Sanity Opinion

Evaluators should review three important areas when rendering an opinion on a defendant's criminal responsibility. First, the evaluator must establish whether the individual had a mental disease or defect at the time of the crime that would qualify for consideration of insanity in the particular jurisdiction. Even if a defendant meets the jurisdictional criteria for a mental disorder or defect, having a mental disorder is not equivalent with the legal definition of insanity.

Second, the evaluator must determine the relationship, if any, between the mental illness or defect and the alleged crime. Understanding the motivation behind the person's actions is a critical component of the insanity evaluation. The evaluator should consider all rational, as opposed to psychotic, motives for the criminal offense. For example, if an individual commits an armed robbery solely to obtain money for a drug purchase, the fact that the individual is depressed is unlikely to be considered a sufficient relationship between the mental state and the criminal behavior for purposes of the insanity defense.

Third, the examiner must apply the relevant insanity test when evaluating the relationship between the person's mental disorder and the alleged acts. For example, under the *M'Naghten* test of insanity (i.e., cognitive standard), the evaluator must determine whether the defendant's mental illness prevented the defendant from knowing what he or she was doing or understanding that his or her actions were wrong. In *M'Naghten* jurisdictions, the examiner should carefully review whether the defendant meets the criteria for each component of this test according to the specific statutory language (AAPL 2014).

Typically, individuals have to be extremely impaired to be unaware or incognizant of their actions. The more easily met component of the *M'Naghten* test involves whether the defendant was able to distinguish right from wrong at the time of the offense. In general, two broad categories relate to the assessment of a defendant's knowledge of the "wrongfulness" of his or her behavior: 1) legal wrongfulness and 2) moral wrongfulness. Jurisdictions vary as to whether both types of wrongfulness are allowed for consideration when determining a defendant's sanity.

An assessment of a person's understanding of the legal wrongfulness of his or her actions involves determining whether defendants understood *at the time of the crime* that what they did was against the law. Examples of potential behaviors that would suggest that a person understands the wrongfulness of his or her behavior are outlined in Table 19–5 (Resnick 2015).

In some jurisdictions, individuals may be found insane if a mental disorder resulted in their being unable to know or understand that their actions were *morally* wrong, even if they knew that their actions were against the law. When evaluating whether defendants' mental disorders rendered them unable to know or understand the moral wrongfulness of their conduct, the examiner should specifically determine whether religious delusions or other symptoms made a defendant believe his or her actions were morally justified at the time of the offense.

In some jurisdictions the insanity standard requires an analysis of defendants' ability to conform their conduct to the requirements of the law at the time of the alleged offense. This analysis focuses on how the mental disorder or defect affected, if at all, the person's ability or capacity to control his or her behavior. In this context, the forensic examiner is evaluating whether the defendant, because of mental illness, could not refrain from his or her behavior or had the ability to refrain from the behavior but chose not to do so. Evidence that may indicate that defendants had the ability to refrain includes stopping their actions when detected by someone during the course of the crime or deferring their actions until the arrival of a more advantageous opportunity.

TABLE 19–5. Evidence regarding knowledge of legal wrongfulness

Efforts to avoid detection

Wearing gloves during a crime

Waiting until the cover of darkness

Taking a victim to an isolated place

Wearing a mask or disguise

Concealing a weapon on the way to a crime

Giving a false name

Threatening to kill witnesses

Giving a false alibi

Disposing of evidence

Wiping off fingerprints

Washing off blood

Discarding a murder weapon

Burying a victim secretly

Destroying incriminating documents

Efforts to avoid apprehension

Fleeing from the scene

Fleeing from the police

Lying to the police

Source. Resnick 2015.

Release of Insanity Acquittees

The majority of individuals found criminally insane are involuntarily committed to a psychiatric facility, where periodic reports regarding their status are forwarded to the responsible court. Individuals found insane may be released when the court has determined that they have met their jurisdictional requirements for a safe release into the community, a process commonly known as "restoration of sanity."

The severity of the underlying crime is theoretically unrelated to the length of time a person is hospitalized. In *Jones v. United States* (1983), Michael Jones pled not guilty by reason of insanity for the misdemeanor offense of attempting to steal a jacket from a department store. The government did not contest Mr. Jones's plea, and he was committed to a psychiatric hospital. Mr. Jones was hospitalized for longer than 1 year, which would have been the maximum sentence had he pled guilty and been sent to prison. Because his hospitalization was longer than the associated prison sentence for his crime, Mr. Jones demanded that he be released or recommitted under the District of Columbia's code for civil commitment.

On appeal, the U.S. Supreme Court held that once persons were found not guilty by reason of insanity, they could be confined to a mental institution until such time as they had regained their sanity or were no longer a danger to themselves or society. The Court noted that the severity of the crime was unrelated to the length of time a person found not guilty by reason of insanity needed to recover from his or her mental illness.

In *Foucha v. Louisiana* (1992), the U.S. Supreme Court further clarified the criteria for continued commitment of a person found not guilty by reason of insanity. Terry Foucha was found not guilty by reason of insanity for aggravated burglary and illegal discharge of a firearm. During his psychiatric hospitalization, his substance-induced psychosis resolved. At his release hearing, his physician testified that although Mr. Foucha no longer had psychotic symptoms, he might pose a danger if released because of his "antisocial personality." Mr. Foucha was recommitted to the hospital and subsequently filed a writ of *habeas corpus* to challenge his continued involuntary hospitalization. On appeal, the U.S. Supreme Court ruled that a person found not guilty by reason of insanity could not be retained in the hospital for potential dangerousness if no mental illness was present.

Diminished Capacity Evaluations

Unlike the insanity defense, which utilizes a specific test to evaluate a defendant's criminal responsibility, a *diminished capacity defense* argues that the defendant lacked the capacity to form the requisite specific intent (i.e., mental state) necessary to prove the crime. Diminished capacity is a partial defense that is only relevant when the legal charge requires that the defendant have specific intent. A diminished capacity defense may still result in the defendant's conviction, but a conviction of a lesser offense.

Diminished capacity defenses are focused on the degree, if any, to which a person's mental disorder impaired his or her ability to form the specific intent to commit a crime. For example, to convict a defendant of first-degree murder, the prosecution generally has to prove some statutorily defined definition of the offense that usually requires the specific intent of premeditation (i.e., malice aforethought). If a mental illness prevented the defendant from being capable of premeditation or malice aforethought, then the defendant may only be guilty of a lesser offense, such as manslaughter. Therefore, a diminished capacity defense requires the forensic expert to evaluate whether the defendant had a particular culpable state of mind.

The doctrine of diminished capacity is controversial, and not all jurisdictions allow mental health testimony that might establish this partial defense. A state's decision to bar such testimony in regard to the effects of intoxication was upheld by the U.S. Supreme Court in the case of *Montana v. Egelhoff* (1996). In this case, James Egelhoff had been camping and partying with friends in the Yaak region of northwestern Montana. Later that evening, Mr. Egelhoff was found severely intoxicated in the back seat of a car, with his two friends dead in the front seat as a result of single gunshot wounds to the backs of their heads. He was subsequently charged with two counts of deliberate homicide.

At trial, Mr. Egelhoff was not allowed to present evidence regarding the impact of his intoxication on his specific intent to kill. After he was found guilty on both counts, he appealed his case to the Supreme Court of Montana, which reversed his conviction, arguing that his due process had been violated when his evidence of intoxication was not allowed in consideration of intent. On appeal, the U.S. Supreme Court upheld that trial court's decision to exclude mental health testimony related to the effects of intoxication on Mr. Egelhoff's specific intent. The Court held that defining *mens rea* (the defendant's "guilty mind") to eliminate the exculpatory value of voluntary intoxication does not offend a fundamental principle of justice.

Likewise, testimony on the effects of severe mental disorders on *mens rea* may also be limited. In the case of *Clark v. Arizona* (2006), the U.S. Supreme Court was asked to review an Arizona trial court decision that prohibited mental health testimony regarding the impact of a psychotic disorder on a defendant's ability to form the required specific intent to kill. Eric Clark, who suffered from paranoid schizophrenia, was charged with the first-degree murder of a police officer in the line of duty. He believed that aliens had invaded Flagstaff, Arizona, and some were posing as government officials. At trial, Mr. Clark was not allowed to present evidence regarding the impact of his psychosis on his alleged intent to kill a police officer. On appeal, the U.S. Supreme Court upheld the trial court's decision to prohibit any mental health testimony regarding Mr. Clark's intent to kill the officer.

Alternative Approaches to Manage Offenders With Mental Illness

Guilty but Mentally Ill

Some states allow a separate verdict of guilty but mentally ill (GBMI) that may be used for individuals who do not meet the legal criteria for insanity but who were mentally ill at the time of the crime. Michigan passed the first GBMI statute in 1975, and 12 states now have some form of a GBMI verdict. Several criticisms of GBMI statutes have arisen since their passage. In particular, defendants found to be GBMI typically receive the same punishment as defendants found guilty, may actually receive longer sentences than had they not pled GBMI, and are not guaranteed mental health treatment when incarcerated as a result of their GBMI finding (Palmer and Hazelrigg 2000). Furthermore, the availability of a GBMI verdict option may make it easier for the trier of fact to choose a GBMI verdict rather than insanity, under the incorrect assumptions that the defendant with mental illness will receive psychiatric treatment in prison or that a person adjudicated legally insane may go free without hospitalization (Sloat and Frierson 2005).

Mental Health and Drug Court Diversion

Rather than forwarding an individual who is facing charges further into the criminal justice system, a number of jurisdictions provide alternative pathways for offenders with mental illness. These pathways are referred to as "diversion" programs because they seek to move persons with mental illness away from jail or prison and into programs that provide mental health treatment.

Diversion programs are generally classified into two categories: prebooking and postbooking diversion programs. *Prebooking* diversion allows the officer to take individuals with mental illness or signs of substance use intoxication who are facing arrest to hospitals or specialized reception centers instead of jail. Under this model, the person avoids being charged with a criminal offense (Sirotich 2009).

Postbooking diversion programs include three basic models: jail-based diversion, court-based diversion, and specialized mental health courts. In the jail-based diversion model, detainees who are identified with a mental illness are diverted to a community-based mental health program with the consent of the judge, district attorney, and defense attorney. In this model, pretrial service evaluators or jail-based mental health clinicians are responsible for identifying those offenders appropriate for diversion.

Under the court-based postbooking diversion model, mental health clinicians who work for the court are responsible for identifying those offenders with mental illness deemed appropriate for community treatment. These court mental health evaluators propose a treatment plan and negotiate community placement and monitoring requirements with the judge, district attorney, and defense attorney. This model involves multiple courts that are individually responsible for diverting those offenders assigned to its particular docket.

In contrast, mental health courts are designed to handle all offenders with mental illness who are identified as appropriate for diversion in one specialized court. Key participants (e.g., judge, court staff, defense attorney, district attorney) in this model typically receive specialized training related to working with persons who are seriously mentally ill. Participation in mental health court is completely voluntary for offenders. Mental health courts mandate community treatment and monitor the offenders' progress. Incentives to participate in treatment include dismissal of charges or avoidance of incarceration upon successful program completion (Lattimore et al. 2003; Sirotich 2009). Drug courts, which operate in a similar fashion to mental health courts, focus on offenders whose primary mental health issues are related to substance use disorders.

In his review of diversion programs, Sirotich (2009) found that jail diversion programs were successful in decreasing the total amount of jail time for persons with mental illness but were not effective in reducing recidivism. In their study specific to mental health courts, Aldigé Hiday et al. (2016) followed participants for 2 years after mental health court completion and compared their outcome to participants who were eligible for mental health court but did not enter the program. Their findings indicated that mental health court participation can reduce recidivism, even after completion of the mental health court program and beyond the provision of treatment and services.

Conclusion

The effect of mental illness on human behavior has been recognized for centuries. Assessments of criminal responsibility involve an in-depth understanding not only of psychiatric diagnoses but also of how a diagnosis may diminish a person's criminal culpability. With the increasing numbers of individuals with mental illness entering the criminal justice system, mental health professionals will play an increasingly prominent role in assessing criminal responsibility, diminished capacity, and appropriateness for diversion of the offender from punishment to community treatment.

Key Concepts

- Evaluations of legal insanity require an assessment of the person's mental state at the time of the offense.

- *Insanity* is a legal definition, and legal tests of insanity vary across jurisdictions and set the standard for evaluating the impact of a defendant's mental illness or defect on his or her criminal behavior.

- Individuals found not guilty by reason of insanity can be involuntarily committed until they are no longer mentally ill and dangerous.

- The evaluation of diminished capacity assesses the impact of a person's mental illness, defect, or substance use on his or her ability to form the requisite specific criminal intent that defines some crimes.

- system include prebooking and postbooking diversion programs and mental health or drug courts.

References

Aldigé Hiday V, Ray B, Wales H: Longer-term impacts of mental health courts: recidivism two years after exit. Psychiatr Serv 67(4):378–383, 2016 26567933

American Academy of Psychiatry and the Law: AAPL Practice Guideline for forensic psychiatric evaluation of defendants raising the insanity defense. J Am Acad Psychiatry Law 42(4)(Suppl):S3–S76, 2014 25492121

American Law Institute: Model Penal Code, § 4.01 (1955)

Clark v Arizona, 548 U.S. 735, 126 S.Ct. 2709 (2006)

Crotty HD: This history of insanity as a defense to crime in English Criminal Law. Calif Law Rev 12:105–123, 1924

Durham v United States, 94 U.S. App. D.C. 228, 214 F.2d 862 (1954)

Foucha v Louisiana, 504 U.S. 71,112 S.Ct. 1780 (1992)

Frendak v United States, 408 A.2d 364 (1979)

Hunsley J, Lee CL, Wood JM: Controversial and questionable assessment techniques, in Science and Pseudoscience in Clinical Psychology. Edited by Lilienfeld SO, Lynn SJ, Lohr JM. New York, Guilford, 2012, pp 42–82

Ibn-Tamas v United States, 407 A.2d 626 (D.C. 1979)

Insanity Defense Reform Act: Pub. L. no. 98-473, 98 Stat. 2057 (1984)

Jones v United States, 463 U.S. 354, 103 S.Ct. 3043 (1983)

Lattimore PK, Broner N, Sherman R, et al: A comparison of prebooking and postbooking diversion programs for mentally ill substance-using individuals with justice involvement. J Contemp Crim Justice 19:30–64, 2003

Montana v Egelhoff, 518 U.S. 37,116 S.Ct. 2013 (1996)

Palmer CA, Hazelrigg M: The guilty but mentally ill verdict: a review and conceptual analysis of intent and impact. J Am Acad Psychiatry Law 28(1):47–54, 2000 10774841

Powell v Texas, 392 U.S. 514, 88 S.Ct. 2145 (1968)

R. v McNaughten (Daniel M'Naghten's Case), 8 E.R. 718 (1843)

Resnick PJ: The detection of malingered psychosis. Psychiatr Clin North Am 22(1): 159–172, 1999 10083952

Resnick PJ: American Academy of Psychiatry and the Law Forensic Review Course Syllabus. Presented at the 46th annual meeting of the American Academy of Psychiatry and the Law, Fort Lauderdale, FL, October 22–25, 2015

Resnick PJ, Noffsinger S: Competency to stand trial and the insanity defense, in The American Psychiatric Publishing Textbook of Forensic Psychiatry. Edited by Simon RI, Gold LH. Washington, DC, American Psychiatric Publishing, 2004, pp 329–347

Robinson v California, 370 U.S. 660, 82 S.Ct. 1417 (1962)

Sirotich F: The criminal justice outcomes of jail diversion programs for persons with mental illness: a review of the evidence. J Am Acad Psychiatry Law 37(4):461–472, 2009 20018995

Sloat LM, Frierson RL: Juror knowledge and attitudes regarding mental illness verdicts. J Am Acad Psychiatry Law 33(2): 208–213, 2005 15985664

Taylor S: Forensic psychology and the role of the forensic psychologist, in Forensic Psychology: The Basics. Edited by Taylor S. New York, Routledge, 2015, pp 1–28

United States v Brawner, 153 U.S. App. D.C. 1, 471 F. 2d 969 (1972)

Walker LEA: Battered woman syndrome: empirical findings. Ann NY Acad Sci 1087:142–157, 2006 17189503

Washington v United States, 129 U.S. App. D.C. 29, 390 F.2d 862 (1967)

Whalen v United States, 445 U.S. 684, 100 S.Ct. 1432 (1980)

CHAPTER 20

Psychiatry and the Death Penalty

Richard L. Frierson, M.D.

Landmark Cases

Estelle v. Smith, 451 U.S. 454, 101 S.Ct. 1866 (1981)

Barefoot v. Estelle, 463 U.S. 880, 103 S.Ct. 3383 (1983)

Ake v. Oklahoma, 470 U.S. 68, 105 S.Ct. 1087 (1985)

Ford v. Wainwright, 477 U.S. 399, 106 S.Ct. 2595 (1986)

Payne v. Tennessee, 501 U.S. 808, 111 S.Ct. 2597 (1991)

State v. Perry, 610 So.2d 746 (1992)

Atkins v. Virginia, 536 U.S. 304, 122 S.Ct. 2242 (2002)

Roper v. Simmons, 543 U.S. 551, 125 S.Ct. 1183 (2005)

Panetti v. Quarterman, 551 U.S. 930, 127 S.Ct. 2842 (2007)

Hall v. Florida, 572 U.S. __, 134 S.Ct. 1986 (2014)

The death penalty has a long and established history, dating back to the eighteenth century B.C. in the Code of Hammurabi, king of Babylon, which codified the death penalty for 25 different crimes. It was also prominent in the Draconian Code of Athens in the seventh century B.C. and in the Roman Laws of the Twelve Tables in the fifth century B.C. (Death Penalty Information Center 2017a). In Great Britain, 288 separate crimes were punishable by death in the eighteenth and early nineteenth centuries under the Bloody Code. However, fewer people were hanged under the Bloody Code than before it (United Kingdom National Archives 2017).

The use of the death penalty in the United States was largely shaped by the laws in Great Britain. The first person executed in what later became the United States was a man at the Jamestown colony who was convicted of espionage in 1608. Dr. Benjamin Rush of Pennsylvania,

TABLE 20–1.   U.S. jurisdictions with the death penalty

Alabama	Louisiana	Pennsylvania
Arizona	Mississippi	South Carolina
Arkansas	Missouri	South Dakota
California	Montana	Tennessee
Colorado	Nebraska	Texas
Florida	Nevada	Utah
Georgia	New Hampshire	Virginia
Idaho	North Carolina	Washington
Indiana	Ohio	Wyoming
Kansas	Oklahoma	U.S. Government
Kentucky	Oregon	U.S. Military

a signer of the Declaration of Independence, was an early opponent of the death penalty, and in 1794 Pennsylvania repealed the death penalty for all offenses except first-degree murder. In the nineteenth century, Rhode Island and Wisconsin abolished the death penalty for all crimes, and between 1907 and 1917 six additional states abolished the death penalty altogether.

However, there was a resurgence in the use of the death penalty between 1920 and 1940, largely due to the invention of cyanide gas, and there were more executions in the 1930s than in any other decade (Death Penalty Information Center 2017b). In the 1960s, interest in the death penalty was declining. In *Furman v. Georgia* (1972), the U.S. Supreme Court declared existing death penalty laws unconstitutional because jurors were given total discretion and arbitrary sentencing could result, thus violating the Eighth Amendment's prohibition against cruel and unusual punishment.

The Modern Death Penalty

After *Furman*, many states enacted new death penalty laws that included bifurcated trials (i.e., separate guilt and sentencing phases) and established aggravating and mitigating circumstances that jurors could apply in their sentencing decision. Four years after *Furman*, the U.S. Supreme Court declared these new laws constitutional because jurors were now given adequate guidance and sentencing would no longer be arbitrary (*Gregg v. Georgia* 1976). Currently, 31 states, the U.S. Government, and the U.S. Military allow for capital punishment (Table 20–1). However, the use of the death penalty in U.S. jurisdictions appears to be on the decline; six states abolished its use between 2007 and 2015: New York (2007), New Mexico (2009), Illinois (2011), Connecticut (2012), Maryland (2013), and Nebraska (2015). The Delaware Supreme Court recently declared the state death penalty law unconstitutional (*Rauf v. State* 2016). As of 2016, governors in four additional states (Colorado, Pennsylvania, Oregon, and Washington) have called for a moratorium. All 31 states listed in Table 20–1 authorize execution by lethal injection. In addition to lethal injection, many states have alternatives: eight states authorize electrocution; three states, lethal gas; three states, hanging; and two states, firing squad (U.S. Department of Justice 2013).

For a capital defendant to be sentenced to death, there must be a finding that one

---

TABLE 20–2. Examples of aggravating circumstances that enable a death sentence

The murder was especially heinous, atrocious, cruel, or depraved (or involved torture).

The defendant knowingly created a grave risk of death for one or more persons in addition to the victim.

The capital offense was committed during the commission of, attempt of, or escape from a specified felony (e.g., armed robbery, burglary, sexual assault, kidnapping).

The defendant committed or attempted to commit more than one murder at the same time.

The murder was committed for pecuniary gain or pursuant to an agreement that the defendant would receive something of value.

The defendant has been convicted of, or committed, a prior murder, a felony involving violence, or other serious felony.

The victim was a government employee, such as a peace officer, police officer, federal agent, firefighter, correctional officer, judge, juror, defense attorney, or prosecutor, in the course of his or her duty.

The murder was committed against a person under age 12 years (or a number of years specified by the jurisdiction).

The murder was committed to avoid or prevent arrest, to effect an escape, or to conceal the commission of a crime.

The murder was committed by means of any weapon of mass destruction.

The murder was an act of terrorism.

The defendant is a future danger (in one of these states: Idaho, Oklahoma, Oregon, Texas, Virginia, Washington, Wyoming).

---

or more aggravating circumstances existed. Each state has the authority to decide aggravating factors, and the numbers of such factors range from 6 (Kentucky) to 20 (Tennessee). Although these factors differ by jurisdiction, common aggravating factors (circumstances) are listed in Table 20–2. Additionally, the sentencing authority must consider the presence of mitigating circumstances and determine whether mitigating circumstances outweigh the aggravating circumstance(s). Examples of common mitigating factors are listed in Table 20–3.

In capital litigation, evaluators may be asked to assess a defendant's competency to stand trial, the defendant's mental state at the time of the alleged offense, the potential presence of intellectual disability, future dangerousness, or mitigating factors to be considered by the jury in sentencing. Additionally, forensic experts may be asked to evaluate a death row inmate's competency to be executed after the execution date is set. The use of forensic psychiatrists in death penalty cases was solidified by the U.S. Supreme Court in *Ake v. Oklahoma* (1985). In this case, a capital defendant, Glen Burton Ake, behaved so bizarrely in court that the judge ordered a competency to stand trial evaluation. After the evaluation the defendant was adjudicated incompetent and committed to a hospital for restoration. After successful restoration, Ake requested the funds to retain a defense psychiatrist in the preparation of an insanity defense. The judge denied this request, and Ake was subsequently convicted and sentenced to death. On appeal to the U.S. Supreme Court, the Court held that an indigent defendant was entitled to the assistance of a psychiatrist on the issues of insanity and future dangerousness and that the denial of that assistance deprived him of due process.

TABLE 20–3.   **Examples of mitigating circumstances that weigh against consideration of a death sentence**

The defendant has no significant history of prior criminal activity.

The capital offense was committed while the defendant was under the influence of extreme mental or emotional disturbance.

The degree of the defendant's participation in the crime was minor, although not so minor as to constitute a defense to prosecution.

The victim was a participant in the defendant's homicidal conduct or consented to the homicidal act.

At the time of the offense, the capacity of the defendant to appreciate the criminality of his conduct or to conform his conduct to the requirements of law was impaired as a result of mental disease or defect, or the effects of intoxication.

The defendant cooperated with law enforcement officers or agencies and with the office of the prosecuting district attorney.

The defendant was under the influence of drugs or alcohol.

The defendant acted under extreme duress or under the substantial domination of another person.

The defendant is not a continuing threat to society.

Epidemiology

Since the U.S. Supreme Court declared in 1976 that the new death penalty laws were constitutional, 1,448 executions have been carried out and 2,902 prisoners currently reside on death row (Death Penalty Information Center 2017b). The vast majority of those currently sentenced to death (98.5%) are men (U.S. Department of Justice 2013).

There is evidence of racial disparity in capital punishment. Jurors may be more likely to convict black defendants than white defendants in death penalty cases (Glaser et al. 2015). Most notably, there is a greater likelihood of a death sentence when the victim was white (Peirce and Radelet 2005, 2011). Moreover, blacks are overrepresented on death row when compared with the general population and the non–death row prison population (Ford 2014). Racial bias, whether by race of offender or race of victim, appears to be a historical legacy, a continuing societal problem, and one of the most significant arguments in the ongoing debate in the United States about use of the death penalty.

Research regarding mental illness among capital defendants and death row inmates is limited, in part because access to prisoners for research purposes is difficult to obtain. Although death row inmates appear to have a disproportionate rate of serious psychiatric disorders when compared with the general prison population, the rates of psychosis in different studies have varied tremendously, from 5% to 60% (Cunningham and Vigen 2002). It appears that many death row inmates experience the onset of serious mental illness after conviction, perhaps precipitated by the stark environment and adverse conditions (i.e., isolation and sensory deprivation) of death row found in many jurisdictions. Additionally, substance use disorders have been found at very high rates among death row inmates, many of whom were under the influence at the time of their capital offense (Frierson et al. 1998). Finally, a significant minority of death row inmates (25%–30%)

have some degree of intellectual impairment, even if they do not qualify for a diagnosis of intellectual disability (Cunningham and Vigen 2002). However, they are not necessarily more likely to be intellectually impaired than persons convicted of murder who receive a different sentence (Frierson et al. 1998).

Ethics

Although the use of the death penalty in the United States appears to be on the decline, the fact that capital punishment still is used at all continues to generate controversy. In fact, the United States remains the only Western industrialized nation that has not abolished the death penalty. Approximately 102 countries have abolished the death penalty, 58 carry out executions, and an additional 32 countries have retained the death penalty but not carried out an execution in over 10 years (Amnesty International 2015).

The participation of psychiatrists or other physicians in the legal process involving capital punishment has been a topic of considerable discussion among professional groups. The American Medical Association's Council on Ethical and Judicial Affairs has held that a physician should not be a participant in a legally authorized execution. *Participation* has been defined as being involved in one of the following (American Medical Association 2007):

1. An action that would directly cause the death of the condemned
2. An action that would assist, supervise, or contribute to the ability of another individual to directly cause the death of the condemned
3. An action that could automatically cause an execution to be carried out on a condemned prisoner

The American Medical Association specifically states that the forensic evaluation of capacity to stand trial, criminal responsibility, aggravating and mitigating circumstances, and competency to be executed does not constitute participation in a legally authorized execution. In fact, no U.S. professional associations prohibit a psychiatrist from evaluating and testifying on these issues. Even testimony for the prosecution during the sentencing phase has been ethically defended as long as the psychiatrist does not testify on the ultimate issue of future dangerousness (Kermani and Drob 1988).

The American Medical Association also prohibits physicians from treating prisoners for the sole purpose of restoring competency to be executed. However, psychiatrists may ethically treat a death row inmate for the purpose of relieving significant suffering or preventing significant injury to self or others. As a result of this treatment, an inmate's competency to be executed may be improved or restored, but treatment specifically to restore competency to be executed is unethical. Psychiatrists practicing in a death row setting are functioning in a complex ethical arena. They should weigh their decision to participate in or abstain from various activities with great care and pay close attention to the circumstances of individual cases (Matthews and Wendler 2006).

Psychiatric Evaluations in Death Penalty Cases

Regardless of the type of evaluation being conducted, psychiatrists should inform defendants or inmates that they are not establishing a treatment relationship. Additionally, the defendant or inmate must be informed of the evaluator's role, the purpose of the evaluation, the party who requested the evaluation, and the limitations of confidentiality (i.e., who will receive information obtained during the evaluation and/or the evaluation report). Prosecution experts must inform the defense attorney of the scheduled evaluation. Psychiatrists should not perform forensic evaluations for the prosecution or the government on persons who have not consulted with legal counsel (American Academy of Psychiatry and the Law 2005).

The evaluation of capacity to stand trial for capital defendants is similar to that for other criminal defendants (see Chapter 18, "Evaluation of Competencies in the Criminal Justice System"). However, a few notable differences exist. In capital cases, the defendant should be capable of understanding the separate guilt and sentencing phases of a death penalty trial and the types of evidence that are presented in each phase. The defendant should be capable of providing the attorney with information that could be used in mitigation; this would include a list of persons who might be called to testify—childhood friends, former teachers or employers, family members, and so forth. Also, because the attorney in capital cases is expected to engage in ongoing dialogue about all matters that could have a material impact on the case, including the factual investigation, legal issues, defense theories, presentation of the defense case, relevant aspects of the client's life, deadlines and schedules, and courtroom presentation and demeanor (Freedman 2009), a capital defendant needs to be able to engage in a more intense and lengthy dialogue and to establish a working relationship with an attorney in ways not required of noncapital defendants.

Due Process, Psychiatric Testimony in Sentencing, and Victim Impact Testimony

In states where future dangerousness is an aggravating factor (i.e., Idaho, Oklahoma, Oregon, Texas, Virginia, Washington, and Wyoming), prosecutors may seek expert mental health testimony to assist with proving this issue. Many death penalty appeals have resulted from the unethical or poor practices by prosecution psychiatrists in death penalty trials. When evaluating defendants facing a potential death sentence, the psychiatrist must clearly understand the parameters that govern these assessments, as well as the numerous clinical, ethical, and legal issues that may arise in the course of the evaluation.

The U.S. Supreme Court addressed some of these issues in *Estelle v. Smith* (1981), a Texas death penalty case in which a prosecution psychiatrist evaluated a capital defendant's capacity to stand trial but did not inform the defendant about the limitations of confidentiality. The psychiatrist specifically failed to inform the defendant that information gathered in the capacity to stand trial evaluation could also be used against the defendant in the sentencing phase of his trial. The prosecution expert also did not notify the defendant's attorney of the scheduled evaluation. The psychiatrist who conducted the capacity to stand trial evaluation was subsequently allowed to testify about the defendant's future dangerousness in the sentencing phase, over the defendant's objection. From information gathered in the capacity to stand trial evaluation, the prosecution psychiatrist declared the defendant a "very severe sociopath" who would "with one hundred percent and absolute certainty" commit future criminal acts if afforded the opportunity. After hearing this testimony, the jury imposed a death sentence. The defendant appealed.

In their ruling in *Estelle v. Smith* (1981), the U.S. Supreme Court affirmed the lower federal courts' decisions that the admission of the doctor's testimony at the sentencing phase violated the defendant's Fifth Amendment privilege against compelled self-incrimination, because the defendant was not advised before the pretrial psychiatric examination that he had a right to remain silent and that any statement he made could be used against him at a capital sentencing proceeding. Additionally the Court found that the failure of the psychiatrist to notify the defendant's attorney of the capacity to stand trial evaluation was a violation of the defendant's Sixth Amendment right to effective assistance of counsel.

In the states that include future dangerousness as an aggravating factor, prosecution evidence concerning the presence of antisocial personality disorder in capital defendants is quite prevalent. Most capital defense attorneys believe that evidence concerning antisocial personality disorder, sociopathy, or psychopathy has a considerable impact on trial outcome (Edens and Cox 2012). Unfortunately, predictions by capital juries that future prison violence is probable have considerable error rates—up to 90% (Reidy et al. 2013). Thus, the confidence of legislators and courts in the ability of capital jurors to predict future violence is likely misplaced.

Psychiatrists are often asked to opine about a defendant's potential for future violence during the sentencing phase.

Such determinations are highly controversial because long-term predictions of violence are difficult and false-positive rates in violence prediction are high. Psychiatrists, like jurors, are more likely to overpredict than underpredict violent behavior. The consequences of an overprediction of future violence in death penalty cases are extremely detrimental to the capital defendant. Therefore, psychiatric experts who agree to provide this type of testimony should consider limiting their testimony to the identification of static and dynamic risk factors and protective factors in regard to a defendant's future dangerousness, without stating a particular likelihood that the individual will behave violently in the future.

Additionally, many lawyers and experts attempt to sway juries through the use of pseudoscientific evidence. The use of neuroscience (e.g., genetics, hormonal studies, brain imaging) in violence risk assessment has not yet achieved scientific acceptance (Glenn and Raine 2014). However, lawyers and experts have sometimes strived to establish tenuous links between brain features and criminal behaviors, especially through the use of neuroimaging. Because clinical and functional imaging techniques are still largely used for research, neuroimaging is particularly susceptible to inappropriate use in the courtroom (Patel et al. 2007).

The use of actuarial instruments, such as the Psychopathy Checklist—Revised (PCL-R; Hare 2003), the Violence Risk Appraisal Guide (VRAG; Quinsey et al. 2006), or others in violence prediction (see Chapter 28, "Violence Risk Assessment"), is equally controversial in capital trials. Although these instruments may identify low-risk individuals with high levels of accuracy, their use as sole determinants of detention, sentencing, and release is not supported by the current evidence (Fazel et al. 2012). Moreover, these instruments were often developed to describe, and were normed using, the general population and do not take into account the low base rate of violent incidents in prison. The presentation of statistics that show the rate of serious violent behavior in prison to be low overall and typically lower than in free society may help jurors place actuarial instrument findings in context (Davis and Sorensen 2013).

Many savvy capital defense attorneys have refused to allow their defendant to be evaluated by non–defense experts for purposes other than the determination of the defendant's capacity to stand trial. However, such refusals have not necessarily stopped prosecution experts from providing testimony in the sentencing phase. In *Barefoot v. Estelle* (1983), a capital jury had been asked to decide whether a defendant convicted of capital murder would commit future acts of violence that would constitute a continuing threat to society. The prosecution entered the defendant's criminal record into evidence and then called two psychiatric experts who had not personally examined Barefoot to testify on this issue. Both experts, in response to hypothetical questions posed by the prosecution, testified that Barefoot would probably commit further acts of violence and represent a continuing threat to society. He was subsequently sentenced to death.

During his habeas appeal, Barefoot argued that psychiatrists, individually and as a class, are not competent to predict future dangerousness and that their testimony in his case violated his due process. He further argued that the use of experts who had not personally examined him was a constitutional error. The U.S. Supreme Court rejected the argument that psychiatrists, "out of the entire universe of persons who might have an opinion on the issue," would know so little about the subject that they should not be permitted to testify. Additionally, the Court rejected the argument against hypothetical testimony and held that expert testimony, whether in the form of an opinion based on hypothetical questions or otherwise, is commonly admitted as evidence where it might help the fact finders do their assigned job.

Despite this legal holding, psychiatrists should be aware that the adequacy of their clinical evaluations may be called into question when expert opinions are offered without personal examinations. Ethical standards regarding the provision of psychiatric expert testimony hold that an expert should make appropriate effort to conduct a personal examination. If, after appropriate effort, obtaining a personal examination is not possible, the expert must clearly state that there was no personal examination and note any resulting limitations to their opinions (American Academy of Psychiatry and the Law 2005).

In almost all death penalty states, the presence of mental illness or intellectual impairment (whether or not there is intellectual disability) may be a mitigating factor in sentencing. Frequently, these mitigating factors will be statutorily defined as "the capital offense was committed while the defendant was under the influence of extreme mental or emotional disturbance." Many state statutes urge jurors to consider the effect of mental illness on the defendant's ability to distinguish right from wrong or to conform his or her behavior to the requirements of the law, even if the defendant did not fully meet the statutory requirement for a verdict of insanity. Additionally, five states (Arkansas, Colorado, Indiana, Kentucky, and Louisiana) include consideration of the effect of alcohol or drug use at the time of a murder.

Most states grant the judge tremendous leeway in determining whether to allow other issues in mitigation. In fact, the U.S. Supreme Court has held that the Eighth and Fourteenth Amendments require that jurors should consider all mitigating factors surrounding the accused murderer before applying the death penalty (*Lockett v. Ohio* 1978). These factors are not limited to those that are statutorily defined, and include the defendant's character or record as well as any circumstances of the offense proffered as a reason for a sentence less than death.

Forensic psychiatrists are frequently called to testify about these issues and to explain to jurors the role of mental illness or intellectual impairment in the defendant's participation in the crime. In multiple-codefendant cases in which intellectual impairment is an issue, the expert may be asked to explain the susceptibility of an individual with intellectual impairment to be unduly influenced or more easily persuaded by nonimpaired codefendants. Experts may also be asked to explain the role of mental illness or substance use on an individual's ability to perceive reality, to apply good judgment, and to control impulses when angry and potentially disinhibited by brain injury, alcohol, or drugs.

Expert psychiatric testimony presented in mitigation may actually be helpful in securing a sentence of life imprisonment rather than death. One study of actual jurors found a significant correlation between the presence of a defense psychiatrist or psychologist in the sentencing phase and the likelihood of jurors having the impression that the defendant was mentally disturbed (Montgomery et al. 2005). A study of death-penalty-qualified mock jurors found that jurors were more likely to sentence a defendant to death when there was no mental health testimony presented in mitigation (Barnett et al. 2004). Jurors were less likely to assign a death sentence when four specific types of mitigation are present:

1. When the defendant was diagnosed with schizophrenia and was unmedicated and psychotic at the time of the alleged offense
2. When the defendant was drug addicted and high at the time of the murder
3. When the defendant had intellectual impairment
4. When there was severe childhood physical and verbal abuse

Sometimes, however, testimony about childhood abuse may lead jurors to assign a death sentence. Some jurors may view such evidence as indicating a lack of rehabilitation potential and may question why all children with strong family histories of abuse do not grow up to commit horrendous crimes (McPherson 1995).

In addition to hearing aggravating and mitigating circumstances, jurors in death penalty cases may hear victim impact testimony. Traditionally, such testimony was excluded from consideration in death penalty cases because it created "a constitutionally unacceptable risk that the jury may impose the death penalty in an arbitrary and capricious manner" (*Booth v. Maryland* 1987). However, in *Payne v. Tennessee* (1991), the U.S. Supreme Court overturned its previous ruling on this issue and declined to declare a *pro se* ban on victim impact testimony. Payne murdered a 28-year-old woman and her 2-year-old daughter. He also attempted to murder her 3-year-old son, but the son survived a brutal stabbing. At trial, the judge allowed the surviving child's grandmother to testify regarding the impact of this crime on her grandson (i.e., that he cries out for his mother and cries for his sister).

Payne was sentenced to death and appealed to the U.S. Supreme Court, alleging that the testimony of the grandmother violated his Eighth Amendment right as outlined in *Booth*. In *Payne*, the Court reversed its earlier decision, stating that the *Booth* decision unfairly weighted the scales in a capital trial because the defense may introduce evidence about the defendant's character and the state cannot counteract such evidence. The Court held that victim impact testimony could be used to show each victim's "uniqueness as a human being."

Competency to Be Executed

As death row inmates approach execution, competency to be executed evaluations may be requested. As of December 2013, the average death row prisoner had been on death row 14.6 years and the average time from sentencing to execution was 137 months (over 11 years) (Bureau of Justice Statistics 2013). Confinement on death row is typified by marked interpersonal isolation and activity deprivation, with human contact restricted to brief interactions with corrections officers, health care providers, or attorneys. These conditions may lead to a host of psychological consequences, including depression, anxiety, and, in some cases, frank psychosis.

Additionally, these harsh conditions lead some death row inmates to waive their appeals and proceed with execution. The U.S. Supreme Court has ruled that such waivers must be granted when they are made knowingly, intelligently, and voluntarily (*Whitmore v. Arkansas* 1990). Frequently in these cases, competency evaluations are ordered to assure that the decision to waive appeals is not the re-

sult of mental illness, especially suicidal ideation associated with depression.

In *Ford v. Wainwright* (1986), Ford had been sentenced to death in Florida in 1974 for murdering a police officer. While on death row he began to display bizarre behavior. Two defense psychiatrists evaluated him and determined he was incompetent to be executed; however, three state psychiatrists found him competent after a joint 30-minute interview. The governor signed the death warrant, and Ford appealed. The U.S. Supreme Court ruled that the Eighth Amendment prohibits the execution of an insane person and that Florida procedures were unconstitutional because Ford was not afforded an opportunity to be heard or to challenge the state experts. Further, the Court stated, Florida procedures placed too much power in the executive branch.

The Court stopped short, however, of defining a specific standard to be used in determining competency to be executed. Justice Lewis Powell, in a concurring opinion, suggested that a narrow cognitive standard would suffice: that the inmate is aware of the punishment he or she is about to suffer and the reason for the punishment. The standard for competency to be executed has been left to the individual states to decide. Whereas some have adopted a narrow cognitive standard, others have also included the ability to rationally communicate with counsel and assist in the appellate process.

The U.S. Supreme Court in *Panetti v. Quarterman* (2007) further clarified the competency to be executed standard and held that a prisoner must have a rational understanding of his execution, not merely an awareness of his upcoming execution. In this case, Panetti, a Texas death row inmate, believed that the state's reason he was being executed (for killing his wife's parents) was a sham, and that he was actually being executed as a part of spiritual warfare to prevent him from preaching the Gospel. The Court held that delusions may prevent a death row inmate from rationally understanding the reason for his execution. Having held that an inmate must have a "rational understanding," the Court declined to further clarify what this actually means (Appelbaum 2007).

For death row inmates adjudicated incompetent to be executed, it is unclear whether administration of forced medication for competency restoration would survive constitutional scrutiny. As mentioned earlier, the American Medical Association considers such treatment unethical. In *State v. Perry* (1992), a death row inmate had been found incompetent to be executed and the trial court issued an order for forced medication to restore his competency. Perry appealed, and the U.S. Supreme Court remanded the case to the trial court for consideration in light of *Washington v. Harper* (1990), which outlined procedures necessary to involuntarily medicate inmates in general but not inmates facing a death sentence. On remand, the trial court once again ordered forced medication for Perry. On appeal, the Louisiana Supreme Court held that forcible medication for restoration of competency to be executed was a violation of the right to privacy contained in the Louisiana State Constitution. Federal courts are silent on this issue. However, in *Singleton v. Norris* (2003), the Eighth Circuit Court of Appeals held that forced medication of a death row inmate who is gravely disabled or poses a likelihood of serious harm to himself or others is not unconstitutional, even if it results in restoration of competency. The court held that the best medical interest of an inmate must be determined without regard to a pending execution date.

Exceptions for Special Populations

The U.S. Supreme Court has now banned capital punishment for several distinct populations, including those with intellectual disability and those younger than 18 years at the time of the commission of the capital offense. Additionally, the American Psychiatric Association (2014) has issued a position statement calling for a ban on capital punishment for individuals who lacked the ability to appreciate the nature, consequences, or wrongfulness of their conduct; who could not exercise rational judgment in relationship to their conduct; or who could not conform their conduct to the requirements of the law. However, this position has yet to be supported by an appellate court.

Chief Justice Earl Warren first coined the phrase *evolving standards of decency* in *Trop v. Dulles* (1958), a case in which a military deserter was appealing his expatriation. It has been used to illustrate that the Eighth Amendment's protections are dynamic and are subject to growth in a maturing society. In *Penry v. Lynaugh* (1989), the U.S. Supreme Court held that an individual could not be excluded from execution on the sole basis of mental retardation (now referred to as intellectual disability). However, in the years that followed, the federal court system and 17 states passed statutes barring the execution of persons with intellectual disability.

Finally, in *Atkins v. Virginia* (2002), the U.S. Supreme Court, citing consistency of the direction of change on this issue, reversed its *Penry* decision. The Court ruled that evolving standards of decency demonstrate that the Eighth

Amendment now precludes the execution of persons with intellectual disability. The Court also held that persons with intellectual disability may unwittingly confess to crimes they did not commit, have poor ability to assist counsel at trial, and appear to lack remorse due to an impression created by their demeanor in court.

A similar reversal had occurred in the case of *Stanford v. Kentucky* (1989), in which the U.S. Supreme Court previously upheld the constitutionality of executing 16- and 17-year-old offenders. In ***Roper v. Simmons*** (2005), the U.S. Supreme Court noted that a national consensus had developed against the execution of juvenile offenders, as 18 states had barred such executions, 12 other states had barred executions altogether, and no state had lowered its age of execution below 18 since *Stanford*. The Court noted that youths lack maturity and have an underdeveloped sense of responsibility, which can result in impetuous and ill-considered actions and decisions. The Court held that evolving standards of decency indicate that the Eighth Amendment now prohibits the execution of those under age 18 at the time of their criminal act.

Since *Atkins*, psychiatrists are frequently asked to determine whether a death row inmate or capital defendant has intellectual disability. The diagnostic criteria for intellectual disability have undergone significant revisions in the *Diagnostic and Statistical Manual of Mental Disorders*, 5th Edition (DSM-5; American Psychiatric Association 2013), with an emphasis on the need to assess adaptive functioning in addition to cognitive limitations. Notably, DSM-5 does not even mention a standardized IQ measurement of approximately 70 or below, but rather requires "deficits in intellectual functioning" as confirmed by clinical assessment and "individualized, standardized intelligence testing." IQ scores that would meet the definition of "deficits in intellectual functioning" are suggested to be those that fall approximately two standard deviations below the mean. On IQ tests with a standard deviation of 15 and a mean of 100, this involves an IQ score ranging from 65 to 75 (70±5).

However, DSM-5 places an emphasis on the importance of using clinical judgment in score interpretation and consideration of the margin of error in measurement and factors that may artificially lower IQ scores. In ***Hall v. Florida*** (2014), the U.S. Supreme Court held that Florida's requirement that a score of 70 or less on an IQ test is necessary to prove intellectual disability violates the Eighth and Fourteenth Amendments of the Constitution. Specifically, if an IQ test score falls within the test's acknowledged and inherent margin of error, the defendant must be able to present additional evidence of intellectual disability, including testimony regarding adaptive deficits.

Additionally, examiners should be aware of the Flynn effect, an upward drift in mean cognitive abilities (and measured IQ) in the population over time (Flynn 1987). This rise in IQ scores over time has been observed with both the Wechsler and Stanford-Binet IQ tests to be approximately three points per decade. Therefore, as scores rise across time, fewer and fewer individuals have intelligence measured in the intellectually disabled range. In contrast, when a new IQ test is developed and published, along with new normative data, there is a significant increase in the proportion of the population with scores falling in the disabled range (i.e., 70 or below).

Unfortunately, the assessment of adaptive functioning in incarcerated individuals is difficult. Adaptive functioning must be assessed in three domains: conceptual, social, and practical. The *conceptual* domain involves abstract thinking, executive functioning, memory, and functional use of academic skills. Assessing this in incarcerated individuals involves examining reading ability, ability to work with an appellate attorney and understand legal principles, ability to manage a canteen fund, and ability to problem solve. To assess vocabulary and basic conceptual abilities, evaluators may find it useful to examine letters that the inmate writes to home or to others.

The *social* domain involves communication and conversational skills, social judgment, and the ability to interact socially and perceive social cues. Assessing this domain involves examining how the inmate interacts with other inmates and correctional officers. Persons with intellectual disability, because of their naiveté or gullibility, may be easily victimized or taken advantage of by other inmates. Deficits in the social domain would be manifest by other inmates easily taking advantage of the inmate or feeling a need to protect the inmate because of a perceived social vulnerability. Gathering information about relationships may involve talking to numerous prison officials who are familiar with the daily activities on death row.

The *practical* domain involves an ability to function in age-appropriate personal care. This is the hardest domain to assess among incarcerated individuals because on death row, other inmates prepare meals, complete laundry, and so forth. Medical records may reveal evidence of the inmate's ability to make medical decisions and maintain compliance with treatment. An inmate who requires assistance when completing medical requests or canteen orders may have deficits in the practical domain. Because adaptive functioning is difficult to assess in incarcerated individuals, information about an individual's level of adaptive functioning prior to incarceration may be more revealing than trying to assess adaptive functioning in prison (Frierson 2015).

Conclusion

Psychiatrists who are involved in the forensic evaluation of capital defendants or death row inmates should be aware of the statutory laws regarding the death penalty in the particular jurisdiction as well as the ethical issues that can arise in capital cases. At trial, experts should be prepared for their opinions and personal ethics to be vigorously challenged. Consequently, opinions should be based on objective evidence and not influenced by personal bias.

Key Concepts

- Physicians cannot ethically participate in legally authorized executions; however, the forensic mental health evaluation of capital defendants or death row inmates does not constitute participation.

- Capital defendants must be informed of the purpose of the psychiatric evaluation, the role of the evaluator, the party requesting the evaluation, and the limitations of confidentiality.

- In most states, the presence of mental illness or intellectual impairment (whether or not there is intellectual disability) may be a mitigating factor in sentencing.

- Testimony on future dangerousness should only be provided after attempting a personal examination of a defendant and should be limited to the identification of risk factors and protective factors without stating a particular likelihood that an individual will or will not behave violently in the future.

- Competency to be executed requires that the inmate is aware of the nature of the punishment and the reason for the punishment; in some jurisdictions it also involves the ability to rationally assist counsel.

- Evolving standards of decency have led to the elimination of the death penalty for persons with intellectual disabilities and for juveniles.

References

Ake v Oklahoma, 470 U.S. 68, 105 S.Ct. 1087 (1985)

American Academy of Psychiatry and the Law: Ethics guidelines for the practice of forensic psychiatry. May 2005. Available at: http://www.aapl.org/ethics.htm. Accessed December 19, 2016.

American Medical Association: Code of medical ethics: opinion 2.06—capital punishment. August 23, 2007. Available at: https://www.law.berkeley.edu/clinics/dpclinic/LethalInjection/LI/QA/docs/AMA. Accessed January 8, 2017.

American Psychiatric Association: Diagnostic and Statistical Manual of Mental Disorders, 5th Edition. Arlington, VA, American Psychiatric Association, 2013

American Psychiatric Association: Position statement on diminished responsibility in capital sentencing. November 2014. Available at: http://www.psychiatry.org/home/policy-finder. Accessed January 8, 2017.

Amnesty International: Death sentences and executions in 2015. 2015. Available at: https://www.amnesty.org/en/latest/research/2016/04/death-sentences-executions-2015/. Accessed January 8, 2017.

Appelbaum PS: Law and psychiatry: Death row delusions: when is a prisoner competent to be executed? Psychiatr Serv 58(10):1258–1260, 2007 17913998

Atkins v Virginia, 536 U.S. 304, 122 S.Ct. 2242 (2002)

Barefoot v Estelle, 463 U.S. 880, 103 S.Ct. 3383 (1983)

Barnett ME, Brodsky SL, Davis CM: When mitigation evidence makes a difference: effects of psychological mitigating evidence on sentencing decisions in capital trials. Behav Sci Law 22(6):751–770, 2004 15386561

Booth v Maryland, 482 U.S. 496, 107 S.Ct. 2529 (1987)

Bureau of Justice Statistics: United States Department of Justice: capital punishment, 2013—statistical tables. 2013. Available at: http://www.bjs.gov/content/pub/pdf/cp13st.pdf. Accessed January 8, 2017.

Cunningham MD, Vigen MP: Death row inmate characteristics, adjustment, and confinement: a critical review of the literature. Behav Sci Law 20(1–2):191–210, 2002 11979498

Davis J, Sorensen JR: Using base rates and correlational data to supplement clinical risk assessments. J Am Acad Psychiatry Law 41(3):391–400, 2013 24051592

Death Penalty Information Center: Death penalty history. 2017a. Available at: http://www.deathpenaltyinfo.org/part-i-history-death-penalty#intro. Accessed January 8, 2017.

Death Penalty Information Center: Facts about the death penalty. 2017b. Available at: http://www.deathpenalty-info.org/documents/FactSheet.pdf. Accessed April 25, 2017.

Edens JF, Cox J: Examining the prevalence, role and impact of evidence regarding Antisocial Personality, sociopathy and psychopathy in capital cases: a survey of defense team members. Behav Sci Law 30(3):239–255, 2012 22374708

Estelle v Smith, 451 U.S. 454, 101 S.Ct. 1866 (1981)

Fazel S, Singh JP, Doll H, et al: Use of risk assessment instruments to predict violence and antisocial behaviour in 73 samples involving 24 827 people: systematic review and meta-analysis. BMJ 345: e4692, 2012 22833604

Flynn JR: Massive IQ gains in 14 nations: what IQ tests really measure. Psychol Bull 101:171–191, 1987

Ford M: Racism and the execution chamber. The Atlantic, June 23, 2014

Ford v Wainwright, 477 U.S. 399, 106 S.Ct. 2595 (1986)

Freedman D: When is a capitally charged defendant incompetent to stand trial? Int J Law Psychiatry 32(3):127–133, 2009 19303637

Frierson RL: DSM-5 and psychiatric evaluations of individuals in the criminal justice system, in DSM-5 and the Law: Changes and Challenges. Edited by Scott C. New York, Oxford University Press, 2015, pp 77–100

Frierson RL, Schwartz-Watts DM, Morgan DW, et al: Capital versus noncapital murderers. J Am Acad Psychiatry Law 26(3):403–410, 1998 9785284

Furman v Georgia, 408 U.S. 23, 92 S.Ct. 2726 (1972)

Glaser J, Martin KD, Kahn KB: Possibility of death sentence has divergent effect on verdicts for black and white defendants. Law Hum Behav 39(6):539–546, 2015 26146816

Glenn AL, Raine A: Neurocriminology: implications for the punishment, prediction and prevention of criminal behaviour. Nat Rev Neurosci 15(1):54–63, 2014 24326688

Gregg v Georgia, 428 U.S. 153, 96 S.Ct. 2909 (1976)

Hall v Florida, 572 U.S. ___, 134 S.Ct. 1986 (2014)

Hare RD: Manual for the Revised Psychopathy Checklist, 2nd Edition. Toronto, ON, Canada, Multi-Health Systems, 2003

Kermani EJ, Drob SL: Psychiatry and the death penalty: dilemma for mental health professionals. Psychiatr Q 59(3):193–212, 1988 3070607

Lockett v Ohio, 438 U.S. 586, 98 S.Ct. 2954 (1978)

Matthews D, Wendler S: Ethical issues in the evaluation and treatment of death row inmates. Curr Opin Psychiatry 19(5):518–521, 2006 16874127

McPherson SB: Psychosocial investigation in death penalty mitigation: procedures, pitfalls, and impact, in Psychology, Law, and Criminal Justice: International Developments in Research and Practice. Edited by Davies G, Lloyd-Bostock M, McMurran M, et al. Berlin, De Gruyter, 1995, pp 286–295

Montgomery JH, Ciccone JR, Garvey SP, et al: Expert testimony in capital sentencing: juror responses. J Am Acad Psychiatry Law 33(4):509–518, 2005 16394228

Panetti v Quarterman, 551 U.S. 930, 127 S.Ct. 2842 (2007)

Patel P, Meltzer CC, Mayberg HS, et al: The role of imaging in United States courtrooms. Neuroimaging Clin N Am 17(4): 557–567, x, 2007 17983970

Payne v Tennessee, 501 U.S. 808, 111 S.Ct. 2597 (1991)

Peirce GL, Radelet ML: Impact of legally inappropriate factors on death sentencing for California homicides, 1990–1999, the empirical analysis. Santa Clara Law Rev 46:433–483, 2005

Peirce GL, Radelet ML: Death sentencing in east Baton Rouge Parish 1990–2008. LA Law Rev 71:658–673, 2011

Penry v Lynaugh, 492 U.S. 302, 109 S.Ct. 2934 (1989)

Quinsey VL, Harris GT, Rice ME, et al: Violent Offenders: Appraising and Managing Risk, 2nd Edition. Washington, DC, American Psychological Association, 2006

Rauf v State, Delaware Supreme Court. August 2, 2016. Available at: http://courts.delaware.gov/Opinions/Download. aspx? id=244410. Accessed January 8, 2017.

Reidy TJ, Sorensen JR, Cunningham MD: Probability of criminal acts of violence: a test of jury predictive accuracy. Behav Sci Law 31(2):286–305, 2013 23613146

Roper v Simmons, 543 U.S. 551, 125 S.Ct. 1183 (2005)

Singleton v Norris, 319 F.3d 1018 (8th Cir. Ark. 2003)

Stanford v Kentucky, 492 U.S. 361, 109 S.Ct. 2969 (1989)

State v Perry, 610 So.2d 746 (1992)

Trop v Dulles, 356 U.S. 86, 78 S.Ct. 590 (1958)

United Kingdom National Archives: Crime and punishment: the bloody code. 2017. Available at: http://www.nationalarchives.gov.uk/education/candp/punishment/g06/g06cs1.htm. Accessed January 8, 2017.

U.S. Department of Justice: Bureau of Justice Statistics. Capital Punishment, 2013—Statistical Tables. Available at: http://www.bjs.gov/content/pub/pdf/cp13st.pdf. Accessed January 8, 2017.

Washington v Harper, 494 U.S. 210, 110 S.Ct. 1028 (1990)

Whitmore v Arkansas, 495 U.S. 149, 110 S.Ct. 1717 (1990)

PART V

Correctional Psychiatry and
Sex Offenders

CHAPTER 21

Correctional Settings and Prisoner Rights

Robert D. Morgan, Ph.D.

Stephanie A. Van Horn, Ph.D.

Joel A. Dvoskin, Ph.D., ABPP

Landmark Cases

Baxstrom v. Herold, 383 U.S. 107, 86 S.Ct. 760 (1966)

Estelle v. Gamble, 429 U.S. 97, 97 S.Ct. 285 (1976)

Vitek v. Jones, 445 U.S. 480, 100 S.Ct. 1254 (1980)

Washington v. Harper, 494 U.S. 210, 110 S.Ct. 1028 (1990)

Sell v. United States, 539 U.S. 166, 123 S.Ct. 2174 (1997)

United States v. Georgia, 546 U.S. 151, 126 S.Ct. 877 (2006)

Brown v. Plata, 563 U.S. 493, 134 S.Ct. 436 (2011)

As of 2013, over 10 million people were incarcerated worldwide (Walmsley 2013), with over 1.6 million in U.S. prisons alone (Guerino et al. 2011). The goals of corrections are twofold: 1) to improve public safety by removing offenders from the community and by providing oversight of offenders allowed to remain in society, and 2) to "correct" offending behavior so that inmates desist from committing future crimes. A myriad of legal mandates direct the manner in which correctional agencies must operate and establish standards for the services that must be provided. In this chapter, we review the various types of correctional settings, the impact of imprisonment and prison culture on inmate functioning, and offender rights.

Corrections and Landmark Cases

Corrections is a broad term that includes both community corrections (e.g., probation, parole) and institutional corrections (e.g., jail, prison). *Jails* house inmates either awaiting trial or convicted of misdemeanor or low-level felony offenses (i.e., usually with sentences of 2 years or less). *Prisons*, on the other hand, house inmates convicted of felonies with sentences typically greater than 2 years. Most prison systems also have so-called supermax facilities, in which inmates have more restrictions; these segregated inmates are typically confined to their cells except for approximately 1 hour per day for exercise and showers. Other than to keep appointments (e.g., medical or legal visits), they remain in their cells. The specific circumstances of incarceration (e.g., single vs. double cells, property and television allowance, staff attitudes) vary significantly from one facility to another.

Regardless of the institutional setting, corrections departments are responsible for providing basic mental health services. *Basic mental health services*, which are distinguished from rehabilitative services, have been described as analogous to services provided in a community mental health center model (Dvoskin and Morgan 2010; Fagan 2003; Morgan 2003); the aim is to assess needs and provide services that alleviate distress, reduce psychiatric symptomatology, and improve individual functioning and coping. In contrast, *rehabilitative services* are intended to alter criminal behaviors, tendencies, and lifestyles so as to reduce

criminal recidivism and to increase desistence and prosocial behavior, all aimed at successful community reentry.

Basic mental health services must be available to all offenders in criminal justice settings, as mandated by public policy initiatives and litigation at state and federal levels (e.g., ***Estelle v. Gamble*** 1976; *Ruiz v. Estelle* 1982). In *Ruiz v. Estelle* (1982), a class action lawsuit brought against the Texas Department of Criminal Justice in 1972, inmates alleged that the agency's management policies amounted to cruel and unusual punishment. Specifically, the claims were based on overcrowding (i.e., two or three inmates in cells designed for one), insufficient security staffing (e.g., not enough officers, use of inmates to supervise other inmates), insufficient medical staffing, unsafe working conditions, and excessive and arbitrary disciplinary procedures.

In 1980, the U.S. District Court held that the conditions constituted cruel and unusual punishment due to overcrowding, lack of sufficient officers or medical professionals, deprivation of due process rights in disciplinary proceedings, inadequate physical and mental health care, and excessive physical force by correctional officers. The court required the Texas Department of Criminal Justice to correct these issues. The state of Texas appealed, but the district court's ruling was upheld by the appellate court in 1982. The ensuing legal battle lasted two decades, and the resulting difficulties of enforcing similar rulings led to the Prison Litigation Reform Act of 1996 (1996a). This act attempted to limit the court's ability to require institutional-level changes that would be unnecessarily difficult for prisons to make by requiring the court 1) to use the "least restrictive means necessary" (Prison Litigation Reform Act 1996b) and 2) to weigh the effect any injunctions may have on public safety (e.g., the mass release of inmates to accommodate mandatory population controls).

Although progress had been made toward securing inmates' rights to timely, quality physical and mental health care, *Ruiz v. Estelle* set forth objective means for meeting those goals. At a minimum, correctional systems must meet the following six requirements (Metzner 2002):

1. A system must be in place for the screening and evaluation of mental illness.
2. Treatment may not solely consist of seclusion or intensive supervision.
3. Trained mental health professionals must be involved in these processes.
4. Complete, accurate, and confidential records must be maintained.
5. Systematic safeguards against inappropriate or dangerous use of psychotropic medication must exist.
6. Suicide prevention programs must be established.

Shortly after the *Ruiz v. Estelle* case was filed, another Texas inmate filed suit alleging that inadequate medical care violated his Eighth Amendment rights against cruel and unusual punishment. In 1976, J. W. Gamble sustained an injury on his prison work assignment. Over the next 3 months, he was seen by several doctors to attend to this injury, although his requests were denied on occasion. Throughout this time, physicians failed to reach a consensus on the exact nature of Gamble's injury. Furthermore, he was disciplined more than once (i.e., placed in segregation) for refusing to work due to the severity of his pain.

The district court dismissed Gamble's claim; however, the U.S. Court of Appeals for the Fifth Circuit reversed that decision. In *Estelle v. Gamble* (1976), the U.S. Supreme Court reversed the decision of the court of appeals and held that the care

Gamble received, although inadequate, did not constitute cruel and unusual punishment (e.g., deliberate indifference or malicious infliction of pain). Despite that outcome, the case made clear that prison (and later jail) systems are prohibited from exhibiting "deliberate indifference" to the serious medical needs of inmates.

In *Brown v. Plata* (2011), a class action lawsuit was brought against the California Department of Corrections and Rehabilitation alleging that inadequate medical resources also violated the prisoners' Eighth Amendment rights. After years of unsuccessful efforts to remedy these deficiencies, federal judges eventually ruled that these violations were primarily due to overcrowding and ordered each facility to release enough prisoners to keep the inmate population within a certain percentage of its design capacity. The state appealed this decision, claiming that the mandated release violated the Prison Litigation Reform Act. The U.S. Supreme Court affirmed the lower court's decision and held that judicial interference was necessary in order to protect the Eighth Amendment rights of the prisoners.

Inmates with mental illness are also afforded some protections similar to civil psychiatric patients. The details leading up to the U.S. Supreme Court case of *Baxstrom v. Herold* (1966) are that Johnnie Baxstrom, while incarcerated, was found to have mental illness and was subsequently transferred to Dannemora State Hospital, a forensic psychiatric hospital in New York. His sentence expired while at Dannemora; however, the Department of Mental Hygiene believed he was too dangerous to be transferred to a civil hospital. State courts dismissed Baxstrom's writs of *habeas corpus*, and his requests for transfer to a civil facility were denied as being outside the court's authority.

The U.S. Supreme Court held that Baxstrom was denied equal protection because he was not afforded a jury review of his sanity (as afforded others who were civilly committed). Additionally, other individuals who were civilly committed to hospitals run by the Department of Corrections were committed only after judicial determination that they were too dangerous to be committed to a civil facility. Because Baxstrom's placement in Dannemora occurred at the behest of administrative officials, the Court determined that Baxstrom had been denied equal protection in this regard as well.

In addition to providing adequate medical and mental health services, jails and prisons are responsible for providing inmates with disability accommodations under the Americans With Disabilities Act (ADA; 1990a). In *United States v. Georgia* (2006), Tony Goodman, who required the use of a wheelchair, sued the state of Georgia, alleging that certain prison conditions (e.g., placement in a cell not wide enough for maneuvering his wheelchair, denial of access to classes and programs) violated his Title II rights (to be protected from discrimination on the basis of disability) under ADA. The state of Georgia claimed "sovereign immunity." The U.S. Supreme Court ruled that Title II supersedes Eleventh Amendment claims to sovereign immunity when violations of the Eighth Amendment are involved.

Imprisonment and Prison Culture

Although it was once generally accepted that incarceration adversely affects inmates' psychological functioning (Cohen and Taylor 1972; Mitford 1973), studies have demonstrated that inmates' mental health functioning can actually improve over the course of incarceration (Bonta and Gendreau 1995; Bukstel and Kilmann 1980; Harding and Zimmermann 1989; Hassan et al. 2011; Taylor et al. 2010; Walker et al. 2014; Zamble and Porporino 1990). In fact, although inmates typically experience anxiety and depression immediately following incarceration, these symptoms generally dissipate after a period of adjustment (MacKenzie and Goodstein 1985).

Thus, imprisonment is not necessarily psychologically harmful, and some system and individual factors, such as the correctional environment, presence of mental illness, and individual resilience, likely influence an offender's ability to adjust to his or her incarceration (Bukstel and Kilmann 1980; Gendreau and Bonta 1984; Gendreau and Thériault 2011). Offenders with mental illness are the exception, because the length of incarceration appears to be negatively associated with these individuals' mental health functioning (Bauer 2012).

Even if prisoners are able to adjust to prison, the effects of that adjustment (i.e., institutionalization) on inmate functioning after release are less clear. For example, gang membership may lead to a safer prison experience (i.e., adjustment) but may create or reinforce skills such as increased violence and prison misconduct that do not translate to community success (Gaes et al. 2001; Griffin and Hepburn 2006). Furthermore, exposing low-risk offenders to correctional interventions with moderate- to high-risk offenders essentially puts low-risk offenders at higher risk for reoffending (Latessa et al. 2010; Smith and Gendreau 2012). These findings led to the recommendation that interventions be tailored to an offender's level of risk. Avoiding the exposure of low-risk offenders to correctional interventions (including incarceration) with moderate- to high-risk offenders decreases the former's future criminal risk (Andrews and Bonta 2010).

The reliance on administrative segregation for disciplining and managing inmate behavior has potential adverse and harmful effects (Grassian 2006; Haney 2009; Kupers 2008). Opponents to the use of segregation suggest that segregation is harmful and can cause lasting emotional damage (Kupers 2008). Although some researchers had described a constellation of symptoms and mental health deficits alleged to result from long-term placement in segregated housing (Grassian 1983), many studies have failed to demonstrate significant adverse effects resulting from the use of administrative segregation (Bonta and Gendreau 1995; Gendreau and Bonta 1984; Suedfeld et al. 1982; Zinger et al. 2001). O'Keefe et al. (2013) report compelling findings from the most sophisticated segregation study to date. Contrary to the researchers' hypotheses, results indicated that administrative segregation confinement of 1 year was generally not associated with the onset of psychological symptoms or cognitive impairment for inmates with or without mental illness, and that inmates with mental illness did not fare worse in administrative segregation than their peers without mental illness. On the other hand, there was no evidence that inmates with serious mental illness (SMI) improved while in segregated housing. Small to moderate effects have been found across a variety of mental health and behavioral domains, suggesting that administrative segregation may not produce any more negative effects than those produced by incarceration more generally (Morgan et al. 2016).

The questions regarding potential harm caused by long-term segregated housing remain ripe for continued investigation, but such research is difficult to conduct. For example, ethics precludes random assignment of inmates to segregation. Few studies have adequately controlled for preexisting mental illness or allowed for a determination of the degree to which distress is caused by incarceration itself as opposed to segregation. Also, significant individual differences in how inmates respond to segregation are likely. Some inmates appear to have an extremely negative response to segregation, whereas others appear to prefer this form of incarceration for various reasons, including personal safety. Finally, the specific conditions of segregation (e.g., staff attitudes, cleanliness and noise of the environment, presence of individual television sets) vary widely across institutions, making it difficult to directly compare inmates' experiences in different facilities.

Increasingly, states have created secure treatment units for inmates with SMI who pose a serious risk of harm to others. In New York and Oregon, for example, these programs were voluntary or negotiated as settlements of class actions. In California, these units were created by court order. Although these programs differ across states, they tend to have a number of common characteristics, including significant increases in out-of-cell time and group therapy.

Some states, such as Michigan, have made significant changes in how segregated housing units are managed. For example, increasing prosocial stimulation and use of contingency management strategies to reinforce prosocial behavior have significantly reduced lengths of stay in segregation, resulting in reduced populations of segregated prisoners (C. Bauman, Warden, Alger Correctional Facility, personal communication, July 7, 2015). Finally, the National Commission on Correctional Health Care (2016) has issued a position statement indicating that prolonged solitary confinement (lasting longer than 15 consecutive days) is cruel, inhumane, and degrading treatment, as well as harmful to an individual's health.

Prisoner Rights

Right to Die

Although capital punishment has been a controversial legal issue, an inmate's right to die has been less frequently debated. Nevertheless, the right to die appears to be an increasingly common request, whether for inmates on death row (Schildkraut 2013) or those suffering from terminal illness (Stone et al. 2012). Questions regarding the right to die in prison remain to be settled, and court rulings on this subject for nonincarcerated populations will likely provide a foundation for future legal decisions regarding incarcerated individuals. As this chapter is being written, physician-assisted suicide is allowed in five states: California, Montana, Oregon, Vermont, and Washington (see Chapter 8, "Physician–Patient Relationship in Psychiatry").

Prison Rape Elimination Act

Rape is sufficiently prominent in popular media portrayals of life in prison (e.g., in the films *The Shawshank Redemption*, *American Me*, and *American History X*) that most individuals sentenced to prison have concerns about being sexually assaulted. In the United States, up to 30% of male inmates may be exposed to unwanted sexual contact (Mariner 2001), an unacceptable situation necessitating governmental intervention. As a result, the Prison Rape Elimination Act of 2003 was passed. This act was designed to "provide for the analysis of the incidence and effects of prison rape in Federal, State, and local institutions and to provide information, re-

sources, recommendations and funding to protect individuals from prison rape" (Prison Rape Elimination Act 2003).

A number of factors have been identified as increasing inmates' risk of sexual assault while incarcerated. These include prior sexual victimization, small stature or appearing physically weak, and identification as gay or transgender (Dumond 2003). Of particular concern is that inmates with a history of mental illness are particularly vulnerable. Prior treatment for any of a range of mental disorders (e.g., depression, anxiety, posttraumatic stress disorder, schizophrenia, bipolar disorder) has been associated with an increased likelihood of abusive sexual contact for both male and female inmates (Wolff et al. 2007).

Due Process Issues

Prisoners with SMI, whether held in jails or in prisons, are typically entitled to the same due process protections as other inmates and detainees, with some exceptions. These exceptions affect due process rights in two opposing directions. On one hand, SMI can result in abrogation of rights routinely granted to other prisoners. On the other hand, some due process rights are specifically afforded to prisoners with SMI and are not available to prisoners without mental illness.

Abrogated Rights

A fact that is seldom mentioned in legal or mental health literature is that having an SMI can dramatically limit a person's rights to a speedy trial, pretrial release (e.g., bail, bond, personal recognizance), and in some cases the right to file motions or agree to plea bargains. According to a study by Axelson and Wahl (1992), psychotic defendants remain in jail 6.5 times longer than other detainees, despite having fewer and less serious charges. Although this study is dated, few indications suggest that these results would be any different today, except perhaps in jurisdictions with mental health courts.

For example, defendants with SMI are often viewed as less likely to appear for court proceedings. Although this belief is unfounded (Council of State Governments 2015b), this criterion is often used by pretrial release agencies in denying pretrial release to people with SMI. Subsequent studies in Franklin County, Ohio (Council of State Governments 2015a), and New York City (Council of State Governments 2012) have confirmed that jail detainees and inmates remain in jail significantly longer if they have a serious mental disorder. Fortunately, efforts are currently under way by organizations such as the Council on State Government's Justice Center and the Arnold Foundation to improve pretrial release possibilities for defendants with SMI (Council of State Governments 2015b).

Ironically, prisoners' rights are especially likely to be affected when a defendant is found to be incompetent to stand trial. Although this finding stems from a defendant's rights to counsel and a fair trial, the consequences of a finding of incompetence often work very much to the defendant's disadvantage. For example, in many jurisdictions, defendants found incompetent to stand trial are precluded from filing pretrial motions. Most importantly, they are denied the ability to agree to a plea bargain, which in many cases, particularly those involving misdemeanors and low-level felonies, could result in sentences of "time served" that would have resulted in immediate release from custody. In addition, the trial process is stalled for the entire time that the defendant is held as incompetent. States may hold incompetent defendants in jail for months or even years, in spite of a court order requiring their transfer to a psychiatric hospital for treatment.

Rights Specific to Prisoners With Serious Mental Illness

Although a prisoner's rights to treatment may include access to inpatient care, inmates also have a right to refuse transfer to outside psychiatric hospitals absent certain requirements. In 1976, in *Meachum v. Fano* (1976), the U.S. Supreme Court ruled that inmates could be transferred from one institution to another without due process, deferring to the discretion of prison officials. However, *Vitek v. Jones* (1980) afforded inmates a right to administrative due process when the intended transfer was to a psychiatric hospital.

The *Vitek* decision has become less and less important over time, for several reasons. First, prisons throughout the United States have implemented routine classification committee hearings for transfers from prison to prison. These hearings typically meet a test for administrative due process. Second, inpatient beds are typically too few in number to accommodate all of the prisoners who might profit from inpatient treatment. In fact, the rights of prisoners are far more likely to be violated by the absence of inpatient psychiatric beds than by involuntary transfer to a hospital. Third, inmates who adamantly refuse inpatient transfers all too often end up in various forms of segregated housing, despite the fact that this form of housing is often countertherapeutic and unlikely to meet the inmate's clinical needs. Fourth, as discussed below, prisons now have other mechanisms by which they can involuntarily medicate some psychotic inmates, which reduces some institutional motivation for transfer to an inpatient hospital.

Prisoners also have rights to due process before they can be forced to take psychotropic medications on a nonemergency basis. However, these rights do not necessarily extend to judicial review. In *Wash-*

ington v. Harper (1990), the U.S. Supreme Court ruled that the due process clause allows states to involuntarily medicate an inmate with SMI, as long as the inmate is deemed dangerous to self or others and the medication is in the inmate's best medical interests. The decision to medicate over an inmate's objection does not require a judicial hearing, only an administrative due process hearing conducted by a special committee consisting of a psychiatrist, a psychologist, and a correctional official, none of whom may be currently involved in the inmate's diagnosis or treatment. Additionally, the inmate has the right to notice of the hearing; the right to attend, present evidence, and cross-examine witnesses; the right to representation by a disinterested lay adviser versed in the psychological issues; and the right to periodic review of any involuntary medication ordered.

Pretrial detainees can also be involuntarily medicated, even if they do not pose a risk to self or others. In *Sell v. United States* (1997), the U.S. Supreme Court opined that involuntarily medicating nondangerous, incompetent defendants could be an appropriate means of furthering the state's interest in bringing to trial those charged with serious crimes. However, the level of due process in such cases under *Sell* is significantly greater (i.e., judicial due process) than under a *Harper* analysis, which requires only administrative due process. Furthermore, *Sell* requires that the following conditions be met:

1. An important government issue must be at stake. Only a case-by-case inquiry can determine whether the government's interest is mitigated by the possibility of a long civil commitment for the treatment of the mental illness or by the fact that long periods of confinement have already been served, as this would be subtracted from any criminal sentence.

2. A substantial probability must exist that the medication will enable the defendant to become competent without substantial side effects that will interfere significantly with the defendant's ability to assist counsel in conducting a defense.

3. The medication must be medically appropriate and necessary to restore the defendant's competency, with no alternative, less intrusive procedures available that would produce the same results.

Other rights may also be due to prisoners with SMI under ADA (*Pennsylvania DOC v. Yeskey* 1998; **United States v. Georgia** 2006). Specifically, ADA requires that qualified individuals with disabilities, including prisoners, not be excluded from participation in or be denied the benefits of the services, programs, or activities of a public entity, or be subjected to discrimination by any public entity (Americans With Disabilities Act 1990b). Furthermore, among others mandates, ADA's Title II regulations also require correctional entities to administer services, programs, and activities in the most integrated setting appropriate to the needs of qualified prisoners with disabilities and to make reasonable modifications to policies, practices, and procedures when necessary to avoid discrimination on the basis of disability (Americans With Disabilities Act 1991; *Chisolm v. McManimon* 2001). Nevertheless, to date, the contours of ADA as applied to mental disabilities in prisons and jails have yet to be fully articulated by courts.

Conclusion

Correctional agencies have a clear constitutional duty to provide treatment for prisoners with SMIs and those in psychiatric crises, regardless of whether these illnesses and crises preexisted incarceration or were caused or exacerbated by incarceration. Additionally, statutory law prohibits discrimination against these prisoners and mandates accommodation of psychiatric disabilities. More importantly, public policy mandates adequate treatment of mental illness and psychiatric crises in jails and prisons. Although the Constitution establishes a "floor" for inmate rights, improving conditions in jails and prisons well beyond the constitutional minimum is good public policy.

Despite the increasing recognition and enforcement of prisoners' rights, correctional facilities have never been held to require a standard of care comparable to optimal care available in the community. The fact remains that jails and prisons are not particularly good places to treat SMI. Under the best of circumstances, jail and prison psychiatrists have extremely large caseloads, and creating a truly therapeutic environment in jails and prisons is extremely difficult. Unfortunately, these conditions, when untreated or undertreated, can interfere with an inmate's ability to profit from correctional programs, and in extreme cases can endanger inmates, detainees, officers, and eventually the community.

Key Concepts

- Prisons and jails have a constitutional duty to avoid being deliberately indifferent to serious medical and psychiatric problems.

- Correctional agencies have a clear constitutional duty to provide treatment for prisoners with serious mental illnesses (SMIs) and those in psychiatric crises.

- Treatment of SMI must not consist solely of psychotropic medication.

- Sexual assault is a significant problem in correctional facilities, particularly for vulnerable populations such as those with SMI.

- Inmates have a right to treatment, including both physical and mental health treatment.

- Research regarding the effects of segregation on the mental health of prisoners is inconclusive. Significant variance in the conditions of segregation contributes to the difficulty in drawing conclusions about the practice. More studies of the effects of long-term segregation are needed.

- In spite of their prisoner status, inmates share many rights with their nonincarcerated peers and have a right to safety and freedom from sexual assault while incarcerated.

References

Americans With Disabilities Act, 42 U.S.C. § 12101 (1990a)

Americans With Disabilities Act, 42 U.S.C. § 12132; 28 C.F.R. § 35.130(a) (1990b)

Americans With Disabilities Act, 28 C.F.R. §§ 35.130(b)(7), (d) (1991)

Andrews DA, Bonta J: The Psychology of Criminal Conduct, 5th Edition. Cincinnati, OH, Anderson, 2010

Axelson GL, Wahl OF: Psychotic versus nonpsychotic misdemeanants in a large county jail: an analysis of pretrial treatment by the legal system. Int J Law Psychiatry 15(4):379–386, 1992 1428421

Bauer R: Implications of long-term incarceration for persons with mental illness. Unpublished doctoral dissertation, Texas Tech University, Lubbock, TX, 2012

Baxstrom v Herold, 383 U.S. 107, 86 S.Ct. 760 (1966)

Bonta J, Gendreau P: Reexamining the cruel and unusual punishment of prison life. Law Hum Behav 14:347–372, 1990

Bonta J, Gendreau P: Reexamining the cruel and unusual punishment of prison life, in Long-Term Imprisonment: Policy, Science, and Correctional Practice. Edited by Flanagan TJ. Thousand Oaks, CA, Sage, 1995, pp 75–94

Brown v Plata, 563 U.S. 493, 134 S.Ct. 436 (2011)

Bukstel LH, Kilmann PR: Psychological effects of imprisonment on confined individuals. Psychol Bull 88(2):469–493, 1980 7422755

Chisolm v McManimon, 275 F.3d 315, 324–25 (3d Cir. 2001)

Cohen S, Taylor L: Psychological Survival: The Experience of Long-term Imprisonment. Harmondsworth, UK, Penguin, 1972

Council of State Governments: Improving outcomes for people with mental illnesses involved with New York City's criminal court and correction systems. December 2012. Available at: https://csgjusticecenter.org/mental-health/publications/improving-outcomes-for-people-with-mental-illnesses-involved-with-new-york-citys-criminal-court-and-correction-systems/. Accessed January 8, 2017.

Council of State Governments: Franklin County, Ohio: A county justice and behavioral health systems improvement project. 2015a. Available at: https://csgjusticecenter.org/mental-health/publications/franklin-county-ohio-a-county-justice-and-behavioral-health-systems-improvement-project/. Accessed January 8, 2017.

Council of State Governments: On the overvaluation of risk for people with mental illnesses. 2015b. Available at: https://csgjusticecenter.org/mental-health/publications/on-the-over-valuation-of-risk-for-people-with-mental-illnesses/. Accessed January 8, 2017.

Dumond RW: Confronting America's most ignored crime problem: the Prison Rape Elimination Act of 2003. J Am Acad Psychiatry Law 31(3):354–360, 2003 14584536

Dvoskin JA, Morgan RD: Correctional psychology, in Corsini Encyclopedia of Psychology, Vol 1. Edited by Weiner I, Craighead WE. New York, Wiley, 2010, pp 417–419

Estelle v Gamble, 429 U.S. 97, 97 S.Ct. 285 (1976)

Fagan TJ: Introduction, in Correctional Mental Health Handbook. Edited by Fagan T, Ax RK. Thousand Oaks, CA, Sage, 2003, pp xiii–xvi

Gaes G, Wallace S, Gilman E, et al: The influence of prison gang affiliation on violence and other prison misconduct. Washington, DC, Federal Bureau of Prisons, March 2001. Available at: https://searchworks.stanford.edu/view/8255626. Accessed January 8, 2017.

Gendreau P, Bonta J: Solitary confinement is not cruel and unusual punishment: people sometimes are. Can J Criminol 26:467–478, 1984

Gendreau P, Thériault Y: Bibliotherapy for cynics revisited: commentary on a one-year longitudinal study of the psychological effects of administrative segregation. Corrections and Mental Health: An Update of the National Institute of Corrections. 2011. Available at: http://www.nicic.gov. Accessed January 8, 2017.

Grassian S: Psychopathological effects of solitary confinement. Am J Psychiatry 140(11):1450–1454, 1983 6624990

Grassian S: Psychiatric effects of solitary confinement. Wash J Environ Law Policy 22:325–383, 2006

Griffin M, Hepburn J: The effect of gang affiliation on violent misconduct among inmates during the early years of confinement. Crim Justice Behav 33:419–466, 2006

Guerino P, Harrison PM, Sabol WJ: Prisoners in 2010. Bureau of Justice Statistics, 2011. Available at: https://www.bjs.gov/content/pub/pdf/p10.pdf. Accessed January 8, 2017.

Haney C: The social psychology of isolation: why solitary confinement is psychologically harmful. Prison Serv J 181:12–20, 2009

Harding T, Zimmermann E: Psychiatric symptoms, cognitive stress and vulnerability factors: a study in a remand prison. Br J Psychiatry 155:36–43, 1989 2605430

Hassan L, Birmingham L, Harty MA, et al: Prospective cohort study of mental health during imprisonment. Br J Psychiatry 198(1):37–42, 2011 21200075

Kupers T: What to do with the survivors? Coping with the long-term effects of isolated confinement. Crim Justice Behav 35:1005–1016, 2008

Latessa E, Lovins LB, Smith P: Final Report: Follow-up evaluation of Ohio's community based correctional facility and halfway house programs—Outcome study. Cincinnati, OH, Center for Criminal Justice Research, February 2010. Available at: https://www.uc.edu/ccjr/reports.html. Accessed January 8, 2017.

MacKenzie DL, Goodstein L: Long-term incarceration impacts and characteristics of long-term offenders: an empirical analysis. Crim Justice Behav 12:395–414, 1985

Mariner J: No Escape: Male Rape in U.S. Prisons. New York, Human Rights Watch, 2001

Meachum v Fano, 427 U.S. 215, 96 S.Ct. 2532 (1976)

Metzner JL: Class action litigation in correctional psychiatry. J Am Acad Psychiatry Law 30(1):19–29, discussion 30–32, 2002 11931366

Mitford J: Kind and Unusual Punishment. New York, Knopf, 1973

Morgan RD: Basic mental health services: services and issues, in Correctional Mental Health Handbook. Edited by Fagan T, Ax RK. Thousand Oaks, CA, Sage, 2003, pp 59–72

Morgan RD, Gendreau P, Smith P, et al: Quantitative syntheses of the effects of administrative segregation on inmates' well-being. Psychol Public Policy Law August 9, 2016 [Epub ahead of print]

National Commission on Correctional Health Care: Position statement on solitary confinement. 2016. Available at: http://www.ncchc.org/solitary-confinement. Accessed January 8, 2017.

O'Keefe ML, Klebe KJ, Metzner J, et al: A longitudinal study of administrative segregation. J Am Acad Psychiatry Law 41(1):49–60, 2013 23503176

Pennsylvania DOC v Yeskey, 524 U.S. 206, 118 S.Ct. 1952 (1998)

Prison Litigation Reform Act, 42 U.S.C. § 1997e (1996a)

Prison Litigation Reform Act. Appropriate remedies with respect to prison conditions. 18 U.S.C. § 3626(a)(1)(A) (1996b)

Prison Rape Elimination Act, P.L. 108–79 (2003)

Ruiz v Estelle, 679 F.2d 1115 (1982)

Sell v United States, 539 U.S. 166, 123 S.Ct. 2174 (1997)

Schildkraut J: An inmate's right to die: legal and ethical considerations in death row volunteering. Crim Justice Stud 26:139–150, 2013

Smith P, Gendreau P: Treatment programs in prison: prison adjustment, recidivism and the risk hypothesis. Unpublished manuscript, 2012

Stone K, Papadopoulos I, Kelly D: Establishing hospice care for prison populations: an integrative review assessing the UK and USA perspective. Palliat Med 26(8): 969–978, 2012 21993807

Suedfeld P, Ramirez C, Deaton J, et al: Reactions and attributes of prisoners in solitary confinement. Crim Justice Behav 9:303–340, 1982

Taylor PJ, Walker J, Dunn E, et al: Improving mental state in early imprisonment. Crim Behav Ment Health 20(3):215–231, 2010 20549784

United States v Georgia, 546 U.S. 151, 126 S.Ct. 877 (2006)

Vitek v Jones, 445 U.S. 480, 100 S.Ct. 1254 (1980)

Walker J, Illingworth C, Canning A, et al: Changes in mental state associated with prison environments: a systematic review. Acta Psychiatr Scand 129(6):427–436, 2014 24237622

Walmsley R: World Prison Population List, 10th Edition. Essex, UK, International Centre for Prison Studies, 2013. Available at: http://www.prisonstudies.org/research-publications?shs_term_node_tid_depth=27. Accessed January 8, 2017.

Washington v Harper, 494 U.S. 210, 110 S.Ct. 1028 (1990)

Wolff N, Shi J, Blitz CL, et al: Understanding sexual victimization inside prisons: factors that predict risk. Criminol Public Policy 6:535–564, 2007

Zamble E, Porporino F: Coping, imprisonment, and rehabilitation: some data and their implications. Crim Justice Behav 17:53–70, 1990

Zinger I, Wichmann C, Andrews DA: The psychological effects of 60 days in administrative segregation. Can J Criminol 43:47–83, 2001

CHAPTER 22

Psychiatric Treatment in Correctional Settings

Robert L. Trestman, Ph.D., M.D.
Jeffrey L. Metzner, M.D.
Kenneth L. Appelbaum, M.D.

Landmark Cases

Baxstrom v. Herold, 383 U.S. 107, 86 S.Ct. 760 (1966)

Estelle v. Gamble, 429 U.S. 97, 97 S.Ct. 285 (1976)

Vitek v. Jones, 445 U.S. 480, 100 S.Ct. 1254 (1980)

Washington v. Harper, 494 U.S. 210, 110 S.Ct. 1028 (1990)

Farmer v. Brennan, 511 U.S. 825, 114 S.Ct. 1970 (1994)

Brown v. Plata, 563 U.S. 493, 131 S.Ct. 1910 (2011)

Treatment of incarcerated individuals with mental illness or substance use disorders (SUDs) shares many characteristics with community-based care. However, given the unique and challenging circumstances of incarceration, treatment obligations, context, and management are substantially different from those in community settings. In addition, "transinstitutionalization" has resulted in ever-increasing numbers of individuals with mental illness being housed in correctional settings. As a result, psychiatrists are more likely to confront some of the issues associated with correctional care, even if they do not practice primarily in correctional settings.

Epidemiology

Although the United States comprises only 5% of the world's total population, the country holds 25% of the world's prisoners (Nagin 2014). One of every 110 U.S. adults is incarcerated at any given time (Glaze and Kaeble 2014) due to the increasing use of incarceration over the past several decades. The United States holds about 1.6 million people in its state and federal prisons (Carson 2015) and an additional 745,000 people in county jails (Minton and Zeng 2015).

The U.S. carceral population is about 90% male (Carson 2015). People from ethnic minorities are disproportionately incarcerated, representing a significant sociological issue. While African Americans constitute about 13% of the U.S. population, they make up 37% of prisoners and 35% of detainees (Carson 2015; Minton and Zeng 2015). The incarcerated are also aging. The number of U.S. prisoners age 65 or older expanded 94 times more rapidly than did the overall prison population between 2007 and 2012 (Human Rights Watch 2012). In 2011, about 8% of state and federal prisoners were age 55 or older (Carson and Sabol 2012).

Although definitions vary and epidemiological methodologies differ, the prevalence of mental illness among incarcerated individuals is unquestionably high. Approximately 15% of incarcerated men and 30% of incarcerated women have a serious mental illness (Fazel and Danesh 2002; Fazel and Seewald 2012; Prins 2014; Steadman et al. 2009; Trestman et al. 2007). One large review study (Fazel and Danesh 2002) found that rates of psychotic disorders among prisoners in 12 countries were 3.7% for males and 4.0% for females, and major depression was observed in 10% of male and 12% of female prisoners. Another large review in-

volving prisoners in 24 countries (Fazel and Seewald 2012) yielded estimated rates of psychotic disorders of 3.6% in men and 3.9% in women; estimated rates of depression were 10.2% in men and 14.1% in women. A U.S. study observed that the 12-month prevalence rate of major mental illness in female prisoners (31%) was twice that in male prisoners (14.5%) (Steadman et al. 2009).

A study of newly admitted U.S. detainees reported that 69.7% of prisoners (77% females vs. 69.4% males) met criteria for a lifetime SUD or other mental disorder (Trestman et al. 2007). Prevalence rates of SUDs are estimated to be between 50% and 70% (Fazel et al. 2006). Mental illness also carries a burden of functional impairment: 31% of newly admitted jail detainees with mental illness had demonstrably impaired physical functioning (Barry et al. 2014).

Screening, Referral, and Assessment

In *Ruiz v. Estelle* (1980), the U.S. Supreme Court established minimum requirements for prison-based mental health care; similar expectations exist in jail settings. These requirements emphasized the need for screening and evaluation to identify inmates needing mental health intervention or treatment. Jails and prisons typically have some form of mental illness and SUD screening, referral, and assessment processes. Screening instruments and processes should be brief and clear, have appropriate psychometric properties, and become part of the mental health record (Ford et al. 2007). Generally, the initial screening on admission to the facility should have a referral rate to a qualified mental health professional of 25%–33% (Maloney et al. 2015).

Evidence-based mental illness screening tools have been developed for jails and prisons (Martin et al. 2013). Two scales in use are the Brief Jail Mental Health Screen (Steadman et al. 2007) and the Correctional Mental Health Screen (Ford et al. 2009). Referrals for mental health assessment occur at intake or through subsequent self-referral or referral by custody staff, clinical staff, family members, lawyers, or others (American Psychiatric Association 2015). Referrals must be timely, be reviewed by a clinician, receive professional clinical judgment, and deliver the care that is ordered (National Commission on Correctional Health Care 2015). The assessment by a qualified mental health professional should follow clinically appropriate standards (Maloney et al. 2015).

Levels of Care

The community mental health model provides a useful guide for the required levels of correctional mental health care. A comprehensive correctional system includes outpatient treatment services, crisis intervention services, a residential treatment program (also known as a special needs program, intermediate care unit, etc.), and inpatient level of care (Metzner and Appelbaum 2015).

Outpatient services typically include clinics with a psychiatrist or psychiatric nurse practitioner for psychotropic medication management, access to time-limited mental health counseling or longer-term monitoring with assessments at least every 90 days, and limited access to group therapies. Individual counseling sessions in a jail are more likely to focus on initial adjustment issues and discharge planning. Prisons are more likely than jails to provide group therapy treatments due to longer lengths of stay and available resources.

Crisis intervention services generally consist of emergent or urgent assessments with interventions that may include transfer to a mental health crisis bed (usually in an infirmary with around-the-clock nursing), time-limited crisis-focused counseling or psychotherapy, referral to a psychiatrist for further assessment and/ or medication management, and other appropriate referrals (e.g., referral to a correctional officer regarding housing or property issues). Mental health crisis beds are commonly used for inmates who are at high risk for suicide or self-harming behaviors, are acutely psychotic, need a comprehensive diagnostic evaluation, and/or require a higher level of care than is available in their current housing unit. Crisis bed units, with an average length of stay between 4 and 10 days, are not designed to provide an inpatient psychiatric level of care.

Residential treatment programs (e.g., special needs units) are usually restricted to inmates with a serious mental illness who need more than an outpatient level of care but less than an inpatient hospitalization. Regardless of the custody level, each inmate in these units should be offered at least 10 hours per week of out-of-cell structured therapeutic activities in addition to at least another 10 hours of out-of-cell unstructured recreation. The out-of-cell structured therapeutic activities often use a psychosocial rehabilitation approach, emphasizing group activities and therapies to promote social skills (Metzner and Appelbaum 2015). Many inmates in these units, especially in higher-security settings, require nonemergency involuntary psychotropic medications to reduce symptom burden and to participate in psychosocial rehabilitation.

Psychiatric hospitalization is the most intensive level of care and the least accessible in correctional settings. Inpatient care is limited because of cost, bed availability, and security concerns. In practice, correctional systems, especially jails, commonly have limited or no access to inpatient psychiatric beds. Prison mental health systems may have memoranda of understanding with their state mental health authority to provide a limited number of forensic hospital beds. A smaller number of prison systems operate their own psychiatric hospital or contract with hospital systems to provide such care.

Regardless of the level of care, an individualized treatment plan should be developed in a timely fashion by the primary clinician and reviewed in a team setting with the patient wherever possible (American Psychiatric Association 2015; National Commission on Correctional Health Care 2015). A quality improvement process should be developed to monitor medication management, continuity of care, access to adequate office and programming space, and the adequacy of staffing. Adequate programming space is necessary to implement the various treatment services in a safe and confidential manner; adequate staffing facilitates continuity of care and meeting of treatment needs (Metzner and Dvoskin 2006).

Special Treatment Programs

Substance Use Disorder Programs

Incarceration provides an opportunity to treat inmates' SUDs. Unfortunately, although 56% of state prisoners met criteria for SUDs in the United States in the early 2000s, only 40% of them received treatment because of limited resources.

Furthermore, most programming is limited to educational models and self-help groups (Taxman et al. 2007). Only 10% of individuals with SUDs typically receive psychotherapeutic residential interventions (Belenko and Peugh 2005), and less than 1% receive medication-assisted treatment (Mumola and Karberg 2006). Expanded access to evidence-based SUD treatment, such as Aggression Replacement Training, which addresses anger management, social skill development, and moral reasoning (Goldstein et al. 1998), or Thinking for a Change, which incorporates cognitive restructuring, social skills, and problem solving (Lowenkamp et al. 2009), is needed.

Therapeutic communities, a very intensive SUD treatment model, were developed and implemented in community settings but are now also in use in correctional settings. Therapeutic communities generally require 6–12 months of residential treatment. A meta-analysis suggests that a therapeutic community increases success rate and duration (as measured by sustained abstinence following program completion and release into the community) but found that in-prison therapeutic communities are more effective when followed by community aftercare (Mitchell et al. 2007). Moreover, despite the substantial resource investment in creating and running a therapeutic community, these programs can result in a net benefit in prison management costs (Zhang et al. 2009).

Coordination Issues for Treatment Programs for Dually Diagnosed Inmates

Although recommended addiction treatments for patients with mental illness and SUD diagnoses are generally the same as for patients with uncomplicated SUDs, growing evidence suggests that treatment for dual diagnosis should combine medication and psychosocial interventions (Taxman 2015). Psychosocial interventions, including cognitive-behavioral therapy for dual diagnosis, need to be adapted to meet the level of functioning of the patients, incorporate criminal lifestyle issues, and address relapse. The optimal timing of treatments, whether sequential (one after the other), parallel (separately but contemporaneously), or integrated by a coordinated team (Mueser et al. 2003), remains an unresolved issue. Each approach has pragmatic limitations that influence local implementation. Limited data are currently available to definitively address this process issue (Taxman 2015).

Management of Inmates Who Self-Harm

The environmental and individual characteristics that lead to nonlethal self-injurious behavior in jails and prisons often differ from those in the community context. Inmates often have motives for self-harm that are unrelated to symptoms of a primary psychiatric disorder (Power et al. 2016). Self-injury can represent an expression of autonomy when few other options exist. It may also function as a coping mechanism or an attempt to get a desired object or outcome (e.g., medical response, relocation to another housing unit).

The highest rate of self-injurious behavior occurs in restricted, segregated, or punitive housing environments where inmates have little to do and little control over activity. One study of U.S. prisons found that about 2% of inmates engage in self-injurious behavior, and 70% of facilities reported multiple episodes each week requiring intervention (Appelbaum et al. 2011). Another study reported a similar 2.4% prevalence rate (Smith and Kaminski 2011).

Effective management of self-injurious behavior in jails and prisons requires cooperation between health care and custody staff, and effective intervention requires an understanding of underlying causes or factors. When a psychiatric disorder contributes to self-injurious behavior, the inmate should receive treatment appropriate to that disorder. Behavioral interventions may be elements of an individualized treatment plan or a behavioral management plan, or may occur during placement on a specialized residential treatment unit (Power et al. 2016). In effective management of self-injurious behavior in correctional institutions, reduction in the frequency or severity of self-injurious behavior (not necessarily cessation of the behavior) is a successful outcome, and reward generally works better than punishment to shape prosocial behavior.

Programs for Inmates With Developmental Disabilities

The management of inmates with developmental disabilities in correctional systems presents challenges, including the fact that such inmates are more vulnerable to exploitation and mistreatment by other inmates. Such vulnerabilities are extensive and range from theft of their property to extortion, assault, and rape (McDermott 2015). The goal of specialized programs for those with developmental disabilities is to provide training and skills enhancement targeted to specific individual and institutional needs. Unfortunately, little work has been done to develop evidence-based correctional programs for persons with developmental disabilities (Nøttestad and Linaker 2005).

Geriatric Inmates

Correctional institutions lack the infrastructure and staffing to meet the demands of geriatric care (Ahalt et al. 2013). Physiological aging is accelerated in the inmate population for many reasons (Human Rights Watch 2012), and individuals over age 50 in correctional settings are commonly referred to as elderly. Given the increasing and substantial population of elderly inmates across many countries (Maschi et al. 2013), specific attention to treatment is critical.

Typical correctional practices create risks for elderly inmates. Such risks derive from architectural and design issues, such as housing, sleeping in bunk beds, walking substantial distances for activities and meals, and the potential to be abused by younger more aggressive inmates (Stojkovic 2007). The United Nations has issued a series of recommendations for managing the incarcerated elderly (United Nations Office on Drugs and Crime 2009). The need for end-of-life care for older adults in prison is also receiving increased attention. Although at least 69 prison-based hospice programs exist in the United States (Hoffman and Dickinson 2011), the size, quality, and standards of such programs are inconsistent.

Suicide Prevention Programs

The rates of suicide in incarcerated populations are higher than in the community because of increased risk factors such as high rates of mental illness and substance abuse and the stressors inherent in incarceration. Successful implementation of suicide prevention programs has resulted in a decrease in the rates of suicide in both jails and prisons during the past 20 years (Hayes 2013). Nevertheless, suicide was the most common cause of death for jail inmates during 2012 (40 suicides per 100,000 inmates) and the fifth most common cause of death for prison

inmates (16 per 100,000 inmates) (Noonan 2014). Inmates in jail who are age 55 or older are more likely to commit suicide than other inmates; in prisons, age is not a distinguishing risk factor (Noonan 2014). Hanging is the most common method of carceral suicide (Hayes 2010). Fifty percent of suicides in jails occurred within the first 4 months of incarceration (Hayes 2012), whereas 65% of suicides in prisons occurred after the first year of incarceration (Mumola 2005). Common risk factors for suicide are presented in Table 22–1.

Key components of an adequate suicide prevention program are training, identification, referral, evaluation, housing and monitoring, communication, intervention, notification, review, and debriefing (Hayes 2013). All staff having direct contact with inmates should have annual, appropriate incarceration-specific training relevant to suicide prevention. A key identification opportunity occurs during the initial screening process, which should take place in a setting that facilitates sound confidentiality of the conversation while still allowing for visual oversight and security by custody staff.

The need for a suicide risk assessment may occur at any point during incarceration and is usually triggered by a referral to mental health services related to various stressors (e.g., receiving a "Dear John" letter, being sentenced) (Hughes and Metzner 2015). A formalized process for referral to mental health staff should be in place for timely evaluations of at-risk inmates. Mental health providers need to be trained in the use of acceptable suicide risk assessment instruments.

Inmates assessed as acutely suicidal require housing in a health care setting with placement in a suicide-resistant cell with appropriate observation and daily out-of-cell clinical interventions by staff (Hughes and Metzner 2015). An inmate's

---

TABLE 22–1. **Risk factors associated with suicide in correctional facilities**

Caucasian

Male gender

Charged with committing or convicted of a violent offense

History of mental illness and/or substance abuse

History of suicidal behavior

Single-cell housing (especially if in a lockdown setting)

---

clothing should be replaced with a suicide-resistant gown only when the inmate is engaging in self-destructive behavior. However, belts and shoelaces should be removed when an inmate is placed on suicide precautions. Clear communication among all involved staff is critical to assure appropriate observation and interaction. A targeted treatment plan should outline appropriate clinical interventions (Metzner and Appelbaum 2015).

Institutions need procedures that address notifications following a suicide, the subsequent review process (i.e., psychological autopsy and mortality review), and a debriefing process for staff and affected inmates. For optimum management, each correctional facility should have a suicide prevention committee that meets regularly and includes mental health, medical, and custody staff to review implementation of the suicide prevention plan's policies and procedures (Hughes and Metzner 2015).

Due Process Issues

Correctional clinicians and administrators need to know and comply with the standards for due process in their own jurisdictions. The Constitution sets a floor for, but not a ceiling on, liberty protections. States can provide procedural and substantive due process protections that exceed constitutionally mandated minimums but cannot fall below minimal standards set by the Constitution. For example, some state constitutions and laws require full judicial reviews for involuntary commitment or treatment of prisoners. However, a number of cases have challenged state practices on the basis of due process, claiming that state laws regarding treatment of prisoners with mental illness violate the Fourteenth Amendment.

Several U.S. Supreme Court cases address equal protection and due process rights of inmates. ***Baxstrom v. Herold*** (1966) involved a challenge to a New York statute governing civil commitment of inmates at the expiration of their penal sentences. All other civilly committed persons in the state were provided access to a jury review, but this statute did not provide inmates with the same access. The Court found that this disparate procedure denied equal protection to inmates who had completed their sentences and would otherwise be released. Thus, civil commitment of released inmates, with the exception of sex offenders (see Chapter 23, "Forensic Assessment of Sex Offenders"), requires the same judicial process as commitment of those who have not been previously incarcerated.

The case of ***Vitek v. Jones*** (1980) also involved the standard for involuntary commitment of an inmate to a mental hospital. In contrast to ***Baxstrom***, ***Vitek*** involved an inmate who still had time to serve in his prison sentence; the alternative to commitment in *Vitek* was remaining in prison, not being released into the community. Nevertheless, the Court found that involuntary transfer of a prisoner to a mental hospital implicates a liberty interest protected by the due process clause of the Fourteenth Amendment.

In the Court's view such transfers expose the inmate to additional stigmatization and to mandatory behavior modification as a treatment for mental illness. Although these deprivations of liberty require protection under the due process clause, they do not necessitate all of the protections afforded to other civilly committed individuals. The Court held that inmates have a right to written notice of the transfer, legal counsel, a hearing before an independent decision maker, written findings from that hearing, and effective and timely notification of these rights.

In *Washington v. Harper* (1990), the Court considered both substantive and procedural due process requirements for treating a prison inmate involuntarily with antipsychotic medications. The Court held that the state could involuntarily treat with antipsychotic medications a prison inmate who has a serious mental illness if the inmate is dangerous to self or others and the treatment is in the inmate's medical interest. Regarding the procedural protections, the Court held that the due process clause of the Fourteenth Amendment did not require a judicial hearing. In the Court's view, the inmate's interests could be "adequately protected, and perhaps better served, by allowing the decision to medicate to be made by medical professionals rather than a judge" (*Washington v. Harper* 1990, at 231).

In *Sandin v. Conner* (1995), the Supreme Court held that an inmate's confinement in disciplinary segregation did not require a separate hearing process.

Despite the *Sandin* decision, correctional systems have continued to provide a due process hearing to inmates who have been charged with a disciplinary infraction that could result in transfer to a disciplinary segregation housing unit or loss of privileges. Such hearings commonly involve one or more hearing officers who decide whether the prisoner is guilty or not guilty of the alleged misconduct following an administrative hearing in which the prisoner can present evidence in a rather informal manner.

Prisoners with mental illnesses are commonly overrepresented in disciplinary segregation units, especially in correctional systems that have inadequate mental health systems. As a result, legal remedies in response to class action suits have included developing policies and procedures that mandate mental health considerations in the disciplinary process for inmates demonstrating behaviors suggestive of a mental illness. A clinician who is not directly involved in the prisoner's treatment should provide this assessment to avoid compromising the therapeutic alliance. The mental health review should address whether mitigating factors related to the prisoner's mental illness existed at the time of the alleged misconduct (i.e., whether the prisoner's mental illness related to the behaviors that led to the rule infraction) and provide dispositional recommendations if the prisoner is found guilty of the alleged infraction. The goal of these assessments is to reduce the number of inmates with a mental illness in segregation units and/or limit the amount of time they are placed in such units.

Security Versus Treatment

Despite occasional conflicts, good institutional security and effective patient treatment support each other. Historically, mental health services were often seen as peripheral to the mission of correctional facilities and were expected to adapt to security practices even when those practices led to violations of basic clinical standards. Now, however, medical and mental health services are integral components of constitutionally acceptable correctional facilities. The legal obligation to provide timely and appropriate services has been reiterated in several Supreme Court decisions. For example, in *Estelle v. Gamble* (1976), the Court held that deliberate indifference to a prisoner's serious medical needs constitutes cruel and unusual punishment that contravenes the Eighth Amendment.

In *Farmer v. Brennan* (1994), the Supreme Court extended this principle to include deliberate indifference to an inmate's safety in a case involving the alleged beating and rape of a preoperative transsexual inmate by another inmate. Prior to *Farmer*, court decisions were inconsistent in regard to whether a finding of deliberate indifference required actual knowledge by an official of a danger to the inmate (i.e., a subjective test) or whether this finding could be based on an objective test of what the official "should have known." The Court held in *Farmer* that prison officials could be liable under the Eighth Amendment for denying an inmate humane conditions of confinement, but only if officials had had actual knowledge that inmates faced a substantial risk of serious harm and failed to take reasonable measures to abate that risk. Such humane conditions include adequate food, clothing, shelter, medical care, and safety. The Court also cautioned prison officials against using the subjective test to ignore dangers to inmates because a fact finder could conclude that a prison official knew of a substantial risk from the very fact that the risk was obvious.

Correctional mental health professionals' extreme deference to custody staff preferences has at times led to unjustified practices, such as routinely conducting clinical assessments and interventions at the cell fronts of inmates in segregation settings. Appropriate mental health care, however, requires a confidential setting, just as surgery requires a sterile field. Exigent circumstances may warrant exceptions to providing a confidential setting, but convenience or cost does not. Correctional facilities must provide adequate space, inmate movement, and security for mental health care to occur in confidential settings, just as facilities must provide an adequate supply of sterile equipment for nursing, medical, and dental procedures.

Abuse of controlled substances by inmates can pose significant problems because of the high rates of substance abuse in correctional populations and because of security concerns associated with diversion and misuse of the medications (Tamburello 2015). Even medications not typically considered substances of abuse, such as quetiapine, can develop nicknames associated with abuse (e.g., Susie Q) in the community and especially in prisons (Tamburello et al 2012). Existing guidelines (American Psychiatric Association 2015), however, do not support complete prohibitions of controlled substances for inmates who can benefit from them. Detailed prescribing protocols can help correctional settings to limit misuse of medications while ensuring access for inmates with legitimate needs (Appelbaum 2009; Tamburello et al 2012).

In *Brown v. Plata* (2011), the U.S. Supreme Court upheld a decision by a lower court empowered by the Prison Litigation Reform Act of 1996 that ordered reductions in the prison population within the California Department of Corrections and Rehabilitation (CDCR). The lower court had determined that a remedy for the unconstitutional state of medical and mental health care could not be achieved without reducing the excessive overcrowding within the CDCR. In other words, the U.S. Supreme Court determined that providing constitutionally adequate health care was not possible unless the overcrowding was reduced to a level that did not exceed 137.5% of the design capacity of the CDCR's prison facilities.

Use of Force

Prisoners with mental illness are commonly overrepresented in incidents involving a planned (i.e., nonemergent) use of force (Human Rights Watch 2015). Before implementing a planned use of force involving a prisoner with a mental illness or suspected mental illness, appropriately trained custody staff should try deescalation techniques and contact mental health staff for consultation and intervention. A cooling-off period (often lasting several hours) is frequently effective and may facilitate resolution of the inci-

dent without the use of force and allow the inmate or staff to "save face," depending on the events that led to the incident.

The use of force in a health care setting is particularly problematic if it involves the use of pepper spray or Tasers, because of the negative impact on the therapeutic milieu. All use-of-force incidents involving inmates with a mental illness or bizarre behaviors need a timely quality improvement review by a multidisciplinary team of medical, mental health, and custody leadership staff.

Conclusion

Understanding the framework, obligations, and context of mental health treatment in jails and prisons is critical for many forensic psychiatrists. The evolution of psychiatric care in correctional settings has been driven and shaped by litigation. The current status of correctional psychiatric treatment presents significant opportunities for improving the lives of incarcerated individuals with mental illness.

Key Concepts

- Suicide risk is elevated in jails and prisons.

- The prevalence of mental illness and substance use disorder is elevated in jails and prisons.

- Detainees and prisoners have constitutionally guaranteed rights to mental health care.

- Minimum standards for treatment access and treatment in jails and prisons have been developed as a result of litigation.

- Levels of mental health care in corrections follow a community model.

References

Ahalt C, Trestman RL, Rich JD, et al: Paying the price: the pressing need for quality, cost, and outcomes data to improve correctional health care for older prisoners. J Am Geriatr Soc 61(11):2013–2019, 2013 24219203

American Psychiatric Association: Psychiatric Services in Correctional Facilities. Arlington, VA, American Psychiatric Publishing, 2015, pp 29–32

Appelbaum KL: Attention deficit hyperactivity disorder in prison: a treatment protocol. J Am Acad Psychiatry Law 37(1):45–49, 2009 19297632

Appelbaum KL, Savageau JA, Trestman RL, et al: A national survey of self-injurious behavior in American prisons. Psychiatr Serv 62(3):285–290, 2011 21363900

Barry LC, Ford JD, Trestman RL: Comorbid mental illness and poor physical function among newly admitted inmates in Connecticut's jails. J Correct Health Care 20(2):135–144, 2014 24659760

Baxstrom v Herold, 383 U.S. 107, 86 S.Ct. 760 (1966)

Belenko S, Peugh J: Estimating drug treatment needs among state prison inmates. Drug Alcohol Depend 77(3):269–281, 2005 15734227

Brown v Plata, 563 U.S. 493, 131 S.Ct. 1910 (2011)

Carson EA: Prisoners in 2014 (Report No NCJ 248955). Washington, DC, U.S. Department of Justice, Bureau of Justice Statistics, 2015

Carson EA, Sabol WJ: Prisoners in 2011 (Report No NCJ 239808). Washington, DC, U.S. Department of Justice, Bureau of Justice Statistics, 2012

Estelle v Gamble, 429 U.S. 97, 97 S.Ct. 285 (1976)

Farmer v Brennan, 511 U.S. 825, 114 S.Ct. 1970 (1994)

Fazel S, Danesh J: Serious mental disorder in 23000 prisoners: a systematic review of 62 surveys. Lancet 359(9306):545–550, 2002 11867106

Fazel S, Seewald K: Severe mental illness in 33,588 prisoners worldwide: systematic review and meta-regression analysis. Br J Psychiatry 200(5):364–373, 2012 22550330

Fazel S, Bains P, Doll H: Substance abuse and dependence in prisoners: a systematic review. Addiction 101(2):181–191, 2006 16445547

Ford JD, Trestman RL, Wiesbrock V, et al: Development and validation of a brief mental health screening instrument for newly incarcerated adults. Assessment 14(3):279–299, 2007 17690384

Ford JD, Trestman RL, Wiesbrock VH, et al: Validation of a brief screening instrument for identifying psychiatric disorders among newly incarcerated adults. Psychiatr Serv 60(6):842–846, 2009 19487358

Glaze LE, Kaeble D: Correctional Populations in the United States, 2013 (Report No NCJ 248479). Washington, DC, U.S. Department of Justice, Bureau of Justice Statistics, 2014

Goldstein A, Glick B, Gibbs J: Aggression Replacement Training, Revised Edition. Champaign, IL, Research Press, 1998

Hayes LM: National Study of Jail Suicide: 20 Years Later (NIC Accession No 024308). Washington, DC, U.S. Department of Justice, National Institute of Corrections, 2010

Hayes LM: National study of jail suicide: 20 years later. J Correct Health Care 18(3):233–245, 2012 22569904

Hayes LM: Suicide prevention in correctional facilities: reflections and next steps. Int J Law Psychiatry 36(3–4):188–194, 2013 23664363

Hoffman HC, Dickinson GE: Characteristics of prison hospice programs in the United States. Am J Hosp Palliat Care 28(4):245–252, 2011 20834030

Hughes K, Metzner JL: Suicide risk management, in The Oxford Textbook of Correctional Psychiatry. Edited by Trestman R, Appelbaum K, Metzner J. New York, Oxford University Press, 2015, pp 237–244

Human Rights Watch: Old behind bars: the aging prison population in the United States, 2012. 2012. Available at: https://www.hrw.org/report/2012/01/27/old-behind-bars/aging-prison-population-united-states. Accessed January 9, 2017.

Human Rights Watch: Callous and cruel: use of force against inmates with mental disabilities in U.S. jails and prisons, 2015. Available at: https://www.hrw.org/report/2015/05/12/callous-and-cruel/use-force-against-inmates-mental-disabilities-us-jails-and. Accessed January 9, 2017.

Lowenkamp CT, Hubbard DJ, Makarios MD, Latessa EJ: A quasi-experimental evaluation of thinking for a change: a "real-world" application. Criminal Justice and Behavior 36(2):137–146, 2009

Maloney MP, Dvoskin J, Metzner JL: Mental health screening and brief assessments, in The Oxford Textbook of Correctional Psychiatry. Edited by Trestman R, Appelbaum K, Metzner J. New York, Oxford University Press, 2015, pp 57–61

Martin MS, Colman I, Simpson AI, et al: Mental health screening tools in correctional institutions: a systematic review. BMC Psychiatry 13:275, 2013 24168162

Maschi T, Viola D, Sun F: The high cost of the international aging prisoner crisis: well-being as the common denominator for action. Gerontologist 53(4):543–554, 2013 23042691

McDermott BE: Developmental disabilities, in The Oxford Textbook of Correctional Psychiatry. Edited by Trestman RL, Appelbaum KL, Metzner JL. New York, Oxford University Press, 2015, pp 299–304

Metzner JL, Appelbaum KL: Levels of care, in The Oxford Textbook of Correctional Psychiatry. Edited by Trestman RL, Appelbaum KL, Metzner JL. New York, Oxford University Press, 2015, pp 112–116

Metzner J, Dvoskin J: An overview of correctional psychiatry. Psychiatr Clin North Am 29(3):761–772, 2006 16904510

Minton TD, Zeng Z: Jail Inmates at Midyear 2014 (Report No NCJ 248955). Washington, DC, U.S. Department of Justice, Bureau of Justice Statistics, 2015

Mitchell O, Wilson D, MacKenzie D: Does incarceration-based drug treatment reduce recidivism? A meta-analytic synthesis of research. J Exp Criminol 3:353–375, 2007

Mueser KT, Noordsy DL, Drake RE, et al: Integrated Treatment for Dual Disorders: A Guide to Effective Practice. New York, Guilford, 2003

Mumola CJ: Suicide and Homicide in State Prisons and Local Jails (Report No NCJ 210036). Washington, DC, U.S. Department of Justice, Bureau of Justice Statistics, 2005

Mumola C, Karberg J: Drug Use and Dependence, State and Federal Prisoners, 2004 (Report No NCJ 213530). Washington, DC, U.S. Department of Justice, Bureau of Justice Statistics, 2006

Nagin DS: Reinventing sentencing in the United States. Criminol Public Policy 13:499–502, 2014

National Commission on Correctional Health Care: Standards for Mental Health Services in Correctional Facilities. Chicago, IL, National Commission on Correctional Health Care, 2015

Noonan M: Mortality in Local Jails and State Prisons, 2000–2012: Statistical Tables (Report No NCJ 247448). Washington, DC, U.S. Department of Justice, Bureau of Justice Statistics, 2014

Nøttestad JA, Linaker OM: People with intellectual disabilities sentenced to preventive supervision—mandatory care outside jails and institutions. J Policy Pract Intell Disabil 2:221–228, 2005

Power J, Smith HP, Trestman RL: "What to do with the cutters?"–Best practices for offender self-injurious behaviors. Crim Justice Stud 29:57–76, 2016

Prins SJ: Prevalence of mental illnesses in U.S. state prisons: a systematic review. Psychiatr Serv 65(7):862–872, 2014 24686574

Prison Litigation Reform Act, 42 U.S.C. § 1997e (1996)

Ruiz v Estelle, 503 F. Supp. 1265 (S.D. Tex. 1980)

Sandin v Conner, 515 US 472 (1995)

Smith HP, Kaminski RJ: Self-injurious behaviors in state prisons: findings from a national survey. Crim Justice Behav 38:26–41, 2011

Steadman HJ, Robbins PC, Islam T, et al: Revalidating the Brief Jail Mental Health Screen to increase accuracy for women. Psychiatr Serv 58(12):1598–1601, 2007 18048564

Steadman HJ, Osher FC, Robbins PC, et al: Prevalence of serious mental illness among jail inmates. Psychiatr Serv 60(6):761–765, 2009 19487344

Stojkovic S: Elderly prisoners: a growing and forgotten group within correctional systems vulnerable to elder abuse. J Elder Abuse Negl 19(3–4):97–117, 2007 18160383

Tamburello AC: Prescribed medication abuse, in The Oxford Textbook of Correctional Psychiatry. Edited by Trestman RL, Appelbaum KL, Metzner JL. New York, Oxford University Press, 2015, pp 165–172

Tamburello AC, Lieberman JA, Baum RM, et al: Successful removal of quetiapine from a correctional formulary. J Am Acad Psychiatry Law 40(4):502–508, 2012 23233472

Taxman FS: Dual diagnosis, in The Oxford Textbook of Correctional Psychiatry. Edited by Trestman RL, Appelbaum KL, Metzner JL. New York, Oxford University Press, 2015, pp 254–259

Taxman FS, Perdoni ML, Harrison LD: Drug treatment services for adult offenders: the state of the state. J Subst Abuse Treat 32(3):239–254, 2007 17383549

Trestman RL, Ford J, Zhang W, et al: Current and lifetime psychiatric illness among inmates not identified as acutely mentally ill at intake in Connecticut's jails. J Am Acad Psychiatry Law 35(4):490–500, 2007 18086741

United Nations Office on Drugs and Crime: Handbook for Prisoners With Special Needs. Vienna, Austria, United Nations Office on Drugs and Crime, 2009

Vitek v Jones, 445 U.S 480, 100 S.Ct. 1254 (1980)

Washington v Harper, 494 U.S. 210, 110 S.Ct. 1028 (1990)

Zhang SX, Roberts RE, McCollister KE: An economic analysis of the in-prison therapeutic community model on prison management costs. J Crim Justice 37:388–395, 2009

CHAPTER 23

Forensic Assessment of Sex Offenders

John Bradford, M.D., D.P.M., FRCPC
Giovana V. de Amorim Levin, M.D., FRCPC
Brad D. Booth, M.D., FRCPC
Michael C. Seto, Ph.D., C.Psych.

Landmark Cases

Specht v. Patterson, 386 U.S. 605, 87 S.Ct. 1209 (1967)

Allen v. Illinois, 478 U.S. 364, 106 S.Ct. 2988 (1986)

Kansas v. Hendricks, 521 U.S. 346,117 S.Ct. 2072 (1997)

Kansas v. Crane, 534 U.S. 407, 122 S.Ct. 867 (2002)

McKune v. Lile, 536 U.S. 24, 122 S.Ct. 2017 (2002) (AAPL only)

United States v. Comstock, 560 U.S. 126, 130 S.Ct. 1949 (2010)

Sexual offending is, unfortunately, a common occurrence. Although child sexual abuse is likely underreported, international rates range from 7% to 36% for girls and from 3% to 29% for boys (Finkelhor 1994; Stoltenborgh et al. 2011). Rates of rape and sexual assault are similarly high: in 2012 and 2013, over 1 in 1,000 persons in the United States over age 12 was sexually assaulted (Truman and Langton 2014).

Sexual offenses include noncontact offenses such as indecent exposure, being a peeping Tom, and possession of child pornography. They may also involve contact sexual crimes against children, sexual assault of adults, and sexual homicide. Although some sex offenders may have a variety of psychiatric diagnoses, including paraphilic disorders, some may not have a diagnosis.

The focus of this chapter is on the forensic assessment of sex offenders involved in sexually violent predator and dangerous offender proceedings, which can be extended in a simplified form to any other sex offender assessment. We discuss the legal background and basic issues involved and review specific key issues related to providing assessments of sex offenders for the courts, including standardized testing, the role of paraphilic disorders in offending, risk assessment, concerns regarding special populations, and the role of treatment in reducing and managing risk and recidivism.

Legal Background

Although one of the purposes of the legal system is to deter individuals from committing offenses, some individuals do not seem to respond to legal consequences for socially proscribed behavior. Repeat sex offenders appear to fall into this category. Despite repeated incarceration and attempts at treatment, some high-risk individuals continue to offend. Repeat sex offenders are "neither deterred nor changed by incarceration because their actions were driven by an uncontrollable impulse to commit their horrible crime" (Chenier 2003, p. 76).

Michigan, in 1937, was the first of many states to enact sexual psychopath laws to deal with these individuals. Minnesota, which followed suit in 1939, enacted the "psychopathic personality" law. This allowed the commitment of people with "emotional instability" or "lack of customary standards of good judgment" that rendered them irresponsible for conduct related to sexual matters and thereby dangerous (Minnesota Statute 26.10 1941).

Early sexual psychopath laws such as these were premised on the idea that deviant behavior was caused by illness and that repeat sex offenders could be treated and cured, allowing them to return to society safely (La Fond 1998). However, U.S. Supreme Court decisions did not support these statutes. For example, in *Specht v. Patterson* (1967), the Court unanimously held that the Fourteenth Amendment due process clause was violated when Mr. Specht was denied the rights to be present with counsel, to confront the evidence against him, to cross-examine witnesses, and to offer his own evidence and be heard. Early sexual psychopath laws were therefore, for the most part, repealed.

Despite the fate of these early laws, a second generation of "sexually violent predator" laws in the United States has evolved. These statutes allow indefinite civil commitment of individuals after they have served their prison sentences for committing multiple or particularly heinous sexual crimes. A series of landmark cases demonstrates that the courts consider the current sexually violent predator laws to be constitutional. These rulings also indicate that the role of psychiatric forensic assessment of sex offenders is likely to continue.

In *Allen v. Illinois* (1986), for example, Terry Allen was charged with unlawful restraint and deviant sexual assault. The state of Illinois filed a petition to have him declared a sexually dangerous person under the Illinois Dangerous Persons Act. Pursuant to the act, Mr. Allen was required to undergo two psychiatric examinations. Based in part on the psychiatrists' testimony, Mr. Allen was found to be a sexually dangerous person under the Illinois statute. Mr. Allen appealed, claiming his Fifth Amendment right against self-incrimination had been violated.

The U.S. Supreme Court, in a 5–4 decision, found that the Illinois Act's goal was to provide treatment, not punishment, for sexually dangerous persons. The Court ruled that forcing Mr. Allen to submit to psychiatric evaluation that could be used against him in a sexually dangerous person commitment hearing did not violate his Fifth Amendment right against self-incrimination. Because the law was civil in nature, and not criminal, the Fifth Amendment protections did not apply.

Similarly, Leroy Hendricks, diagnosed with pedophilia, was civilly committed under the Kansas Sexually Violent Predator (SVP) Act after his release from prison. This act states that persons who are likely to engage in "predatory acts of sexual violence" due to "mental abnormality" or "personality disorder" can be indefinitely confined. Mr. Hendricks appealed the validity of his commitment. In *Kansas v. Hendricks* (1997), the U.S. Supreme Court held that the Kansas SVP Act was constitutional and that the rather vague term "mental abnormality" used in the Kansas statute did not violate the right to substantive due process. The Court also ruled that Mr. Hendricks's civil commitment after serving most of his prison sentence did not violate double jeopardy because the Kansas SVP Act was civil in nature and not punitive.

In *Kansas v. Crane* (2002), the U.S. Supreme Court again upheld the Kansas SVP Act. Michael Crane, who had a history of exhibitionism and antisocial personality disorder, was adjudicated as a sexual predator under the Kansas SVP Act. The Kansas Supreme Court reversed this ruling, finding that these diagnoses did not of themselves constitute a "volitional impairment," as the act required. The U.S. Supreme Court held that mental illness and dangerousness were essential requirements for finding that a person met the Kansas SVP Act; however, a finding of total volitional impairment was not necessary. Nevertheless, the Court held that the Constitution required some proof of lack of control to distinguish a dangerous sexual predator's behavior from typical criminal recidivism.

In another Kansas case, *McKune v. Lile* (2002), the U.S. Supreme Court considered whether required admission of guilt to past sexual offenses as a prerequisite for participating in a sex offender program violated the Fifth Amendment right against compelled self-incrimination. Participation in the state's Sexual Abuse Treatment Program required that inmates fill out a form detailing their prior sexual activities, including illegal sexual conduct, regardless of whether the activities included uncharged criminal offenses. Inmates who refused to participate automatically had a reduction in prison privileges (canteen, television, visitation, etc.) and could be transferred to a maximum security unit. The Court ruled that the policy requiring disclosure of sexual crimes did not violate the Fifth Amendment because consequences for not participating in the program did not lengthen the sentence; it only altered conditions of confinement.

The U.S. Supreme Court addressed similar issues in federal law in *United States v. Comstock* (2010). The Adam Walsh Child Protection and Safety Act of 2006 authorizes the federal government to order civil commitment of sexually dangerous persons who are already in the custody of the Federal Bureau of Prisons but who are coming to the end of their sentences. In *Comstock*, federally convicted sex offenders in North Carolina moved to dismiss petitions requesting their indefinite civil commitment. The Supreme Court held that federal law allowed Congress the constitutional authority to enact this legislation and to pursue civil commitment of federally convicted sex offenders on the basis of "sexual dangerousness."

Basic Issues in the Forensic Assessment of Sex Offenders

Preparation for the Psychiatric Interview

The psychiatrist may be called on by the defense or prosecution or appointed by the court to evaluate individuals charged with sexual offenses. As in any forensic evaluation, assessors should initially clarify the nature of the legal question and the relevant statutory or case law. The forensic evaluator should be familiar with definitions of *mental condition* and *reduced capacity to resist* and other pertinent terminology.

Forensic psychiatrists must be appropriately qualified for and experienced in conducting these specialized evaluations. Qualifications for conducting sexually violent predator or dangerous offender evaluations usually include completion of a fellowship in forensic psychiatry with participation in and supervised completion of this type of assessment. Psychiatrists should also be familiar with the literature and current methods used within the field to conduct evaluations, including the limitations of diagnostic and predictive measures.

The qualified evaluator should obtain and review *all* available information prior to meeting with the evaluee. Sources of information include official details of current and previous offenses, institutional records, transcripts from court proceedings, collateral information, mental health and treatment records, school records, and other information that might be available. Often, lawyers will attempt to send only partial records, which can adversely affect the accuracy of the assessment. Experienced evaluators would notice whether the documentation was incomplete. If this is the case, a precondition of completing the assessment would be the full disclosure of all relevant documentation.

In addition, individuals who have known the evaluee, such as family members, should be contacted when possible to gain insight about lifelong patterns of behavior. The psychiatrist should bear in mind that some of these individuals may be advocating on behalf of the person being evaluated rather than providing accurate reports.

Prior to starting the evaluation, the psychiatrist should obtain the evaluee's informed consent and warn the evaluee about the limitations of confidentiality of the assessment (e.g., whether defense assessments are discoverable). Routine information imparted to the evaluee includes the fact that the psychiatrist will be completing an independent assessment that may be harmful, neutral, or helpful to the person's legal case and that the information disclosed should not be considered confidential.

The Psychiatric Interview

The interview should include enough details to allow completion of the Hare Psychopathy Checklist—Revised (PCL-R; Hare 2003), which should be part of any sexually violent predator or dangerous offender assessment if possible. This instrument is particularly helpful because of the importance of psychopathy in considering risk of reoffending and potential response to treatment (Barbaree 2005; Bradford et al. 2008; Langton et al. 2006). The evaluee's history should include a review of early childhood issues, sexual and physical abuse history, academic history that encompasses behavioral problems, relationship history, occupational history, substance use history, financial history, and medical history.

The evaluee's legal history should also be considered in detail. Each previous and current offense should be reviewed with the evaluee. Evaluees not uncommonly disagree with parts of the "official version" of their offense history, often minimizing the seriousness of the offenses. Nevertheless, glaring differences should be explored. Additionally, psychiatric evaluators should be certain to review a complete sexual history with the evaluee. This should include discussion of sexual outlets and frequency of sexual outlets, evidence of "hypersexuality" (Bradford 2001; Kafka 2001; Långström and Hanson 2006), and an exploration of paraphilic interests.

Clarifying the evaluee's motivations for offending and the potential role of substance use is important. Evaluators should also assess for the presence of mental illness and consider how this might affect the evaluee's risk to the community or management needs. Although often overlooked, rates of severe mental illness among sex offenders can be substantial (Table 23–1).

The offender's institutional behavior should also be reviewed, including misconduct or offenses committed while incarcerated. Evaluators should be certain to explore whether evaluees have previously been under supervision, whether they were compliant with expectations, and whether they were successfully supervised without reoffending.

The details of treatment obtained by the offender for mental illness, sexual offending, substance abuse, and anger management problems should be reviewed. Discussion should include who provided the treatment, what specifically the treatment involved, whether the treatment led to improvements, and whether the offender is willing to pursue further treatment. This information can be important for assessing the offender's risk and mak-

ing recommendations about what strategies may assist in safely managing the person in the community. For example, arguments that the person's risk cannot be reduced to a manageable level for the community are difficult to support if the offender has never received an evidence-based treatment.

Specific Issues in the Forensic Assessment of Sex Offenders

Psychological Testing

"Deviant" sexual arousal is an important factor in sex offender risk assessment. If individuals are aroused by children, their risk of offending against a child is higher than if they are not aroused by children (Hanson and Bussière 1998; Hanson and Morton-Bourgon 2005). Deviant sexual arousal to nonsexual violence and sexual violence (sexual sadism) has been documented, and if present this significantly increases the risk of future sexual violence (Hanson and Morton-Bourgon 2005). The Sex Offender Risk Appraisal Guide includes deviant sexual arousal as a predictor of future recidivism; the results of this assessment have face validity (Quinsey et al. 2015).

Measuring sexual preference is primarily accomplished by one of two methods. The first is *penile plethysmography* (PPG), also known as *penile tumescence testing* or *phallometric testing*. This procedure involves measuring arousal circumferential changes in the penis while the evaluee is exposed to visual or auditory stimuli of children or nonconsensual sexual situations. PPG testing has been adapted to assist in the diagnosis of pedophilia (Blanchard et al. 2001; Freund and Blanchard 1989; Looman and Mar-

TABLE 23–1.   Rates of severe mental illness among sex offenders

Disorder	Dunsieth et al. (2004)	Kafka and Hennen (2002)	Booth (2010)
Mood disorder	58%	72%	56%
Anxiety disorder	23%	38%	28%
Alcohol or substance abuse issues	85%	41%	55%
Personality disorder	56%	—	47%
Psychotic disorder	—	4%	16%
Paraphilic disorder	74%	100%	65%
Impulse-control disorder or ADHD	38%	36%	20%
Mental retardation or developmental delay	—	—	31%
Dementia	—	—	10%

Note. ADHD=attention-deficit/hyperactivity disorder.

shall 2001) with some success. Similarly, the method has been used to assist in the evaluation of rapists.

The literature on PPG is extensive and highlights several controversies. Clinicians using this technique must be aware of this literature to be able to assist the court appropriately. For example, some nonoffenders and some nonparaphilic men will have significant arousal to rape and pedophilic stimuli. Similarly, nonresponse is not uncommon and may incorrectly suggest that the individual does not experience deviant arousal. Thus, caution should be used when administering testing prior to a conviction because PPG may inappropriately bias the criminal proceedings.

Evaluators should be familiar with the sensitivity and specificity of the PPG. The literature on PPG indicates potentially troubling issues with cost, availability, faking, instrumentation differences, nonstandard stimuli, the use of low-level arousal to determine sexual preference, and psychometric properties (Lalumière and Harris 1998; Lalumière et al. 2005; Marshall and Fernandez 2003; Seto 2008; Seto et al. 2008). Despite these limitations, PPG allows for objective assessment of arousal and is recommended, when available, for evaluating deviant sexual arousal and therefore the risk to sexually reoffend.

In some jurisdictions, evaluators using PPG will not be able to use visual stimuli depicting children in sexual situations as a result of federal or state child pornography laws. An alternative option is to conduct testing with audio stimuli of stories describing sex with children.

Although conducting PPG testing as part of a sex offender evaluation is the preferred method, many clinicians will not have access to PPG testing. When PPG is not available, *visual reaction time* (Abel et al. 1998) may provide valuable information regarding risk (Gray et al. 2015). This procedure is based on the premise that individuals will look at stimuli they find arousing for a much shorter or longer time than nonarousing stimuli. In the test, individuals look at a series of clothed individuals of various ages, genders, and ethnicity. They also self-rate their interest in these images and complete a set of questionnaires. Visual reaction time results have reliability similar to that of PPG (Abel et al. 1998). In addition, this testing does not use nude photos of children, making it preferable in some circumstances. Visual reaction time measures are also faster and easier to administer, although evaluators cannot score the results themselves and the test must be administered and interpreted by trained evaluators.

Sexual preference testing is always recommended in evaluations of sex offenders; however, test results do not provide the evaluator with sufficient information to understand the individual's offending and risk to the community. Clinicians may need to access additional testing to address clinical issues that may be relevant to this determination. For example, IQ testing may be appropriate for individuals with developmental delay. Neuropsychological testing may be helpful for individuals with a history of stroke or traumatic brain injury. Tests for malingering or personality disorder may be administered. Scales and continuous performance testing may identify attention-deficit/hyperactivity disorder.

Paraphilic Disorders and Sexual Offending

The link between paraphilic disorders and sexual offending is both intuitive and empirical (Laws and O'Donohue 2008). Paraphilic disorders predispose some individuals to committing certain sexual offenses. However, paraphilic disorders are not necessary or sufficient factors, because nonparaphilic individuals sometimes commit sexual offenses and because not all paraphilic individuals commit sexual offenses.

The link between paraphilic disorders and sexual offending can be misleading. Some laypeople (and clinicians) assume that a person who has molested a child must be a pedophile and that all pedophiles will molest children. Some pedophiles, however, have never had any known sexual contact with children, and a substantial proportion of child molesters would not meet diagnostic criteria for pedophilic disorder (Seto 2008; Seto et al. 2008).

Nonetheless, paraphilic disorders represent an important motivation for sexual offending. Pedophilic disorder is linked with child pornography and sexual offending against children, sexual sadism disorder is linked with rape, exhibitionistic disorder is associated with indecent exposure, voyeuristic disorder is associated with trespassing and related crimes, and so on. In some cases, fetishistic disorder is associated with ostensibly nonsexual crimes (e.g., someone with an underwear fetish who breaks into women's residences to obtain more underwear).

Identified sex offenders not uncommonly have more than one paraphilic disorder. In fact, having a paraphilic disorder significantly increases the likelihood of having another paraphilic disorder (Abel et al. 1988; Bradford et al. 1992; Freund et al. 1997). This may reflect common vulnerabilities in the etiology of paraphilic disorders, such as prenatal insults and childhood head injury.

The belief that reoffending sex offenders tended to commit only the same type of offenses is now known to be false. Some offenders with a history of sexual offenses against children might subsequently commit a sexual offense against an adult, and vice versa. Similarly, offenders with a history of sexual offenses against girls between ages 10 and 13 years might subsequently offend against younger or older girls or boys (English et al. 2000; Heil et al. 2003). Evidence suggests that "crossover" offenders engage in more high-risk behaviors and are more likely to reoffend. Therefore, risk management for this group cannot be as focused as it might be for "noncrossover" offenders. For example, a probation or parole officer cannot decrease risk of reoffending for a crossover offender simply by prohibiting unsupervised contact with children if the individual has some risk of offending against adults as well (Abel et al. 1988; Bradford et al. 1992).

Risk Assessment

Forensic psychiatrists and other professionals who assess sex offenders should appraise the risk posed for future offenses. Accurate knowledge about an offender's risk informs legal decision making and assists in decision making about security level, treatment intensity, and the identification of potential targets for supervision. Meaningful variation exists in the risk for reoffending posed by sex offenders (Hanson and Bussière 1998). Most sex offenders do not fall into a high-risk category, and those who do can be identified for more intensive intervention and treatment, more secure detention, and enhanced supervision when released.

Current models of sexual offending suggest two major dimensions of risk of reoffending. The first is often labeled *sexual deviance* and encompasses paraphilic disorders, sexual preoccupation, and a preference for impersonal sex. The second is often labeled *antisocial tendencies* and encompasses personality traits, negative attitudes and beliefs, negative associations, and unstable lifestyles that increase the likelihood of antisocial and criminal behavior (Hanson and Morton-Bourgon 2005; Lalumière et al. 2005; Seto 2008). Sexual deviance "drives" sexual offending, whereas antisocial tendencies represent the lack of inhibition or control over the motivation to sexually offend (Pullman et al. 2016). Examples of variables representing the two major risk dimensions are provided in Table 23–2.

Sex offenders with high scores on measures of antisocial tendencies are at greater risk of committing either nonsexual or sexual offenses in the future. Sex offenders whose scores are high on measures of deviant sexual interests are at greater risk of committing sexual offenses

in the future. Offenders whose scores are high in both dimensions are at particularly high risk to reoffend.

Traditionally, decisions about risk of reoffending were made on the basis of unstructured clinical judgment. This approach has been highly criticized as incorrectly overestimating risk (Quinsey et al. 2015). Current evidence-based practice supports the use of actuarial measures or structured professional guides to assess sex offender risk (see Chapter 28, "Violence Risk Assessment"). Actuarial measures are composed of mathematically identified static (nonchangeable) risk factors that help to predict the outcome of interest. Although such measures are helpful, they cannot account for evaluee-specific factors (e.g., disinhibition from dementia causing an offense) and changes in the evaluee (e.g., successful treatment). Structured clinical guides comprise lists of empirically or theoretically identified risk factors and often include dynamic (changeable) factors. They do not, however, provide probabilistic estimates of the likelihood of recidivism.

Professional guidelines and case law support the use of actuarial measures or structured professional guides in sex offender risk assessment. Evaluators should be aware of the benefits and limitations of the methods they choose and be able to explain these to the court. Moreover, evaluators should be aware of whether courts have accepted the method as valid under *Frye v. United States* (1923) or *Daubert v. Merrell Dow Pharmaceuticals* (1993) (see Chapters 1, "The Expert Witness," and 2, "Introduction to the Legal System").

Some risk assessment measures have undergone multiple, independent validation studies examining their predictive accuracy with regard to sexual recidivism (Hanson 2002; Hanson and Mor-

TABLE 23–2. **Variables indicating antisocial tendencies or sexual deviance, the two major risk dimensions identified in sex offender follow-up research**

Antisocial tendencies	Sexual deviance
Psychopathy	Phallometrically assessed sexual arousal by children or coercive sex
Antisocial personality disorder	
Childhood behavior problems	Self-reported interests in paraphilic activities or targets
Criminal history	
Substance abuse	Early sexual behavior problems
Antisocial attitudes, beliefs, and values	Sexual offense history
Associations with criminal peers	Sexual victim age and gender

ton-Bourgon 2005). Reviews of these validation studies indicate that actuarial measures produced the highest accuracies, followed by structured professional guides and then unstructured judgments (Hanson 2002; Hanson and Morton-Bourgon 2009; Kingston et al. 2008). The Static-99R (Harris et al. 2003), an actuarial measure, has undergone many successful cross-validations in both forensic mental health and correctional settings. The Sexual Violence Risk–20 (Quinsey et al. 2015), a structured professional guide, has also undergone cross-validation, though not to the same extent as the Static-99R. The Sex Offender Risk Appraisal Guide (Hart and Boer 2010) has demonstrated good validity for predicting violent recidivism by sex offenders, an outcome measure that includes nonsexually violent and contact sexual offenses.

Special Populations

When performing forensic assessment of sex offenders, the clinician should be aware of the current literature regarding any special categories of offenders (Seto and Eke 2005, 2015; Seto et al. 2006). A growing literature is available on these special populations, including sex offenders with mental disorders (Booth 2010) or developmental delays (Harris and Tough 2004; Riches et al. 2006), as

well as elderly sex offenders (Fazel et al. 2002; Hanson 2002). Also, Internet offenders are increasingly being sent for forensic psychiatric evaluation.

Recidivism and Treatment

Completing sex offender assessments requires a fundamental knowledge of sex offender recidivism. Studies of recidivism provide important information that complements the formal risk assessment, because they provide the background on how the risk assessment instruments have been developed and studied. Courts often appreciate "base-rate" formulations—that is, information about how many sex offenders overall will recidivate and whether the evaluee is at a higher or lower risk when compared with the base rate.

Differences in the base rates of recidivism among different types of sex offenders are well established. For example, sex offenders against adult females ("rapists"), extrafamilial child molesters, and incest perpetrators—the usual categories studied—have different rates of recidivism (American Psychiatric Association 1999). In general terms, rapists have the highest rates of recidivism, followed by extrafamilial child molesters, and incest perpetrators have the lowest rates. The strongest predictors of sexual offense recidivism relate to variables associated with sexual deviance and, in particular, deviant sexual arousal, followed by variables associated with antisocial tendencies such as antisocial personality disorder (Furby et al. 1989; Hanson and Bussière 1998).

Studies have also found a significant relationship between increasing age and a reduced risk of sexual offense recidivism. The risk of recidivism tended to approach 0% in individuals at age 60 years (Hanson et al. 2002). In addition, studies have indicated that a mental disorder diagnosis was not predictive of recidivism either alone or in multivariate categories, although comorbid substance use disorders and personality disorders showed some predictive validity (Kingston et al. 2015).

Base recidivism rate studies generally focus on untreated individuals. However, assessments of risk must include evaluations of whether the individual has received appropriate trials of evidence-based treatments, including psychotherapy and medications. Evaluators should be familiar with the literature regarding the effectiveness of treatments, the relationship to risk, and the treatments that might be available or have been tried for sex offenders.

Psychological and pharmacological treatment is believed to reduce the recidivism rate (Alexander 1999; Hanson et al. 2002). Nevertheless, some controversy and disagreement continue among experts about the effectiveness of treatment outcome for sex offenders (Seto et al. 2008). A combination of cognitive-behavioral and hormonal treatments is the most promising of available treatments (Losel and Schmucker 2005; Schmucker 2015). Treatment programs using a cognitive-behavioral approach, as well as those using a defined systemic approach, were also associated with re-

ductions in sexual recidivism and general recidivism (Hanson et al. 2002).

Some evidence indicates that deviant sexual arousal can be reduced by pharmacological treatment (Thibaut et al. 2010). This treatment involves the use of agents to reduce sex drive, which is specifically associated with a reduction in sexual fantasies, sexual urges, and behavior that includes deviant sexual behavior. Pharmacological treatment has also been shown to have effects on recidivism similar to the effects found in surgical castration studies (American Psychiatric Association 1999).

Pharmacological treatment of sex offenders commonly involves one of three types of agents: selective serotonin reuptake inhibitors (SSRIs), hormonal agents, or antiandrogens. SSRIs act through the increase in central serotonin levels, whereas hormonal agents and antiandrogens reduce available testosterone (Thibaut et al. 2010). The hormonal agents in common usage are medroxyprogesterone acetate and various luteinizing hormone–releasing hormone agonists, such as leuprolide acetate (Bradford 2000). Luteinizing hormone–releasing hormone agonists produce a pharmacological castration state, with the plasma testosterone levels falling to castration levels (Bradford 2000; Thibaut et al. 2010). Cyproterone acetate, widely used in Canada and Europe but unavailable in the United States, blocks the intracellular androgen receptors throughout the body.

Bradford (2000, 2001) proposed an algorithm for the pharmacological treatment of sex offenders based on a paraphilia severity model taken from the *Diagnostic and Statistical Manual of Mental Disorders*, 3rd Edition, Revised (DSM-III-R; American Psychiatric Association 1987). The algorithm advocates the use

TABLE 23–3. **World Federation of Societies of Biological Psychiatry: algorithm for treatment of paraphilias in adult males**

Level	Indications	Treatment
1	"Hands-off" paraphilias, low risk of sexual violence	Cognitive-behavioral therapy
2	"Hands-off" paraphilias, low risk of sexual violence No satisfactory results at Level 1	Selective serotonin reuptake inhibitors (SSRIs)
3	"Hands-on" paraphilias but without penetration Paraphilic sexual fantasies without sexual sadism No satisfactory results at Level 2	SSRIs combined with low-dose oral antiandrogen, such as cyproterone acetate

4	Moderate and high risk of sexual violence, i.e.,
	   Severe paraphilias with more intrusive fondling
	   No sexual sadism fantasies and/or behavior
	No satisfactory results at Level 3
		Full-dose oral antiandrogen, such as cyproterone acetate, with or without SSRIs

5	High risk of sexual violence and severe paraphilic disorders Sexual sadism fantasies and/or behavior or physical violence No compliance or no satisfactory results at Level 4	Long-acting luteinizing hormone–releasing hormone agonists such as leuprolide acetate or triptorelin, with or without cyproterone acetate
6	Most severe paraphilic disorders No satisfactory results at Level 5	Full pharmacological castration, with or without SSRIs

Source. Thibaut et al. 2010

of psychological treatment as the first level of treatment for all sex offenders, regardless of severity of paraphilic disorders. It proceeds through various levels of pharmacological treatment, leading ultimately to pharmacological castration for catastrophic severity and some severe categories of paraphilic disorders. In 2010, the World Federation of Societies of Biological Psychiatry (WFSBP) established evidence-based guidelines for the pharmacological/biological treatment of the paraphilic disorders in adult males (Thibaut et al. 2010). The WFSBP has also recommended an algorithm for treatment of adolescent sex offenders (Thibaut et al. 2016) (Table 23–3).

Conclusion

Evaluation of sex offenders requires specialized training and expertise. Evaluators should be able to demonstrate that their opinions are based on an understanding of principles of risk assessment, sex offender recidivism, and the potential effects of treatment. They should also understand the strengths and limitations of the assessment tools and available treatments.

The assessment of sex offenders includes consideration of psychiatric diagnoses and the role of paraphilic interests. Risk assessment should include the Hare Psychopathy Checklist—Revised and actuarial or structured risk assessment, as well as an evaluation of the treatments provided in the past to the offender and a review of any supervision failures that have occurred.

Key Concepts

- Psychiatrists conducting sex offender evaluations should be familiar with relevant legal definitions and standards in their jurisdictions.

- Psychiatric evaluations of sex offenders may be used for legal and treatment purposes, including assessing risks of reoffending.

- Not all sex offenders are at increased risk of reoffending; assessments of potential recidivism should be made on a case-by-case basis.

- Risk assessments should include dynamic and static factors associated with recidivism and the limitations of the instruments used.

- Psychological and biological treatments can be effective in reducing risk of recidivism.

References

Abel GG, Becker JV, Cunningham-Rathner J, et al: Multiple paraphilic diagnoses among sex offenders. Bull Am Acad Psychiatry Law 16(2):153–168, 1988 3395701

Abel GG, Huffman J, Warberg B, et al: Visual reaction time and plethysmography as measures of sexual interest in child molesters. Sex Abuse 10:81–95, 1998

Adam Walsh Child Protection and Safety Act, Public Law 109-248, 2006

Alexander MA: Sexual offender treatment efficacy revisited. Sex Abuse 11(2):101–116, 1999 10335563

Allen v Illinois, 478 U.S. 364, 106 S.Ct. 2988 (1986)

American Psychiatric Association: Diagnostic and Statistical Manual of Mental Disorders, 3rd Edition, Revised. Washington, DC, American Psychiatric Association, 1987

American Psychiatric Association: Task Force on Sexually Dangerous Offenders: Dangerous Sex Offenders: A Task Force Report of the American Psychiatric Association. Washington, DC, American Psychiatric Association, 1999

Barbaree HE: Psychopathy, treatment behavior, and recidivism: an extended follow-up of Seto and Barbaree. J Interpers Violence 20(9):1115–1131, 2005 16051730

Blanchard R, Klassen P, Dickey R, et al: Sensitivity and specificity of the phallometric test for pedophilia in nonadmitting sex offenders. Psychol Assess 13(1):118–126, 2001 11281033

Booth BD: Special populations: mentally disordered sexual offenders (MDSOs), in Managing High-Risk Sex Offenders in the Community: Risk Management, Treatment, and Social Responsibilities. Edited by Harrison K. Devon, UK, Willan, 2010, pp 193–208

Bradford J: The treatment of sexual deviation using a pharmacological approach. J Sex Res 37:248–257, 2000

Bradford JM: The neurobiology, neuropharmacology, and pharmacological treatment of the paraphilias and compulsive sexual behaviour. Can J Psychiatry 46(1):26–34, 2001 11221487

Bradford JM, Boulet J, Pawlak A: The paraphilias: a multiplicity of deviant behaviours. Can J Psychiatry 37(2):104–108, 1992 1562953

Bradford J, Firestone P, Ahmed AG: The paraphilic disorders and psychopathy, in International Handbook of Psychopathic Disorders and the Law, Vol 1. Edited by Felthous A, Sass H. West Sussex, UK, Wiley, 2008, pp 275–290

Chenier E: The criminal sexual psychopath in Canada: sex, psychiatry and the law at mid-century. Can Bull Med Hist 20(1): 75–101, 2003 13678043

Daubert v Merrell Dow Pharmaceuticals, Inc, 509 U.S. 579, 113 S.Ct. 2786 (1993)

Dunsieth NW Jr, Nelson EB, Brusman-Lovins LA, et al: Psychiatric and legal features of 113 men convicted of sexual offenses. J Clin Psychiatry 65(3):293–300, 2004 15096066

English K, Jones L, Pasini-Hill D, et al: The Value of Polygraph Testing in Sex Offender Treatment. Washington, DC, National Institute of Corrections/National Institute of Justice, 2000

Fazel S, Hope T, O'Donnell I, et al: Psychiatric, demographic and personality characteristics of elderly sex offenders. Psychol Med 32(2):219–226, 2002 11866317

Finkelhor D: The international epidemiology of child sexual abuse. Child Abuse Negl 18(5):409–417, 1994 8032971

Freund K, Blanchard R: Phallometric diagnosis of pedophilia. J Consult Clin Psychol 57(1):100–105, 1989 2925958

Freund K, Seto MC, Kuban M: Frotteurism and the theory of courtship disorder, in Sexual Deviance: Theory, Assessment, and Treatment. Edited by Laws D, O'Donohue WT. New York, Guilford, 1997, pp 111–130

Frye v United States, 54 App.D.C. 46, 293 F. 1013 (D.C. Cir. 1923)

Furby L, Weinrott MR, Blackshaw L: Sex offender recidivism: a review. Psychol Bull 105(1):3–30, 1989 2648438

Gray SR, Abel GG, Jordan A, et al: Visual Reaction Time™ as a predictor of sexual offense recidivism. Sex Abuse 27(2):173–188, 2015 24058094

Hanson RK: Recidivism and age: follow-up data from 4,673 sexual offenders. J Interpers Violence 17:1046–1062, 2002

Hanson RK, Bussière MT: Predicting relapse: a meta-analysis of sexual offender recidivism studies. J Consult Clin Psychol 66(2):348–362, 1998 9583338

Hanson RK, Morton-Bourgon KE: The characteristics of persistent sexual offenders: a meta-analysis of recidivism studies. J Consult Clin Psychol 73(6):1154–1163, 2005 16392988

Hanson RK, Morton-Bourgon KE: The accuracy of recidivism risk assessments for sexual offenders: a meta-analysis of 118 prediction studies. Psychol Assess 21(1):1–21, 2009 19290762

Hanson RK, Gordon A, Harris AJ, et al: First report of the collaborative outcome data project on the effectiveness of psychological treatment for sex offenders. Sex Abuse 14(2):169–194, discussion 195–197, 2002 11961890

Hare R: Hare Psychopathy Checklist—Revised (PCL-R). Toronto, ON, Multi-Health Systems, 2003

Harris A, Phenix A, Hanson RK, et al: STATIC-99 Coding Rules Revised, 2003. Ottawa, ON, Canada, Solicitor General Canada, Government of Canada, 2003. Available at: http://www.static99.org/pdfdocs/static-99-coding-rules_e.pdf. Accessed January 9, 2017.

Harris AJ, Tough S: Should actuarial risk assessments be used with sex offenders who are intellectually disabled? J Appl Res Intellect Disabil 17:235–241, 2004

Hart SD, Boer DP: Structured professional judgment guidelines for sexual violence risk assessment: the Sexual Violence Risk-20 (SVR-20) and Risk for Sexual Violence Protocol (RSVP), in Handbook of Violence Risk Assessment. Edited by Otto RK, Douglas KS. New York, Routledge/Taylor & Francis Group, 2010, pp 269–294

Heil P, Ahlmeyer S, Simons D: Crossover sexual offenses. Sex Abuse 15(4):221–236, 2003 14571530

Kafka MP: The paraphilic–related disorders: a proposal for a unified classification of nonparaphilic hypersexuality disorders. Sexual Addiction & Compulsivity 8:227–239, 2001

Kafka MP, Hennen J: A DSM-IV Axis I co-morbidity study of males (n=120) with paraphilias and paraphilia-related disorders. Sex Abuse 14:349–366, 2002 12375492

Kansas v Crane, 534 U.S. 407, 122 S.Ct. 867 (2002)

Kansas v Hendricks, 521 U.S. 346, 117 S.Ct. 2072 (1997)

Kingston DA, Yates PM, Firestone P, et al: Long-term predictive validity of the risk matrix 2000: a comparison with the static-99 and the sex offender risk appraisal guide. Sex Abuse 20(4):466–484, 2008 18840901

Kingston DA, Olver M, Harris M, et al: The relationship between mental disorders and recidivism in sexual offenders. Int J Forensic Ment Health 14:10–22, 2015

La Fond JQ: The costs of enacting a sexual predator law. Psychol Public Policy Law 4:468–504, 1998

Lalumière ML, Harris GT: Common questions regarding the use of phallometric testing with sexual offenders. Sex Abuse 10:227–237, 1998

Lalumière ML, Harris GT, Quinsey VL, et al: The Causes of Rape: Understanding Individual Differences in Male Propensity for Sexual Aggression. Washington, DC, American Psychological Association, 2005

Långström N, Hanson RK: High rates of sexual behavior in the general population: correlates and predictors. Arch Sex Behav 35(1):37–52, 2006 16502152

Langton CM, Barbaree HE, Harkins L, et al: Sex offenders' response to treatment and its association with recidivism as a function of psychopathy. Sex Abuse 18(1):99–120, 2006 16598661

Laws D, O'Donohue WT (eds): Sexual Deviance: Theory, Assessment, and Treatment. New York, Guilford, 2008

Looman J, Marshall W: Phallometric assessments designed to detect arousal to children: the responses of rapists and child molesters. Sex Abuse 13:3–13, 2001

Losel F, Schmucker M: The effectiveness of treatment for sexual offenders: a comprehensive meta-analysis. J Exp Criminol 1:117–146, 2005

Marshall WL, Fernandez Y: Phallometric Testing with Sexual Offenders: Theory, Research, and Practice. Brandon, VT, Safer Society Press, 2003

McKune v Lile, 536 U.S. 24, 122 S.Ct. 2017 (2002) (AAPL only)

Pullman L, Stephens S, Seto MC: A motivation-facilitation model of adult male sexual offending, in The Wiley Handbook on the Psychology of Violence. Edited by Cuevas CA, Rennison CM. Hoboken, NJ, Wiley-Blackwell, 2016, pp 482–500

Quinsey VL, Harris GT, Rice M, et al: Violent Offenders: Appraising and Managing Risk, 3rd Edition. Washington, DC, American Psychological Association, 2015

Riches VC, Parmenter TR, Wiese M, et al: Intellectual disability and mental illness in the NSW criminal justice system. Int J Law Psychiatry 29(5):386–396, 2006 16793136

Schmucker MLF: The effects of sexual offender treatment on recidivism: An international meta-analysis of sound quality evaluations. J Exp Criminol 11:597–630, 2015

Seto MC: Pedophilia and Sexual Offending Against Children: Theory, Assessment, and Intervention. Washington, DC, American Psychological Association, 2008

Seto MC, Eke AW: The criminal histories and later offending of child pornography offenders. Sex Abuse 17(2):201–210, 2005 15974425

Seto MC, Eke AW: Predicting recidivism among adult male child pornography offenders: Development of the Child Pornography Offender Risk Tool (CPORT). Law Hum Behav 39(4):416–429, 2015 25844514

Seto MC, Cantor JM, Blanchard R: Child pornography offenses are a valid diagnostic indicator of pedophilia. J Abnorm Psychol 115(3):610–615, 2006 16866601

Seto MC, Marques JK, Harris GT, et al: Good science and progress in sex offender treatment are intertwined: a response to Marshall and Marshall (2007). Sex Abuse 20(3):247–255, 2008 18775837

Specht v Patterson, 386 U.S. 605, 87 S.Ct. 1209 (1967)

Stoltenborgh M, van Ijzendoorn MH, Euser EM, et al: A global perspective on child sexual abuse: meta-analysis of prevalence around the world. Child Maltreat 16(2):79–101, 2011 21511741

Thibaut F, De La Barra F, Gordon H, et al; WFSBP Task Force on Sexual Disorders: The World Federation of Societies of Biological Psychiatry (WFSBP) guidelines for the biological treatment of paraphilias. World J Biol Psychiatry 11(4):604–655, 2010 20459370

Thibaut F, Bradford JM, Briken P, et al; WFSBP Task Force on Sexual Disorders: The World Federation of Societies of Biological Psychiatry (WFSBP) guidelines for the treatment of adolescent sexual offenders with paraphilic disorders. World J Biol Psychiatry 17(1):2–38, 2016 26595752

Truman JL, Langton L: Criminal Victimization 2013 (Report No NCJ 247648). Washington, DC, U.S. Department of Justice, Bureau of Justice Statistics, 2014. Available at: http://www.bjs.gov/content/pub/pdf/cv13.pdf. Accessed January 8, 2017.

United States v Comstock, 560 U.S. 126, 130 S.Ct. 1949 (2010)

PART VI

Children and Families

CHAPTER 24

Forensic Evaluations of Children and Adolescents

Peter Ash, M.D.

Elissa Benedek, M.D.

Landmark Cases

Board of Education v. Rowley, 458 U.S. 176, 102. S.Ct. 3034 (1982)

Irving Independent School District v. Tatro, 468 U.S. 883, 104 S.Ct. 3371 (1984)

General Principles

Forensic work in child and adolescent psychiatry tends to have a different thrust from forensic work with adults. In a case involving adults, the psychiatric expert is typically retained by a party to the case (although in court-ordered evaluations, the expert works directly for the court). Therefore, the expert is on one side or the other of an adversarial process. Moreover, the well-being of the evaluee typically is not the court's prime consideration.

In contrast, regardless of which adult or agency is paying the bill, the psychiatric expert in both civil and criminal matters involving juveniles is often expected to evaluate and advocate for the well-being of the child. In cases involving child placement, the child is generally not even formally a party in the case. The emphasis on the child's interests may give forensic work with children a more therapeutic focus and may be more familiar to clinicians who view themselves primarily as therapists. However, the primary emphasis of a forensic evaluation of a child or adolescent remains a dedication to striving for objectivity in the interest of truth.

Another key difference in forensic work with children and adolescents is that interviewing young persons requires different techniques from evaluating adults. The accreditation guidelines for forensic psychiatry training programs specifically state that forensic fellows who have not completed a child and adolescent psychiatry training program should not independently conduct forensic evaluations of children under age 14 years (Accreditation Council for Graduate Medical Education 2016).

Because there is a national shortage of child and adolescent psychiatrists (American Academy of Child and Adolescent Psychiatry 2016), however, in underserved, nonurban areas, some general psychiatrists have considerable experience working with youth and conducting forensic evaluations involving children. In addition, even if clinicians do not evaluate or treat children, adult patients in their role as parents may become involved in litigation concerning their children. Thus, the range of issues in child and adolescent forensic psychiatry that may affect the work of a general psychiatrist is very wide.

The specialized interviewing techniques required to form the relationship necessary to conduct a productive interview of a child, such as play and drawing techniques, are beyond the scope of this chapter. The interested reader or child and adolescent psychiatrist is referred to standard reference works on forensic child and adolescent psychiatry (Benedek et al. 2010; Haller 2002). The evaluation of adolescents is a different matter. Many general psychiatrists have had training and experience working with adolescents and also conduct forensic evaluations on this population. Nevertheless, general psychiatrists should think carefully before agreeing to conduct such an evaluation and anticipate that their expertise in working with this age group will be the subject of cross-examination.

Many of the differences in cases involving minors, when compared with adults, follow from two legal presumptions: 1) minors are considered less responsible for their actions than are adults, and 2) minors are legally held to be less competent than adults. Salient differences in child and adolescent cases in which the forensic issues are similar to adult cases are listed in Table 24–1.

Some types of cases involving minors have no clear adult parallels. This group of cases arises from the different standing of adults and children under the law. Forensic cases involving minors without clear adult analogues arise in situations in which the parents are not in a position to speak appropriately for the child. These can include circumstances such as when the parents themselves disagree (custody in divorce), when the parents have interests opposed to the child's interests (abuse and neglect, termination of parental rights), or when the child acts outside the parents' control (delinquency, some medical care issues). In these civil cases, an attorney, generally referred to as a guardian *ad litem* (from the Latin "for the suit"), commonly is appointed to represent the best interests of the minor. Some legal controversy has arisen as to what a guardian *ad litem* should do if his or her view of the child's best interest differs from that of the minor. Some jurisdictions allow for the additional appointment of a child-directed attorney whose duty is to advocate for the child's expressed position.

Forensic evaluations focus on whether or not the individual's condition meets a forensic test specific to the matter at issue. Forensic tests in similar cases vary from state to state and in federal jurisdictions. Nevertheless, certain general principles cut across jurisdictions. Typical forensic tests in cases involving minors that have no clear counterpart in adult forensic work are listed in Table 24–2.

TABLE 24–1. **Key differences in cases involving minors in which the forensic issue is the same as for adults**

Issue	Difference from adult cases
Civil cases	
Malpractice	Because minors are less responsible than adults, clinicians have a greater duty to protect them from other patients, from committing suicide, and so on.
Personal injury	Minors are more sympathetic plaintiffs. Minors are held to a lesser degree of responsibility, which tends to shift responsibility to defendants.
Civil commitment	Minors are less commonly committed because in most states it is only required if parents refuse to voluntarily admit minor.
Civil competency	Minors are presumed legally incompetent except in specific situations authorized by state law.
Disability	Social Security disability criteria for children are worded slightly differently. School-related issues are mostly governed by education legislation.
Threat assessment	School threat assessment uses different techniques than workplace violence assessment.
Criminal cases	
Competency to stand trial	Almost all states now require competency to stand trial in juvenile court, but the statutory test may be somewhat different. Incompetence in most states may be due to developmental immaturity.
Criminal responsibility	Insanity is not usually a defense in juvenile court and is rare in adolescents waived to adult court.
Competency to waive a constitutional right (e.g., confess, waive counsel, plead guilty)	Developmental considerations affect whether waiver is knowing, intelligent, and voluntary.
Sex offenders	Minors are more treatable than adults.

Beginning a Forensic Evaluation

Clarification of Role

The differences between adult and child forensic work require that psychiatrists clearly define the consultant's role at the beginning of a case. Clarity at the start of a case goes a long way toward preventing problems down the road. Before beginning the evaluation, the forensic consultant should consider the following questions:

1. What is the forensic question that needs to be answered?
2. Who is requesting the evaluation: the minor, a parent, a guardian *ad litem*, an attorney, an agency, a school, a court?
3. Who is to be interviewed?
4. If a minor is being interviewed, who will give informed consent for the evaluation?

TABLE 24–2. Forensic child and adolescent cases without clear adult analogues

Issue	Typical forensic test
Abuse/neglect proceedings	Varies according to the stage of the proceeding:
	Was the child abused or neglected?
	Are the parents fit to raise the child?
	Should protective services pursue reunification?
	Is termination of parental rights in the best interests of the child?
Adoption	Is termination of parental rights in the best interests of the child?
	If mother is a minor, is she competent to give up child for adoption?
Custody in the context of divorce	What is in the best interests of the child?
Medical care	
Provide own consent	When minors can provide their own consent varies according to state law. Although the general rule is that minors cannot provide consent, state law may give some minors authority to provide consent in certain situations (e.g., outpatient therapy, treatment of sexually transmitted diseases, contraception, abortion) or a right to object (e.g., to psychiatric hospitalization). Some states allow a mature minor to provide consent.
Consent to an abortion without parental consent	Is the girl a mature minor?
Participation in research that will not benefit minor	Assent is required if the minor can understand general nature of participation, in addition to parental consent.
Special education services	Is child seriously emotionally disturbed? If so, what special education services are appropriate?
Delinquency	
Study and report	What mental health issues are relevant in rehabilitating and planning a disposition for the child?
Waiver to adult court	What is the risk of future violence and likelihood of rehabilitation?

5. What are the limits on confidentiality in the evaluation?
6. To whom will the report be sent (including to what extent will a parent control whether the report is sent at all)?
7. What are the arrangements for paying the fees?

These issues are frequently more complex in cases involving minors than in cases involving adults. First, minors have limited formal decision-making author-

ity, so although the minor may be the subject of a case, others will often be speaking for the minor in court. Second, in child placement cases, both in divorce/custody and in abuse/neglect proceedings, the child is typically not a formal party to the case at all. In such cases, the consultant should consider in advance how (or whether) the report will be brought to the attention of the court in the event a parent does not like the outcome.

Fees should generally be agreed on in principle and may be paid prior to conducting the work. In any event, fees should be paid prior to completing the evaluation or testifying, unless the retaining agent is a corporate defendant or state agency. During cross-examination, physicians are often asked how much they have been paid. A parent who is disappointed in an evaluation is easily tempted to withhold payment, either to save money or to prevent distribution of the report. Evaluators concerned that they might not be paid their full fees may be subject to a subtle source of bias, which may be brought out on cross-examination (e.g., "Now Doctor, do you really think you'll be paid for your testimony today if it's not favorable to Mr. X?").

Forensic Evaluations of One's Own Patients

Not uncommonly, a minor or a parent in treatment will become the subject of a legal proceeding. This most often occurs in custody cases. The attorney for either the child or a parent may wish to use the treating clinician as the expert on the grounds that the clinician knows the child or parent best. However, treating clinicians are best advised to avoid becoming the expert in such cases. By conducting a forensic evaluation, clinicians take on a duty toward the court, in addition to their continuing duty to the patient.

This potential dual role conflict is known as the *double-agent problem*: being the agent of the child, as therapist, and being an agent of the court or parent, as forensic evaluator. The ethical principle of striving for objectivity is difficult to achieve when wearing two hats (Strasburger et al. 1997). Conflicting duties give rise to a host of difficulties (see Chapters 3, "Ethics in Forensic Psychiatry," and 4, "Forensic Evaluations and Reports"). Even if psychiatrists believe that the double-agent problem can be

surmounted, the court is likely to see treating psychiatrists as biased toward their patients and discount the weight given to the expert's opinions. Treating psychiatrists are generally advised to refer their patients to another clinician for forensic evaluation.

Such a referral is also advisable because the expert role usually is quite disruptive of treatment. Conducting a forensic assessment will generally require going outside the established treatment relationship. Once the child (or parent) knows that the therapist is a route to the judge, confidentiality goes out the window, the patient has a motive to distort what he or she tells the therapist, and the parameters of the treatment change. Furthermore, the clinician may not have a wellformed opinion on the particular forensic issue. For example, a divorcing parent may want the clinician to give an opinion on postdivorce custody arrangements, but the clinician may not have assessed the parents' parenting capacity or compared their relationships with the child.

An attorney for a parent may nevertheless subpoena the treating psychiatrist or the psychiatrist's records. Such actions can sometimes be discouraged. For example, in a child custody case in which a mother's attorney threatens to subpoena the child's treating psychiatrist, the therapist may point out that such an action will disrupt the child's treatment, and thus may serve as evidence that the mother is not acting in the best interest of the child.

Consent for Evaluation

If a forensic evaluation of a minor is ordered by the court, parental consent is not required. If an evaluation is requested by a parent, then the evaluator should obtain the informed consent of the parent, which should include a signed release to send the report to designated recipients. In limited situations, an adolescent can provide consent for the evaluation. Such situations arise if the adolescents are emancipated (because they are married, are in the military, or are self-supporting and living independently) or waived to adult criminal jurisdiction. Adolescents may also be able to consent to treatment (e.g., when a girl is seeking to obtain an abortion without her parents' knowledge or when an adolescent lives in a state that allows certain classes of minors to consent to medical treatment). In any event, the evaluator should explain to the child or adolescent, in developmentally appropriate terms, the nature of the evaluation and indicate with whom information will be shared. In child cases, optimal practice includes explaining to the child the reasons for the evaluation and obtaining the assent (rather than consent) of the child.

Exceptions to Confidentiality

As a general rule, confidentiality is controlled by the person or agency that provides legal consent for the evaluation. In some instances, most often to protect a child, legal and ethical obligations compel a treating clinician to disclose forensically relevant information to outside agencies without a release from the consenting party, such as when a clinician suspects child abuse (see Chapter 25, "Evaluations of Juveniles in Civil Law").

In the unenviable necessity of reporting their own patients as suspected child abusers, clinicians face the challenge of conforming to their duty to report while attempting to maintain a therapeutic alliance. Under such circumstances, notifying the patient that a report is being made and the reason for making the report is almost always the best course of action. Many therapists fear that a patient

reported for suspected child abuse will become angry and either quit therapy or mistrust the therapist in the future. An open acknowledgment of the difficulty and an offer to help the patient resolve the difficulties that gave rise to the reported behaviors often allow the patient to continue to see the therapist as an ally. Clinicians who do not tell the patient about the report run the risk that the patient will think the therapist is complicit with the abuse (many patients know about reporting duties) or that the patient will later find out (the anonymity of reports is not all it might be) and feel betrayed.

Ethical Issues

The general principles of forensic ethics discussed in Chapter 3 apply to forensic work with minors, although the control of consent and confidentiality is different, as discussed in the previous two subsections. The published commentary that is part of the ethics code of the American Academy of Psychiatry and the Law (2005) is intended to apply to forensic evaluations involving minors and specifically addresses issues of special expertise for those who interview children and the importance of interviewing all parties before opining about child custody.

The American Academy of Child and Adolescent Psychiatry (2014) states that its ethics code "should be used by all practitioners of this specialty in every professional context," and therefore it applies to forensic work. This ethics code is organized around keeping a developmental perspective and upholding the principles of beneficence, nonmaleficence, autonomy, confidentiality, fidelity, and justice. The code explicitly recognizes that evaluations that take place in a context other than treatment, such as forensic work, proceed from somewhat different principles than those that apply to treatment encounters, and so are consistent with the American Academy of Psychiatry and the Law's (2005) ethics code for forensic work.

Evaluation of Personal Injury Cases Involving PTSD

The *Diagnostic and Statistical Manual of Mental Disorders,* 5th Edition (DSM-5; American Psychiatric Association 2013), made a number of changes to the criteria for the diagnosis of posttraumatic stress disorder (PTSD) in children. The criterion for trauma was expanded from actual or threatened death or serious injury to include sexual violence. Because PTSD often presents differently in children than in adults, DSM-5 also gives notes under some of the other criteria regarding alternative presentations in children; it also gives a separate list of complete criteria for the diagnosis of PTSD for children younger than age 7. Although DSM-5 is a categorical diagnostic system, according to which a patient either has or does not have PTSD, the symptoms actually lie on a continuum. Some children may exhibit some symptoms but not enough to meet full diagnostic criteria.

Although estimates vary widely, exposure to trauma in childhood is fairly common. Nevertheless, only about one third of children exposed to trauma go on to develop PTSD (Cohen et al. 2010). The likelihood of developing PTSD following a trauma is correlated with the type and severity of exposure (McLaughlin et al. 2013).

Forensic assessment of the impact of trauma on children is more complex than assessment of trauma's impact on adults

due to a variety of factors. First, obtaining a clear history of what a young child experienced may be difficult. Young children are less likely to talk about what happened to them. If extrinsic evidence of what occurred is not available, the history given by the child is key. Because children, especially preschool children, are more suggestible than adolescents or adults, the examiner needs to be careful not to ask suggestive questions that might lead the child to distort the history, contaminate future evaluations, and potentially lead to the evaluator's report being discredited.

Second, youth of different developmental stages will react to the same trauma in very different ways. For example, young children may lack an understanding of certain threats or sexual behaviors that would be traumatic to adolescents, and young children are much more likely to have their responses to trauma affected by the degree of stress their parents show.

Third, a child's coping strategies in response to a trauma will vary depending on the child's developmental level. A number of structured interviews and rating scales have been developed for childhood PTSD, and selecting appropriate measures may be helpful in clarifying the types and severity of the child's symptoms (for examples, see U.S. Department of Veterans Affairs, National Center for PTSD 2017).

In addition to assessing the child's reaction to trauma, the forensic psychiatrist must assess the parent's response to the trauma. In evaluating the source of a plaintiff's complaint, the examiner should consider confounding variables, including a parent's reaction or overreaction or a parent's wish to exaggerate or embellish symptomatology for secondary gain.

The forensic clinician may be asked the impact of the trauma on the child's future development. Group data about outcomes following childhood or adolescent trauma may be difficult to apply to an individual case because of the wide variation in children's responses, and the particular circumstances of the case may not match the traumas experienced by the subject group in the study. The forensic expert therefore often must resort to applying general developmental theories to particular fact situations, while remaining ever cognizant of the difficulties in making accurate predictions.

Special Education

Special education is regulated primarily by a series of federal laws that began with the Education for All Handicapped Children Act, first passed in 1975 and subsequently amended, and then reauthorized by the Individuals With Disabilities Education Act of 1990 (IDEA) and subsequently amended. These laws are complex, but the central idea is that all children are entitled to "free appropriate public education" and that children with special needs are to be given an Individualized Education Program (IEP), which includes parental input, by the school to address those needs. Given that such services are expensive and many school districts lacked resources, considerable litigation ensued in which parents have attempted to push school systems to provide services for their children beyond those the school offered to provide.

In the case of *Board of Education v. Rowley* (1982), Rowley was a deaf child whose parents requested that the school provide a qualified sign language interpreter to assist her communication in her regular education classes. She was performing better than average in her classes, although the U.S. District Court of Appeals found that she also understood less than she would have if she were not deaf. The U.S. Supreme Court found that the schools were providing free appropriate public education by virtue of Rowley having access to and receiving educational benefit. The court's decision stated that this did not entitle the child to the best program or one that would "maximize potential" as long as she was progressing normally from grade to grade.

The extent of services that a school was required to provide was again raised in *Irving Independent School District v. Tatro* (1984). The parents of Tatro, an 8-year-old girl with spina bifida that left her unable to empty her bladder, brought suit to have the school provide urinary catheterization. The U.S. Supreme Court held that catheterization was a "related service" rather than a "medical service" and therefore the school must provide it. The Court differentiated between "related services," which could be provided by a nurse in school health services, and "medical services," which needed to be provided by a licensed physician.

The *Rowley* and *Tatro* cases, as well as most special education cases, are interpretations of federal statutes, not of the Constitution. Therefore, if the statute is amended or repealed by Congress, the Supreme Court's holding may no longer be valid. Since 1975, the general trend of the amendments to special education laws has been to increase groups covered. For example, the 2004 amendments to IDEA extended services for children with autism and some other developmental disabilities into the prekindergarten years. Section 504 of the Rehabilitation Act of 1973 and the Americans With Disabilities Act of 1990 are civil rights statutes that require some services for disabled people, and therefore also have some effect on educational institutions; however, because IDEA provides funding whereas these civil rights statutes do not, most educational litigation revolves around interpretation of IDEA.

Psychiatric evaluators who become involved in special education cases need to be aware of the law that affects the particular case as well as the interpretation of that law in their jurisdiction. Evaluations of a child's needs for special education services tend to be extensive and include psychological testing, observation of the school milieu, observation of the child in the classroom, and collateral reports from school and parents, in addition to interviews of the child. Reports of evaluations for special education depart from the general rule that legal jargon should be avoided in a forensic report; in such evaluations, terms that have special legal meanings need to be used correctly. For example, in discussing a child with conduct disorder or oppositional defiant disorder, the evaluator should be aware that in most jurisdictions, children with an "emotional disability" qualify for services, whereas those with "social maladjustment" do not.

Suicide Risk Assessment

Suicide is currently the second leading cause of death, after accidents, for youth ages 15–19 years. In 2013, the suicide rate in this age group in the United States was 8.69 per 100,000 (Centers for Disease Control and Prevention 2016). Suicide is much less common for early adolescents, ages 10–14 years (1.99 per 100,000 in 2013), and is rare for prepubertal children. Many of the principles pertinent to the assessment of adults discussed in Chapter 27, "Suicide Risk Assessment," are relevant to the assessment of suicidal adolescents. Nevertheless, approaches to younger patients are somewhat dif-

ferent from those used with adults because of youths' developmental differences, different living circumstances, and different legal status. Key differences between suicidal adults and suicidal adolescents are listed in Table 24–3.

The Centers for Disease Control and Prevention (CDC) conducts an annual survey of adolescent risky behavior. According to the CDC's 2013 Youth Risk Behavior Survey, in the previous 12 months, 17% of high school students had seriously considered suicide, 13.6% had made a plan, 8% had made a suicide attempt, and 2.7% had made an attempt of sufficient severity as to receive medical attention (Kann et al. 2014). Girls had about twice the rate of boys in each of these categories. The rate of suicidal ideation is about 2,000 times the rate of completed suicide. This high ratio reveals the limitation of using ideation as a strong predictive risk factor for completed suicide. Studies have not identified factors that allow a clinician to accurately predict which adolescents will commit suicide. Research on adolescent suicide risk factors has identified many different factors that increase risk when compared with normal subjects (American Academy of Child and Adolescent Psychiatry 2001; Cash and Bridge 2009; Dervic et al. 2008; Gould et al. 2003). Risk factors commonly cited in the literature are listed in Table 24–4.

In boys, previous attempts appear to be the strongest risk factor, increasing the risk about 30 times over that of the normal population (Brent et al. 1999; Shaffer et al. 1996). Marttunen et al. (1993) identified a precipitant in 70% of a series of completed adolescent suicides, and half the precipitants occurred in the 24 hours preceding the suicide. The close proximity of the precipitant to the suicide clearly implies a very short window for intervention. Protective factors include the na-

TABLE 24–3. **Key differences between suicidal adults and suicidal adolescents**

Category	Compared with adults, for adolescents:
Risk factors	Suicide accounts for a higher proportion of all deaths.
	Suicidal ideation is more common.
	Suicide attempts are more common.
	Disruptive behavior disorders increase risk.
	Contagion effects are more powerful.
Diagnostic differences	Psychotic disorder is much less common.
Symptoms	Although suicidal ideation is more common, suicidal ideation is more likely to be denied when asked about.
	Lethality of means is more commonly misjudged.
Treatment	SSRIs require more monitoring.
	Family involvement in treatment is more important.
Legal status	Legal consent for treatment needs to be provided by someone other than patient.
	Hospitalization over the patient's objection can often be accomplished without resorting to civil commitment.
	Patient's responsibility for treatment compliance is reduced.
Aftermath of completed suicide	Full discussion with parents less constrained by confidentiality limitations because parents control record release.

Note. SSRI=selective serotonin reuptake inhibitor.
Source. Reprinted from Ash P: "Suicidal Children, Adolescents, and College Students," in *The American Psychiatric Publishing Textbook of Suicide Assessment and Management,* 2nd Edition. Edited by Simon RI, Hales RE. Washington, DC, American Psychiatric Publishing, 2012, pp. 349–366. Copyright © 2012 American Psychiatric Association. Used with permission.

ture of available social support from family and peers; internal resistances to suicide, such as religious objections; the extent to which stressors in the environment can be ameliorated; and the usefulness of the family in monitoring the youth's thinking and behavior.

An assessment of depressive feelings and symptoms, suicidal ideation, and a history of attempts of self-harm should be a routine component of the initial evaluation of any adolescent or depressed child. Suicide assessment is an ongoing process, however, and should not be restricted to the initial evaluation. The assessment focuses on the risk and protective factors identified in the previous paragraphs. Because many suicidal adolescents may be reluctant to disclose suicidal ideation, information from collateral sources and prior psychiatric records helps round out the clinical picture. In the event of an adverse outcome and resulting malpractice litigation, liability often turns on the adequacy of the initial documentation and documentation of continuing suicide assessments.

The American Academy of Child and Adolescent Psychiatry (2001) has developed a practice parameter for the assessment and treatment of suicidal behaviors. In a clinical assessment, suicidal ideation, especially when coupled with a plan involving lethal means or a recent attempt, is the most common trigger for a judgment of imminent danger requiring hospitalization. The clinician should assess what the youth thought the outcome of the attempt would be. Younger adolescents and preadolescents com-

TABLE 24–4. **Summary of leading risk factors for adolescent suicide**

Individual factors

Previous suicide attempt

High intent/lethality of method

Psychopathology

    Major depression

      Helplessness and hopelessness

    Bipolar disorder

    Substance abuse comorbid with other psychopathology

    Schizophrenia

    Conduct or personality disorder, especially with impulsive characteristics

Demographic factors

Over age 14 years, risk increases with age

Male

White

Unwed adolescent with unwanted pregnancy

Family and environmental factors

Firearm in the home

Family pathology/discord

Abuse (physical or sexual)

History of violence

Recent stressors

    Separation

    Arrest/legal problems

Source. Reprinted from Ash P: "Suicidal Children, Adolescents, and College Students," in *The American Psychiatric Publishing Textbook of Suicide Assessment and Management,* 2nd Edition. Edited by Simon RI, Hales RE. Washington, DC, American Psychiatric Publishing, 2012, pp. 349–366. Copyright © 2012 American Psychiatric Association. Used with permission.

monly misjudge the lethality of means, such as by overestimating the lethality of a selective serotonin reuptake inhibitor (SSRI) overdose or underestimating the lethality of an aspirin overdose. Assessing dynamic factors, including which stressors have precipitated previous suicidal thinking or past attempts, and assessing the likelihood of recurrence of such stressors helps in determining risk and possible treatment interventions.

Malpractice

Forensic evaluators may be asked to review the care of other psychiatrists in mal-practice litigation involving youth. The general principles of malpractice are discussed in Chapter 12, "Professional Liability in Psychiatric Practice," and reviews of liability issues affecting child and adolescent psychiatrists are available in the literature (Ash 2010; Ash and Nurcombe 2018; Caudill 2006). Because insurers maintain their data in categories derived from plaintiffs' complaints, accurate data regarding claims are difficult to obtain. An analysis of recent data from one insurer revealed that the most common cause of loss was for "incorrect treatment," a category that could include any aspect of treatment, and accounted for 36% of cases, followed by medication issues (16%) and suicide or attempted suicide (16%) (Professional Risk Management Services 2015).

Malpractice cases involving the treatment of minors may raise issues that differ somewhat from otherwise similar fact situations that involve adult patients. The following list describes the most commonly occurring differences.

- *Psychopharmacology.* Minors generally cannot consent to medication treatment, so the consent process with parents will be scrutinized. Drug companies that receive U.S. Food and Drug Administration (FDA) approval for indications in adults often do not do the research necessary to get approval for use in children and adolescents, so more medications commonly prescribed to minors are used off-label, which can raise questions about their appropriateness. The FDA's black box warning regarding risk of suicide with the use of SSRIs in minors means that increased monitoring of those medications is necessary.
- *Lessened patient responsibility.* Because minors are presumed legally incompetent, they are seen as less responsible for their actions, so in the event of an outpatient suicide, a jury may apportion more blame to the treating clinician than they would for a similar suicide by a competent adult. Child plaintiffs are likely to be seen by a jury as more sympathetic victims.
- *Child abuse.* The requirement to report child abuse or neglect is an additional duty, and failure to recognize abuse may be seen as negligent.
- *Definition of the patient.* Most child

treatment involves seeing parents in addition to the child, and seeing a child in the context of family treatment is also common. Unless the doctor–patient relationship is clearly defined at the outset of treatment, the clinician may be liable for issues related to the "treatment" of a family member.

Despite these differences, child and adolescent psychiatrists are at lower risk of being sued than their adult counterparts (Ash 2002), and when they are sued, they are most often not found liable. From a clinical perspective, good patient care and good documentation are the key protective factors for avoiding an adverse verdict.

Conclusion

Forensic evaluations of children and adolescents follow the same general principles as forensic evaluations of adults. The differences in the evaluation process flow from the fact that a youth under age 18 is, with rare exceptions, legally incompetent, which then requires an adult to speak for him or her on questions of consent and confidentiality. The content differences flow from the fact that a youth's developmental stage creates differences across many domains, including appropriate interviewing techniques, symptom expression, and subjective experience. In addition, because minors are not independent in their choice of family constellation or school, they may be involved in legal cases involving custody and education that have no adult analogue.

Key Concepts

- Forensic evaluations of preadolescents usually require specialized training in child and adolescent psychiatry.

- Many of the differences in cases involving minors, when compared to adults, follow from the legal presumptions that minors are less responsible for their actions than are adults and are less legally competent than adults.

- Issues of confidentiality and consent need to take into account that in most cases, some adult speaks legally for the child.

- Posttraumatic stress disorder often presents with different symptoms in children than in adolescents or adults.

- Special education services are tailored to a child's needs through the Individualized Education Program (IEP) devised for that child. Mental health evaluations used in creating an IEP need to take into account the particular requirements of applicable special education law.

- Among adolescents, suicidal ideation is overwhelmingly more common than completed suicide. Nevertheless, although suicide in children and prepubertal children is rare, suicide is the second leading cause of death among adolescents ages 15–19.

References

Accreditation Council for Graduate Medical Education: ACGME Program Requirements for Graduate Medical Education in Forensic Psychiatry, 2016. Available at: http://www.acgme.org/Portals/0/PFAssets/ProgramRequirements/406_forensic_psych_2016_1-YR.pdf. Accessed December 29, 2017.

American Academy of Child and Adolescent Psychiatry: Practice parameter for the assessment and treatment of children and adolescents with suicidal behavior. J Am Acad Child Adolesc Psychiatry 40(7)(Suppl):24S–51S, 2001 11434483

American Academy of Child and Adolescent Psychiatry: Code of ethics, 2014. Available at: https://www.aacap.org/App_Themes/AACAP/docs/about_us/transparency_portal/aacap_code_of_ethics_2012.pdf. Accessed December 29, 2017.

American Academy of Child and Adolescent Psychiatry: Workforce issues. 2016. Available at: http://www.aacap.org/aacap/resources_for_primary_care/Workforce_Issues.aspx. Accessed December 29, 2017.

American Academy of Psychiatry and the Law: Ethics guidelines for the practice of forensic psychiatry. May 2005. Available at: http://www.aapl.org/ethics.htm. Accessed December 19, 2016.

American Psychiatric Association: Diagnostic and Statistical Manual of Mental Disorders, 5th Edition. Arlington, VA, American Psychiatric Publishing, 2013

Americans With Disabilities Act Pub. L. No. 101-336, 1990

Ash P: Malpractice in child and adolescent psychiatry. Child Adolesc Psychiatr Clin N Am 11(4):869–885, 2002 12397903

Ash P: Malpractice and professional liability, in Principles and Practice of Child and Adolescent Forensic Mental Health. Edited by Benedek EP, Ash P, Scott CL. Washington, DC, American Psychiatric Publishing, 2010, pp 419–430

Ash P: Suicidal children, adolescents, and college students, in The American Psychiatric Publishing Textbook of Suicide Assessment and Management, 2nd Edition. Edited by Simon RI, Hales RE. Washington, DC, American Psychiatric Publishing, 2012, pp 349–366

Ash P, Nurcombe B: Malpractice and professional liability, in Lewis's Child and Adolescent Psychiatry: A Comprehensive Textbook, 5th Ed. Edited by Martin A, Bloch MH, Volkmar FR. Philadelphia, PA, Wolters Kluwer, 2018, pp 996–1010

Benedek EP, Ash P, Scott CL (eds): Principles and Practice of Child and Adolescent Forensic Mental Health. Washington, DC, American Psychiatric Publishing, 2010

Board of Education v Rowley, 458 U.S. 176, 102. S.Ct. 3034 (1982)

Brent DA, Baugher M, Bridge J, et al: Age- and sex-related risk factors for adolescent suicide. J Am Acad Child Adolesc Psychiatry 38(12):1497–1505, 1999 10596249

Cash SJ, Bridge JA: Epidemiology of youth suicide and suicidal behavior. Curr Opin Pediatr 21(5):613–619, 2009 19644372

Caudill OB Jr: Avoiding malpractice in child forensic assessment, in Forensic Mental Health Assessment of Children and Adolescents. Edited by Sparta SN, Koocher GP. New York, Oxford University Press, 2006, pp 74–87

Centers for Disease Control and Prevention: WISQARS fatal injury reports, national and regional, 1999–2013. 2016. Available at: http://www.cdc.gov/injury/wisqars/fatal_injury_reports.html. Accessed December 29, 2017.

Cohen JA, Bukstein O, Walter H, et al; AACAP Work Group On Quality Issues: Practice parameter for the assessment and treatment of children and adolescents with posttraumatic stress disorder. J Am Acad Child Adolesc Psychiatry 49(4):414–430, 2010 20410735

Dervic K, Brent DA, Oquendo MA: Completed suicide in childhood. Psychiatr Clin North Am 31(2):271–291, 2008 18439449

Gould MS, Greenberg T, Velting DM, Shaffer D: Youth suicide risk and preventive interventions: a review of the past 10 years. J Am Acad Child Adolesc Psychiatry 42(4):386–405, 2003 12649626

Haller LH (ed): Forensic psychiatry. Child Adolesc Psychiatr Clin N Am 11:(entire issue), 2002

Individuals With Disabilities Education Act (IDEA). Pub. L. No. 101-476, 1990

Irving Independent School District v Tatro, 468 U.S. 883, 104 S.Ct. 3371 (1984)

Kann L, Kinchen S, Shanklin SL, et al; Centers for Disease Control and Prevention (CDC): Youth risk behavior surveillance—United States, 2013. MMWR Suppl 63(4):1–168, 2014 24918634

Marttunen MJ, Aro HM, Lönnqvist JK: Precipitant stressors in adolescent suicide. J Am Acad Child Adolesc Psychiatry 32(6):1178–1183, 1993 8282662

McLaughlin KA, Koenen KC, Hill ED, et al: Trauma exposure and posttraumatic stress disorder in a national sample of adolescents. J Am Acad Child Adolesc Psychiatry 52(8):815–830.e14, 2013 23880492

Professional Risk Management Services: The Psychiatrists' Program cause of loss (2005–2014). Rx for Risk 23:7, 2015

Rehabilitation Act. Pub. L. No. 93-112, 1973

Shaffer D, Gould MS, Fisher P, et al: Psychiatric diagnosis in child and adolescent suicide. Arch Gen Psychiatry 53(4):339–348, 1996 8634012

Strasburger LH, Gutheil TG, Brodsky A: On wearing two hats: role conflict in serving as both psychotherapist and expert witness. Am J Psychiatry 154(4):448–456, 1997 9090330

U.S. Department of Veterans Affairs National Center for PTSD: Child measures of trauma and PTSD, 2017. Available at: https://www.ptsd.va.gov/PTSD/professional/assessment/child/index.asp. Accessed June 3, 2017.

CHAPTER 25

Evaluations of Juveniles in Civil Law

Cheryl D. Wills, M.D.

Landmark Cases

Painter v. Bannister, 258 Iowa 1390, 140 N.W.2d 152 (1966)

Landeros v. Flood, 17 Cal.3d 399, 551 P.2d 389 (1976)

Parham v. JR and JL, 442 U.S. 584, 99 S.Ct. 2493 (1979)

Santosky v. Kramer, 455 U.S. 745, 102 S.Ct. 1388 (1982)

People v. Stritzinger, 34 Cal. 3d 505, 668 P.2d 738 (1983)

State v. Andring, 342 N.W. 2d 128 (Minn. 1984)

DeShaney v. Winnebago County Department of Social Services,
489 U.S. 189, 109 S.Ct. 998 (1989)

Child forensic psychiatrists conduct developmentally informed evaluations to address legal and/or policy matters salient to the mental health of minors. Although child forensic psychiatrists may restrict their practice to forensic consultations involving minors, their training in general, forensic and child psychiatry also qualifies them to conduct forensic examinations of adults. Forensi- cally trained child psychiatrists are in short supply in North America. Therefore, a subgroup of forensic psychiatrists, who have not completed a residency in child psychiatry but have substantial interest and clinical experience in working with older adolescents, also provide forensic consultations in matters involving older adolescents. However, when conducting forensic evaluations of minors, both child psychiatrists and adult forensic psychiatrists who are not child trained are required to meet the duty of care and practice standards expected of child and adolescent forensic psychiatrists.

Children and adolescents mature into adults through distinct physiological, cognitive, social, and adaptive transformations or developmental stages. Toward the end of the nineteenth century, courts and legislators in the United States began to recognize that this developmental process makes juveniles different from adults. Prior to that time, no statutory protections or judicial standards existed for minors in most areas, including education, custody, adoption, labor, maltreatment, and incarceration. This chapter examines the evolution of policy, legislation, and case law in civil (i.e., nondelinquency) matters involving children and adolescents and how this informs the practice of child forensic psychiatry.

The Well-Being of Children

Until relatively recently, children were thought of as miniature adults, considered the property of their fathers, and treated as a source of cheap labor. The movement to change these perceptions gained ground in 1912, when President William Howard Taft established the Federal Children's Bureau (Lindenmeyer 1997). This agency, the first of its type in the world, was charged with oversight of matters including policy and legislation that pertained to the well-being of children. The Federal Children's Bureau, which established state bureaus in 1921, focused on maternal-infant health, child and adolescent development, education, and child labor laws.

U.S. courts also weighed in on matters involving the well-being of children. In 1944, the U.S. Supreme Court, in *Prince v. Massachusetts* (1944), granted states the authority to protect children by intervening in the family unit to monitor the family's actions. This case involved parents who invoked religious doctrine to justify ignoring child labor laws. The Court reasoned that parental authority is not absolute and can be restricted by the government in the interests of a youth's welfare. Also, Title IV of the Social Security Act of 1935, known as Aid to Dependent Children (and later renamed Aid to Families with Dependent Children [AFDC]), was established to provide resources to indigent parents for their children (Cauthen and Amenta 1996).

Meanwhile, child and adolescent psychiatry was developing as a specialized field that offered outpatient and residential models of care. Children and adolescents needed clinical interventions conducive to healthy development. In 1959, the American Board of Psychiatry and Neurology recognized child psychiatry as a subspecialty and introduced a certifying examination in child psychiatry (see American Board of Psychiatry and Neurology 2015).

Progressive legislative, policy, and judicial actions on behalf of children changed social perceptions. Children were increasingly acknowledged to be developmentally distinct individuals who needed to be supported, educated, and nurtured to foster their maturation into healthy adults. The role of health care professionals in child welfare litigation changed precipitously after the publication of "The Battered Child Syndrome" (Kempe et al. 1962) in the *Journal of the American Medical Association*. This article, in which child maltreatment was described as a traumatic experience with physical, mental, and sometimes fatal consequences for children, catalyzed medical guidelines and legal policy development involving child abuse and neglect.

Child Abuse and Mandated Reporting

In 1971, the U.S. Senate established a Subcommittee on Children and Youth that increased awareness of and brought increased attention to the problem of child maltreatment (Gil 1973). That year, the California Court of Appeals determined that expert testimony about the battered child syndrome was admissible in court (*People v. Jackson* 1971). By 1973, all states had mandatory child abuse reporting laws that required various professionals, including teachers, child care workers, clergy, health care and mental health providers, and law enforcement professionals, among others, to report suspected child abuse and neglect. States that fail to enforce the statutes risk losing federal funding.

The mandated reporter's obligation to report is based on the *reasonable professional standard*—that is, what a professional of similar education, skill, and experience believes would reasonably indicate abuse or neglect of the child. In some jurisdictions, the mandated reporting requirement for child abuse and neglect also covers individuals with developmental disabilities, intellectual disabilities, or physical impairment until they turn age 21 (e.g., Ohio Revised Code § 2151.421 2016). Mandated reporters who make a good faith effort to comply with the statute receive immunity from liability, whereas those who fail to fulfill the state-mandated duty can be subjected to legal sanctions (Singley 1998). Additionally, persons who willfully or intentionally make a false report of child abuse or neglect can face criminal and civil sanctions (Child Welfare Information Gateway 2016).

A physician's obligation to recognize and treat battered child syndrome was examined in *Landeros v. Flood* (1976). In 1971, Dr. A.J. Flood, an emergency room physician, treated 11-month-old Gita Landeros for nonaccidental leg and skull fractures and bruises, injuries for which her mother proffered no explanation. Dr. Flood sent the child home, where she incurred additional injuries. Three months later, a different physician diagnosed Gita with battered child syndrome and reported the findings to child protective and law enforcement officials. Gita was removed from her mother's custody, and Gita's mother and stepfather were convicted of child abuse.

Gita's state-appointed guardian sued Dr. Flood and his employer for malpractice. The plaintiff sought to introduce expert testimony to show that Dr. Flood's management of Gita's health (including his failure to diagnose battered child syndrome and to report Gita's injuries to the appropriate authorities) fell below the standard of care and resulted in her subsequent injuries. The trial court dismissed the case. The California Supreme Court reversed the trial court's decision and held that the plaintiff's petition was actionable because the standard of care requires physicians to diagnose, treat, and report abused children to the proper authorities as a matter of law. The court also decided that medical expert testimony regarding battered child syndrome and the standard of care was admissible.

Some mandated reporters are obligated to protect children whom they suspect are being abused. However, a state's failure to protect children from abuse by third parties was not found to be a constitutional violation in *DeShaney V. Winnebago County Department of Social Services (DSS)* (1989). Randy DeShaney had full custody of his 4-year-old son Joshua, who was hospitalized due to injuries consistent with abuse. The case was reviewed by a child protection team consisting of health care, mental health care, social services, law enforcement, and legal professionals. The team formulated a care plan for Joshua that included periodic monitoring of his well-being by the DSS. Mr. DeShaney agreed to comply with the plan, the abuse charges against him were dismissed, and he was permitted to take Joshua home.

During two subsequent home visits, Joshua's DSS caseworker documented that Joshua had newer bruises and that she suspected Mr. DeShaney was not following the care plan. When the caseworker attempted a third visit, Mr. DeShaney told her Joshua was unavailable. The DSS did not recommend removal of Joshua from the home, and his injuries eventually resulted in permanent brain damage and profound mental retardation[1] for which Joshua required lifetime institutionalization.

Joshua's mother sued the DSS on her son's behalf under 42 U.S.C. §1983. This federal statute permits filing of civil actions against "state actors"—that is, persons acting with legal authority, often referred to as "acting under color of law." She alleged that the DSS deprived Joshua of his liberty interest in bodily integrity under the Fourteenth Amendment's substantive due process clause by failing to protect him from his father's aggression. The district court granted summary (or pretrial) judgment for the DSS, and the Seventh Circuit Court of Appeals affirmed the lower court's decision.

The U.S. Supreme Court affirmed the appellate court's decision. The Court held that a state does not have a constitutional obligation to protect a minor child from violence committed by a private citizen such as a parent. The Court reasoned that the substantive due process clause applies only to special classes of individuals, such as institutionalized persons, including children, who have limitations on their freedoms to act on their own behalf. Thus, because Joshua was not part of a special class, the Fourteenth Amendment did not apply in his case. Nevertheless, the Court also indicated that the DSS may have violated its duty under tort law, in states with relevant law, because the state did not provide Joshua adequate protection against his father. This left the door open for Joshua's mother to file a malpractice suit against the DSS.

States have a compelling interest in prosecuting individuals who allegedly have abused children (*Maryland v. Craig* 1990). At times, this interest conflicts with the need to protect a defendant's mental health treatment records, as was demonstrated in **State v. Andring** (1984). David Andring was voluntarily hospitalized in a mental health crisis unit after he was charged with three counts of second-degree criminal sexual conduct with minors. He admitted to the behavior during what he thought were confidential individual and group therapy sessions. Minnesota State attorneys learned about Mr. Andring's confession and moved for discovery disclosure of the medical record. The trial court granted the state access to all of the defendant's group therapy records.

Prior to trial, Mr. Andring petitioned the Minnesota Supreme Court to review the trial court's decision regarding the admissibility of his mental health records.

---

[1]Termed *intellectual disability* in the *Diagnostic and Statistical Manual of Mental Disorders*, 5th Edition [American Psychiatric Association 2013])

The Minnesota Supreme Court, considering issues related to criminal confessions and the limitations of privilege in inpatient psychiatric treatment, reversed the lower court's decision. The *Andring* court held that the physician–patient privilege under the federal Alcoholism Prevention, Treatment, and Rehabilitation Act Amendments of 1974 extends to confidential group psychotherapy sessions because they are an integral and necessary part of the patient's mental health treatment.

The court, however, also reasoned that the federal law did not preclude limited use of a patient's records in child abuse proceedings if reporting such abuse is mandated by state law. The Minnesota law mandating reporting of child abuse required reporting the name of the child, the parent or guardian, the nature and extent of the child's injuries, and the name and address of the reporter. Thus, the information mandated by Minnesota law needed to be reported, but the therapist-client privilege protected by the federal Alcohol Rehabilitation Act prohibited release of additional information, including specific information about the offenses disclosed by the perpetrator.

The federal Alcohol Rehabilitation Act affords greater federal protection for the confidentiality of substance use treatment records than for medical or mental health records to reduce privacy barriers to obtaining substance use treatment. Substance use treatment data therefore have a higher level of privilege than do mental health treatment records. Nevertheless, privilege is automatically waived in accordance with child abuse reporting statutes when children disclose that they have been abused or neglected.

In *People v. Stritzinger* (1983), the California Supreme Court reviewed the limitation of privilege in outpatient psychotherapy when the evaluee confesses to criminal behavior. In this case, 13-year-old Sarah told her mother that Sarah's stepfather, Carl Stritzinger, had been sexually abusing Sarah for 15 months. Sarah's mother suggested that Sarah and Mr. Stritzinger meet with a psychologist, Dr. Walker. Sarah disclosed the abuse to Dr. Walker, who reported it to the child welfare agency. Dr. Walker separately interviewed Mr. Stritzinger, who acknowledged abusing Sarah. Dr. Walker reluctantly disclosed Mr. Stritzinger's confession to the investigating sheriff, who insisted that therapist-client privilege did not protect the information.

Mr. Stritzinger was convicted of abusing Sarah. He appealed the decision to the California Supreme Court, which held that Mr. Stritzinger's communications with Dr. Walker were privileged and should not have been admitted at trial. The court determined that Dr. Walker had discharged the statutory duty to report Sarah's alleged abuse when he reported her statements to child welfare officials, and a second report was not necessary.

Testimonial Capacity

The stress of testifying can impede a witness's effort to convey critical information that may alter the outcome of a trial. In the United States, there is a presumption of testimonial competence and a standard for testimonial competence that must be met whenever a witness's capacity to testify is questioned. In *Wheeler v. United States* (1895), the U.S. Supreme Court determined that a boy age 5½ years was competent to take an oath and to testify as long as he understood the difference between the truth and a lie, the consequences of telling a lie, and the duty to tell the truth. In making the determination of testimonial competence, the trial judge observes the child's physical and intellectual presentation and may question the child to determine his or her intelligence, ability to communicate, and ability to understand the requirements and liability of the oath.

At times, the judge may determine that an assessment of testimonial capacity should be conducted privately *in camera* (in chambers) instead of a courtroom. The U.S. Supreme Court determined in *Kentucky v. Stincer* (1987) that a judge who conducts an *in camera* assessment of a child to determine the child's testimonial capacity is not violating the defendant's Sixth Amendment right to confront witnesses because testimonial capacity is a pretrial determination. In contrast, the standard for testimonial capacity does not take into consideration how facing the abuser during courtroom testimony may affect the child witness during and after the trial.

In *People v. Stritzinger* (1983), Mr. Stritzinger also contended in his appeal to the California Supreme Court that his Sixth Amendment Right to confront his accuser was violated because Sarah failed to testify at trial. Sarah had a history of hallucinations and self-injurious behavior and feared testifying. Sarah's mother testified that Sarah's testimony would jeopardize her mental stability. The trial court invited the state to present medical testimony to corroborate the mother's concerns; this did not occur, and Sarah did not testify. Instead, Sarah's pretrial testimony was used during the trial.

The California Supreme Court held that because Sarah's mother was not a mental health expert, her statements about Sarah's mental fitness and the potential emotional consequences of testifying were not sufficient to exclude Sarah's testimony. The *Stritzinger* court acknowledged that testimony by a victim of child abuse can be detrimental to the child's development and recovery process and suggested that expert testimony and the judge's observation of and interaction with the child can inform the court's decision regarding whether or not the child should testify.

Testifying under direct examination and cross-examination, in front of a room of strangers, while facing one's abuser can be stressful. Victims of child abuse have been exploited in relationships in which they were less powerful. They may blame themselves for the abuse, may fear for their lives (or for the safety of loved ones), and/or may not realize or accept that what happened to them was wrong. The onus of testifying sometimes can result in altered or unintelligible testimony for many reasons, including fear and stress, the desire not to upset the perpetrator, and not wanting to relive the trauma. Nevertheless, witnesses should not fear for their safety when they testify under oath.

When a state has a modified testimonial procedure to protect child witnesses of abuse, the protocol must pass constitutional muster. The U.S. Supreme Court examined this matter in *Maryland v. Craig* (1990). Maryland had a statute that permitted a child abuse victim to testify indirectly, if testimony in the direct presence of the defendant would subject the child to serious emotional distress such that it would hamper the child's communication ability and therefore the child's testimonial capacity. The prosecutor used expert witness testimony to successfully invoke this statute in the case of Sandra Ann Craig, a preschool and kindergarten operator who was the defendant in a child sexual abuse case. The child testified in the presence of the prosecutor and the defense attorney, who was in constant communication with the defendant. The child's oath, examination, and cross-examination were transmitted via closed circuit television to the courtroom, where the judge, jury, and defendant viewed them. The judge ruled on any objections. Ms. Craig was convicted of several abuse-related charges.

Ms. Craig appealed the conviction on the grounds that the proceedings violated her Sixth Amendment right to confront her accuser. The Maryland Court of Appeals reversed and remanded the case to the district court. The appellate court held that the Sixth Amendment confrontation clause was not absolute. The appellate court also determined that the trial court, prior to ruling on the Maryland statute, was required to determine whether the child would experience serious emotional stress caused by face-to-face confrontation with the defendant.

Ms. Craig then appealed to the U.S. Supreme Court, which affirmed the appellate court decision. The Court held that the state had a compelling interest in protecting child witnesses from being traumatized during testimony and in prosecuting child abusers. Maryland's procedure for indirect testimony fostered promulgation of reliable evidence as is required by the adversarial process and thus satisfied the confrontation clause of the Sixth Amendment.

Children and Legal Status

Foster Care

When caretakers fail to provide proper care for and supervision of minors, the courts may intervene to find suitable placements in the least restrictive alternative setting for the minors until matters can be remedied. Foster care placement aspires to allow children to thrive in a healthy family setting. When a child has specialized needs, such as complex medical or mental health concerns, a therapeutic foster home may be the least restrictive residential alternative for that child. Therapeutic foster parents receive additional training on how to meet the child's individualized needs, and the child receives intensive treatment interventions. Therapeutic residential placement represents the next level of care for youths who are unable to thrive in foster care placements.

Child Custody

Divorce can be stressful for children and for parents who strive to put their emotional interests aside while focusing on financial, residential, and parenting matters. When divorcing parents cannot agree on a suitable child custody plan, the matter is usually settled in family court. Custodial adjudication has come a long way since Roman law, when children were the property of their fathers, mothers had no legal rights, and fathers were given custody of the children in the case of divorce.

This state of affairs changed in the nineteenth century with the application of the so-called tender years doctrine. This English common law principle held that mothers were better suited to caring for children during a child's "tender" years (generally regarded as age 4 years and younger) (Blakesley 1981). In 1839, the British Parliament enacted the Custody of Infants Act, which instituted a presumption of maternal custody of children under age 7 years and also gave discretion to judges in child custody adjudication. In 1873, Parliament extended the presumption of maternal custody to children under age 16 years (Bookspan 1993). Exceptions were made when the father convinced the court that the mother was morally unfit.

The tender years doctrine was adopted by U.S. courts but gradually lost favor in the twentieth century as the courts began to apply the principle of child rights known as the "best interests of the child" standard (Child Welfare Information Gateway 2013a). This standard requires evaluating and balancing the specific circumstances and needs of the individual child. The best interests standard, when implemented effectively, informs adjudication of a custodial arrangement that ideally provides children with the support and guidance they need to mature into healthy, self-supporting adults. The standard leaves room for interpretation; it is sufficiently flexible to allow judges to adjust to the fluidity and inevitable changes in a child's development as well as changes in social and cultural circumstances, including consideration of what constitutes a family unit.

The best interests standard does not delineate a hierarchy of interests or suggest how evidence should be refined, interpreted, or weighed. Each individualized custodial determination should consider the preferences of the parents and the child while deemphasizing biases, including stereotypes, historical precedent, socioeconomic status, parental disability, and alternate or nontraditional lifestyles. The mental and physical health of the parents and child are factors, as are the child's developmental and psychological needs. Also, the court can distinguish between the custodial parent, with whom the child lives, and the psychological parent, with whom the child has an attachment. Additionally, the child's interactions within various systems, including family, education, community, and health care, are taken into consideration.

Child forensic psychiatrists have a challenging role in custody evaluations. They must ascertain and interpret data that may inform the retaining attorney and court about what custodial arrangements may be in the child's best interests. The evaluation proceeds more smoothly when parents objectively focus on the child's needs, but unfortunately this often does not occur. In more serious cases, one parent may engage in parental alienation, which unreasonably undermines the relationship of the child with the other parent. This is detrimental to the child and can worsen emotional problems, including mental disorders, in the child and the victimized parent. The child forensic psychiatric expert can help the court understand these dynamics and may, if so requested, make recommendations to address the problem (Sauber 2013).

The best interests standard was first adopted in *Painter v. Bannister* (1966). Harold Painter, a freelance writer and photographer, lost his wife and 2-year-old daughter in a tragic car accident. Afterward, he asked his deceased wife's parents, the Bannisters, to temporarily take custody of his 5-year-old son Mark until Mr. Painter was able to get his life back in order. Sixteen months later, Mr. Painter remarried and asked the Bannisters to return Mark, but the Bannisters would not relinquish custody. Mr. Painter filed suit in state district court and was awarded custody of his son.

The Bannisters appealed the case to the Supreme Court of Iowa, which reversed the lower court's decision. The court held that it was not in Mark's best interests to live with his father, establishing that the best interests doctrine was the legal standard for custody decisions. The court reasoned that the Bannisters, who were well educated and financially stable, provided a conventional and consistent lifestyle for Mark. Although Mr. Painter was Mark's biological parent, Mr. Bannister had become Mark's psychological parent. In making this decision, the court relied heavily on the expert testimony of a child psychologist and concluded that Mr. Painter, who had a Bohemian approach to life and negligible income, would provide Mark a life with less structure and security than the Bannisters. The *Painter* decision was controversial because Mr. Painter, although a fit parent, lost custody of his son to adults who were not Mark's biological parents.

Termination of Parental Rights

Termination of parental rights (TPR) ends the legal relationship between the parent and child, thereby rendering the child eligible for adoption. Terminating parental rights is intended to increase the likelihood of placing youths with caretakers who will meet their long-term developmental needs. TPR can be voluntary, occurring, for example, when parents decide to place a child for adoption. Involuntary TPR requires the court to sever the relationship over the parent's objection. Parents can be adjudicated unfit in cases of severe or chronic child abuse, neglect, or abandonment involving the identified child or another child in the home. Parents also may have parental rights severed for the identified child if they have involuntarily lost parental rights to another child (Child Welfare Information Gateway 2013b).

The Adoption and Safe Families Act of 1997 requires a state seeking involuntary TPR to show that it has made reasonable efforts, via implementing a social service plan, to preserve and reunify the family (Civic Impulse 1997). The social services agency must provide services to the parent(s) conducive to achieving reunification. Exceptions to this requirement are made for cases involving par-

ents who have participated in extreme torture or abandonment of the identified child or who have committed homicide of another biological child, or in other statutorily specified circumstances or situations.

The legal standard of proof for TPR was reviewed by the U.S. Supreme Court in *Santosky v. Kramer* (1982). In this case, child neglect by the Santoskys resulted in the removal of three of their children from their home in a 5-year period. Despite numerous efforts by social services staff to reunite the family, the Santoskys repeatedly failed to have supportive and meaningful interactions with their children. New York State petitioned the family court for a termination of the Santoskys' parental rights. The defendants challenged New York's "preponderance of the evidence" standard for proving permanent parental neglect and terminating parental rights. The trial court determined that the Santoskys were incapable of taking appropriate care of their children, even with supervisory intervention, and that TPR was in the children's best interests.

The Santoskys appealed to the New York Supreme Court, which affirmed the lower court decision, and to the New York Court of Appeals, which dismissed the petition. The case was reviewed by the U.S. Supreme Court, which determined that the preponderance of the evidence standard violates procedural due process protected by the Fourteenth Amendment. The Court reasoned that TPR is final and irrevocable and the preponderance standard introduces a significant risk for error that would unnecessarily destroy the family unit. Thus, the Court held that in TPR cases, due process requires application of the higher standard of clear and convincing evidence.

Notably, the clear and convincing evidence standard does not apply to Native

American children who disproportionately have been adopted by non–Native American families, often without due process or recognition of tribal customs and standards (Wills and Norris 2010). The Indian Child Welfare Act of 1978, which assigned jurisdiction of custody matters involving Native American children to tribal courts, was reviewed by the U.S. Supreme Court in *Mississippi Choctaw Indians v. Holyfield* (1989). In this case, a Native American woman who lived on a reservation tried to avoid tribal jurisdiction over the adoption of her twins by giving birth away from the reservation and allowing a non–Native American family to adopt the twins in state court. The U.S. Supreme Court held that regardless of where a Native American child is born, the tribal court has jurisdiction over the child's custody if the child or the natural parents reside on the reservation. The tribal court also has concurrent jurisdiction in other cases involving the custody of Native American children, and most of these cases can be transferred to tribal court.

Emancipation of Mature Minors

Emancipation of minors, also known as "divorcing one's parents," is a variation of TPR that in some jurisdictions can be initiated by the child (Barnett 2013). Emancipated minors are recognized as independent adults prior to the statutory age of majority. They are responsible for their finances, housing, health care, education, and safety. They can enter into contracts and can inherit, buy, and sell property. The parents of an emancipated minor are no longer obligated to provide for the child, cannot require the minor's obedience, and cannot control the minor's earnings. Emancipated minors, however, are not free to vote, consume alcohol, or drive until they reach the statutorily determined minimum legal age (National Conference of Commissioners on Uniform State Laws 2015).

Emancipation statutes exist in 32 states, each of which restricts emancipation to specific situations (Barnett 2013; Cornell University Law School 2017). For example, some states emancipate youths of a certain age so that they may independently seek medical treatment for sexual health or mental disorders. The age at which youths may seek inpatient or outpatient psychiatric care or psychotropic medication is also statutorily determined. Forensic psychiatrists should be familiar with the legal standards for youth emancipation for mental health care services in the jurisdictions in which they practice.

At times, child forensic psychiatrists may be asked to provide consultations to the court or to attorneys in emancipation cases. The best interests standard generally applies in emancipation proceedings. Emancipation may be a beneficial option for a healthy, self-sufficient youth. In contrast, emancipation may be detrimental for an adolescent whose parents pursue TPR to avoid financial responsibility (Barnett 2013).

States that allow emancipation generally require minors to show that they have residential and financial independence from their caretakers; have social, emotional, and intellectual maturity; have completed school; and are capable of making decisions about their well-being (Cornell University Law School 2017). A minor who enlists in the military or gets married is usually considered to be legally emancipated. Courts also take into consideration any extenuating circumstances, such as abuse and neglect.

Due Process and Psychiatric Hospitalization

In the managed care climate of the twenty-first century, psychiatric hospital administrators and physicians are relatively unlikely to hospitalize or warehouse psychiatrically stable minors in an effort to keep inpatient beds full. In the 1970s, however, concerned parties feared that hospitals were allowing children, whose parents or guardians sought voluntary psychiatric hospitalization for them, to be kept in psychiatric hospitals, in some cases for years, without due process. *Parham v. JR and JL* (1979), a class action lawsuit, was brought against the administrators of a state psychiatric hospital in Georgia. The plaintiffs contended that the state's voluntary hospitalization procedures for minors, which required an initial psychiatric assessment but no adversarial or fact-finding hearing by a court, violated the due process clause of the Fourteenth Amendment.

The federal district court held that the minors had a right to a hearing before an impartial fact finder at the time of hospitalization. The court was concerned that some parents might be using the hospital to avoid having to raise their behaviorally or emotionally challenging children. The case was appealed to the U.S. Supreme Court, which reversed the lower court finding and remanded the case for further review. The Court held that an objective examination by a staff psychiatrist was sufficient to ascertain if the statutory criteria for admission were met. The Court also held that periodic review of the need for continued hospitalization, which reduces the risk of error in the initial admission determination, is required. The case was remanded to the district court to determine whether sufficient periodic review had occurred.

Conclusion

Child forensic psychiatrists provide expert consultation in civil litigation involving child abuse, child custody, and child policy development that may affect the emotional well-being of minors. The skill set of a child forensic psychiatrist is suited to the challenge of conducting dispassionate developmentally informed expert examinations of children and adolescents. The need for child forensic psychiatric consultation will continue to grow in the twenty-first century. Experts should remain cognizant of advancements in medicine, technology, society, culture, and legal thinking that are salient to litigation involving the well-being of children and adolescents.

Key Concepts

- The Sixth Amendment right of an alleged child abuser to directly confront the testifying victim is not absolute.

- States do not have a constitutional obligation to protect children from abuse and neglect by third parties, but failure to do so could result in tort litigation.

- Courts use the "best interests of the child" standard in child custody litigation cases.

- Voluntary hospitalization of a minor is subject to initial and periodic review by qualified professionals and does not require an adversarial or fact-finding hearing.

- The age at which a minor may voluntarily consent to psychiatric care is statutorily determined.

- The legal standard of proof for termination of parental rights in the United States is clear and convincing evidence.

- The duty to maintain the confidentiality of a minor is automatically waived when a mandated reporter suspects that a child or adolescent has been abused or neglected.

- States may intervene on behalf of abused children to facilitate testimonial capacity.

References

American Board of Psychiatry and Neurology: Initial certification statistics. 2015. Available at: http://www.abpn.com/about/facts-and-statistics/. Accessed January 9, 2017.

American Psychiatric Association: Diagnostic and Statistical Manual of Mental Disorders, Fifth Edition. Arlington, VA, American Psychiatric Association, 2013

Barnett LC: Having their cake and eating it too? Post-emancipation child support as a valid judicial option. Chicano Law Rev 80:1799–1840, 2013

Blakesley C: Child custody and parental authority in France, Louisiana and other states of the United States: a comparative analysis. Boston College International and Comparative Law Review 283:285–359, 1981

Bookspan PT: From a tender years presumption to a primary parent presumption: has anything really changed—should it? BYU J Pub L 8:75–89, 1993

Cauthen NK, Amenta E: Not for widows only: institutional politics and the formative years of Aid to Dependent Children. Am Sociol Rev 61:427–448, 1996

Child Welfare Information Gateway: Determining the best interests of the child. Washington, DC, U.S. Department of Health and Human Services, Children's Bureau, 2013a. Available at: https://www.childwelfare.gov/pubPDFs/best_interest.pdf. Accessed January 9, 2017.

Child Welfare Information Gateway: Grounds for involuntary termination of parental rights. Washington, DC, U.S. Department of Health and Human Services, Children's Bureau, 2013b. Available at: https://www.childwelfare.gov/pubPDFs/groundtermin.pdf. Accessed January 9, 2017.

Child Welfare Information Gateway: Penalties for failure to report and false reporting of child abuse and neglect, 2016. Washington, DC, Department of Health and Human Services, Children's Bureau, 2016. Available at: https://www.childwelfare.gov/pubPDFs/report.pdf#page=2andview=Penalties%20for%20false%20reporting. Accessed January 9, 2017.

Civic Impulse: H.R. 867—105th Congress: Adoption and Safe Families Act of 1997. 1997. Available at: https://www.govtrack.us/congress/bills/105/hr867. Accessed January 9, 2017.

Cornell University Law School: WEX Legal Dictionary LII—Emancipation of Minors: Laws. 2017. Available at: https://www.law.cornell.edu/wex/table_emancipation. Accessed January 9, 2017.

DeShaney v Winnebago County Department of Social Services, 489 U.S. 189, 109 S.Ct. 998 (1989)

Gil D: Hearing before the United States Senate Subcommittee on Children and Youth on the Child Abuse Prevention Act. J Clin Child Adolesc 2:7–10, 1973

Indian Child Welfare Act of 1978 25 U.S.C. §§ 1901–63 (1978)

Kempe CH, Silverman FN, Steele BF, et al: The battered-child syndrome. JAMA 181:17–24, 1962 14455086

Kentucky v Stincer, 482 U.S. 730, 107 S.Ct. 2658 (1987)

Landeros v Flood, 17 Cal.3d 399, 551 P.2d 389 (1976)

Lindenmeyer K: A Right to Childhood: The U.S. Children's Bureau and Child Welfare, 1912–46. Champaign, IL, University of Illinois Press, 1997

Maryland v Craig, 497 U.S. 836, 110 S.Ct. 3157 (1990)

Mississippi Choctaw Indians v Holyfield, 490 U.S. 30, 109 S.Ct. 1597 (1989)

National Conference of Commissioners on Uniform State Laws: Termination of support—age of majority, 2015. Available at: http://www.ncsl.org/research/human-services/termination-of-child-support-age-of-majority.aspx. Accessed January 9, 2017.

Ohio Revised Code § 2151.421 Reporting child abuse or neglect. 2016. Available at: http://codes.ohio.gov/orc/2151.421. Accessed January 9, 2017.

Painter v Bannister, 258 Iowa 1390, 140 N.W.2d 152 (1966)

Parham v JR and JL, 442 U.S. 584, 99 S.Ct. 2493 (1979)

People v Jackson, 18 Cal. App. 3d 504, 95 Cal. Rptr. 919 (1971)

People v Stritzinger, 34 Cal. 3d 505, 668 P.2d 738 (1983)

Prince v Massachusetts, 321 U.S. 158, 64 S.Ct. 438 (1944)

Santosky v Kramer, 455 U.S. 745, 102 S.Ct. 1388 (1982)

Sauber SR: Reunification planning and therapy, in Parental Alienation: The Handbook for Mental Health and Legal Professionals. Edited by Lorandos D, Bernet W, Sauber SR. Springfield, IL, Charles C Thomas, 2013, pp 190–231

Singley SJ: Failure to report suspected child abuse: civil liability of mandated reporters. J Juv L 19:236, 1998

State v Andring, 342 N.W. 2d 128 (Minn. 1984)

Wheeler v United States, 159 U.S. 523, 16 S. Ct. 93 (1895)

Wills CD, Norris DM: Custodial evaluations of Native American families: implications for forensic psychiatrists. J Am Acad Psychiatry Law 38(4):540–546, 2010 21156915

CHAPTER 26

Evaluations of Juveniles in the Criminal Justice System

Peter Ash, M.D.

Landmark Cases

Application of Gault, 387 U.S. 1, 87 S.Ct. 1428 (1967)

Fare v. Michael C., 442 U.S. 707, 99 S.Ct. 2560 (1979) (AAPL only)

Graham v. Florida, 560 U.S. 48, 130 S.Ct. (2010)

Miller v. Alabama, 567 U.S. ___, 132 S.Ct. 2455 (2012)

Working with juveniles involved in juvenile or adult criminal court cases differs from working with adults in criminal cases. These differences arise from the developmental immaturity of juvenile defendants, from the juvenile courts' explicit mandate to provide rehabilitation for youths who come before them, and from procedural differences in both juvenile and adult courts. The vast majority of juvenile criminal cases that are referred for forensic evaluation involve adolescents; cases involving children and preadolescents are typically handled with less formal procedures.

Most forensic evaluations of juveniles have adult counterparts. Key differences are shown in Table 26–1. However, evaluations of juveniles for waivers to adult court and for the so-called "study and report," an evaluation to assist with rehabilitation treatment planning, do not have clear adult analogues. Forensic tests relevant to those evaluations are shown in Table 26–2.

TABLE 26–1.   Key differences in criminal cases involving minors in which the forensic test is the same as for adults

Issue	Difference from adult cases
Competency to waive a constitutional right (e.g., competency to confess, waive right to counsel, or plead guilty)	Developmental considerations affect whether waiver is knowing, intelligent, and voluntary.
Competency to stand trial	Incompetence in some states may be due to developmental immaturity.
Criminal responsibility	Insanity defenses are not allowed as a defense in juvenile court in many jurisdictions and are rare when adolescents are waived to adult court.
Mitigation/sentencing	Developmental considerations are highly relevant.

The large increase in adolescent juvenile violent offenses in the 1980s and early 1990s led to a heightened concern about public safety and a trend toward treating adolescent offenders more like adults, as clarified by the comment, "do the crime, do the time." The spate of juvenile mass murders in school settings in the 1990s further exacerbated public safety concerns about violent adolescents and led to the adoption of new state statutes and procedures that had the effect of moving more youth into the adult criminal justice system.

As it became clear in the 2000s that the juvenile crime rate had dropped significantly from its height in 1993, the pendulum began to swing in the opposite direction, exemplified in legal changes that emphasized that adolescents were different from adults, having less competence, less culpability, and less developmentally mature judgment.

Prearrest Evaluations

Adolescents in Treatment

Evaluations of minors who seek the services of a psychiatrist in a treatment context but who are in a situation that may lead to arrest need to be approached carefully. Sometimes, a parent may take a youth to a psychiatrist because the parent suspects the child has been involved in conduct that may lead to arrest. For example, if a father takes an adolescent to a psychiatrist because he suspects his son has sexually abused a child, the clinician owes a duty to the minor as his or her patient, not to the police. Although the evaluation is confidential, the psychiatrist will have an obligation to notify child protective services if he or she forms a reasonable suspicion that child abuse took place. Thus, the clinician should inform both the father and the patient of this duty prior to asking about material that may lead to such a report.

The psychiatrist who anticipates that a juvenile might be arrested should recommend strongly that the parent obtain the services of an attorney for the child, if such action has not yet been taken. The psychiatrist should seriously consider deferring the clinical evaluation until an attorney has been retained or appointed. In most cases, psychiatrists should not ask anything about the circumstances of an alleged crime until they have a clear sense of what questions the attorney will ask. Following this course of action will help the psychiatrist avoid the possibil-

TABLE 26–2. **Forensic child and adolescent cases without clear adult analogues: delinquency**

Issue	Typical forensic test
Study and report	What mental health issues are relevant in rehabilitating and planning a disposition for the delinquent?
Waiver to adult court	What is the risk of future dangerousness and amenability to rehabilitation?

ity that the psychiatric evaluation will be used to incriminate the patient.

In addition, if no attorney has been obtained or appointed, the psychiatrist should discuss with the parent what to do if the youth is questioned by the police. Without giving legal advice, the psychiatrist should help the parent and adolescent understand their options and some of the possible consequences of cooperating with the police. As is the case for any criminal suspect, talking to the police without first consulting with an attorney is seldom in the youth's best interest.

Once a youth has an attorney, the psychiatrist can be helpful to the patient by working with the attorney. The authorities have wide discretion in juvenile cases in regard to the charge (e.g., manslaughter rather than murder) and disposition (e.g., probation with conditions rather than incarceration). This discretion includes whether to arrest the youth at all. Rapid institution of treatment may decrease the likelihood of arrest. A skilled attorney can have considerable impact on the course of a case by negotiating with the authorities without resorting to formal criminal procedures. A youth's attorney can often make effective use of mental health information and treatment plans in such negotiations.

The cautions about obtaining incriminating information, mentioned above, become even more imperative when the youth is unaccompanied by a parent. For example, a general psychiatrist providing coverage to an emergency department may become involved in a case when the police accompany a distressed, just-arrested youth, to an emergency room. The psychiatrist should provide limited treatment for acute distress (assuming appropriate informed consent can be obtained); however, the psychiatrist should keep in mind that any information obtained during evaluation and treatment may not remain confidential. Clinicians unfamiliar with juvenile criminal processes all too often begin an interview in the emergency room by asking, "What happened?" They then might obtain highly incriminating information that later gets passed along, formally or informally, to law enforcement. Even if the obtained information remains privileged, legal consequences may follow from the fact that the youth has told a narrative of events without a clear understanding of the implications of doing so. For example, the youth might believe that he or she has already "confessed," after talking to the clinician, and therefore be ready to repeat the story to the police before obtaining the advice of counsel ("After all, I already told the doctor what happened…").

School Threat Assessments

Mass shootings (defined here as involving three or more murders with no cooling off period in between) by students in

K–12 schools generate enormous amounts of media coverage and grave concerns about school safety. Although there had been isolated incidents of multiple killings involving targeted victims (e.g., a student angry with a teacher) and fights at school that resulted in multiple deaths, the first mass shooting in the United States by a K–12 student during school hours involving random victims occurred in Moses Lake, Washington, in 1996 (Wikipedia 2017). In the next 3 years, six additional incidents were committed by students in K–12 schools, culminating with the shooting in Littleton, Colorado, in which 15 individuals were killed and 21 wounded. Research on these incidents in the late 1990s and on incidents of mass shootings by nonstudents found no clear profile of a school shooter that prospectively identified the killers. The one commonality found was that all shooters had told others of their plan but were not taken seriously (Ash 2016). This finding led schools to strongly urge students and staff to report any threat, and the resulting heightened surveillance has led to more evaluation of threats and a marked reduction in episodes of school shootings.

Threat evaluation research has grown largely out of law enforcement work focused on adults, but similar principles likely apply to adolescents. Many psychiatrists tend to think about the assessment of potential violence as similar to the assessment of suicidal thinking, with its emphasis on identifying risk factors, violent ideation, and plan. However, such evaluations have been recognized to be fairly ineffective in predicting planned predatory violence. For example, the most robust general risk factor for future violence, a history of past violence, has not been found in school shooters (Vossekuil et al. 2002). Threat evaluation has moved away from profiling the subject toward

evaluating pathways that lead to violent action. Such evaluations focus less on the characteristics of the subject and more on any recent behavior that suggests the subject is moving on a path toward violence.

Because individuals frequently deny planning predatory violence, other indicators of violent thinking are important. A key concept in these evaluations is "leakage": fantasies of thinking and planning violence that may spill out in identifiable ways. These can include, for example, communicating a fascination with weapons and assassinations with peers, writing in diaries, drawing pictures, Internet chatting on violence-related themes, and making veiled threats to peers.

Federal law enforcement agencies have developed threat assessment procedures for schools (Vossekuil et al. 2002). These approaches emphasize that an attack is the consequence of an understandable and discernible process of thinking and behavior. In evaluating a pathway toward violence, actions that indicate planning, such as practice with a weapon or surveillance of a victim, are especially worrisome. A youth will frequently deny planning violence in interviews. Therefore, collateral information, particularly from peers, is vital.

The best way to obtain a comprehensive picture of recent student actions involves working as part of a team with school personnel and law enforcement. Many school districts have established multidisciplinary threat assessment teams, which include school personnel, law enforcement, and mental health clinicians, to evaluate threats. A lone clinician should be very cautious, once a serious threat has been made, about concluding that the risk of violence is low based solely on findings from an individual interview. Findings from a psychiatric evaluation need to be integrated with information from other sources to develop an assessment of the level of risk and a prevention plan.

Waiving Constitutional Rights: *Miranda* Warnings and Confessions

Many states require that a parent or legal guardian be present before a minor can be interrogated. However, parents who have raised their child to be honest and admit mistakes may advise their children to confess to the police. In all U.S. jurisdictions, a detained youth must be given a *Miranda* warning before an interrogation. Younger adolescents may cognitively understand what a *Miranda* warning is but are nevertheless more likely to waive their rights and confess than are older adolescents or adults unless special precautions are used to assure that the youth understands (Grisso 2013). Juveniles may also misunderstand what it takes to assert their *Miranda* rights.

In *Fare v. Michael C.* (1979), 16-year-old Michael, who was already on probation, was implicated in a murder. During interrogation, after receiving his *Miranda* warnings, he asked for his probation officer, someone he knew and trusted, instead of a lawyer. This request was denied. On appeal, the California Supreme Court held that Michael's request to see his probation officer at the commencement of interrogation negated any possible willingness on his part to discuss his case, and therefore further interrogation violated his Fifth Amendment right against self-incrimination. On further appeal the U.S. Supreme Court held that a juvenile asking for his probation officer is not the same as asking for a lawyer

and therefore Michael's request was not an assertion of his *Miranda* rights.

Although a majority of adolescents have a basic understanding when read a *Miranda* warning, a majority of 11- to 15-year-olds have significant deficits in appreciating the importance of their right against self-incrimination (Viljoen et al. 2007). Further complicating assessment of youths' understanding of their rights are the facts that jurisdictions vary in how *Miranda* warnings are worded and that such evaluations are typically retrospective, often occurring considerably after arrest and after a youth has had discussions with his or her attorney. After individuals waive their *Miranda* rights, pressured interrogations are considerably more likely to lead to false confessions by youths than by adults (Malloy et al. 2014).

Juvenile Court

The Illinois Juvenile Court Act of 1899 first established juvenile courts. Chicago Juvenile Judge Julian Mack, an early proponent of juvenile courts, described their purpose as follows: "To get away from the notion that the child is to be dealt with as a criminal; to save it from the brand of criminality, the brand that sticks for life; to take it in hand and instead of first stigmatizing and then reforming it, to protect it from the stigma—this is the work which is now being accomplished by dealing even with most of the delinquent children through the court that represents the *parens patriae* power of the state, the court of chancery [juvenile court]" (Mack 1909, p. 109).

The juvenile court model caught on, and within several decades practically all states had juvenile courts. Minor defendants' criminal due process rights were traded for rehabilitation. Lawyers were seen as unnecessary because the juvenile court system was not an adversarial system. Treatment plans were to be made by psychologists and psychiatrists, who were becoming more mainstream. Rehabilitation would prevent youth from becoming adult criminals.

Many historians trace the beginning of child psychiatry to the forces set in motion by that 1899 Juvenile Court Act. In Chicago, a group of women on the board of directors of Jane Addams's Hull House wanted to investigate the causes of juvenile delinquency, and in 1909 they established the Juvenile Psychopathic Institute, with "its avowed object being to investigate, to ascertain if possible, the causes of delinquency in children" (Patrick 1915). Dr. Healy, its first director, was a neurologist interested in studying the delinquents' brain functioning, and the board, which included Jane Addams and the juvenile judge Julian Mack, was interested in delinquents' personalities and the effects of social factors. Healy formed multidisciplinary teams to study these multiple facets. The institute was the first child guidance clinic and set the pattern for later such clinics to follow. Child psychiatry thus began in the community, rather than in medical schools, with colleagues who were more likely to be teachers, judges, and social workers than physicians (Schowalter 2003).

By the mid-1960s, the mental health community had developed an increasing sense of hopelessness regarding delinquency, feeling that "nothing worked" (U.S. Department Health and Human Services 2001). The U.S. Supreme Court was increasingly attending to defendants' rights, holding in *Gideon v. Wainwright* (1963) that indigent defendants had the right to an attorney, and holding in *Miranda v. Arizona* (1966) that adult defendants needed to be informed of their right against self-incrimination and their right to an attorney before interrogation. In 1966, the Court found that juveniles had to be granted a hearing before being waived to adult criminal jurisdiction, stating that "there may be grounds for concern that the child receives the worst of both worlds: that he gets neither the protections accorded to adults nor the solicitous care and regenerative treatment postulated for children" (*Kent v. United States* 1966). A year later, the Supreme Court decision in ***Application of Gault*** (1967) recognized that juvenile courts functioned very much as criminal courts and juvenile defendants required a number of criminal due process protections. Gerald Gault, age 15, was taken into custody without parental notification after a neighbor complained that Gault made an offensive phone call. After coming home from work and not finding Gault, his mother located him at the local juvenile detention facility. At trial a week later, Gault, without a lawyer, was sentenced to a juvenile industrial school until he turned age 21. His accuser did not appear in court. On appeal, the U.S. Supreme Court, in an 8–1 decision, held that Gault's constitutional rights had been violated because he had been denied the right to an attorney, had not been formally notified of the charges against him, had not been informed of his right against self-incrimination, and had no opportunity to confront his accusers. Subsequent court decisions brought most other adult criminal due process requirements (except trial by jury) to juvenile procedures, but rehabilitation remains a primary mission of the juvenile court.

State laws, which vary considerably, govern which cases are heard in juvenile court; there are no federal juvenile courts. Status offenses—those actions that would not be crimes if committed by adults—include running away, truancy, curfew violations, and incorrigibility (being beyond the control of one's parents). Delinquency cases are those cases that would be prosecuted in adult criminal court if the offense had been committed by an adult. A juvenile who commits a serious offense may be waived to adult criminal court (see section "Waivers to Adult Court" later in this chapter). In 2013, juvenile courts handled about 109,000 status offense cases and about 10 times as many delinquency cases (Hockenberry and Puzzanchera 2015).

Status Offenses

In some states, status offense cases are heard in family court, but in an increasing number of states, status offenses are processed in social service agencies or family crisis agencies rather than courts. In many cases that begin with a petition in juvenile court, youth are diverted out of the juvenile court system to such agencies for treatment or case management. Those status cases heard in juvenile or family court may result in a youth being found, depending on the jurisdiction, as a "person in need of supervision," a "child in need of supervision," or a somewhat more expanded category, a "child in need of services." The Juvenile Justice and Delinquency Prevention Act of 1974, which set federal standards for state juvenile courts, prohibits incarceration of status offenders in detention facilities. In 2013, about 44% of petitioned cases were adjudicated as status offenses; of the offenders in those cases, 54% were put on probation, and 8% were sent to out-of-home placements (Hockenberry and Puzzanchera 2015).

The most common mental health evaluation ordered by judges in status offense cases is the "study and report," which is intended to assist in formulating a disposition. A *study and report* is a general psychological evaluation that often includes psychological testing and concludes with recommendations for mental health and psychosocial interventions. If the defendant youth was in treatment prior to arrest, the treating clinician may be contacted to provide collateral information.

Competency to Stand Trial

Juveniles have generally been presumed incompetent in many contexts (e.g., voting, ability to enter into a contract). As recently as the beginning of the twenty-first century, only a handful of states required juveniles to be competent to stand trial in juvenile court. Since then, through statutes and court decisions, all states have come to require that juveniles be competent to stand trial. State statutes vary with regard to many factors, including whether immaturity constitutes grounds for incompetency, whether different standards for competency exist depending on the severity of the offense, whether different procedures are allowable (e.g., pausing the proceedings to provide education to the juvenile defendant about what is occurring), and what qualifications are required of juvenile examiners.

Lower age and lower intelligence are two robust factors in predicting incompetence to stand trial. About half of adolescents below age 15 years are estimated to be sufficiently limited as to be considered incompetent (Grisso et al. 2003). Below-average intelligence amplifies the effects of lower age, and studies of juvenile justice populations suggest that the mean IQ of this population is below 85, or, in one study, in the 70s (Ficke et al. 2006). Although adolescents of normal intelligence who are ages 15 and older tend to perform about as well as adults of normal intelligence on most competency measures, the high percentage of older juvenile defendants who have below-average intelligence serves to increase the likelihood that such a defendant is incompetent.

Other developmental factors may also affect competence through their effects on adolescent judgment, particularly in making decisions about whether to take a plea offer or go to trial. Adolescents, compared with adults, tend to give less weight to risk and more weight to immediate rewards when compared to long-term consequences. Adolescents also are more susceptible to pressure and influence from peers (see section "Adolescents Waived to Adult Criminal Court" later in this chapter). Although in many respects the assessment of competence in a juvenile is similar to the evaluation of an adult (see Chapter 18, "Evaluation of Competencies in the Criminal Justice System"; Mossman et al. 2007), the developmental differences call for increased attention to aspects of adolescent judgment. In those states that allow developmental immaturity to be a basis for a finding of incompetency, explaining the basis for a finding of incompetency often requires an analysis of the juvenile defendant's development.

Although a forensic psychiatric or psychological examination is the best way to assess competence in a particular case under a jurisdiction's rules, competence assessment instruments may provide useful additional information. The Mac-Arthur Competence Assessment Tool—Criminal Adjudication (MacCAT-CA; Otto et al. 1998), originally developed for adults, has some comparative data for adults and juveniles (Grisso et al. 2003). The Juvenile Adjudicative Competence Interview (JACI; Grisso 2005) more specifically attempts to assess adolescents' developmental problems in decision making.

Insanity Evaluations in Juvenile Court

Insanity pleas are far less common in cases involving adolescents than in cases involving adults. Because psychotic disorders are found less frequently in adolescents than in adults, relatively few adolescent defendants have a psychotic illness that would provide the grounds for an insanity defense based on mental illness. Because one of the missions of juvenile court is rehabilitation, those adolescents with a mental illness sufficient to substantiate an insanity plea typically have a treatment plan for their mental illness as part of their disposition. In part, for this reason, only a minority of states allow insanity pleas in juvenile court (Pollock 2001).

Treatment Following Adjudication

A general psychiatrist who accepts a patient for whom psychiatric treatment is made a condition of probation may be required to share certain information that would normally be confidential. The treating clinician should have a clear understanding with both the probation officer and the patient regarding the nature of the information that will be provided to the probation officer. Clinicians vary in how they structure such understandings.

As a general rule, clinicians treating adult patients on probation can attempt to maintain the confidentiality by making clear that they will only advise the probation officer whether the patient is attending sessions and whether the psychiatrist believes treatment is completed. The patient should also be advised that if payment for treatment sessions is not made, the patient will not be seen and this will be reported to the probation officer as nonattendance. The clinician treating a juvenile may wish to broaden this stance to some degree. A juvenile probation officer often can be a useful ally in assisting the clinician to obtain court and community services for a patient. The psychiatrist may appreciate being able to release to the probation officer information that will justify additional services.

Waivers to Adult Court

When minors are arrested on serious criminal charges involving serious violent crimes, they may be waived to adult court. State laws govern which of the three general types of waiver will apply to an individual case.

1. *Judicial waivers* are those in which a hearing is conducted before a juvenile court judge, who will typically consider the nature of the crime, the likelihood of future dangerousness, and the youth's amenability to rehabilitation in deciding whether to move the case to adult court.
2. *Direct file* or *prosecutorial waivers* allow the prosecutor to decide in certain cases (e.g., murder committed by a youth over a certain age) to move the case to adult court.
3. *Mandatory* or *legislative waivers* derive from statutes which, based on the defendant's age and the charge, automatically waive the youth to adult court. Waiver statutes typically take this form: "Youth over the age of X, who are charged with one of the following offenses..., may [or shall] be waived to adult court if..."

Practically all states have some form of judicial waiver. The U.S. Supreme Court has held that a judge cannot waive a youth without a hearing (*Kent v. United States* 1966). In response to the upsurge in juvenile crime in the early 1990s, many states adopted direct file or mandatory waivers such that by the end of 2004, a majority of states had such provisions (Snyder and Sickmund 2006). As stated in the previous section, "Juvenile Court," there are no federal juvenile courts: minors arrested on a federal charge have a hearing before a federal district court judge to determine whether they should be prosecuted in federal district court as an adult or remanded to a state juvenile court.

Waiver hearings often use mental health evaluations to assist the judge in making a determination. Judges have considerable discretion as to what factors they consider and how they weigh each factor. The statutory criteria for waiver to federal court (Delinquency Proceedings in District Courts, 2011) are typical of the factors considered and include the age and social background of the juvenile, the nature of the alleged offense, the extent and nature of the juvenile's prior delinquency record, the juvenile's present intellectual development and psychological maturity, the nature of past treatment efforts and the juvenile's response to such efforts, and the availability of programs designed to treat the juvenile's behavioral problems. The increase in mandatory waivers has led to a marked decrease in the number of judicial waivers: in 2011, only 0.4% of defendants who had originally been petitioned in juvenile court were *judicially* waived to adult court (Hockenberry and Puzzanchera 2014).

Adolescents Waived to Adult Criminal Court

If a youth is waived to adult court, the full panoply of adult criminal processes comes into play, including issues of competency to stand trial and insanity or other diminished capacity defenses. Insanity defenses are rare in waived youths because, as noted, the incidence of psychosis is considerably lower in adolescents than in adults and also because severe mental illness provides a strong basis to not waive a youth to adult jurisdiction.

Sentencing

In a series of four decisions since 2005, the U.S. Supreme Court has found that adolescents as a class are less culpable than adults who have committed similar serious crimes. These decisions have markedly changed the landscape regarding sentencing adolescents tried in criminal court for serious offenses. In *Roper v. Simmons* (2005), the Court found that the death penalty constituted cruel and unusual punishment for minors and was thus unconstitutional for all crimes committed by a youth under age 18 (see Chapter 20, "Psychiatry and the Death Penalty"). The Court found that adolescent culpability was reduced because 1) adolescents are developmentally immature, more impulsive, and more likely to respond to peer pressure; 2) some adolescent criminal behavior is affected by adverse environmental circumstances (e.g., their living environment and parents) that they cannot escape; and 3) adolescent character is not fully developed so an adolescent's actions do not reflect enduring character traits. The Court in *Roper* did not explicitly cite the burgeoning research on adolescent brain development; however, this research has served as a basis for an understanding of greater impulsivity among adolescents and is frequently brought up in testimony in adolescent sentencing hearings.

In *Graham v. Florida* (2010), 16-year-old Terrance Graham was arrested for armed burglary and a lesser offense, was waived to adult jurisdiction, and accepted a plea bargain that involved probation but withheld adjudication of guilt. Less than 6 months later, he was arrested for other crimes. The second arrest constituted a probation violation, so a resentencing hearing was held on the initial armed burglary. Despite the fact that both the defense and the prosecution recommended sentences of less than 6 years, the judge gave Graham the maximum sentence of life imprisonment. Because Florida had eliminated parole, the sentence constituted life without parole (LWOP). On appeal, Graham challenged his LWOP sentence as a violation of the Eighth Amendment's prohibition against cruel and unusual punishment. The U.S. Supreme Court, using a culpability analysis similar to that in *Roper*, found that a sentence of LWOP for youth under age 18 was unconstitutional for all crimes less than murder.

In *Miller v. Alabama* (2012), the Court found that even in a case of murder committed by an adolescent, a *mandatory* LWOP sentence was unconstitutional, but that an LWOP sentence could be imposed following a sentencing hearing, although the Court expressed its view that LWOP sentences for adolescents should be rare. The *Miller* ruling left unclear what would happen to those adolescents who had previously received a mandatory LWOP sentence. However, the Court ruled in *Montgomery v. Louisiana* (2016) that *Miller* applies retroactively to all minors sentenced to mandatory LWOP. Therefore, the approximately 2,500 adolescents who were serving mandatory LWOP sentences (Human Rights Watch 2008) that were handed down prior to *Miller* had to be either resentenced or afforded a parole hearing.

The legal principles regarding reduced culpability for adolescents have led to an increase in forensic mental health input into sentencing adolescents (and also

---

TABLE 26–3. **Factors to consider in evaluating adolescent culpability**

Factors pertaining to insanity defenses

Mental illness or mental defect

Appreciation of wrongfulness

Ability to conform to law

Factors pertaining to reduced culpability

Immaturity

    Impulsivity

    Susceptibility to peer pressure

    Risk taking

    Time sense, overweighting immediate rewards compared to long-term costs

    Limited ability to empathize

    Incomplete brain development

    IQ and adaptive functioning

Environmental circumstances

Adverse environmental factors, history of abuse and neglect

Peer group norms

Personality factors

Incomplete personality development

Psychopathy

Out-of-character action

Nature of the crime

Degree of fit with patterns of adolescent crime as opposed to patterns of adult crime

Seriousness of the crime and harm done

Reactive attitudes toward the offense

Other prognostic factors

Future dangerousness

Amenability to rehabilitation

Malingering

Source. Adapted from Ash 2012.

young adults) for serious crimes. In evaluating a particular juvenile defendant, the evaluator should examine the relationship between general factors that may reduce adolescent culpability and the fact situation in a particular case. For example, impulsivity and peer pressure effects are likely to be relevant mitigating factors in a fact pattern in which a group of adolescents was in the process of committing a burglary, the homeowner unexpectedly returned home, one of the adolescents happened to have a handgun, and that adolescent felt threatened and shot the homeowner. In contrast, a fact pattern may rule out mitigating factors such as impulsivity and peer pressure, even if the youth was known to have attention-deficit/hyperactivity disorder and some history of impulsivity. Such might be the case, for example, if an adolescent was angry at his ex-girlfriend's new boyfriend; he announced to friends that he was "going to get him," and his friends tried to dissuade him; but he then stalked the new boyfriend for a week until he found him alone, at which time he shot him. Ash (2012) provides an analysis of factors most relevant to assessing culpability (Table 26–3).

Conclusion

Changes in crime rates, legal principles, and court procedures have brought about significant changes in the nature of criminal forensic work with youth. School threat assessment protocols have come into being; competency evaluations for juvenile courts that once were rare are now routine; and testimony on adolescent culpability, bolstered by major advances in understanding adolescent brain development, is common and relies heavily on neurobiological findings that were unknown 20 years ago. While evaluations of youthful defendants bear many similarities to evaluations of adults, the changing legal landscape and increased appreciation of the effects of developmental immaturity have led to juvenile forensic work being an exciting, rapidly evolving field.

Key Concepts

- In evaluations of youth likely facing imminent arrest, the evaluator should be cautious about encouraging the youth to provide potentially incriminating information.

- Evaluations of students who have made moderate or serious threats of violence at school often utilize a team approach that includes school personnel, law enforcement, and mental health evaluation, and the data gathered should include collateral information from peers and school.

- The rehabilitative mission of the juvenile court broadens the usefulness of mental health input when compared to adult criminal procedures.

- Status offenses—that is, offenses that would not be crimes if committed by an adult (e.g., running away and school truancy)—are increasingly being handled through social service agencies rather than by juvenile courts.

- Evaluations of an adolescent's competency to stand trial differ from similar evaluations of adults in their added focus on issues of developmental immaturity.

- The courts have provided legal analyses of why adolescents as a class are less culpable for serious violent offenses than adults who commit similar crimes.

References

Application of Gault, 387 U.S. 1, 87 S.Ct. 1428 (1967)

Ash P: But he knew it was wrong: evaluating adolescent culpability. J Am Acad Psychiatry Law 40(1):21–32, 2012 22396338

Ash P: School shootings and mental illness, in Gun Violence and Mental Illness. Edited by Gold LH, Simon RI. Arlington, VA, American Psychiatric Association Publishing, 2016, pp 105–126

Delinquency Proceedings in District Courts; Transfer for Criminal Prosecution. 18 U.S.C. § 5032, 2011. Available at: https://www.gpo.gov/fdsys/granule/USCODE-2010-title18/USCODE-2010-title18-partIV-chap403-sec5032. Accessed January 10, 2017.

Fare v Michael C., 442 U.S. 707, 99 S.Ct. 2560 (1979) (AAPL only)

Ficke SL, Hart KJ, Deardorff PA: The performance of incarcerated juveniles on the MacArthur Competence Assessment Tool—Criminal Adjudication (MacCAT-CA). J Am Acad Psychiatry Law 34(3): 360–373, 2006 17032960

Gideon v Wainwright, 372 U.S. 335, 83 S.Ct. 792 (1963)

Graham v Florida, 560 U.S. 48, 130 S.Ct. (2010)

Grisso T: Evaluating Juveniles' Adjudicative Competence: A Guide for Clinical Practice. Sarasota, FL, Professional Resource Press, 2005

Grisso T: Forensic Evaluation of Juveniles, 2nd Edition. Sarasota, FL, Professional Resource Press, 2013

Grisso T, Steinberg L, Woolard J, et al: Juveniles' competence to stand trial: a comparison of adolescents' and adults' capacities as trial defendants. Law Hum Behav 27(4):333–363, 2003 12916225

Hockenberry S, Puzzanchera C: Delinquency Cases Waived to Criminal Court, 2011 (Report No NCJ 248410). Washington, DC, U.S. Department of Justice, Bureau of Justice Statistics, 2014

Hockenberry S, Puzzanchera C: Juvenile Court Statistics 2013. Pittsburgh, PA, National Center for Juvenile Justice, 2015

Human Rights Watch: The Rest of Their Lives: Life Without Parole for Youth Offenders in the United States in 2008. New York, Human Rights Watch, 2008

Juvenile Justice and Delinquency Prevention Act, Pub. L. No. 93–415, 42 U.S.C. § 5601 et seq, 1974, reauthorized, 2002

Kent v United States, 383 U.S. 541, 86 S.Ct. 1045 (1966)

Mack JW: The juvenile court. Harv Law Rev 23:104–122, 1909

Malloy LC, Shulman EP, Cauffman E: Interrogations, confessions, and guilty pleas among serious adolescent offenders. Law Hum Behav 38(2):181–193, 2014 24127891

Miller v Alabama, 567 U.S. ___, 132 S.Ct. 2455 (2012)

Miranda v Arizona, 384 U.S. 436, 86 S.Ct. 1602 (1966)

Montgomery v Louisiana, 577 U.S. __, 136 S.Ct. 718 (2016)

Mossman D, Noffsinger SG, Ash P, et al; American Academy of Psychiatry and the Law: AAPL Practice Guideline for the forensic psychiatric evaluation of competence to stand trial. J Am Acad Psychiatry Law 35(4)(Suppl):S3–S72, 2007 18083992

Otto RK, Poythress NG, Nicholson RA, et al: Psychometric properties of the MacArthur Competence Assessment Tool–Criminal Adjudication. Psychol Assess 10:435–443, 1998

Patrick HT: The Juvenile Psychopathic Institute of Chicago. JAMA LXIV:71–72, 1915

Pollock ES: Those crazy kids: providing the insanity defense in juvenile courts. Minn Law Rev 85:2041–2078, 2001

Roper v Simmons, 543 U.S. 551, 125 S.Ct. 1183 (2005)

Schowalter JE: A history of child and adolescent psychiatry in the United States. Psychiatric Times, September 1, 2003. Available at: http://www.psychiatrictimes.com/articles/history-child-and-adolescent-psychiatry-united-states. Accessed January 10, 2017.

Snyder HN, Sickmund M: Juvenile Offenders and Victims: 2006 National Report. Washington, DC, Office of Juvenile Justice and Delinquency Prevention, 2006

U.S. Department Health and Human Services: Youth Violence: A Report of the Surgeon General. Rockville, MD, U.S. Department Health and Human Services, 2001

Viljoen JL, Zapf PA, Roesch R: Adjudicative competence and comprehension of Miranda rights in adolescent defendants: a comparison of legal standards. Behav Sci Law 25(1):1–19, 2007 17285585

Vossekuil B, Fein R, Reddy M, et al: The Final Report and Findings of the Safe School Initiative: Implications for the Prevention of School Attacks in the United States. Washington, DC, U.S. Department of Education, Office of Elementary and Secondary Education, Safe and Drug-Free Schools Program and U.S. Secret Service, National Threat Assessment Center, 2002

Wikipedia: List of school shootings in the United States, 2017. Available at: https://en.wikipedia.org/wiki/List_of_school_shootings_in_the_United_States. Accessed May 21, 2017.

PART VII

Special Issues in
Forensic Psychiatry

CHAPTER 27

Suicide Risk Assessment

Liza H. Gold, M.D.
Kaustubh G. Joshi, M.D.

When retained in professional liability cases involving patient suicide, forensic evaluators have to provide testimony regarding whether defendant psychiatrists met the standard of care. Appropriate suicide risk assessment (SRA) and treatment interventions based on the level of risk are essential elements of this determination. Although failure to perform an adequate SRA is rarely the only claim of professional negligence made when patients commit suicide, patient suicide is one of the leading causes of professional liability suits against psychiatrists. Since 2006, suicide and attempted suicide have accounted for 15% of malpractice claims in the United States (see Table 12–1 in Chapter 12, "Professional Liability in Psychiatric Practice") (Professional Risk Management Services 2016).

Patient suicide is not necessarily the result of poor treatment or treatment errors, even when these represent deviations from the standard of care. Additionally, patients who receive appropriate and timely treatment may ultimately commit suicide. Nevertheless, whether a patient's suicide occurs in a hospital or in the community, failure to evaluate suicide risk appropriately is a common allegation in professional negligence claims (Scott and Resnick 2012).

SRA and management of suicide risk are core competencies expected of all mental health professionals (Accreditation Council for Graduate Medical Education 2016; Jacobs et al. 2003). In suicide malpractice cases, plaintiffs often claim that the treating psychiatrist failed to meet the standard of care by multiple acts of commission and/or omission. As the gateway to effective treatment, SRA can decrease the risk of suicide. Competent treatment and safety management of potentially suicidal patients is guided by the identification of modifiable or treatable acute, high-risk suicide factors as well as available protective factors (Simon 2012a). Forensic psychiatrists should be familiar with elements that constitute comprehensive SRAs and the appropriate treatment utilization of these assessments in order to provide expert testimony in suicide malpractice cases.

Suicide Risk Assessment: Evidence-Based Evaluations

As in any type of professional malpractice case, the plaintiff bears the burden of proving that the defendant psychiatrist's treatment did not meet the standard of care (see Chapter 12). Conducting SRAs is a core professional competency because patients' treatment needs are best served by assessing levels of suicide risk based on identification and mitigation of risk factors rather than by attempting to predict suicide. Fortunately, despite the relative frequency of suicide deaths, absolute rates of suicide are low. Unfortunately, predicting low-base-rate events is an inherently unreliable endeavor that results in a high number of false-positive predictions (Swanson 2011).

SRA is a process that identifies evidence-based suicide risk factors and protective factors. The gathered data are then synthesized into a clinical formulation of foreseeable risk of suicidal behavior (Jacobs et al. 2003; Silverman 2014; Simon 2012a). The level of risk dictates the need for and types of treatment interventions. Systematic SRA is therefore critical to clinical decision making, safety planning and management, triage decisions, treatment planning regarding voluntary or involuntary hospitalization, and overall risk management (Silverman and Berman 2014; Simon 2012b).

SRA is a process, not an event. A single assessment may have to suffice for a patient in an emergency room, where treatment options may be limited to broad interventions such as hospitalization. In contrast, a patient with major depressive disorder and alcohol use disorder in outpatient treatment will require repeated assessments, particularly in the context of psychosocial stressors or before changes in treatment, such as decreasing the frequency of therapy sessions.

Malleable risk factors identified and prioritized in SRAs include evidence-based acute or short-term risk factors, chronic or long-term risk factors, and protective factors. Short-term risk factors are those found prospectively and statistically significant within 1 year of assessment. These include panic attacks, anxiety, loss of pleasure or interest, agitated depression, decreased concentration, and insomnia. Long-term risk factors are those associated with completed suicides 2–10 years following assessment. They include suicidal ideation, suicide intent, severe hopelessness, and prior attempts. Protective factors, or those factors that decrease risk of suicide, include close, supportive family relationships; treatment compliance; and others (Jacobs et al. 2003).

The distinction between risk factors and warning signs is important when evaluating risk of suicide. A *suicide risk factor* is a factor empirically demonstrated to correlate with suicide, regardless of when it first becomes present. The presence of chronic or long-term risk factors, such as a history of past suicide attempts and major depressive disorder, establishes lifetime vulnerability to suicide risk. In contrast, *suicide warning signs* are the earliest detectable signs that indicate acute heightened risk for suicide. Warning signs such as giving away possessions or calling people to say good-bye, some of which are also short-term risk factors, provide observable markers consistent with potentially increased intent. The presence of one or more warning signs is indicative of acutely increased suicide risk, regardless of the presence or absence of suicide risk factors that confer lifetime vulnerability (Berman and Silverman 2014; Rudd 2014).

Forensic clinicians should bear in mind that no single risk factor is pathognomonic for suicide. A single suicide risk factor, or even a combination of risk factors, does not have the statistical significance on which to base an overall risk assessment due to the low absolute risk of suicide (Jacobs et al. 2003; Simon 2012b). In addition, no SRA method can reliably identify who will die by suicide (sensitivity) and who will not (specificity) (Simon 2012a). Not everyone with a psychiatric disorder has suicidal thoughts or behaviors, and two people with the same psychiatric diagnosis will have varying degrees of risk for suicide. Finally, evaluators should bear in mind that an individual's level of suicide risk can change rapidly and often without notice (Simon 2012a).

A detailed review of all risk and protective factors and the strength of the empirical evidence behind them is beyond the scope of this chapter. Nevertheless, familiarity with some of the most important static and dynamic risk factors and protective factors is essential to an analysis of whether a defendant psychiatrist has conducted an adequate SRA.

Demographics of Suicide

Suicide, which most often occurs in the context of psychiatric illness and/or substance use, is a serious public health problem in the United States (Centers for Disease Control and Prevention 2016a). Suicide has been the tenth or eleventh leading cause of death overall in the United States for at least the last decade (Centers for Disease Control and Prevention 2016b). In 2014, a total of 42,773 people died by suicide, resulting in an annual age-adjusted suicide rate of 12.93 per 100,000 (Centers for Disease Control and Prevention 2016b). From 1999 through 2014, the age-adjusted suicide rate among men and women of all ethnic groups under age 75 increased 24%, from 10.5 to 13.0 per 100,000 population, with a greater pace of increase after 2006 (Curtin et al. 2016).

Demographic information generally identifies static rather than dynamic risk factors but nevertheless is a major component of an SRA. Suicide rates vary by sex, ethnicity, and age. Men accounted for 78% of all suicides in 2014 (Centers for Disease Control and Prevention 2016b). Although women make suicide attempts three times more often than men, the male-to-female ratio of suicide deaths is 3.4:1. In 2014, the suicide rate among men was 21.1 per 100,000; among women, the rate was 6.0 (American Association of Suicidology 2016). White men have the highest rates of suicide (24.1 per 100,000 in 2014), about 3.5 times the rate of white women (6.9 per 100,000). Native Americans have the second highest rate of suicide, 10.8 per 100,000 in 2014; African American women have the lowest rates, at 2.1 per 100,000 (American Association of Suicidology 2016).

Suicide is most common in the elderly and in adolescents and young adults. Men age 75 and older have the highest rates of suicide, at 38.8 per 100,000, followed by men ages 45–64, with a suicide rate of 29.7 per 100,000, an increase in this group of 43% since 1999 (Centers for Disease Control and Prevention 2016b). Of male attempters age 65 or older, 31.6% complete suicide (Bostwick et al. 2016). Suicide is the second leading cause of death for adolescents and young adults, with rates of 11.6 per 100,000 for those ages 15–24 in 2014 (American Association of Suicidology 2016; Centers for Disease Control and Prevention 2016b).

Other groups at high risk of suicide are also identifiable by demographic information. For example, suicide is the second leading manner of death, after accidents (including traffic accidents), among U.S. service members (Corr 2014). Additional groups with higher suicide risk include individuals who are widowed, divorced, or single (Centers for Disease Control and Prevention 2016b); veterans (U.S. Department of Veterans Affairs 2012); persons with particular occupations (e.g., agricultural workers, physicians, veterinarians, attorneys) (Milner et al. 2013); gay, lesbian, transgender, or bisexual populations (Haas et al. 2011); and persons with disabilities or chronic pain (Arsenault-Lapierre et al. 2004; Betz et al. 2016).

Psychiatric Illness and Substance Use

Beyond demographics, the strongest individual risk factors for suicide are psychiatric disorders and substance use disorders (Ilgen et al. 2008). The presence of a psychiatric disorder is among the most consistently reported risk factors for suicidal behavior (Nock et al. 2008). Up to 90% of individuals who commit suicide have a diagnosable psychiatric disorder at the time of death, most commonly depression or substance abuse (Cavanagh et al. 2003; Nock et al. 2008). One meta-analysis (Arsenault-Lapierre et al. 2004) found that, on average, approximately 87% of individuals who committed suicide had a mental disorder, and persons who committed suicide were more likely to have symptoms that met criteria for more than one psychiatric diagnosis.

Affective, substance-related, personality, and psychotic disorders account for most of the diagnoses among suicide completers (Arsenault-Lapierre et al. 2004). Of these, mood disorders are most common, followed closely by alcohol use disorders, with highest risk for individuals with both affective disorders and alcohol use disorders (Arsenault-Lapierre et al.

2004; Cavanagh et al. 2003). Suicide is one of the leading types of injury mortality linked with alcohol consumption (Conner et al. 2014). Individuals with alcohol dependence who come to clinical attention are at approximately nine times higher risk of completed suicide compared with the general population (Kaplan et al. 2013).

Acute use of alcohol in the hours preceding suicidal behavior, regardless of the presence of an alcohol use disorder, is also highly correlated with suicide and is a powerful independent risk factor beyond the risk conferred by chronic alcohol use (Dahlberg et al. 2004; Kaplan et al. 2013). An analysis of the National Violent Death Reporting System data found that alcohol was present at the time of death in one-third of suicides by firearms, hangings, and poisonings (Conner et al. 2014). These three methods constitute over 90% of suicide deaths in the United States. Moreover, blood alcohol concentration levels in suicide decedents were high, with the mean exceeding 80 mg/dL, the legal limit for drinking and driving (Conner et al. 2014).

Notably, firearm suicide decedents had the highest mean levels of blood alcohol concentration compared with hanging or poisoning suicide decedents (Conner et al. 2014). Individuals who had any level of acute alcohol consumption were 5.9 times as likely to commit firearm suicide as those who had no acute alcohol consumption, and in cases of excessive acute alcohol consumption, 77.1 times more likely to commit firearm suicide (Branas et al. 2011).

Suicide Attempts, Suicidal Ideation, and Suicidal Behavior

A prior history of a suicide attempt is considered one of the most robust predictors of eventually completed suicide. Approximately 60% of individuals complete suicide on their first attempt; however, of those who survive a first attempt, 80% of subsequent completed suicides occur within a year of the initial attempt (Bostwick et al. 2016). Risk of suicide, although highest in the first 12 months after a first attempt, is present to a lesser but still significant degree over 5 years (Beautrais 2003) and 10 years (Coryell and Young 2005).

Suicidal ideation and related behaviors, including warning signs and preparation or rehearsal, are also among the most significant suicide risk factors. Evidence of suicide preparation or rehearsal was found to be associated with a significant risk of suicide over a 10-year follow-up period (Coryell and Young 2005). The National Comorbidity Survey found that approximately 90% of unplanned suicide attempts and 60% of planned first attempts occurred within 1 year of the onset of suicidal ideation (Kessler et al. 1999). The probability of transitioning from suicidal ideation to suicidal plan was 34%; the probability of transition from a plan to an attempt was 72% (Kessler et al. 1999).

Therefore, when conducting SRAs, clinicians should consider frequency, specific content, intensity, duration, and prior episodes (Berman and Silverman 2014; Rudd 2014; Simon 2012b). Inquiries into whether the patient has rehearsed or practiced an attempt and about patterns of impulsive behaviors should be documented. Nonspecific suicidal thoughts that have no associated subjective or objective intent and that are fleeting or of short duration are not evidence of risk escalation beyond an individual's chronic baseline level (Rudd 2014; Simon and Gold 2016). However, the presence or absence of suicidal thinking is not a particularly good indicator of escalating sui-

cide risk, particularly when individuals have a history of multiple attempts and/or chronic suicidal ideation (Rudd 2014; Simon 2012b).

Impulsive Suicide and Adverse Life Events

Although suicidal ideation and planning are major risk factors for suicide, many suicide attempts also demonstrate a strong component of impulsivity. For example, the majority of studies of impulsivity and suicide have found an absence of proximal planning or abruptness of attempt in over 50% of cases (Rimkeviciene et al. 2015). Seventy-five percent of attempts occur within 3 hours or less from the time of initial suicidal ideation, planning, or decision to the suicide act. The length of time from first thought to the suicide act has been found to be as little as a few minutes to a few hours (Ilgen et al. 2008; Shenassa et al. 2004; Simon et al. 2001; Yip et al. 2012). The absence of proximal planning and the suddenness of a suicide attempt are associated with the absence of mental disorder, the presence of fewer comorbid conditions, and the presence of alcohol use disorders (Rimkeviciene et al. 2015).

Adverse life events are common precursors to suicide and suicide attempts, particularly after recent alcohol consumption (Powell et al. 2001) and particularly among adults with compromised coping skills such as alcohol use disorders or psychiatric or psychological vulnerabilities (Hawton 2007; Nock et al. 2008; Owens et al. 2003). Examples of such events include loss of a significant relationship, financial or employment setbacks, involvement in legal or disciplinary problems, or perceived public shame or humiliation. In vulnerable individuals, an adverse event may lead to a suicide attempt within a relatively short period of time. Owens et al. (2003) found that half of all suicide decedents suffered at least one adverse life event in their final month of life, most commonly involving relationships, money, and work.

Transient personal crises also can create considerable emotional distress. Combined anger and impulsivity are a combination of traits related to suicide and suicidal behavior, irrespective of diagnosis (Fawcett 2012). Intense negative emotions, specifically anger, rage, shame, and guilt, which may arise quickly in a crisis situation, can lead to an unplanned suicide attempt (Rimkeviciene et al. 2015). Suicidal ideation among impulsive attempters may be more transient and temporary than that experienced by persons with chronic depression (Simon et al. 2001). Notably, however, as the acute phase of a crisis passes, the urge to commit suicide often decreases (Deisenhammer et al. 2009; Miller and Hemenway 2008; Miller et al. 2012; Yip et al. 2012).

Protective Factors

Although less research is available regarding factors that protect against suicide, such factors are critically important because they can decrease the probability of a fatal outcome. Protective factors, like risk factors, vary with the clinical presentation of the individual patient at risk (Simon 2012b), and SRAs should include questions about a patient's reasons for living. Arguably, the most important protective factor is accessible and available family and/or other social supports. Treatment engagement and compliance is also an essential protective factor (Simon and Gold 2016).

Additional examples of protective factors include sense of family responsibility, pregnancy, child-related concerns (Gold 2012), religious beliefs, cultural sanctions against suicide, and a positive

therapeutic relationship with a treatment provider (Nock et al. 2008; Simon 2012b). Notably, having a follow-up appointment scheduled on discharge from either the emergency department or an inpatient service, whether or not the appointment is actually kept, appears to be strongly protective, significantly reducing the risk of dying on a subsequent attempt (Bostwick et al. 2016). Nevertheless, in any individual, a delicate balance may exist between suicide risk and protective factors. Acute high suicide risk may override factors that might otherwise be protective (Berman and Silverman 2014; Simon 2012b).

Suicide Risk Assessment Methodology

Data Collection

No single method for conducting a standardized SRA has been widely agreed on or adopted by a professional organization. A variety of SRA models are available and may be effectively used in systematic SRA (Simon 2012b). All include systematic inquiries and review of demographic risk factors, short-term and long-term risk factors, and the individual's unique risk factors and protective factors (Simon 2012b). Table 27–1 provides a summary of the methods used to collect the data needed for SRA. Of course, not all this information will be available in every case.

Many clinicians continue to rely on unaided clinical judgment based on clinical interview alone in assessing suicide risk. Although clinical experience and judgment are an essential part of SRA, greater experience does not necessarily result in better judgment or improved competence (Berman and Silverman 2014; Silverman

2014). Unaided and unstructured clinical judgment and intuition are highly subject to error and are especially vulnerable to the influence of personal social biases (Simon 2012a).

Many clinicians also rely on structured or semi-structured checklists, which generally list suicide risk factors and sometimes list protective factors. A checklist of risk and protective factors can prompt clinicians to systematically review all relevant factors. Important risk and protective factors are easily overlooked in the absence of systematic assessment (Simon 2012a). However, such checklists alone are also not effective SRA methodologies (Homaifar et al. 2013; Jacobs et al. 2003; Simon 2012b). Checklists are overly sensitive and lack specificity. None of them have been tested for reliability and validity (Silverman 2014; Silverman and Berman 2014; Simon 2009). In addition, checklists cannot encompass all the relevant risk factors present for a given patient (Simon 2012b).

Clinicians may also rely on patient self-surveys asking about suicidal ideation and history. Patient self-report instruments cannot be considered adequate SRA methodology. Patients at risk for suicide, particularly individuals with strong intent, may deny having suicidal thoughts or plans or may conceal or minimize recent or past suicidal behaviors (Nock et al. 2008; Rudd 2014; Silverman 2014; Simon 2012a).

Collateral information may be key, particularly when a patient denies suicidal ideation, intent, or plans. Family members should be consulted if possible, because they may be aware of changes in behavior or warning signs that the patient does not report (Simon 2012b). Additional collateral information can be obtained from the medical record, the patient's medical and mental health providers, friends, and possibly other sources,

such as police records (Silverman and Berman 2014; Simon 2012b) (Table 27–1).

The use of combined methodology increases opportunities for capturing significant information. For example, because suicidal ideation, suicide intent, and suicide planning may be difficult for some patients to disclose directly, the inclusion of self-report measures provides a potential opportunity for detecting thoughts of suicide (Silverman and Berman 2014). Empirically identified risk and protective factors associated with suicide, organized into domains with some descriptive explanations and specifiers, are listed in a sample checklist in Table 27–2. This list, like any SRA checklist, should be considered an aid or a guide to a thorough clinical assessment intended to encourage and facilitate systematic assessment.

Competently performed SRAs reflect that clinicians have used a systematic method of gathering essential data and attempted to gather from multiple sources. Attempting to obtain all necessary information from one source is likely to result in an incomplete assessment. Routine, systematic SRAs should combine semi-structured tools, self-report surveys, and the clinical interview. Semi-structured screening instruments complement and improve routine clinical assessments and can provide support and corroboration for a well-conducted clinical SRA (Silverman 2014; Silverman and Berman 2014; Simon 2009, 2012b).

Data Synthesis

The assessment of overall suicide risk involves an understanding of how risk factors interact, resulting in a heightened or lowered risk of suicide (Berman and Silverman 2014; Simon 2012a, 2012b). As a general rule, suicide risk increases with the emergence of distinct warning signs,

TABLE 27–1.   **Suicide risk assessment methodology: gathering the data**

Identify distinctive individual suicide risk factors.

Identify acute suicide risk factors.

Identify protective factors.

Evaluate medical history, including laboratory data if available.

Obtain information from other clinical care providers such as primary care providers.

Interview patient's significant others.

Speak with current or prior mental health treatment providers, including, if inpatient, treatment team.

Review patient's current and prior hospital records.

Source.   Adapted from Simon 2012a.

increases in symptom severity and complexity, and the presence of associated suicidal behaviors such as preparation, rehearsals, or attempts (Rudd 2014). Many risk factors are not simply present or absent but are present in varying degrees of severity. In addition, certain factors may contribute to risk in some individuals but not in others or may be relevant only when they occur in combination with particular psychosocial stressors (Jacobs et al. 2003). The clinician's judgment is central in identifying and assigning clinical weight to the risk and protective factors identified through systematic assessment (Berman and Silverman 2014; Simon 2012b).

Clinicians should then consider treatment interventions targeted at specific modifiable risk factors. Static and immutable factors, such as demographic characteristics or historical data, are important to identify for purposes of assessing overall risk. However, these cannot be changed and therefore are not useful as targets for treatment interventions. Modifiable and treatable suicide risk factors should be identified as early as possible and treated aggressively. For example, anxiety, depression, insomnia, and psychosis may respond rapidly to medications as well as psychosocial in-

terventions. Clinicians should also identify, support, and, when possible, enhance protective factors. Psychosocial interventions, for example, can help a patient mobilize or reinforce existing social supports (Jacobs et al. 2003; Rudd 2014; Simon 2012b).

The accuracy of any SRA decreases over time as circumstances and clinical risk factors change. Most individuals with suicidal ideation have varying levels of ambivalence about committing suicide. Suicide intent can increase with accumulation of stressors or decrease as effective interventions are implemented. Consequently, SRAs need to be repeated according to the clinical needs of the patient, particularly when a treatment decision, such as discharge from inpatient treatment, is considered (Jacobs et al. 2003; Silverman and Berman 2014; Simon 2012b).

Risk factors, protective factors, and overall suicide risk are weighted on a dimensional scale of low, moderate, or high risk (Berman and Silverman 2014; Rudd 2014; Simon 2012b). Although dimensional rating scales are not precise, most clinicians caution practitioners against relying on models based on quantifiable scores (Berman and Silverman 2014; Simon 2009; Wortzel et al. 2013). Numerical scoring systems are arbitrary

TABLE 27–2.   **Sample checklist: suicide risk assessment factors**

Domain	Specific risk factor
I. Predisposition to suicidal behavior	❏ History of psychiatric diagnoses (including substance abuse): higher risk with recurrent disorders, comorbidity, chronicity
	❏ History of suicidal behavior: higher risk with previous attempts, high lethality; considered chronic risk if two or more attempts have been made
	❏ Recent discharge from inpatient psychiatric treatment: high risk in first year after discharge, higher in first month after discharge, highest during first week after discharge
	❏ Demographic considerations: age, gender, ethnicity
	❏ History of sexual, physical, or emotional abuse
II. Identifiable precipitants or stressors (most can be conceptualized as losses)	❏ Financial
	❏ Interpersonal relationship(s) and relationship instability (loss of social support)
	❏ Professional, identity
	❏ Acute or chronic health problems (can be loss of independence, autonomy, or function)
III. Symptomatic presentation	❏ Depressive symptoms, highest risk associated with comorbid anxiety and substance abuse symptoms
	❏ Bipolar disorder, highest risk early in course of disorder
	❏ Anxiety, especially acute agitation
	❏ Schizophrenia, especially in time periods following active phases
	❏ Borderline and antisocial personality features
IV. Hopelessness	❏ Severity
	❏ Duration
V. Nature of suicidal thinking and behaviors	❏ Current ideation: frequency, intensity, and duration
	❏ Presence of suicidal plan, increased risk with specificity
	❏ Availability of means (consider multiple methods)
	❏ Lethality of means, including both medical and perceived lethality
	❏ Active suicidal behaviors, including preparation and rehearsal behaviors
	❏ Suicide intent, with subjective and objective markers (warning signs)
VI. Previous suicide attempts (and nonsuicidal self-injury)	❏ Frequency
	❏ Perceived lethality and outcome
	❏ Opportunity for rescue and help seeking
	❏ Preparatory behaviors (including rehearsal)
	❏ Reaction to previous attempts (feelings about survival and lessons learned)

TABLE 27–2.   **Sample checklist: suicide risk assessment factors** *(continued)*

Domain	Specific risk factor
VII. Impulsivity and self-control	❑ Subjective self-control
	❑ Objective control (e.g., substance abuse, impulsive behaviors, aggression)
VIII. Presence of suicide warning signs	❑ Active suicidal thinking
	❑ Preparation and rehearsal behavior
	❑ Hopelessness
	❑ Anger
	❑ Recklessness, impulsivity, dramatic mood changes
	❑ Anxiety and agitation
	❑ Feeling trapped
	❑ No reasons for living, no purpose in life
	❑ Increased alcohol or substance abuse
IX. Protective factors	❑ Presence and accessibility of social support
	❑ Problem-solving skills, history of coping skills
	❑ Active participation in treatment
	❑ Presence of hopefulness
	❑ Children present in the home
	❑ Pregnancy
	❑ Religious commitment
	❑ Life satisfaction
	❑ Intact reality testing
	❑ Fear of social disapproval
	❑ Fear of suicide or death

Source.   Adapted from Rudd 2014.

and idiosyncratic, and create an illusion of scientific accuracy that can be misleading (Simon 2009).

Low risk is generally characterized by mild psychiatric symptoms with no associated suicidal intent or features. Moderate risk emerges as symptoms escalate, warning signs start to emerge, and evidence of subjective intent is identified. High risk is characterized by four primary elements: serious psychiatric symptoms, the presence of active intent (subjective or objective), the presence of warning signs, and limited protective factors. Once objective evidence of suicide intent is identified, such as preparation and rehearsal behaviors, a high-risk designa-

tion is more likely to be assigned (Rudd 2014).

Treatment Planning

Treatment planning for patients at risk of suicide should be organized around minimizing risk factors and maximizing protective factors. Whether a patient is treated on an inpatient or outpatient basis, risk of suicide will fluctuate over time. As noted above, SRAs will need to be repeated, particularly when a patient's psychosocial circumstances change significantly or a change in a patient's treatment plan is being considered.

Higher versus lower levels of assessed risk carry greater imperatives for aggressive treatment planning, triage, and intervention (Berman and Silverman 2014). For example, hospitalization is indicated when suicide risk is high and patients present an acute danger to themselves. Patients who refuse collaborative hospitalization may require involuntary hospitalization. Depending on other factors, such as family support or severity of symptoms, moderate- or low-risk patients might require the increased structure and support of an intensive outpatient or day-treatment program; others might benefit more from interventions such as increased medication or attendance at substance use abstinence programs.

Means Restriction

Because suicide is a behavior that is both preventable and multidetermined, many interventions can potentially decrease the number of suicide deaths. However, only two interventions have been empirically demonstrated to be effective in decreasing suicide mortality: mental health treatment and restriction of lethal means (Mann and Michel 2016; Mann et al. 2005; Miller and Hemenway 2008). The latter is relevant to this text. Reducing access to highly lethal and commonly used suicide methods decreases rates of suicide (Mann and Michel 2016; Miller et al. 2016a). When SRAs are able to identify specific plans and means that suicidal individuals intend to use to end their lives, treatment interventions should include consideration of restricting access to lethal means.

Although interventions regarding means restriction for patients at risk of suicide are not necessarily means specific, access to firearms deserves special consideration. First, firearms are the most common means of suicide in the United States (American Association of Suicidology 2016). Between 2003 and 2013, firearm suicide consistently accounted for over 50% of suicide deaths, more than double the number of the next most common method, suffocation (including hanging) (Centers for Disease Control and Prevention 2016b). In contrast, firearms account for only 4.5% of suicides in other high-income countries (World Health Organization 2014). The likelihood that a specific method of suicide will lead to death is related to its accessibility (Yip et al. 2012). Rates of civilian firearm ownership are higher in the United States than in any other high-income country (Graduate Institute of Geneva 2007). Approximately one-third of all U.S. households report having at least one gun in the home (Krouse 2012; Swanson et al. 2015).

Second, firearms are the most lethal means of suicide, with a case fatality ratio of 83%–91% (Miller et al. 2016a). The case fatality ratio for suicide by suffocation is 66%–84%; for drug poisoning (including intentional overdose), the case fatality rate is 2%. Firearm suicide is significantly more common among men (42.8% of all suicide deaths in 2014, compared to only 7% among women) (Centers for Disease Control and Prevention 2016b). Nevertheless, although women are less likely than men to use firearms to commit suicide, when they do, they are equally likely to die (Bostwick et al. 2016).

Third, substantial evidence indicates that, unlike access to other means of suicide, the presence of firearms in the home is associated with significantly increased risk of suicide (Anglemyer et al. 2014; Brent et al. 2013; Miller et al. 2016b). In contrast, rates of suicide from methods other than firearms are not correlated with rates of household firearm ownership (Miller et al. 2016b). The association between higher rates of overall suicide and firearm suicide and higher rates of gun ownership is independent of psychopathology (Betz et al. 2011; Ilgen et al. 2008; Miller et al. 2012, 2013).

Means restriction is all the more important for individuals who have survived a first suicide attempt. As discussed above (see subsection "Suicide Attempts, Suicidal Ideation, and Suicidal Behavior"), a history of a suicide attempt confers significantly elevated risk of suicide in the 12 months following the attempt. Restricting access to lethal means during this time can substantially decrease risk. In addition, the majority of individuals who survive a suicide attempt do not go on to die by suicide. Studies have consistently demonstrated that over time, less than 10% of suicide attempt survivors go on to die by suicide (Owens et al. 2002). Although these low rates may be an underestimate of the rate of subsequent suicide deaths in survivors of attempts (Bostwick et al. 2016), even doubling or tripling the rates indicates that a substantial number of individuals who survive a first attempt will not go on to die by suicide.

Despite the common belief that individuals who are intent on committing suicide and who lack access to their preferred means will find another means to commit suicide, most studies have demonstrated that restriction of one method does not inevitably lead to substitution of another means (Yip et al. 2012). In addition, when method substitution occurs, particularly if the preferred method would have been firearms, chances of surviving a suicide attempt increase (Conner and Zhong 2003) because other methods are less lethal (Miller et al. 2016a).

Reducing the availability of lethal means during a crisis can prolong the period between the decision to commit suicide and the suicidal act. This provides time during which suicidal impulses and intent may decrease and opportunities to access assistance increase, thereby averting fatal outcomes (Miller et al. 2016a; Yip et al. 2012). Initiatives targeted at reducing access to guns in attempts to reduce rates of suicide are relatively new; outcome studies are limited. Nevertheless, the data indicating that reducing availability and access to firearms have lowered suicide rates are robust (Mann and Michel 2016).

Because firearms are highly available, highly lethal, and commonly used in suicide, evaluators conducting SRAs should specifically ask about access to firearms. Important inquiries include whether the patient owns guns, has access to guns owned by someone else, and has plans to purchase any firearms (Simon 2012a; Wintemute et al. 1999). If a suicidal patient has access to firearms, regardless of the presence or absence of other risk factors, steps should be taken to separate the individual at risk from the firearms. Psychiatrists can work with high-risk patients and their families or support networks to remove firearms from a patient's immediate environment, even if temporarily (Simon and Gold 2016).

SRA inquiries about access to means should not be limited to firearms. Other types of individual- and population-type means restrictions have been suggested and variously implemented (see Lester 2012). For example, clinicians who have concerns about individual patients committing suicide by overdosing on their prescribed medications may limit the quantity of medications dispensed at any one time or have collaboratively allowed willing family members to maintain control of the patient's medication supplies. Population-based forms of means restrictions, such as placing fences or barriers on bridges and other high structures, have also been implemented, with evidence of reducing mortality rates (see, e.g., Beautrais 2007).

Suicide and Professional Liability

Patient suicide is an unavoidable occupational hazard in psychiatric practice. "A clinical axiom states that there are three kinds of psychiatrists: 1) those who have had a patient die by suicide, 2) those who will have a patient die by suicide, and 3) those who will have more than one patient die by suicide" (Simon 2012b, p. 555). The distress clinicians experience when a patient commits suicide may be compounded by concerns that a professional malpractice claim based on their treatment of a deceased patient will be brought against them.

Just as treatment errors do not necessarily result in a patient's suicide, a patient's suicide does not necessarily result in professional liability claims. However, when suicides do result in malpractice claims, such claims generally are brought under theories of negligence, including the following (Simon 2012b):

- Failure to diagnose the patient's condition properly
- Failure to assess suicide risk adequately
- Failure to implement an appropriate treatment plan using reasonable treatment interventions and safety precautions

Evidence of the clinician's failure to conduct an SRA or to intervene in a manner indicated by the level of risk can be used to demonstrate required elements in a negligence claim, including "deviation" from the standard of care and "dereliction of duty" that "directly" resulted in the patient's death (see Chapter 12).

The forensic evaluations in such claims often turn on whether the treating clinician conducted reasonable SRAs and whether the patient's suicide attempt or suicide was foreseeable. *Foreseeability* is a legal term meaning "the quality of being reasonably anticipatable" (Garner 2014, p. 764). Foreseeability is not equivalent to predictability or preventability. Although clinicians cannot predict or prevent a patient's suicide, a reasonable clinical basis exists for assessing the patient's suicide risk. The assessment of suicide risk is determinable and, therefore, foreseeable (Simon 2012b).

Medical malpractice cases require that plaintiffs demonstrate deviation from the standard of care (see Chapter 12). In claims involving completed suicides, certain factors are reviewed to determine whether the actions of the psychiatrist met the standard of care in treating the deceased patient. These include the following (Frierson 2007):

- Adequate identification and evaluation of risk and protective factors
- A reasonable treatment plan developed on the basis of the patient's clinical needs
- Appropriate implementation and modification of the treatment plan based on ongoing clinical assessment
- The psychiatrist's level of current knowledge in the assessment and treatment of suicidal patients
- Adequate documentation in the record to support that appropriate care was provided

The *standard of care*, a legal concept defined by state law, is the standard measure applied to negligence claims. The standard of care is determined by expert testimony, practice guidelines, the psychiatric literature, hospital policies and procedures, and other authoritative sources (Simon 2012b). Experts retained by both plaintiff and defense provide testimony regarding the practice of a reasonable physician and whether the defendant provided care that was consistent with such practice.

Many psychiatrists continue to rely on "suicide prevention contracts" as interventions that mitigate the risk of suicide. No evidence indicates that such contracts prevent suicide (Edwards and Sachmann 2010). In fact, suicide prevention contracts may increase patients' risk for suicide by falsely reassuring clinicians, who may then fail to conduct SRAs and make therapeutic interventions (Simon 2012b; Wettstein 2017). These contracts may also increase risk of liability, because such contracts establish that the patient is a suicide risk but do not establish that the risk has been assessed. No-suicide contracts cannot substitute for repeated SRAs and treatment planning and do not protect psychiatrists from liability. If used, no-suicide contracts should be adjuncts to comprehensive evaluations, ongoing SRA, and safety management planning (Simon 2012b).

Documentation

Forensic psychiatric evaluations in suicide malpractice cases rely on available documentation of the patient's treatment. Documentation of SRAs that inform treatment and management interventions substantiates the defendant psychiatrist's clinical judgment and supports arguments that the defendant psychiatrist provided good patient care (Simon 2012b).

Failure to document SRAs does not cause patient suicide; however, failing to provide such documentation is, of itself, a deviation from standard of care and can support plaintiffs' arguments of negligence. When SRAs and treatment interventions are not documented, courts are less able to evaluate the clinical complexities and ambiguities inherent in the assessment, treatment, and management of patients at risk for suicide (Simon 2012a). Documentation limited to "patient denies HI, SI, CFS" (homicidal ideation, suicidal ideation, contracts for safety), often found in record reviews in suicide malpractice cases, does not serve as a substitute for documentation of an adequate SRA (Simon 2012a).

Documentation that supports defense arguments that appropriate care was provided should include ongoing and repeated assessment, treatment, and safety management decisions. It should reflect consideration of factors that increase risk; factors that mitigate risk; treatment interventions and the outcome of those interventions; changes in circumstances that affect level of risk or treatment planning; and discussions with the patient and family regarding risk and steps that can be taken to mitigate risk. Documentation of consultation with colleagues can also support a defendant psychiatrist's position (Simon 2012a, 2012b).

Documentation that includes a patient's comments indicating decreased suicide risk can also support defense arguments. In addition, patient quotes often carry significant weight with jurors (Frierson 2007). In contrast, changes made by defendant psychiatrists to the medical records after a patient commits suicide create significant suspicion as a suicide malpractice case goes to trial.

Conclusion

Expert testimony in suicide malpractice cases requires forensic clinicians to understand that competent SRAs are an essential element in determining whether a defendant psychiatrist's treatment met the standard of care. Psychiatrists cannot predict suicide; they are, however, required to assess the risk of suicide through systematic SRA and to implement a treatment plan to mitigate risk of suicide through interventions appropriate and proportional to the level of risk. SRAs should routinely include consideration of means restrictions, particularly when patients have access to firearms. Contemporaneous documentation of SRAs, treatment, and intervention outcomes in mitigating suicide risk represents both good clinical care and evidence that a defendant psychiatrist's treatment met the standard of care despite the unfortunate outcome of patient suicide.

Key Concepts

- Expert testimony is required to establish the standard of care in suicide malpractice cases. An expert's determination of whether a defendant psychiatrist's treatment of a patient who later committed suicide requires a familiarity with the principles and utilization of suicide risk assessments (SRAs).

- SRAs do not predict suicide; rather, they represent assessment of evidence-based risk and protective factors, which, when taken together, provide identification of low, moderate, or high risk of suicide.

- A single SRA is typically not sufficient; adequate use of SRAs reflects a defendant psychiatrist's understanding that SRA is a process, not an event, and should occur prior to significant treatment interventions, especially those that affect patient safety, such as inpatient discharge.

- Treatment interventions should be based on identification of dynamic risk factors as well as protective factors that can be put into place or increased.

- Failure to document SRAs does not cause suicide; however, evaluation of whether the treatment provided met the standard of care is more difficult when contemporaneous documentation is unavailable or when documentation has been altered after the patient's suicide.

References

Accreditation Council for Graduate Medical Education: ACGME Program Requirements for Graduate Medical Education in Psychiatry, 2016. Available at: http://www.acgme.org/Portals/0/PFAssets/ProgramRequirements/400_psychiatry_2016.pdf?ver=2016-09-30-123700-277. Accessed April 25, 2017.

American Association of Suicidology: Facts and statistics, 2016. 2016. Available at: http://www.suicidology.org/resources/facts-statistics. Accessed January 11, 2017.

Anglemyer A, Horvath T, Rutherford G: The accessibility of firearms and risk for suicide and homicide victimization among household members: a systematic review and meta-analysis. Ann Intern Med 160(2): 101–110, 2014 24592495

Arsenault-Lapierre G, Kim C, Turecki G: Psychiatric diagnoses in 3275 suicides: a meta-analysis. BMC Psychiatry 4:37, 2004 15527502

Beautrais AL: Subsequent mortality in medically serious suicide attempts: a 5-year follow-up. Aust NZ J Psychiatry 37(5): 595–599, 2003 14511088

Beautrais A: Suicide by jumping. Crisis 28(Suppl 1):58–63, 2007 26212196

Berman AL, Silverman MM: Suicide risk assessment and risk formulation, part II: suicide risk formulation and the determination of levels of risk. Suicide Life Threat Behav 44(4):432–443, 2014 24286521

Betz ME, Barber C, Miller M: Suicidal behavior and firearm access: results from the second injury control and risk survey. Suicide Life Threat Behav 41(4):384–391, 2011 21535097

Betz ME, Wintersteen M, Boudreaux ED, et al: Reducing suicide risk: challenges and opportunities in the emergency department. Ann Emerg Med 68(6):758–765, 2016 27451339

Bostwick JM, Pabbati C, Geske JR, et al: Suicide attempt as a risk factor for completed suicide: even more lethal than we knew. Am J Psychiatry 173(11):1094–1100, 2016 27523496

Branas CC, Richmond TS, Ten Have TR, et al: Acute alcohol consumption, alcohol outlets, and gun suicide. Subst Use Misuse 46(13):1592–1603, 2011 21929327

Brent DA, Miller MJ, Loeber R, et al: Ending the silence on gun violence. J Am Acad Child Adolesc Psychiatry 52(4):333–338, 2013 23571100

Cavanagh JT, Carson AJ, Sharpe M, et al: Psychological autopsy studies of suicide: a systematic review. Psychol Med 33(3):395–405, 2003 12701661

Centers for Disease Control and Prevention, National Center for Injury Prevention, Division of Violence Prevention: Suicide prevention: a public health issue. 2016a. Available at: http://www.cdc.gov/violenceprevention/pdf/asap_suicide_issue2-a.pdf. Accessed January 11, 2017.

Centers for Disease Control and Prevention: Injury prevention and control: data and statistics (WISQARS). 2016b. Available at: http://www.cdc.gov/injury/wisqars/index.html. Accessed January 11, 2017.

Conner KR, Zhong Y: State firearm laws and rates of suicide in men and women. Am J Prev Med 25(4):320–324, 2003 14580634

Conner KR, Huguet N, Caetano R, et al: Acute use of alcohol and methods of suicide in a U.S. national sample. Am J Public Health 104(1):171–178, 2014 23678938

Corr WP 3rd: Suicides and suicide attempts among active component members of the U.S. Armed Forces, 2010–2012; methods of self-harm vary by major geographic region of assignment. MSMR 21(10):2–5, 2014 25357138

Coryell W, Young EA: Clinical predictors of suicide in primary major depressive disorder. J Clin Psychiatry 66(4):412–417, 2005 15816781

Curtin SC, Warner MA, Hedegaard H: Increase in suicide in the United States, 1999–2014. April 2016. Available at: http://www.cdc.gov/nchs/products/databriefs/db241.htm. Accessed January 10, 2017.

Dahlberg LL, Ikeda RM, Kresnow MJ: Guns in the home and risk of a violent death in the home: findings from a national study. Am J Epidemiol 160(10):929–936, 2004 15522849

Deisenhammer EA, Ing CM, Strauss R, et al: The duration of the suicidal process: how much time is left for intervention between consideration and accomplishment of a suicide attempt? J Clin Psychiatry 70(1):19–24, 2009 19026258

Edwards SJ, Sachmann MD: No-suicide contracts, no-suicide agreements, and no-suicide assurances: a study of their nature, utilization, perceived effectiveness, and potential to cause harm. Crisis 31(6): 290–302, 2010 21190927

Fawcett J: Depressive disorders, in The American Psychiatric Publishing Textbook of Suicide Assessment and Management, 2nd Edition. Edited by Simon RI, Hales RE. Washington, DC, American Psychiatric Publishing, 2012, pp 109–121

Frierson RL: The suicidal patient: risk assessment, management, and documentation. Psychiatric Times, April 15, 2007. Available at: http://www.psychiatrictimes.com/articles/suicidal-patient-risk-assessment-management-and-documentation. Accessed on January 11, 2017.

Garner BA (ed): Black's Law Dictionary, 10th Edition. St. Paul, MN, Thomson West, 2014

Gold LH: Suicide and gender, in The American Psychiatric Publishing Textbook of Suicide Assessment and Management, 2nd Edition. Edited by Simon RI, Hales RE. Washington, DC, American Psychiatric Publishing, 2012, pp 453–478

Graduate Institute of Geneva: Small arms survey. 2007. Available at: http://www.smallarmssurvey.org/publications/by-type/yearbook/small-arms-survey-2007.html. Accessed January 11, 2017.

Haas AP, Eliason M, Mays VM, et al: Suicide and suicide risk in lesbian, gay, bisexual, and transgender populations: review and recommendations. J Homosex 58(1):10–51, 2011 21213174

Hawton K: Restricting access to methods of suicide: rationales and evaluation of this approach to suicide preventions. Crisis 28(Suppl):4–9, 2007

Homaifar B, Matarazzo B, Wortzel HS: Therapeutic risk management of the suicidal patient: augmenting clinical suicide risk assessment with structured instruments. J Psychiatr Pract 19(5):406–409, 2013 24042246

Ilgen MA, Zivin K, McCammon RJ, et al: Mental illness, previous suicidality, and access to guns in the United States. Psychiatr Serv 59(2):198–200, 2008 18245165

Jacobs DG, Baldessarini RJ, Conwell Y, et al: Practice guideline for the assessment and treatment of patients with suicidal behaviors. American Psychiatric Association, November 2003. Available at: https://psychiatryonline.org/pb/assets/raw/sitewide/practice_guidelines/guidelines/suicide.pdf. Accessed January 11, 2017.

Kaplan MS, McFarland BH, Huguet N, et al: Acute alcohol intoxication and suicide: a gender-stratified analysis of the National Violent Death Reporting System. Inj Prev 19(1):38–43, 2013 22627777

Kessler RC, Borges G, Walters EE: Prevalence of and risk factors for lifetime suicide attempts in the National Comorbidity Survey. Arch Gen Psychiatry 56(7):617–626, 1999 10401507

Krouse WJ: Gun control legislation. Congressional Research Service, 2012. Available at: https://fas.org/sgp/crs/misc/RL32842.pdf. Accessed December 2, 2016

Lester D: Suicide prevention by lethal means restriction, in The American Psychiatric Publishing Textbook of Suicide Assessment and Management, 2nd Edition. Edited by Simon RI, Hales RE. Washington, DC, American Psychiatric Publishing, 2012, pp 581–592

Mann JJ, Michel CA: Prevention of firearm suicide in the United States: what works and what is possible. Am J Psychiatry 173(10):969–979, 2016 27444796

Mann JJ, Apter A, Bertolote J, et al: Suicide prevention strategies: a systematic review. JAMA 294(16):2064–2074, 2005 16249421

Miller M, Hemenway D: Guns and suicide in the United States. N Engl J Med 359(10):989–991, 2008 18768940

Miller M, Azrael D, Barber C: Suicide mortality in the United States: the importance of attending to method in understanding population-level disparities in the burden of suicide. Annu Rev Public Health 33:393–408, 2012 22224886

Miller M, Barber C, White RA, Azrael D: Firearms and suicide in the United States: is risk independent of underlying suicidal behavior? Am J Epidemiol 178(6):946–955, 2013 23975641

Miller M, Barber C, Azrael D: Firearms and suicide in the United States, in Gun Violence and Mental Illness. Edited by Gold LH, Simon RI. Washington, DC, American Psychiatric Publishing, 2016a, pp 31–48

Miller M, Swanson SA, Azrael D: Are we missing something pertinent? A bias analysis of unmeasured confounding in the firearm-suicide literature. Epidemiol Rev 38(1):62–69, 2016b 26769723

Milner A, Spittal MJ, Pirkis J, et al: Suicide by occupation: systematic review and meta-analysis. Br J Psychiatry 203(6):409–416, 2013 24297788

Nock MK, Borges G, Bromet EJ, et al: Suicide and suicidal behavior. Epidemiol Rev 30:133–154, 2008 18653727

Owens C, Booth N, Briscoe M, et al: Suicide outside the care of mental health services: a case-controlled psychological autopsy study. Crisis 24(3):113–121, 2003 14518644

Owens D, Horrocks J, House A: Fatal and non-fatal repetition of self-harm: systematic method versus intent. Am J Psychiatry 142:228–231, 2002

Powell KE, Kresnow MJ, Mercy JA, et al: Alcohol consumption and nearly lethal suicide attempts. Suicide Life Threat Behav 32(1)(Suppl):30–41, 2001 11924693

Professional Risk Management Services: The Psychiatrists' Program®: Cause of Loss, 2006–2015. Arlington, VA, Professional Risk Management Services, 2016

Rimkeviciene J, O'Gorman J, De Leo D: Impulsive suicide attempts: a systematic literature review of definitions, characteristics and risk factors. J Affect Disord 171:93–104, 2015 25299440

Rudd MD: Core competencies, warning signs, and a framework for suicide risk assessment in clinical practice, in The Oxford Handbook of Suicide and Self-Injury. Edited by Nock MK. New York, Oxford University Press, 2014, pp 323–336

Scott CL, Resnick PJ: Patient suicide and litigation, in The American Psychiatric Publishing Textbook of Suicide Assessment and Management, 2nd Edition. Edited by Simon RI, Hales RE. Washington, DC, American Psychiatric Publishing, 2012, pp 539–552

Shenassa ED, Rogers ML, Spalding KL, et al: Safer storage of firearms at home and risk of suicide: a study of protective factors in a nationally representative sample. J Epidemiol Community Health 58(10): 841–848, 2004 15365110

Silverman MM: Suicide risk assessment and suicide risk formulation: essential components of the therapeutic risk management model. J Psychiatr Pract 20(5):373–378, 2014 25226200

Silverman MM, Berman AL: Suicide risk assessment and risk formulation, part I: a focus on suicide ideation in assessing suicide risk. Suicide Life Threat Behav 44(4):420–431, 2014 25250407

Simon OR, Swann AC, Powell KE, et al: Characteristics of impulsive suicide attempts and attempters. Suicide Life Threat Behav 32(1)(Suppl):49–59, 2001 11924695

Simon RI: Suicide risk assessment forms: form over substance? J Am Acad Psychiatry Law 37(3):290–293, 2009 19767492

Simon RI: Suicide risk assessment: gateway to treatment and management, in The American Psychiatric Publishing Textbook of Suicide Assessment and Management, 2nd Edition. Edited by Simon RI, Hales RE. Washington, DC, American Psychiatric Publishing, 2012a, pp 3–28

Simon RI: Therapeutic risk management of the suicidal patient, in The American Psychiatric Publishing Textbook of Suicide Assessment and Management, 2nd Edition. Edited by Simon RI, Hales RE. Washington, DC, American Psychiatric Publishing, 2012b, pp 553–577

Simon RI, Gold LH: Decreasing suicide mortality, in Gun Violence and Mental Illness. Edited by Gold LH, Simon RI. Washington, DC, American Psychiatric Publishing, 2016, pp 249–289

Swanson JW: Explaining rare acts of violence: the limits of evidence from population research. Psychiatr Serv 62(11):1369–1371, 2011 22211218

Swanson JW, Sampson NA, Petukhova MV, et al: Guns, impulsive angry behavior, and mental disorders: results from the National Comorbidity Survey Replication (NCS-R). Behav Sci Law 33(2–3):199–212, 2015 25850688

U.S. Department of Veterans Affairs: Suicide data report, 2012. Available at: http://www.va.gov/opa/docs/suicide-data-report-2012-final.pdf. Accessed on January 11, 2017.

Wettstein RM: Specific issues in psychiatric malpractice, in Principles and Practice of Forensic Psychiatry, 3rd Edition. Edited by Rosner R, Scott C. Boca Raton, FL, Taylor & Francis, 2017

Wintemute GJ, Parham CA, Beaumont JJ, et al: Mortality among recent purchasers of handguns. N Engl J Med 341(21):1583–1589, 1999 10564689

World Health Organization: Preventing suicide: a global imperative. Geneva, World Health Organization, 2014. Available at: http://apps.who.int/iris/bitstream/10665/131056/1/9789241564779_eng.pdf?ua=1andua=1. Accessed January 10, 2017.

Wortzel HS, Matarazzo B, Homaifar B: A model for therapeutic risk management of the suicidal patient. J Psychiatr Pract 19(4):323–326, 2013 23852108

Yip PS, Caine E, Yousuf S, et al: Means restriction for suicide prevention. Lancet 379(9834):2393–2399, 2012 22726520

CHAPTER 28

Violence Risk Assessment

Daniel C. Murrie, Ph.D.

Elisha R. Agee, Psy.D.

Interpersonal violence is a leading cause of death and a primary concern for public health and policy. Assessing and managing the risk of violence has become a primary concern of psychiatry, particularly forensic psychiatry. Decades ago in his seminal article, Shah (1978) documented at least 15 contexts in which mental health professionals must assess risk of violence; since then, the number of such contexts has increased. For example, questions of violence risk emerge amid general psychiatric practice, particularly during decisions about hospitalization or discharge. Importantly, widespread deinstitutionalization and disappearing options for inpatient care have left community psychiatrists treating severely ill, and potentially dangerous, patients far more than in previous decades (Buchanan et al. 2012). Questions about violence risk remain central to criminal sentencing proceedings, juvenile disposition and transfer proceed-

ings, and child protection matters. Even in psychiatric evaluations that do not obviously address violence, such as those addressing malpractice, preemployment screening, workplace disability, fitness for duty, university disciplinary proceedings, or even immigration proceedings, concerns about violence risk may be central to certain cases.

Assessments of violence risk are challenging, in part because they involve two fundamental but competing values: individual civil liberties and public safety. Poor practice in violence risk assessment may contribute to unnecessary restriction of freedom for some individuals or physical harm to others. Given this complexity, historical efforts to assess violence risk have been far from perfect, and legal mandates to assess violence risk have evolved. However, the knowledge and procedures underlying violence risk assessments have improved substantially in recent years, such that forensic psychiatrists and psychologists now have meaningful expertise to offer in assessing and reducing violence risk.

Legal Mandates to Address Violence Risk

Although many types of forensic evaluations (e.g., trial competence, legal sanity) are guided by explicit legal standards, no single legal standard defines violence risk or prescribes the steps of violence risk assessment. Violence risk per se is not a specific legal determination like competence or sanity, but rather a consideration underlying a variety of legal questions. Legal developments over the past several decades have expanded the contexts that may prompt a violence risk assessment, and courts have generally upheld expert testimony addressing violence risk.

Violence risk assessment occurs in civil commitment proceedings, as all states have enacted statutes that allow for the involuntary hospitalization of individuals found dangerous to themselves or others. Additionally, violence risk assessments are useful in *Tarasoff* (*Tarasoff v. Regents of University of California* 1976) jurisdictions where psychiatrists may incur liability if their patients harm third parties (see Chapter 8, "Physician–Patient Relationship in Psychiatry"). Just as the courts have seemed to expand the duty for clinicians to identify and intervene in potential violence, the courts have welcomed assessments of violence to inform legal proceedings. In *Barefoot v. Estelle* (1983), the U.S. Supreme Court considered the admissibility of psychiatrists' opinions and held the following: "The suggestion that no psychiatrist's testimony may be presented with respect to a defendant's future dangerousness is somewhat like asking us to disinvent the wheel.…[I]t makes little sense, if any, to submit that psychiatrists, out of the entire universe of persons who might have an opinion on the issue, would know so little about the subject that they should not be permitted to testify" (p. 897).

In the ensuing years, courts continued to uphold the conclusion that mental health professionals can and should assess "dangerousness." The U.S. Supreme Court has rejected the contention that reliably predicting future criminal behavior is impossible (*Schall v. Martin* 1984; *United States v. Salerno* 1987). More recently, the Court ruled that civilly committing previously incarcerated sex offenders as "sexually violent predators" requires a prediction of future dangerousness (*Kansas v. Hendricks* 1997) (see Chapter 23, "Forensic Assessment of Sex Offenders").

Progress in Violence Risk Assessment

Until the 1980s, clinicians answered questions about violence risk in a dichotomous fashion, just as the legal system requested (Heilbrun 2009). Clinicians categorized patients as either "dangerous" or "not dangerous," and the legal system responded accordingly. Clinicians formulated opinions based on their training, experience, theories, or intuition via unguided or unstructured clinical judgment (Monahan 2008). Early research suggested that clinicians making these all-or-none dangerousness predictions tended to be wrong more often than not (Monahan 1981).

Faced with the ongoing demands for violence risk assessment, alongside clear evidence of weaknesses in violence risk assessment practice, scholars began to work toward making violence predictions more empirically rigorous and ethically defensible (Conroy and Murrie 2007). As research progressed, scholars increasingly emphasized what is now commonly understood: violence risk is not solely a fixed personal trait but rather the product of a complex interaction of personal and contextual factors. The paradigm began to shift from the dichotomous "dangerousness prediction" to assessment of the degree of violence risk, or "risk assessment" (Heilbrun 2009). Although clinicians could not perfectly predict violence, they could assess the risk factors for future violence in order to guide interventions.

Epidemiological research has shed light on the base rates of violence in the community, even among people with psychiatric illness (Elbogen and Johnson 2009; Swanson et al. 2006), and a landmark research program has provided unprecedented data on violence base rates and risk factors (Monahan et al. 2001). Such studies have provided foundational knowledge for violence risk assessment.

Foundational Knowledge for Violence Risk Assessment: Base Rates of Violence

A *base rate* is the prevalence of a particular characteristic or behavior within a particular population (Arkes 1989). Without first considering the frequency of a behavior (e.g., violent acts) in a relevant population, clinicians are prone to either underestimate or overestimate the likelihood of a particular person engaging in violent behavior. Monahan (1981) identified knowledge of appropriate base rates as *the* most important piece of information in violence prediction. He also emphasized that ignorance or ne-

glect of base rates is one of the most significant errors clinicians make in violence risk assessment. Considering base rates of violence involves conceptual and practical challenges (Conroy and Murrie 2007). Nevertheless, clinicians should become familiar with base rates of violence, particularly across four dimensions: age, gender, psychiatric status, and location (Heilbrun 2009).

Age

Violent crime peaks in late adolescence or early adulthood, declines after age 30, and continues to decline steadily throughout adulthood (Hirschi and Gottfredson 1983; Sweeten et al. 2013). One-quarter (25%) of high school students reported a physical fight during the past year (Kann et al. 2014), and 30% committed a violent crime during the past year (U.S. Department of Health and Human Services 2001). Although delinquency and certain violent behaviors are statistically normative among youth, they usually desist by adulthood (Moffitt 1993).

Gender

Generally, women commit violence far less frequently than men. For example, 2012 data from the U.S. Census Bureau and the FBI suggest that the base rate of violence was approximately 0.05% among women and approximately 0.2% among men (U.S. Department of Justice 2012). However, *among psychiatric populations*, base rates of violence among women are nearly equivalent to those among men (Lidz et al. 1993; Newhill et al. 1995). Data from the landmark MacArthur Violence Risk Assessment Study revealed similar prevalence rates of violence among male (29.7%) and female (24.6%) discharged psychiatric patients at 1-year follow-up (Robbins et al. 2003).

However, the victims of women's violence were more likely to be family members, and the location of women's violence was more likely to be the home. Women's violence tends to be less visible, and for this reason is often underreported to law enforcement and underappreciated by clinicians. In fact, multiple studies reveal that clinicians tend to underestimate their female patients' risk of violence (e.g., Coontz et al. 1994; Elbogen et al. 2001; Skeem et al. 2005a, 2005b).

Psychiatric Status

Although surveys reveal that the majority of the public assumes that people with mental illness are inevitably "dangerous" (Link et al. 1999), epidemiological studies shed a more nuanced light. In a seminal study of Epidemiological Catchment Area data, Swanson et al. (1990) reported that violent behavior within the previous year was self-reported by 2% of survey respondents with no mental illness, 8% of those with schizophrenia only, and 21% of those with substance abuse only. Generally, epidemiological studies find a small but meaningful increase in violence rates among people with serious mental illness compared to those without such illness, and a much greater increase in rates of violence among those people with substance abuse problems *and* mental illness (Van Dorn et al. 2012). The MacArthur Violence Risk Assessment Study (Monahan et al. 2001; Steadman et al. 1998), which tracked 1,136 patients from psychiatric hospitals in four cities for 1 year, found a 27.5% base rate of violence in the 1-year follow-up period, but the prevalence of violence differed greatly among those who had major mental disorders with (31.1%) and without (17.9%) co-occurring substance abuse. Overall, most rigorous studies find that the relationship between mental illness and violence is best explained by mediating factors such as specific symptoms, situational circumstances, or substance abuse, rather than only mental illness per se (Elbogen et al. 2016).

Location

Base rates of violence also vary by location, particularly in comparisons of community and institutional settings. Violence in community mental health contexts appears fairly rare; one study estimated a 6% prevalence of violent acts in a 6-month period (Shergill and Szmukler 1998). In contrast, base rates of violence within psychiatric hospitals tend to be higher, ranging from 10% to 44% depending on the study (Monahan et al. 2001; Newhill et al. 1995; Soliman and Reza 2001). Rates differ by type of inpatient setting (e.g., acute vs. continuing care) and commitment status (e.g., civil vs. forensic).

Empirically Supported Risk Factors for Violence

A working knowledge of empirically supported risk factors for violence is critical for thorough violence risk assessment. Risk factors are those that precede a particular outcome, although they do not necessarily *cause* the outcome (Kraemer et al. 1997). Clinicians tend to underemphasize empirically supported risk factors and overemphasize factors that have little empirical support (Elbogen et al. 2002), so it is essential that forensic psychiatrists prioritize true, empirically supported risk factors. These factors comprise two basic types: *static risk factors,* which are historical and unlikely (or impossible) to change, and *dynamic risk factors*, which change over time and are potentially amenable to intervention.

Static Risk Factors

Past Violence

Not surprisingly, one of the strongest predictors of future violence is past violence. Across meta-analyses, aspects of criminal history consistently emerge as some of the strongest predictors of violent recidivism (Andrews et al. 2006). The predictive power of past violence holds across groups, including adults with or without mental illnesses (Bonta et al. 1998; Elbogen and Johnson 2009), sexual offenders (Boer et al. 1997), and juvenile offenders (Cottle et al. 2001). However, context matters: violence that is committed in one setting (e.g., the community) does not necessarily translate to risk of violence in a different setting (e.g., prison) (Conroy and Murrie 2007; Cunningham 2010).

Psychopathy

Psychopathy—a personality syndrome distinct from, and less common than, antisocial personality disorder—is characterized by a pattern of interpersonal (e.g., grandiose, manipulative, exploitative), emotional (e.g., shallow or labile emotions, poor empathy), and behavioral (e.g., impulsive, irresponsible) qualities (Hare 2003). In clinical and forensic settings, clinicians assess psychopathy with the Hare Psychopathy Checklist—Revised (PCL-R; Hare 2003), a collection of 20 items scored on the basis of record review plus a semi-structured clinical interview. PCL-R scores predict general antisocial behavior (Leistico et al. 2008), violence (Hemphill et al. 1998), and sexual offending (Hawes et al. 2013). Indeed, psychop-

athy emerged as the strongest risk factor for violence among psychiatric patients in the MacArthur Violence Risk Assessment Study (Monahan et al. 2001; Skeem and Mulvey 2001).

Prior Supervision Failure

Prior supervision failure is another research-identified risk factor for violent recidivism, including supervision failures in correctional contexts (e.g., probation or parole violations, rearrest) or forensic psychiatric contexts (e.g., conditional release plans) (Andrews et al. 2006; Bonta et al. 1996).

Dynamic Risk Factors

Despite being more challenging to assess, dynamic factors are often more predictive of violence in the short term and are promising targets for risk reduction efforts (Douglas and Skeem 2005).

Substance Use

Substance use or abuse alone dramatically increases the odds of violence among individuals without mental disorders (Swanson 1994) but also mediates the relationship between mental illness and violence (Elbogen and Johnson 2009; Fazel et al. 2009). Although substance use or abuse is often treated as a static risk factor, alcohol and drug use changes over time and predicts proximate acts of violence (Mulvey et al. 2006).

Impulsivity

When confronted with frustration or provocation, impulsive individuals are less likely to inhibit or modulate their reaction, and more likely to respond without forethought or planning (Barratt 1994). Empirically, impulsiveness predicts self-reported violent thoughts as well as violent behaviors (Grisso et al. 2000; Monahan et al. 2001).

Anger

Studies reveal modest correlations between anger and violence (e.g., Novaco 1994). For example, anger predicted serious violence the following week among high-risk psychiatric patients, and is more closely related to violence than most psychiatric symptoms (Skeem et al. 2006).

Psychosis

Research spanning decades has reached varied conclusions about the relationship between psychosis and violence. Given discrepant findings, scholars conducted a meta-analysis that now provides the best data regarding psychosis and violence (Douglas et al. 2009). Although psychosis was associated with a 49%–68% increased likelihood of violence across *all* studies, the authors noted, "Perhaps the most important finding... is the extent to which the strength of association between psychosis and violence differed as a function of moderator variables" (p. 693). The odds of violence for individuals with psychosis were *higher* than for people with nonpsychotic mental illnesses or without mental illness; however, the odds of violence associated with psychosis were *lower* when compared to people with personality disorders (i.e., antisocial personality disorder or psychopathy).

Coid et al. (2013) found that three types of delusions—delusions of persecution, conspiracy, and being spied on— were significantly associated with violence. However, all three relationships were mediated by anger. Some studies have found that command hallucinations predict violent behavior (McNiel et al. 2000; Monahan et al. 2001). However, studies of "threat/control-override" symptoms (i.e., hallucinations involving a threat of harm from others, or the perception that one's self-control is overridden by an outside force) have produced mixed results (Appelbaum et al. 2000; Link and Stueve 1994; Swanson et al. 1996). Overall, psychosis appears to precede violence in a few individuals but is not the proximal cause of most violence, even among those with psychiatric illness (Skeem et al. 2015).

Treatment Nonadherence

Medication nonadherence predicts violence among psychiatric patients (Bartels et al. 1991; Monahan et al. 2001). Patients' positive perceptions of their treatment need and treatment effectiveness are associated with reduced odds of violence (Elbogen et al. 2006). Both medication adherence and treatment participation fluctuate over time (Svedberg et al. 2001) and may have both direct and indirect relationships with violence.

Approaches to Violence Risk Assessment

As the foundational knowledge underlying violence risk assessment has evolved over the past few decades, so have the methods to integrate and apply this knowledge in individual cases.

Unstructured Clinical Judgment

Historically, the primary professional approach to violence risk assessment has been unstructured clinical judgment. As Monahan (2008) explained, "In unstructured assessment, risk factors are selected and measured based on the mental health professional's theoretical orientation and prior clinical experience. What these risk factors are, or how they are measured, might vary from case to case depending on which seem most relevant to the professional doing the assessment. At the conclusion of the assessment, risk factors are combined in an intuitive or holistic manner to generate an overall professional opinion about a given individual's level of violence risk" (p. 19).

The process in unstructured clinical judgment is not necessarily transparent, objective, accurate, or reliable (Lidz et al. 1993; Monahan 1981, 2008). Absent structure, assessments are vulnerable to inconsistency across clinicians and even by the same clinician across different cases (Guy et al. 2015). Unstructured approaches have performed particularly poorly when contrasted with the highly structured actuarial approach.

Actuarial Assessment

Actuarial approaches (also known as *mechanical, statistical,* or *mathematical approaches*) use a research-derived formula to estimate the probability of future violence. Actuarial approaches define which data should be considered and what algorithm should be used to weigh and combine that data, leading to a fixed conclusion about risk (Grove and Meehl 1996; Meehl 1954). The most familiar examples of actuarial approaches, for most people, are the algorithms that insurance companies use to set insurance rates.

Researchers have repeatedly compared the unstructured clinical judgment approach with actuarial approaches and have concluded that actuarial approaches are far superior (Dawes et al. 1989; Grove and Meehl 1996; Grove et al. 2000; Hanson and Morton-Bourgon 2009). For example, the authors of a comprehensive meta-analysis comparing clinical versus actuarial prediction across many disciplines concluded that "one area in which the statistical method is most clearly superior to the clinical approach is the prediction of violence" (Ægisdóttir et al. 2006, p. 368).

Most actuarial measures are easy-to-use tools, developed from a specific data set, that allow users to code—for a particular individual—certain clearly defined risk factors that were measured in the original data set, and then examine the frequency of a particular outcome (e.g., violence) among individuals in the data set with the same risk factors, or the same number of identified risk factors. Afterward, a clinician offers a structured conclusion such as, "Mr. Smith has X risk factors, making him similar to group Y, of whom 27% went on to commit violence." The perceived objectivity of actuarial approaches and supportive research have been so compelling that some scholars argue that sole reliance on actuarial measures is the *only* appropriate means to assess risk (Quinsey et al. 2006).

Most clinicians in routine practice appear reluctant to adopt actuarial violence risk assessment instruments (Elbogen et al. 2002; Hilton et al. 2006; Monahan 2008) because they do not allow consideration of some case-specific data, particularly unique or dynamic variables. Also, actuarial instruments have limited utility for guiding specific interventions or risk management strategies.

Structured Professional Judgment

Other modern violence risk assessment measures reflect an approach labeled *structured professional judgment* (SPJ) (Webster et al. 1997). SPJ is intended to capture the strengths but minimize the weaknesses of both actuarial and clinical judgment approaches. Tools based on the SPJ model delineate research-identified risk factors (just as actuarial measures do) but rely on the clinician's judgment to gather, weigh, and combine these risk factors into a final risk formulation. Like actuarial measures, they tend to be more reliable, transparent, and accurate than unstructured assessment; however, unlike actuarial approaches, they allow clinicians the flexibility to consider factors beyond the instrument and/or weigh some factors as more important than others, inviting clinical judgment.

SPJ instruments comprise 1) a list of static and dynamic risk factors to consider and 2) a scheme for coding these factors (usually as absent, partially present, or present). SPJ instrument manuals usually provide recommendations for collecting information, determining final opinions, and communicating these opinions about violence risk. Final opinions about risk are not determined solely by summing the risk factors; clinicians may conclude for qualitative reasons that actual risk is higher or lower than a simple tally of risk factors would suggest (Douglas et al. 2013; Webster et al. 1997). Final risk opinions are not communicated numerically but are conceptualized and communicated in a categorical manner (e.g., low, moderate, or high risk) to reflect the clinician's degree of concern about future violence.

Using Instruments to Assess Violence Risk Assessments

Historically, psychiatrists have not used risk instruments often, perhaps because few instruments were conducive to fast-paced, routine psychiatric practice. However, even psychiatric authorities increasingly emphasize that structured assessment approaches outperform unstructured approaches (Buchanan et al. 2012). Structured approaches are particularly important in forensic contexts, in which assessments must be transparent and defensible. Indeed, most modern fo-

rensic or correctional violence risk assessments are facilitated by a structured instrument (Singh et al. 2014).

Instruments can be categorized by the degree to which they structure four key components, or steps, of the risk assessment process: 1) identifying risk factors, 2) measuring or scoring the risk factors, 3) combining risk factors, and 4) producing a final risk estimate (Monahan 2008; Skeem and Monahan 2011). A written list of research-identified risk factors adds structure to the first step but not to the subsequent steps. Popular SPJ approaches such as the Historical Clinical Risk Management–20 (HCR-20; Webster et al. 1997) structure two of these four components (i.e., identifying risk factors and scoring the risk factors). At the far end of the continuum, the highly structured, purely actuarial measures, exemplified by the Violence Risk Appraisal Guide (VRAG; Quinsey et al. 1998, 2006), structure all four components of the process.

Historical Clinical Risk Management–20

The HCR-20 (Webster et al. 1997), now in its third version (Douglas et al. 2013), is the most widely used and researched violence risk assessment approach using the SPJ model and is probably the most widely used violence risk assessment instrument of any sort (Singh et al. 2014). The HCR-20 was developed to assess risk of violence among adult male and female civil psychiatric patients, forensic psychiatric patients, and criminal offenders (Douglas et al. 2013).

The HCR-20 comprises 20 risk factors grouped into three domains: Historical (past), Clinical (present), and Risk Management (future). Extensive literature supports the instrument's reliability (across raters) and predictive validity (with respect to predicting violent outcomes). Clinician risk judgments based on the HCR-20 appear to perform as well as or better than those based on other risk instruments, according to several large-scale meta-analytic studies (Campbell et al. 2009; Fazel et al. 2012; Guy 2008; Singh et al. 2011).

Classification of Violence Risk

The Classification of Violence Risk (COVR; Monahan et al. 2005, 2006) was developed with data from the seminal MacArthur Violence Risk Assessment Study (Monahan et al. 2001). The COVR is an interactive computer software program that guides the clinician through a chart review and brief patient interview necessary to measure 40 risk factors and calculate a risk estimate following an "iterative classification tree" methodology (Monahan 2010; Monahan et al. 2005). Finally, the COVR generates a report that places the examinee's violence risk into one of five categories based on the violence rates among subsamples of patients in the MacArthur study (e.g., a 1% rate of violence in the lowest-risk subsample, and a 76% rate of violence in the highest-risk subsample). Nevertheless, the clinician using the instrument, not the instrument itself, is responsible for the final risk estimate. The clinician should begin with the instrument-generated violence risk category but also consider the possibility of any factors (beyond those in the instrument) that may raise or lower risk before offering a final risk estimate and developing a risk management plan.

Violence Risk Appraisal Guide

The VRAG (Quinsey et al. 1998, 2006) is a 12-item actuarial instrument developed through an extensive program of research

with mentally ill offenders in Canada. Researchers coded dozens of potential risk factors from the institutional files of a maximum-security forensic psychiatric hospital, and then followed patients for an average of 7 years after release, documenting new criminal charges for violence (or returns to the hospital for similarly violent behavior). The instrument requires evaluators to code 12 risk factors, which are then statistically weighted and summed to produce an overall estimate of violence risk. This instrument-produced estimate *must* be the only final risk estimate; the instrument authors warn that "clinical judgment is too poor to risk contaminating" an objective actuarial estimate (Quinsey et al. 2006, p. 197).

Instrument Selection

No credible argument or data demonstrate that completely unstructured, unguided clinical judgment is better than more structured approaches. However, much room remains for reasonable disagreement about *which* structured approach (i.e., which instrument) is most accurate, and much research has attempted to solve this conundrum (Heilbrun et al. 2010; Singh et al. 2011). A review of such literature is beyond the scope of this chapter, but it can be fairly summarized by stating that *no single structured violence risk assessment tool consistently outperforms all others* (Campbell et al. 2009; Fazel et al. 2012; Singh et al. 2011).

Performing the Violence Risk Assessment

As in all forensic evaluations, the evaluator should begin the violence risk assessment with a clear referral question and authority to proceed (e.g., a court order or engagement letter from counsel). Then the clinician should gather all available, relevant collateral data before interviews with the examinee.

The clinician's goals usually involve violence *prevention* more than violence *prediction*. Therefore, the aim of the assessment is to gain a rich understanding of the examinee's violence risk sufficient to plan risk management strategies. As the examiner proceeds through the evaluation, the distinction between *risk status* and *risk state* provides a helpful framework for organizing risk-relevant information (Douglas and Skeem 2005); the former is crucial to understanding an individual's risk relative to others, and the latter is crucial to understanding changes in an individual's risk over time.

Risk Status

Generally, risk status involves a patient's risk of violent behavior relative to other individuals in a particular population or context (Douglas and Skeem 2005). Some examinees will always remain at higher risk status and warrant closer risk monitoring because of unalterable historical characteristics, such as past violence.

Even at the earliest stages of evaluation, a clinician can obtain information about a patient's psychiatric and criminal history, as well as other personal data, which can be used to identify the patient's population or comparison group for the purpose of considering base rates of violence. This referral information may include some basic static risk factors for violence. During interviews, the clinician can elicit more information about a patient's risk status. By inquiring about the details of psychiatric symptoms, substance abuse, and especially violence history, the clinician further assesses risk status. The clinician must ask questions that are specific to past violence. Such questions include a thorough review of all past instances of violence:

- What were the nature, type, frequency, and severity?
- Who were past victims?
- What was the context or setting for the violence?
- What events preceded and followed the violence?
- How recent was the last instance of violence, and is there any evidence of escalation?

Eliciting all information about past violence is essential to understanding the contexts and situations in which the examinee could most likely commit violence in the future. These details not only help inform risk status but also plant the seeds of future risk management strategies. Finally, the clinician should ask about instances in which the examinee was *nearly* violent but did not proceed with violence. The answers may provide clues to the examinee's strengths and potential risk management strategies that a clinician can use later.

When forming an initial estimate of risk status, the clinician should (in most circumstances) use one of the many well-researched instruments for assessing violence risk, as described in the previous section. An underrecognized benefit of structured risk instruments is helping clinicians to avoid an overemphasis on psychiatric symptoms and to consider the much broader range of (nonpsychiatric) risk factors for violence.

Risk State

In contrast to risk status, *risk state* refers to a person's *current* violence risk compared with his or her own risk in the past. In other words, risk state involves the "individual's propensity to become involved in violence at a given time, based on particular changes in biological, psychological, and social variables in his or her life" (Douglas and Skeem 2005, p. 349). Therefore, assessing risk state involves a focus on the examinee's current clinical status, for example:

- Are there changes in the psychiatric symptoms that seem most relevant to violence risk?
- Is substance use increasing?
- Has conflict with family escalated?

In many ways, these considerations are common in routine psychiatric practice for assessing improvement or decline in clinical functioning and intervening appropriately. Forensic evaluators, however, consider these clinical changes as they relate to violence potential and then explicitly explore with examinees the prospect of violence.

Optimal assessment involves not only addressing an examinee's current risk state but also *anticipating* factors that would change that risk state. For example, the examiner should consider questions such as these: Is the examinee's sobriety tenuous? Is he or she involved in a volatile relationship that could escalate toward violence? Is an otherwise high-risk individual in a stable and protective relationship such that if the person lost the relationship, he or she would likely resume violence without the stability the relationship provides?

Evaluators may perceive a change in risk state because the examinee conveys— whether to the evaluator or to others—a *threat* of violence or a desire to harm someone. Patients may convey threats in a manner that is overt and intentional, or inadvertent and accidental. In either scenario, authorities use the term "threat leakage" to describe situations in which an individual conveys to a third party the intent to harm a target (Meloy and O'Toole 2011). In addition to threatening statements or articulated desires, threat leakage may include behaviors that leave a clinician concerned that the patient poses a threat to one or more particular victims. For instance, an examinee who loses a relationship or a job, increasingly ruminates on a grievance against the ex-partner or ex-supervisor who caused the loss, and increasingly knows the whereabouts of that person, may pose a threat even if he or she has not explicitly articulated a threat.

Conclusion

The field of violence risk assessment has developed extensive data regarding the rates and correlates of violence, particularly among individuals with mental illness. Clinicians now have a wealth of knowledge to inform risk assessments and a range of well-researched assessment techniques to employ. They need not rely on the unstructured and impressionistic judgments that were common in the past. Moving forward, the challenge will be to employ these best practices in consistent and transparent ways that help courts and facilities employ the best risk management practices.

Key Concepts

- Demands for violence risk assessments have increased, both in forensic and clinical contexts.

- At the same time, the field has developed a rich knowledge base detailing the rates and correlates of violence in psychiatric and criminal justice populations.

Though perfect predictions of violence will never exist, this knowledge base allows for responsible assessments of violence risk, rooted in empirical data.

- No credible rationale supports relying on unstructured clinical judgment, but strong rationale supports using one of the many well-developed, well-researched structured instruments that aid in violence risk assessment.

- Administering an instrument, alone, is not conducting a violence risk assessment. Evaluators should select an instrument appropriate to the case at hand, and then employ it along with the careful review of collateral data and a thorough interview.

- Evaluators should consider an examinee's risk status (i.e., risk compared to others in the same population, based on history and static risk factors) and risk state (i.e., current risk level, as evidenced in dynamic risk factors and clinical condition) to form a broad perspective on violence risk.

- The goal of assessment is not violence prediction but rather violence *prevention*. Therefore, risk assessments should lead to detailed, individualized risk management plans.

References

Ægisdóttir S, White MJ, Spengler PM, et al: The meta-analysis of clinical judgment project: fifty-six years of accumulated research on clinical versus statistical prediction. Couns Psychol 34:341–382, 2006

Andrews DA, Bonta J, Wormith SJ: The recent past and near future of risk and/or need assessment. Crime Delinq 52:7–27, 2006

Appelbaum PS, Robbins PC, Monahan J: Violence and delusions: data from the MacArthur Violence Risk Assessment Study. Am J Psychiatry 157(4):566–572, 2000 10739415

Arkes HR: Principles in judgment/decision-making: research pertinent to legal proceedings. Behav Sci Law 7:429–456, 1989

Barefoot v Estelle, 463 U.S. 880, 103 S.Ct. 3383 (1983)

Barratt ES: Impulsiveness and aggression, in Violence and Mental Disorder: Developments in Risk Assessment. Edited by Monahan J, Steadman HJ. Chicago, IL, University of Chicago Press, 1994, pp 61–79

Bartels SJ, Drake RE, Wallach MA, et al: Characteristic hostility in schizophrenic outpatients. Schizophr Bull 17(1):163–171, 1991 2047786

Boer DP, Wilson RJ, Gauthier CM, et al: Assessing Risk of Sexual Violence: Guidelines for Clinical Practice. Edited by Webster CD, Jackson MA. New York, Guilford, 1997

Bonta J, Harman WG, Hann RG, et al: The prediction of recidivism among federally sentenced offenders: a re-validation of the SIR scale. Can J Criminol 38:61–79, 1996

Bonta J, Law M, Hanson K: The prediction of criminal and violent recidivism among mentally disordered offenders: a meta-analysis. Psychol Bull 123(2):123–142, 1998 9522681

Buchanan A, Binder R, Norko M, et al: Psychiatric violence risk assessment. Am J Psychiatry 169(3):340, 2012 22407122

Campbell MA, French S, Gendreau P: The prediction of violence in adult defenders: a meta-analytic comparison of instruments and methods of assessment. Crim Justice Behav 36:567–590, 2009

Coid JW, Ullrich S, Kallis C: Predicting future violence among individuals with psychopathy. Br J Psychiatry 203(5):387–388, 2013 24072757

Conroy MA, Murrie DC: Forensic Evaluation of Violence Risk: A Guide to Risk Assessment and Risk Management. Hoboken, NJ, Wiley, 2007

Coontz PD, Lidz CW, Mulvey EP: Gender and the assessment of dangerousness in the psychiatric emergency room. Int J Law Psychiatry 17(4):369–376, 1994 7890471

Cottle CC, Lee RJ, Heilbrun K: The prediction of criminal recidivism in juveniles: a meta-analysis. Crim Justice Behav 28:367–394, 2001

Cunningham MD: Evaluation for Capital Sentencing. New York, Oxford University Press, 2010

Dawes RM, Faust D, Meehl PE: Clinical versus actuarial judgment. Science 243(4899):1668–1674, 1989 2648573

Douglas KS, Skeem JL: Violence risk assessment: Getting specific about being dynamic. Psychol Public Policy Law 11:347–383, 2005

Douglas KS, Guy LS, Hart SD: Psychosis as a risk factor for violence to others: a meta-analysis. Psychol Bull 135(5):679–706, 2009 19702378

Douglas KS, Hart SD, Webster CD, et al: HCR-20V3: Assessing Risk for Violence: User Guide. Burnaby, BC, Canada, Mental Health, Law, and Policy Institute, Simon Fraser University, 2013

Elbogen EB, Johnson SC: The intricate link between violence and mental disorder: results from the National Epidemiologic Survey on Alcohol and Related Conditions. Arch Gen Psychiatry 66(2):152–161, 2009 19188537

Elbogen EB, Williams AL, Kim D, et al: Gender and perceptions of dangerousness in civil psychiatric patients. Leg Criminol Psychol 6:215–228, 2001

Elbogen EB, Calkins C, Scalora MJ, et al: Perceived relevance of factors for violence risk assessment: a survey of clinicians. Int J Forensic Ment Health 1:37–47, 2002

Elbogen EB, Van Dorn RA, Swanson JW, et al: Treatment engagement and violence risk in mental disorders. Br J Psychiatry 189:354–360, 2006 17012659

Elbogen EB, Dennis PA, Johnson SC: Beyond mental illness: targeting stronger and more direct pathways to violence. Clinic Psychol Sci 2016 [Epub ahead of print]

Fazel S, Långström N, Hjern A, et al: Schizophrenia, substance abuse, and violent crime. JAMA 301(19):2016–2023, 2009 19454640

Fazel S, Singh JP, Doll H, et al: Use of risk assessment instruments to predict violence and antisocial behaviour in 73 samples involving 24 827 people: systematic review and meta-analysis. BMJ 345:e4692, 2012 22833604

Grisso T, Davis J, Vesselinov R, et al: Violent thoughts and violent behavior following hospitalization for mental disorder. J Consult Clin Psychol 68(3):388–398, 2000 10883555

Grove WM, Meehl PE: Comparative efficiency of informal (subjective impressionistic) and formal (mechanical, algorithmic) prediction procedures: the clinical-statistical controversy. Psychol Public Policy Law 2:293–323, 1996

Grove WM, Zald DH, Lebow BS, et al: Clinical versus mechanical prediction: a meta-analysis. Psychol Assess 12(1):19–30, 2000 10752360

Guy LS: Performance indicators of the structured professional judgment approach for assessing risk for violence to others: a meta-analytic survey. Unpublished doctoral dissertation, Simon Fraser University, Burnaby, BC, Canada, 2008

Guy LS, Douglas KS, Hart SD: Risk assessment and communication, in APA Handbook of Forensic Psychology: Vol. 1: Individual and Situational Influences in Criminal and Civil Context. Edited by Cutler BL, Zaph PA. Washington, DC, American Psychological Association, 2015, pp 35–86

Hanson RK, Morton-Bourgon KE: The accuracy of recidivism risk assessments for sexual offenders: a meta-analysis of 118 prediction studies. Psychol Assess 21(1):1–21, 2009 19290762

Hare RD: Manual for the Revised Psychopathy Checklist, 2nd Edition. Toronto, ON, Canada, Multi-Health Systems, 2003

Hawes SW, Boccaccini MT, Murrie DC: Psychopathy and the combination of psychopathy and sexual deviance as predictors of sexual recidivism: meta-analytic findings using the Psychopathy Checklist—Revised. Psychol Assess 25(1):233–243, 2013 23088204

Heilbrun K: Evaluation for Risk of Violence in Adults. New York, Oxford University Press, 2009

Heilbrun K, Yasuhara K, Shah S: Approaches to violence risk assessment: overview and critical analysis, in Handbook of Violence Risk Assessment (International Perspectives on Forensic Mental Health). Edited by Otto R, Douglas KS. New York, Routledge/Taylor & Francis, 2010, pp 1–7

Hemphill JF, Hare RD, Wong S: Psychopathy and recidivism: a review. Leg Criminol Psychol 3:139–170, 1998

Hilton NZ, Harris HT, Rice ME: Sixty-six years of research on the clinical versus actuarial prediction of violence. Couns Psychol 34:400–409, 2006

Hirschi T, Gottfredson M: Age and the explanation of crime. American Journal of Sociology 89:552–584, 1983

Kann L, Kinchen S, Shanklin SL, et al: Youth risk behavior surveillance, United States, 2013. MMWR Surveill Summ 63(4):1–168, 2014

Kansas v Hendricks, 521 U.S. 346, 117 S.Ct. 2072 (1997)

Kraemer HC, Kazdin AE, Offord DR, et al: Coming to terms with the terms of risk. Arch Gen Psychiatry 54(4):337–343, 1997 9107150

Leistico AM, Salekin RT, DeCoster J, et al: A large-scale meta-analysis relating the hare measures of psychopathy to antisocial conduct. Law Hum Behav 32(1):28–45, 2008 17629778

Lidz CW, Mulvey EP, Gardner W: The accuracy of predictions of violence to others. JAMA 269(8):1007–1011, 1993 8429581

Link B, Stueve A: Psychotic symptoms and the violent/illegal behavior of mental patients compared to the community, in Violence and Mental Disorder: Development in Risk Assessment. Edited by Monahan J, Steadman H. Chicago, IL, University of Chicago Press, 1994, pp 137–158

Link BG, Phelan JC, Bresnahan M, et al: Public conceptions of mental illness: labels, causes, dangerousness, and social distance. Am J Public Health 89(9):1328–1333, 1999 10474548

McNiel DE, Eisner JP, Binder RL: The relationship between command hallucinations and violence. Psychiatr Serv 51(10): 1288–1292, 2000 11013329

Meehl P: Clinical Versus Statistical Prediction: A Theoretical Analysis and a Review of the Evidence. Minneapolis, University of Minnesota Press, 1954

Meloy JR, O'Toole ME: The concept of leakage in threat assessment. Behav Sci Law 29(4):513–527, 2011 21710573

Moffitt TE: Adolescence-limited and life-course-persistent antisocial behavior: a developmental taxonomy. Psychol Rev 100(4):674–701, 1993 8255953

Monahan J: The Clinical Prediction of Violent Behavior. Washington, DC, U.S. Government Printing Office, 1981

Monahan J: Structured risk assessment of violence, in Textbook of Violence Assessment and Management. Edited by Simon R, Tardiff K. Washington, DC, American Psychiatric Publishing, 2008, pp 17–33

Monahan J: The classification of violence risk, in Handbook of Violence Risk Assessment (International Perspectives on Forensic Mental Health). Edited by Otto R, Douglas KS. New York, Routledge/Taylor & Francis, 2010, pp 187–198

Monahan J, Steadman HJ, Silver E, et al: Rethinking Risk Assessment: The MacArthur Study of Mental Disorder and Violence. Oxford, UK, Oxford University Press, 2001

Monahan J, Steadman HJ, Robbins PC, et al: An actuarial model of violence risk assessment for persons with mental disorders. Psychiatr Serv 56(7):810–815, 2005 16020812

Monahan J, Steadman HJ, Appelbaum PS, et al: The classification of violence risk. Behav Sci Law 24(6):721–730, 2006 17171769

Mulvey EP, Odgers C, Skeem J, et al: Substance use and community violence: a test of the relation at the daily level. J Consult Clin Psychol 74(4):743–754, 2006 16881782

Newhill CE, Mulvey EP, Lidz CW: Characteristics of violence in the community by female patients seen in a psychiatric emergency service. Psychiatr Serv 46(8):785–789, 1995 7583478

Novaco RW: Anger as a risk factor for violence among the mentally disordered, in Violence and Mental Disorder: Developments in Risk Assessment. Edited by Monahan J, Steadman HJ. Chicago, IL, University of Chicago Press, 1994, pp 21–59

Quinsey VL, Harris GT, Rice ME, et al: Violent Offenders: Appraising and Managing Risk. Washington, DC, American Psychological Association, 1998

Quinsey VL, Harris GT, Rice ME, et al: Violent Offenders: Appraising and Managing Risk, 2nd Edition. Washington, DC, American Psychological Association, 2006

Robbins PC, Monahan J, Silver E: Mental disorder, violence, and gender. Law Hum Behav 27(6):561–571, 2003 14724956

Schall v Martin, 467 US. 253, 104 S. Ct. 2403 (1984)

Shah SA: Dangerousness: a paradigm for exploring some issues in law and psychology. Am Psychol 33(3):224–238, 1978 655477

Shergill SS, Szmukler G: How predictable is violence and suicide in community psychiatric practice? Journal of Mental Health 7:393–401, 1998

Singh JP, Grann M, Fazel S: A comparative study of violence risk assessment tools: a systematic review and metaregression analysis of 68 studies involving 25,980 participants. Clin Psychol Rev 31(3):499–513, 2011 21255891

Singh JP, Desmarais SL, Hurducas C, et al: Use and perceived utility of structured violence risk assessment tools in 44 countries: findings from the IRiS Project. Int J Forensic Ment Health 13:193–206, 2014

Skeem J, Monahan J: Current directions in violence risk assessment. Curr Dir Psychol Sci 20:38–42, 2011

Skeem JL, Mulvey EP: Psychopathy and community violence among civil psychiatric patients: results from the MacArthur Violence Risk Assessment Study. J Consult Clin Psychol 69(3):358–374, 2001 11495166

Skeem JL, Mulvey EP, Odgers C, et al: What do clinicians expect? Comparing envisioned and reported violence for male and female patients. J Consult Clin Psychol 73(4):599–609, 2005a 16173847

Skeem J, Schubert C, Stowman S, et al: Gender and risk assessment accuracy: underestimating women's violence potential. Law Hum Behav 29(2):173–186, 2005b 15912722

Skeem JL, Schubert C, Odgers C, et al: Psychiatric symptoms and community violence among high-risk patients: A test of the relationship at the weekly level. J Consult Clin Psychol 74(5):967–979, 2006 17032100

Skeem J, Kennealy P, Monahan J, et al: Psychosis uncommonly and inconsistently precedes violence among high-risk individuals. Clin Psychol Sci 4:40–49, 2015

Soliman AE, Reza H: Risk factors and correlates of violence among acutely ill adult psychiatric inpatients. Psychiatr Serv 52(1):75–80, 2001 11141532

Steadman HJ, Mulvey EP, Monahan J, et al: Violence by people discharged from acute psychiatric inpatient facilities and by others in the same neighborhoods. Arch Gen Psychiatry 55(5):393–401, 1998 9596041

Svedberg B, Mesterton A, Cullberg J: First-episode non-affective psychosis in a total urban population: a 5-year follow-up. Soc Psychiatry Psychiatr Epidemiol 36(7):332–337, 2001 11606001

Swanson JW: Mental disorder, substance abuse, and community violence: an epidemiological approach, in Violence and Mental Disorder. Edited by Monahan J, Steadman H. Chicago, IL, University of Chicago Press, 1994, pp 101–136

Swanson JW, Holzer CE 3rd, Ganju VK, et al: Violence and psychiatric disorder in the community: evidence from the Epidemiologic Catchment Area surveys. Hosp Community Psychiatry 41(7):761–770, 1990 2142118

Swanson JW, Borum R, Swartz MS, et al: Psychotic symptoms and disorders and the risk of violent behavior in the community. Crim Behav Ment Health 6:309–329, 1996

Swanson JW, Swartz MS, Van Dorn RA, et al: A national study of violent behavior in persons with schizophrenia. Arch Gen Psychiatry 63(5):490–499, 2006 16651506

Sweeten G, Piquero AR, Steinberg L: Age and the explanation of crime, revisited. J Youth Adolesc 42(6):921–938, 2013 23412690

Tarasoff v Regents of University of California, 17 Cal. 3d 425, 551 P.2d 334, 131 Cal. Rptr. 14 (1976)

United States v Salerno, 481 U.S. 739, 107 S.Ct. 2095 (1987)

U.S. Department of Health and Human Services: Youth Violence: A Report of the Surgeon General. Rockville, MD, Office of the Surgeon General, 2001. Available at: https://www.ncbi.nlm.nih.gov/books/NBK44294/. Accessed January 12, 2017.

U.S. Department of Justice, Federal Bureau of Investigation, Criminal Justice Information Services Division: Crime in the United States, 2012. 2012. Available at: https://ucr.fbi.gov/crime-in-the-u.s/2012/crime-in-the-u.s.-2012. Accessed January 12, 2017.

Van Dorn R, Volavka J, Johnson N: Mental disorder and violence: is there a relationship beyond substance use? Soc Psychiatry Psychiatr Epidemiol 47(3):487–503, 2012 21359532

Webster CD, Douglas KS, Eaves D, et al: HCR-20: Assessing Risk for Violence (Version 2). Burnaby, BC, Canada, Mental Health, Law, and Policy Institute, Simon Fraser University, 1997

CHAPTER 29

Geriatric Forensic Psychiatry

Patricia R. Recupero, J.D., M.D.

Marilyn Price, M.D.

Geriatric forensic psychiatry encompasses a broad and diverse variety of issues. Among the most common evaluations in geriatric forensic psychiatry are those for testamentary capacity and guardianship. Forensic psychiatrists or clinicians may also be asked to assess elderly persons' competency or capacity for decision making or activities that may pose a risk to themselves or others, such as living independently or driving. Aging persons can also become involved in the criminal justice system, more commonly as victims but also as perpetrators. Evaluators need to consider the particular vulnerabilities of the geriatric population when performing competence to stand trial and criminal responsibility evaluations (American Bar Association Commission on Law and Aging [ABACLA] and American Psychological Association 2005; ABACLA et al. 2006). Additionally, elder abuse can affect a victim's emotional and financial well-being. This chapter provides starting points to help forensic specialists and clinicians formulate a successful plan for evaluating an elderly person at the intersection of geriatric and forensic psychiatry.

Evaluation of Decision-Making Capacity

As the number of elderly persons with cognitive deficits rises, forensic psychiatrists will increasingly be asked to make evaluations of decision-making capacity (ABACLA and American Psychological Association 2008). Traditionally, decisional capacity was conceptualized as an all-or-none phenomenon. Currently, clinicians and courts recognize that decisional capacity can be retained for some tasks but not for others, resulting in an effort to find areas of retained capacity. In the aging population, a variety of capacities may be questioned, such as the following:

- Capacity to consent to medical care or research participation
- Capacity to consent to sexual relations, to marry, or to divorce
- Financial capacities (capacity to manage property and business, to convey real property, to enter into a contract, testamentary capacity, and donative capacity)
- Fitness to operate a motor vehicle
- Capacity to live independently
- Capacity to execute a durable power of attorney or health care advance directive

Capacity evaluations are context specific, so that evaluees are considered to lack capacity if they fail to maintain the "requisite level and classification of abilities relevant to a specific action or decision" (Arias 2013, p. 140). The task-specific approach recognizes that an individual can exhibit performance differences across functional domains, with the possibility that applying performance-enhancement methods may be effective for certain functions (ABACLA and American Psychological Association 2008).

When the examiner is assessing a specific decision-making capacity in an elderly examinee, it is helpful to address the following nine conceptual elements (ABACLA and American Psychological Association 2008):

1. Identify the applicable legal standard(s) used in the jurisdiction.
2. Identify and evaluate functional elements related to the specific capacities to be assessed.
3. Describe the medical and psychiatric diagnoses that could be contributing to incapacity.

4. Evaluate cognitive functioning, which is particularly relevant in an aging population.
5. Determine the extent to which psychiatric or emotional factors could be playing a role in the presentation.
6. Appreciate the individual's values in assessing why the person may have made certain choices.
7. Identify risks related to the individual and particular circumstances.
8. Consider options that could enhance the individual's capacity.
9. Formulate a clinical judgment of capacity.

Generally speaking, the goal of an assessment for decision-making capacity in an elderly person is to maximize the evaluee's autonomy and dignity while mitigating potential harm that could arise from failing to intervene when cognitive deficits or other factors have rendered the person vulnerable to abuse or from other threats to the evaluee's well-being.

Guardianship and Conservatorship

Definitions

The term *competency* refers to a legal finding, whereas *capacity* usually refers to the clinical findings found on examination. Some states use the terms *legal competency* and *clinical capacity* to differentiate the two concepts. Generally, *guardianship* refers to the appointment of a substitute decision maker with fiduciary responsibility to act in the best personal and financial interests of the ward, whereas *conservatorship* tends to be more narrowly focused on protecting the ward's financial security.

Jurisdictions may differ in the circumstances under which a guardian or conservator can be appointed. Many states have adopted rules based on the Uniform Probate Code, in which a guardian or conservator can be appointed for "an individual who, for reasons other than being a minor, is unable to receive and evaluate information or make or communicate decisions to such an extent that the individual lacks the ability to meet essential requirements for physical health, safety, or self-care, even with appropriate technological assistance" (National Conference of Commissioners on Uniform State Laws 2015, § 5-102 [4]). The Uniform Probate Code's procedural requirements for the appointment of a guardian or conservator are detailed; forensic examiners evaluating an incapacitated person for potential guardianship or conservatorship should be familiar with the laws of the jurisdiction in which the petition has been filed.

Executional capacity refers to the ability to perform a task oneself. Lack of executional capacity does not necessarily imply a loss of decisional capacity, because a task can be delegated to another (Collopy 1988). For example, an elder may have severe arthritis of the hands, making it difficult to write or use a computer; as a result, the task of paying monthly bills might be assigned to an adult child. As long as the elder is able to make and direct the execution of financial decisions, generally there would be no finding of financial incapacity (ABACLA and American Psychological Association 2008).

Some jurisdictions do not use the terms *guardianship* or *conservatorship* but rather employ the terms *guardianship of person* and *guardianship of finances*. A *plenary guardianship* removes all personal decision-making responsibility and authority from an incapacitated person. However, laws in many states require clinicians and the courts to consider whether the person retains capacity in certain areas so that the guardianship can be limited.

Performing Guardianship and Conservatorship Evaluations

The forensic examiner may need to assess whether the elderly evaluee's global deficits are such that a plenary guardianship may be necessary or whether the evaluee has retained capacity in certain areas, such that a limited guardianship can be crafted. For example, in Massachusetts (State of Massachusetts 2016) court-directed inquiries may include whether the evaluee can do some or all of the tasks listed in Table 29–1.

A similar assessment for areas of continued competence may yield information that will allow for a limited conservatorship. For example, Massachusetts recommends that the financial abilities listed in Table 29–2 be evaluated.

The condition that has led to any loss of capacity should be clearly described, as should the examiner's determination of whether existing deficits are likely temporary or permanent. The examiner should consider social factors and risk factors and the examinee's values, religion, and cultural views. The examiner should also identify any reversible factors, such as the presence of delirium or a medication side effect, and offer suggestions for optimizing the level of functioning (ABACLA and American Psychological Association 2008). Courts can order temporary guardianships or conservatorships with limited emergency provisions if the elder is expected to recover.

Consent for Medical Treatment

Informed consent must be obtained prior to providing treatment to a patient (see Chapter 8, "Physician–Patient Relation-

TABLE 29–1.   **Areas of capacity to be assessed when considering limited guardianship**

Maintain adequate hygiene	Be left alone without danger
Prepare meals and eat	Drive or use public transportation
Recognize abuse or neglect	Make and communicate choices about roommates
Give or withhold medical consent	Initiate and follow a daily schedule of leisure activities
Choose and direct caregivers	
Manage medications	Travel
Contact help if ill or experiencing a medical emergency	Establish and maintain personal relationships with friends, relatives, or coworkers
Choose or establish abode and maintain a relatively safe and clean shelter	Determine degree of participation in religious activities
	Use the telephone

Source.   Adapted from State of Massachusetts, Probate and Family Courts. General Information Regarding Guardianships and Conservatorships, 2016. Available at: http://www.mass.gov/courts/docs/forms/probate-and-family/mpc190-general-information.pdf. Accessed March 28, 2016.

ship in Psychiatry"), but neurocognitive deficits may affect the patient's medical decision-making capacity. Elderly people are vulnerable to deficits in processing speed, attention and concentration, working memory, short- and long-term memory, receptive and expressive language, calculations, verbal reasoning, visual-spatial and visuoconstructional reasoning, executive functioning, and motor and sensory acuity. A psychiatric disorder could compromise insight and lead to impulsivity. In some cases, successful treatment can restore capacity.

The ability to consent to medical treatment is dependent on functional abilities related to cognitive processing. Four case-law standards are commonly recognized to convey capacity (ABACLA and American Psychological Association 2008):

1. *Expressing a choice.* Patients may "lack capacity because they cannot communicate a treatment choice, or vacillate to such an extent in their choice that it is seen to reflect a decisional impairment" (p. 53).
2. *Understanding.* The standard of understanding refers to "the ability to comprehend diagnostic and treatment-related information" (p. 53). Under this standard, the evaluator would disclose the nature of a disorder and ask the evaluee to repeat it, and then do the same for the proposed treatment and any alternatives. The evaluee would be asked to repeat or explain the risks and benefits of proposed treatment and alternatives.
3. *Appreciation.* The standard of appreciation "especially reflects the ability to infer the possible benefits of treatment, as well as accept or believe the diagnosis" (p. 53). It therefore involves the concepts of insight and foresight. An evaluator might inquire, for example, as to whether the examinee believes that he or she has a problem and whether the proposed treatment can be helpful.
4. *Reasoning.* "The standard of reasoning involves the ability to state rational explanations or to process information in a logically or rationally consistent manner" (p. 53). The examiner would consider whether the evaluee has demonstrated internal consistency in decisions. The examiner

TABLE 29–2. **Specific financial abilities to be assessed when considering limited conservatorship**

Protect and spend small amounts of money	Pay, settle, prosecute, or contest any claim
Manage and use checks	Enter into a contract, financial commitment, or lease arrangement
Give gifts and donations	Continue or participate in the operation of a business
Buy or sell real property	
Deposit, withdraw, dispose, or invest monetary assets	Employ persons to advise or assist the evaluee
Establish and use credit cards	Resist exploitation, coercion, or undue influence

Source. Adapted from State of Massachusetts, Probate and Family Courts. General Information Regarding Guardianships and Conservatorships, 2016. Available at: http://www.mass.gov/courts/docs/forms/probate-and-family/mpc190-general-information.pdf. Accessed March 28, 2016.

would investigate whether a decision is consistent with the individual's values and whether multiple options have been considered. The evaluation would include discussion about why the selected option was chosen.

Testamentary Capacity

Testamentary capacity refers to the ability to execute a valid last will and testament. In the United States, the threshold for demonstrating testamentary capacity is rather low (Frolik 2001; Scalise 2008). To execute a valid will, the testator must know "the nature and extent of his property," know "the natural objects of his bounty" (presumed beneficiaries such as surviving spouse and children), know "how the will would dispose of his property," and "have the ability to make a rational plan as to the disposition of his property" (Frolik 2001, p. 257). Testators must be aware that they are executing and publishing their last will and testament. In the spirit of maintaining a low threshold for testamentary capacity, courts may uphold a will executed during a "lucid interval," even if the testator is believed to lack capacity at other times; however, experts have raised concerns about the validity of the "lucid interval" legal con-

cept in the context of testators with major neurocognitive disorder (Shulman et al. 2015).

Assessment of Testamentary Capacity

Evaluations to determine whether a person possessed testamentary capacity at the time of a will's execution are among the most common assessments performed in geriatric forensic psychiatry, and will contests appear to be growing more common (Marson et al. 2004; Shulman et al. 2007). These evaluations may be contemporaneous (Shulman et al. 2009) (i.e., a psychiatric examination of a living testator) or retrospective (i.e., an examination of factors relating to a deceased testator's mental state at the time of a will signing). Retrospective assessments of testamentary capacity pose unique challenges due to the necessity of relying on documents and collateral sources rather than direct examination of a testator (Shulman et al. 2005).

Targets of inquiry during the assessment of testamentary capacity vary depending upon the circumstances surrounding the will's execution. When evaluating a testator near the end of life, the examiner should assess for delirium, which is common among individuals with terminal illness (Peisah et al. 2014). Several psychiatric conditions can affect testamentary capacity and vulnerability to undue influence, including major or minor neurocognitive disorder, alcohol abuse, affective disorders, and delusions (Shulman et al. 2007). Wills may also be invalidated on the basis of what the law terms an "insane delusion," even if the testator otherwise possesses testamentary capacity (Shulman et al. 2007).

Undue Influence

Undue influence is a legal term that refers to the subversion of a testator's will, such that the written "last will and testament" document reflects the intent of another person (the influencer) rather than the true intentions of the testator (Peisah et al. 2009). For a will to be invalidated on the basis of undue influence, the testator must possess testamentary capacity (Peisah et al. 2009) but must have been unduly influenced by another person. Undue influence is distinct from duress and fraud, which can also invalidate wills (Madoff 1997). *Duress* refers to the use of coercion or force to cause changes to specific aspects of a will, whereas *fraud* involves the use of lies (Spivack 2010). Undue influence is more nuanced, and will contests based on allegations of undue influence are more likely to require the assistance of a forensic psychiatrist (Recupero et al. 2015).

Scholars have identified factors likely to trigger a testamentary challenge on the basis of undue influence, including unusual distribution schemes and disinheriting spouses or close blood relatives (Frolik 2001). Often, wills are contested by family members of an elderly testator who has left the bulk of his or her estate to a nonrelative, such as a medical caregiver, religious minister, extramarital lover, friend or neighbor, attorney, ac-

countant, or organization or charity important to the alleged influencer.

Although standards vary among jurisdictions, several elements generally are required to establish undue influence (Marson et al. 2004):

1. The testator must have been susceptible to undue influence.
2. There must have been a confidential relationship between the testator and the influencer.
3. The person exerting influence must have used that relationship to effect a change in the will.
4. This change does not represent the true intent or wishes of the testator, but that of the influencer.

Susceptibility to influence is the most difficult element to prove (Frolik 2001), and testimony from a forensic specialist is often necessary to establish this condition.

When performing an assessment of possible undue influence, the forensic psychiatrist should be sensitive to the potential for bias. Personal values, beliefs, and prejudice may affect the way a will is perceived by third parties. Legal scholars have demonstrated the apparent influence of gender stereotype bias and homophobia or heteronormativity in judges' decisions to invalidate wills. For example, historically, wills of female testators were upheld less than half as often as those of male testators despite similar case factors (Murthy 1997), and judges have overturned wills that disinherited estranged blood relatives and bequeathed the bulk of an estate to a long-term same-sex romantic partner (Madoff 1997).

The presence of severe mental illness does not necessarily mean that a will does not represent the true wishes of the testator. The examiner should approach an assessment for undue influence by focusing on functional impairment (if any) and criteria relevant to the legal elements of the claim, not merely the testator's diagnosis and stereotypes about persons carrying such a diagnosis.

Fitness to Drive

Psychiatrists may be asked to assess whether an elderly person possesses the capacity to operate a motor vehicle safely. Carr and O'Neill (2015) provide a detailed review of current research on driving and major neurocognitive disorder, and their findings may be helpful to evaluators who need to learn more about specific factors involved in an individual case. They discuss the correlation between disinhibited behaviors in major neurocognitive disorder due to frontotemporal lobar degeneration and impaired driving, as well as the perception and attention problems posed by major neurocognitive disorder due to Lewy body disease. Different forms of major neurocognitive disorder and different medications used in the treatment of chronic illness can lead to different types of impairments that are relevant to fitness to drive. For example, Alzheimer's disease often carries a loss of insight, and data suggest that "individuals with [Alzheimer's disease] rarely relinquish their driving privileges voluntarily and often cease driving only after being involved in a [motor vehicle collision]" (Moorhouse et al. 2011, p. 61).

A recommendation that a patient or evaluee cease driving should be made carefully and only when supported by objective facts, not merely stereotypes or bias against older drivers. Losing the privilege to drive can result in increased isolation and loneliness and decreased independence for the elderly person. Although a diagnosis of mild neurocognitive

disorder does not in itself render someone unfit to drive, "with any new diagnosis of a progressive neurodegenerative dementia, clinicians should immediately begin a conversation about the inevitability of future driving cessation" (Carr and O'Neill 2015, p. 1615).

Objective factors that may lend support to the clinical or forensic opinion that a patient or evaluee should no longer be permitted to drive might include any of the following:

- Recent motor vehicle accident with the elderly driver at fault
- Recent tickets for moving violations, particularly when these infractions are of recent onset and not consistent with the driver's previous behavior
- Poor performance on a driving simulator or road test
- Documented medical conditions that adversely affect driving performance (Charlton et al. 2010), such as a recent history of seizures or macular degeneration
- Side effects of medications that the person is taking, such as drowsiness, blurred vision, or slowed reaction time (Hetland and Carr 2014)
- Poor performance on psychometric, cognitive, or other neuropsychological testing with domains relevant to driving performance

Collateral information from caregivers and others who believe that the patient or evaluee is no longer able to drive safely may be helpful but should be supported with additional evidence gleaned from more objective sources. Information available to the psychiatrist at the time of the evaluation may not be sufficient for a final determination. Psychometric tests, for example, can help to identify the need for further testing "but should not be the sole determinants in deciding to continue or revoke driving privileges" (Carr and O'Neill 2015, p. 1617). If the evaluee has not yet performed a road test, the psychiatrist can recommend such testing before giving a final opinion.

Several helpful resources are available to guide and facilitate the assessment of driving capacity in elderly people. Some resources are freely available online (see, e.g., American Association of Retired Persons 2015a, 2015b; American Automobile Association 2015; American Medical Association and National Highway Traffic Safety Administration 2010; Keeping Us Safe 2011, 2016).

Problematic Behaviors

Forensic professionals may be asked to evaluate elderly persons whose behavior has become problematic to their families, treatment providers, or third parties. Evaluations may also be requested for an elderly person for whom significant changes later in life (e.g., new romantic relationships following the loss of a spouse) have caused family members or concerned others to question the elder's decision-making capacity or safety.

In the case of a new romantic relationship arising among elderly persons, often third parties, such as caregivers, are concerned with the individuals' ability to consent to sexual activity (Tarzia et al. 2012). When sexual activity occurs between an individual who possesses capacity to consent and one who lacks that capacity due to advanced major neurocognitive disorder, the sexual activity may be viewed by third parties and legal authorities as a form of criminal sexual assault (Tarzia et al. 2012), even when the sexual intimacy occurs in the context of a married couple. Cases may be more complicated when both parties have functional impairments; the "perpetrator" of

an alleged sexual assault, for example, may be impaired such that his or her culpability is questionable. Fortunately, resources are freely available to help guide such capacity evaluations (ABACLA and American Psychological Association 2008).

Disinhibition

Disinhibited behaviors in elderly patients can be troubling to caregivers and may pose problems in social and community settings, such as assisted living or residential care facilities. Especially common in individuals with major neurocognitive disorder due to frontotemporal lobar degeneration, disinhibition is also seen in patients with Alzheimer's disease. Disinhibition may also be related to psychiatric conditions not attributed to aging, such as mania in bipolar disorder, social skills deficits in autism spectrum disorders, and intoxication from substance abuse, or may be due to side effects of a medication.

Disinhibited behaviors may include committing theft or shoplifting, leaving the bathroom door open while using the toilet or shower, disrobing in public, swearing or discussing inappropriate subjects in front of children, violation of social norms (e.g., taking food from another person's plate, use of racial slurs or insulting comments, inappropriate staring at strangers), or problematic sexual behavior. The psychiatrist should consider differential diagnoses when evaluating an elderly person with disinhibited behavior. Even if the person has a neurocognitive disorder, it may be appropriate to screen for comorbid bipolar disorder and substance use, as well as medication side effects, instead of assuming that problematic behaviors are due to organic brain disease. Different underlying causes may require different treatment recommendations.

Psychiatrists should be cognizant of the risk of bias. For example, although the expression of sexual needs is considered healthy and normal in younger populations, sexuality in elderly patients with a neurocognitive disorder is often assumed to be pathological or problematic by caregivers (Villar et al. 2014). Ageism or paternalistic attitudes (e.g., aversion to sexuality in older persons, or assuming that elderly persons with a neurocognitive disorder are necessarily vulnerable and in need of aggressive protection) can impede a successful and accurate forensic evaluation.

Agitation and Aggression

When one is evaluating an elderly person for agitated or violent behavior, it may be helpful to review brain imaging studies for potential structural abnormalities. For example, traumatic brain injury and major neurocognitive disorder due to frontotemporal lobar degeneration can lead to impaired decision making and affect regulation, and prefrontal and temporal lesions have been linked to violent behavior (Bannon et al. 2015). Therefore, brain imaging may provide helpful information if, for example, the evaluee has a history of falls or strokes.

Paranoia may cause a person with Alzheimer's disease to be fearful of caregivers and may lead to violent outbursts when the patient feels threatened or unsafe. Patients with Alzheimer's disease often use physical gestures to communicate distress or basic needs when they have reduced capacity for verbal communication. Similarly, neurocognitive disorder–related disinhibition and agitation can impair anger management and coping skills in persons who were formerly able to restrain themselves when angered or frustrated. Common factors to consider in cases of agitated behavior include mania, difficulties in verbal language, dissociative states, delirium, and others. When aggressive behavior or a physical assault occurs, a forensic mental health evaluation might be recommended in order to assess for the risk of future violent behavior and to provide recommendations to minimize the risk of future incidents.

Criminal Behavior and the Incarcerated Elderly

Problematic behaviors may result in an elderly person's being arrested and charged with a criminal offense. Forensic assessments of elderly persons with new-onset criminal behavior require special inquiries regarding competency to stand trial or criminal responsibility (see Chapters 18, "Evaluation of Competencies in the Criminal Justice System," and 19, "Evaluation of Criminal Responsibility"). The overall increase in the proportion of older adults among the general population and the trend toward stricter and longer sentences in criminal cases have led to an increase in the numbers of elderly persons in the prison system; the Census Bureau has projected that adults over age 50 may represent 20% of the prison population by 2030 (Maschi et al. 2014).

Unfortunately, little published research is available regarding criminal behavior in elderly persons and regarding older adults in correctional settings. Lewis et al. (2006) found that elderly forensic evaluees tended to be "uneducated, unemployed men with significant legal and psychiatric histories" (p. 329), including high rates of substance abuse (particularly alcohol abuse and dependence), recidivism, and multiple comorbidities. Roughly one-third of the elders in their sample were found incompetent to stand trial, and lack of trial competency correlated strongly with the presence of dementia (i.e., major neurocognitive disorder) (Lewis et al. 2006).

The population of offenders with neurocognitive disorders poses particular problems with respect to placement: "Nursing homes may refuse to admit elderly people accused or convicted of felonies, forensic hospitals may not have treatment units geared to their needs, and communities may be reluctant to accept them into group home settings" (Lewis et al. 2006, pp. 329–330). Furthermore, in terms of resources and funding, prisons may be ill equipped to care for elderly inmates with complex medical comorbidities, which are common in this population (Maschi et al. 2014).

Elder Abuse

Forensic psychiatrists may be asked to evaluate elderly persons believed to be victims of abuse. According to the American Medical Association (1994), elder abuse and/or neglect is "an act of commission or omission that results in harm or threatened harm to the health or welfare of an older adult" (p. 5). Five major types of elder abuse have been recognized: "*physical abuse*, or acts carried out with the intention to cause physical pain or injury; *psychological* or *verbal abuse*, defined as acts carried out with the aim of causing emotional pain or injury; *sexual abuse*, defined as nonconsensual sexual contact of any kind; *financial exploitation*, involving the misappropriation of an older person's money or property; and *neglect*, or failure of a designated caregiver to meet the needs of a dependent older person" (Lachs and Pillemer 2015, p. 1947). The prevalence of elder abuse over a 12-month period ranges from 7.6% to 10% (Acierno et al. 2010; Burnes et al. 2015; Laumann et al. 2008; Peterson et al. 2014).

When performing a forensic assessment in the context of suspected elder abuse, the psychiatrist should be cognizant of several factors associated with an increased risk for abuse. Victims are more likely to be female (Laumann et al. 2008) and to be "young old" (Lachs and Pillemer 2015). Other risk factors include a shared living environment, lower income, isolation and lack of social support, the presence of a neurocognitive disorder, functional impairment, and poor physical health (Lachs and Pillemer 2015). Common characteristics of elder abuse perpetrators include being an adult child or spouse of the victim, male gender, past history of substance abuse, existing mental or physical health problems, past contact with police, social isolation, and financial difficulties/unemployment (Lachs and Pillemer 2015). Victims of elder abuse have an increased risk of death, hospitalization, and nursing home placement, as well as development of psychiatric symptoms such as depression and anxiety (Lachs and Pillemer 2015). The psychiatric evaluation of a suspected victim of elder abuse should include assessment for these problems.

Most states have laws that require physicians to report suspected elder abuse to adult protective services, law enforcement, or a regulatory agency. If an investigation finds that elder abuse has occurred, several interventions are available. Lachs and Pillemer (2015) provide an excellent summary of potential strategies for intervention by physicians for each of the types of elder abuse; interventions often proceed even before abuse has been verified. Multidisciplinary teams, including physicians, social workers, attorneys, and law enforcement, are best suited to deal with the complexities of elder abuse (Lachs and Pillemer 2015). Elder abuse may also occur in long-term-care facilities, and every state has a system in place to report suspected elder abuse in a nursing home (Lachs and Pillemer 2015).

Neurocognitive disorders are prevalent in the elderly population and may contribute to a victim becoming susceptible to the abuse. An evaluation may also uncover whether the victim retains decision-making capacity and can competently consent to recommended interventions to deal with the abuse. In addition to undergoing a neurocognitive assessment, victims should be screened for the presence of depression or psychosis, which can affect decisional capacity (Read 2016).

Physicians may have a role in the prosecution of abusers by interpreting medical records, reviewing and performing cognitive assessments, and assessing decision-making ability and susceptibility to undue influence (Navarro et al. 2013).

Conclusion

Evaluations in the area of geriatric forensic psychiatry vary significantly depending on factors in individual cases. Therefore, forensic mental health specialists and geriatric clinicians alike are encouraged to consult additional resources for guidance in performing competent assessments.

Fortunately, several excellent guidelines are available online, such as the American Academy of Psychiatry and the Law's "Practice Guideline for the Forensic Assessment" (Glancy et al. 2015) and a detailed handbook published by the American Bar Association Commission on Law and Aging and the American Psychological Association (2008).

Key Concepts

- The goal of an assessment for decision-making capacity in an elderly person is to maximize the evaluee's autonomy and dignity while mitigating potential harm that could arise from failing to intervene.

- A guardian is a substitute decision maker with fiduciary responsibility to act in the best personal and financial interests of the ward, while a conservator is more narrowly focused on protecting the ward's financial security.

- Assessments in geriatric forensic psychiatry should focus on task-specific capacities; an elderly evaluee may have impairments in one area but retain skills in other important domains.

- Unintentional bias (such as paternalism) is a significant risk in geriatric forensic assessments; objective factors and evidence should support any recommendation that a patient or evaluee lose some freedom or independence.

- Undue influence refers to the subversion of a testator's will, such that the written "last will and testament" document reflects the intent of another person (the influencer) rather than the true intentions of the testator.

- It is important to understand the potential causes of behaviors, such as agitation and disinhibition, that others may characterize as problematic in elderly people.

- Five major types of elder abuse have been recognized: 1) physical abuse, 2) psychological or verbal abuse, 3) sexual abuse, 4) financial exploitation, and 5) neglect.

References

Acierno R, Hernandez MA, Amstadter AB, et al: Prevalence and correlates of emotional, physical, sexual, and financial abuse and potential neglect in the United States: the National Elder Mistreatment Study. Am J Public Health 100(2):292–297, 2010 20019303

American Association of Retired Persons: AARP driver safety course: classroom and online classes. 2015a. Available at: http://www.aarp.org/home-garden/transportation/driver_safety/. Accessed January 13, 2017.

American Association of Retired Persons: We Need to Talk (online seminar), 2015b. Available at: http://www.aarp.org/home-garden/transportation/we_need_to_talk/. Accessed January 13, 2017.

American Automobile Association: Senior Driving (Web page), 2015. Available at: http://seniordriving.aaa.com/. Accessed January 13, 2017.

American Bar Association Commission on Law and Aging, American Psychological Association: Assessment of Older Adults With Diminished Capacity: A Handbook for Lawyers. 2005. Available at: https://www.apa.org/pi/aging/resources/guides/diminished-capacity.pdf. Accessed January 13, 2017.

American Bar Association Commission on Law and Aging, American Psychological Association: Assessment of Older Adults With Diminished Capacity: A Handbook for Psychologists. 2008. Available at: http://www.apa.org/pi/aging/programs/assessment/capacity-psychologist-handbook.pdf. Accessed January 13, 2017.

American Bar Association Commission on Law and Aging, American Psychological Association, National College of Probate Judges: Judicial Determination of Capacity of Older Adults in Guardianship Proceedings. 2006. Available at: http://www.apa.org/pi/aging/resources/guides/judges-diminished.pdf. Accessed January 13, 2017.

American Medical Association: Diagnostic and Treatment Guidelines on Elder Abuse and Neglect (Publ No AA22:92-698-20M). Chicago, IL, American Medical Association, 1994

American Medical Association, National Highway Traffic Safety Administration: Physician's Guide to Assessing and Counseling Older Drivers, 2nd Edition. Chicago, IL, American Medical Association, 2010. Available at: http://www.aarp.org/content/dam/aarp/livable-communities/plan/transportation/older-drivers-guide.pdf. Accessed January 13, 2017.

Arias JJ: A time to step in: legal mechanisms for protecting those with declining capacity. Am J Law Med 39(1):134–159, 2013 23678789

Bannon SM, Salis KL, O'Leary KD: Structural brain abnormalities in aggression and violent behavior. Aggress Violent Behav 25:323–331, 2015

Burnes D, Pillemer K, Caccamise PL, et al: Prevalence of and risk factors for elder abuse and neglect in the community: a population-based study. J Am Geriatr Soc 63(9):1906–1912, 2015 26312573

Carr DB, O'Neill D: Mobility and safety issues in drivers with dementia. Int Psychogeriatr 27(10):1613–1622, 2015 26111454

Charlton J, Koppel S, Odell M, et al: Influence of Chronic Illness on Crash Involvement of Motor Vehicle Drivers: 2nd Edition (Monash University Accident Research Centre, Report No 300). 2010. Available at: http://www.monash.edu/__data/assets/pdf_file/0008/216386/muarc300.pdf. Accessed January 13, 2017.

Collopy BJ: Autonomy in long term care: some crucial distinctions. Gerontologist 28(Suppl):10–17, 1988 3139498

Frolik LA: The strange interplay of testamentary capacity and the doctrine of undue influence: are we protecting older testators or overriding individual preferences? Int J Law Psychiatry 24(2–3):253–266, 2001 11436629

Glancy GD, Ash P, Bath EP, et al: AAPL practice guideline for the forensic assessment. J Am Acad Psychiatry Law 43(2, suppl):S3–S53, 2015 26054704

Hetland A, Carr DB: Medications and impaired driving. Ann Pharmacother 48(4):494–506, 2014 24473486

Keeping Us Safe: Family driving agreement. Keeping Us Safe, 2011. Available at: http://keepingussafe.org/linked/familydrivingagreement100111.pdf. Accessed January 12, 2017.

Keeping Us Safe: Keeping Us Safe, 2016. Available at: http://www.keepingussafe.org/. Accessed January 12, 2017.

Lachs MS, Pillemer KA: Elder Abuse. N Engl J Med 373(20):1947–1956, 2015 26559573

Laumann EO, Leitsch SA, Waite LJ: Elder mistreatment in the United States: prevalence estimates from a nationally representative study. J Gerontol B Psychol Sci Soc Sci 63(4):S248–S254, 2008 18689774

Lewis CF, Fields C, Rainey E: A study of geriatric forensic evaluees: who are the violent elderly? J Am Acad Psychiatry Law 34(3):324–332, 2006 17032956

Madoff RD: Unmasking undue influence. Minn Law Rev 81:571–629, 1997

Marson DC, Huthwaite JS, Hebert K: Testamentary capacity and undue influence in the elderly: a jurisprudent therapy perspective. Law Psychol Rev 28:71–96, 2004

Maschi T, Viola D, T Harrison M, et al: Bridging community and prison for older adults: invoking human rights and elder and intergenerational family justice. Int J Prison Health 10(1):55–73, 2014 25763985

Moorhouse P, Hamilton L, Fisher T, et al: Barriers to assessing fitness to drive in dementia in Nova Scotia: informing strategies for knowledge translation. Can Geriatr J 14(3):61–65, 2011 23251315

Murthy VK: Note: Undue influence and gender stereotypes: legal doctrine or indoctrination? Cardozo Women's Law J 4:105–135, 1997

National Conference of Commissioners on Uniform State Laws: Uniform Probate Code (last amended or revised 2010). Chicago, IL, Uniform Law Commission, 2015

Navarro AE, Gassoumis ZD, Wilber KH: Holding abusers accountable: an elder abuse forensic center increases criminal prosecution of financial exploitation. Gerontologist 53(2):303–312, 2013 22589024

Peisah C, Finkel S, Shulman K, et al; International Psychogeriatric Association Task Force on Wills and Undue Influence: The wills of older people: risk factors for undue influence. Int Psychogeriatr 21(1):7–15, 2009 19040788

Peisah C, Luxenberg J, Liptzin B, et al: Deathbed wills: assessing testamentary capacity in the dying patient. Int Psychogeriatr 26(2):209–216, 2014 24182357

Peterson JC, Burnes DP, Caccamise PL, et al: Financial exploitation of older adults: a population-based prevalence study. J Gen Intern Med 29(12):1615–1623, 2014 25103121

Read SL: The four categories of elder abuse: evaluation approaches. Psychiatric Times, January 11, 2016, pp 32–34, 2016. Available at: http://www.psychiatrictimes.com/geriatric-psychiatry/four-categories-elder-abuse-evaluation-approaches. Accessed January 13, 2017.

Recupero PR, Christopher PP, Strong DR, et al: Gender bias and judicial decisions of undue influence in testamentary challenges. J Am Acad Psychiatry Law 43(1):60–68, 2015 25770281

Scalise RJ Jr: Undue influence and the law of wills: a comparative analysis. Duke J Comp Int L 19:41–106, 2008

Shulman KI, Cohen CA, Hull I: Psychiatric issues in retrospective challenges of testamentary capacity. Int J Geriatr Psychiatry 20(1):63–69, 2005 15578664

Shulman KI, Cohen CA, Kirsh FC, et al: Assessment of testamentary capacity and vulnerability to undue influence. Am J Psychiatry 164(5):722–727, 2007 17475729

Shulman KI, Peisah C, Jacoby R, et al: Contemporaneous assessment of testamentary capacity. Int Psychogeriatr 21(3):433–439, 2009 19323871

Shulman KI, Hull IM, DeKoven S, et al: Cognitive fluctuations and the lucid interval in dementia: implications for testamentary capacity. J Am Acad Psychiatry Law 43(3):287–292, 2015 26438805

Spivack C: Why the testamentary doctrine of undue influence should be abolished. Kansas Law Rev 58:245–308, 2010

State of Massachusetts, Probate and Family Courts: General information regarding guardianships and conservatorships, 2016. Available at: http://www.mass.gov/courts/docs/forms/probate-and-family/mpc190-general-information.pdf. Accessed January 13, 2017.

Tarzia L, Fetherstonhaugh D, Bauer M: Dementia, sexuality and consent in residential aged care facilities. J Med Ethics 38(10):609–613, 2012 22736582

Villar F, Celdrán M, Fabà J, et al: Staff attitudes towards sexual relationships among institutionalized people with dementia: does an extreme cautionary stance predominate? Int Psychogeriatr 26(3):403–412, 2014 24331234

CHAPTER 30

Forensic Psychiatry and Law Enforcement

Debra A. Pinals, M.D.
Marilyn Price, M.D.

The relationship between psychiatric services and law enforcement has evolved along many fronts. Psychiatrists are called on for consultation, training, or assessment as treatment providers and as forensic experts. In this chapter, we review areas of intersection and highlight unique aspects of psychiatric work with law enforcement.

Systems Integration and Prearrest Jail Diversion

Persons with mental illness are often involved in police encounters. For example, in a cohort of state mental health service consumers tracked over 10 years, 28% had experienced at least one arrest (Fisher et al. 2006). One oft-cited survey of police departments found that about 7% of all police contacts involved persons thought to have mental illness (Deane et al. 1999). One in four persons with men-

tal disorders report having had a police arrest, and 1 out of 100 police dispatches and encounters involve a person with mental illness (Livingston 2016). Though a small percentage of total law enforcement contacts involve persons with mental illness, police consider these encounters common and routine (Reuland et al. 2009). Closure of state hospitals is often cited as one of the reasons for the frequency of these encounters, although the causes are far more complicated (Pinals 2014).

Given the overrepresentation of persons with mental illness in the justice system, Munetz and Griffin (2006) described the *sequential intercept model,* a strategy for identifying individuals with mental illness at multiple points along the criminal justice continuum and linking them to services. *Jail diversion* is a broad term that describes redirecting people from the criminal justice system and into treatment, a process that can occur before arrest, after booking, during court processes, at the point of reentry from incarceration, or at any other point in the justice continuum.

At the police intercept point, varying models are used to enhance opportunities for diversion and better outcomes (Deane et al. 1999; Dupont and Cochran 2000). These strategies are labeled based on the agency responsible (i.e., police or mental health agency) and the primary discipline of the responder (i.e., specially trained police officer or mental health professional). For example, the crisis intervention team (CIT), a model that has grown exponentially across police departments, uses a police-based, specialized response (Reuland et al. 2009). These teams comprise a department's select group of officers who receive 40 hours of intensive training to respond to mental health–related police calls and link to mental health services, which may involve prearranged sites for police to "drop off" individuals for further mental health assessment.

Alternatively, in a police-based, specialized mental health response, mental health consultants embedded in police departments are available for on-site and telephone consultations and may respond to crisis calls in a *joint "co-responder" model*. A third model involves the use of *mental health crisis teams* that function as mobile crisis intervention units, which have shown some positive outcomes (Kirst et al. 2015). Often, these teams represent an arm of local community mental health centers or public agencies whose mission is to provide evaluations, treatment, and triage decisions.

Police Mental Health Training

With increasing attention to encounters of police with persons with mental ill-

ness, adequate mental health training for police has been a recognized area of concern (see, e.g., Cotton 2004). When linked to specialized CIT services, police training had a positive impact on case outcomes with regard to disposition and other factors (Teller et al. 2006). CIT training has been shown to decrease stigmatizing attitudes of law enforcement personnel toward people with schizophrenia (Compton et al. 2006; National Alliance on Mental Illness 2017). Cross-training between police and mental health professionals (e.g., ride-alongs, tours of work sites) may improve communication and interagency satisfaction and is highly desirable (Price and Pinals 2006).

Setting a mental health training agenda for police can be complex (Price 2005; Vermette et al. 2005). Standardized training programs, such as Mental Health First Aid (http://www.mentalhealthfirstaid.org), may be adopted for first responders, and/or specialized trainings may be developed. For example, in Massachusetts, an expanded 2-day curriculum was established for new recruits (Reilly 2014).

Although more training can help, education alone will not change all attitudes or provide solutions to all challenges that officers face in managing mental health crises (Dupont and Cochran 2000). A survey using vignettes (Watson et al. 2004) found that police officers considered individuals identified as having mental illness to be less responsible for their situation, more deserving of pity, and more worthy of help. At the same time, officers thought these persons were more dangerous than persons for whom no mental illness information was available. These results led the researchers to question how these perceptions would translate into behavior during a police contact.

Departments providing training face difficult choices when determining how many hours and what information to provide for police officers in addition to training on basic signs and symptoms of mental illness. Some states mandate or qualify training for police, and this can have the effect of a more standardized approach across communities. In terms of specific topics to be covered, however, there may be variability. Important mental health training topics identified by police surveyed in one study included dangerousness, suicide by cop, liability for bad outcomes, and decreasing suicide risk (Vermette et al. 2005). Borum (2000) identified mediation skills, anger control, and verbal conflict deescalation as other areas of important focus. Opportunities for "stigma-busting," including hearing first-hand accounts of people with mental illness, are increasingly common training elements. Also, trauma and the prevalence of traumatic experiences among justice-involved individuals and implicit bias training are emerging topics highlighted in many jurisdictions. Role-play scenarios have been shown to be an effective teaching method as well (Silverstone et al. 2013).

Scrutiny of police actions is a delicate issue given the high stress and potential lethal circumstances of a police encounter with an individual whose emotions or behavior may be out of control. The U.S. Supreme Court has debated police use of force and the need for special accommodations for persons with mental illness who encounter police (*City and County of San Francisco v. Sheehan* 2015). With regard to scrutiny of officer actions, the Supreme Court has held that claims alleging officers used excessive force in the course of their work should be analyzed using an "objective reasonableness" standard (*Graham v. Connor* 1989). Such a standard would take into account the facts and circumstances confronting the officer at the time, rather than data learned retrospectively.

In Australia, a review of fatal officer shootings showed that a high proportion involved individuals with mental illness (Kesic et al. 2010). Similarly, a more recent Australian study found that more than one-third of nonfatal police encounters using force involved a person with a mental disorder, and that individuals with psychoses and schizophrenia were significantly overrepresented (Kesic et al. 2013). Despite some arguments that "nonlethal" weapons, such as pepper spray and Tasers, are "safe," they may not be as safe as originally thought (Edinger and Boulter 2011), and persons with mental illness are at disproportionate risk for being tased (O'Brien et al. 2011). Overall, the data support the need for further research on use of force in police encounters with persons with impaired mental states and point toward implications for future training to reduce the chance of injury to officers and others.

Forceful, command-officer type approaches can paradoxically lead to an escalation of emotions and behavior, whereas patient, one-on-one communication with minimal distraction from others at the scene may more likely lead to a positive outcome (Fyfe 2000). Officers traditionally trained to use their authority as a means of control are now learning strategies of deescalation as alternatives. Mental health professionals working with police in developing and delivering training should be familiar with the police protocols for use of force, and can assist in training on techniques of deescalation based on clinical experience and familiarity with acute signs of mental illness. That said, mental health professionals should defer to police for training in complex police use of force tactics.

Providing training to police about the local mental health system can also be helpful. Police generally attempt to reserve arrest for more violent actions but face difficulties in involuntarily hospitalizing persons with mental illness who have engaged in some type of potentially criminal act. Individual officer discretion and practical solutions may drive decisions (Green 1997). Enhanced collaboration and information about mental health resources through training and systems integration can assist in the management of persons with mental illness in crisis and can maximize safety for all.

Suicide by Cop

Individuals who engage in behaviors intended to provoke police to use lethal force as a means of suicide create another complex interaction for law enforcement. This situation has become known as "suicide by cop," also called "victim-precipitated homicide" (Wolfgang 1959), "law enforcement–forced assisted suicide" (Hutson et al. 1998), and "law enforcement officer–assisted suicide" (Homant and Kennedy 2000). The incidence of suicide by cop may be increasing, although this may be related, in part, to better reporting (Mohandie and Meloy 2000, Mohandie et al. 2009). The following circumstances may indicate suicide-by-cop situations (Lindsay and Lester 2004):

- Subject forces confrontation.
- Event is designed to ensure police response.
- Subject advances toward officer.
- Deadly weapon is present.
- Subject has experienced a recent stressor.

Categorizing these incidents as homicides (based on the police intent in the moment) or suicides (based on the victim intent in the moment) is complicated. Aborted attempts of suicide by cop (by the victim) or attempts representing near-misses (by law enforcement) may not be recognized. Police may not be aware that they are being used to accomplish an individual's suicide. Forensic pathologists do not always agree on the best approach to manner of death designations in these circumstances (Wilson et al. 1998). Some medical examiners have advocated that incidents should be classified as a suicide when the situation is clear with regard to self-intent to die (Neitzel and Gill 2011).

In a review of 707 officer-involved shootings, 36% were found to involve suicide by cop, and the suicide-by-cop incidents were more likely to result in death or injury of the subjects than other officer-involved shootings (Mohandie et al. 2009). Suicide by cop appears to be more commonly associated with males. Persons involved range from late teens to almost 60 years, although average ages tended to be in the 20s and 30s. Many of these individuals had histories of psychiatric problems, including suicidal ideation and depression (Hutson et al. 1998; McKenzie 2006; Mohandie and Meloy 2000; Wilson et al. 1998), and often had histories of substance use and prior arrests (Dewey et al. 2013).

One typological construct of suicide by cop (Mohandie and Meloy 2000) divided the goals of the victim into instrumental and expressive subtypes. The *instrumental* subtype is distinguished by the individual's intent to achieve some secondary aim, whereas the *expressive* subtype describes the behavior as a means of communicating emotions. To achieve these goals, individuals initiate varying degrees of physical threat to police.

Based on a review of 143 incidents, Homant and Kennedy (2000) proposed a different typological model. They divided suicide-by-cop behavior into three categories: 1) direct confrontation, 2) disturbed intervention, and 3) criminal intervention. *Direct confrontation* involves situations in which the subject plans ahead of time to attack law enforcement in order to be killed. Disturbed intervention, the most common category, involves a subject who appears to be acting irrationally and who was suicidal before or became suicidal at the time of police arrival. Individuals may also become suicidal during a *criminal intervention*.

Psychiatrists may be called to examine suicide by cop from a number of different perspectives. In forensic contexts, collateral data and a comprehensive review of an individual's premorbid functioning are critical in an analysis of such incidents. In treatment settings, officer-involved shootings can be highly traumatic and may require mental health services response protocols after the event to help manage and work with the police officer involved (Miller 2006). Psychiatrists also may be involved in assessing police fitness after the development of overt traumatic symptoms or even in treating a police officer involved in the shooting. Given the seriousness of these encounters, further research related to suicide by cop could help with prevention and intervention.

Law Enforcement Fitness-for-Duty Evaluations

Law enforcement is a dangerous, stressful, and health-threatening occupation that places officers at risk of physical injury, homicide, and accidents, as well as psychological injury (International Association of Chiefs of Police [IACP] 2014a). Exposure to death, human misery, inconsistencies in the criminal justice system, and negative public image contribute to the development or exacerbation of posttraumatic stress disorder, depressive and anxiety disorders, suicide, and alcohol abuse (IACP 2014a; Pinals and Price 2013; Violanti and Paton 2000). Impairment of performance due to a mental illness potentially can place the officer, the public, and fellow officers at risk (Glancy et al. 2015). As of 2013, thirty-eight states had statutes or regulations requiring screening of applicants (Cory and Borum 2013).

The IACP (2014b) has advocated that officers' mental health be considered an issue of officer safety. Mental health, particularly suicide risk, has become a priority for law enforcement agencies. According to Federal Bureau of Investigation (FBI) statistics, deaths of law enforcement officers due to suicide exceeded those due to traffic accidents and felonious assaults in 2012 (Clark and O'Hara 2012; U.S. Department of Justice et al. 2012). The profile of an officer who commits suicide is that of a male with an average age of 38, with an average of 12.2 years of experience, and generally below the rank of sergeant (IACP 2014b).

Efforts are growing to change law enforcement culture to encourage officers to seek help early and for leadership to provide avenues for confidential referral and treatment before issues arise that lead to a formal fitness-for-duty evaluation (FFDE). Many departments provide officer training on mental health awareness and stress management, as well as use employment assistance programs, peer support groups (peers trained to recognize early warning signs of mental illness and make referrals) or consortiums, cooperative wellness groups, and regional support teams to intervene early and support officers with mental health issues. Special provisions for officers exposed to "critical incidents"—such as those involving death, suicide, or serious injury of coworker; a line-of-duty shooting; homicides of children or friend or family; and hostage situations—may include a requirement to see a mental health professional confidentially outside the police department (Glancy et al. 2015). A law enforcement agency may consider other options to ensure safety prior to ordering a formal FFDE (IACP 2013).

The IACP (2013) defines an FFDE as a "formal specialized examination of an incumbent employee that results from (1) objective evidence that the employee may be unable to safely or effectively perform a defined job and (2) a reasonable basis for believing that the cause may be attributable to a psychological condition or impairment. The central purpose of an FFDE is to determine whether the employee is able to safely and effectively perform his or her essential job functions" (p. 2).

In ordering an FFDE, a police agency should have "direct evidence of impairment, a credible third party report, or other reliable evidence" (IACP 2013, p. 2). An officer failing to appear for a mandated FFDE may face disciplinary actions (Fischler et al. 2011).

A department's policy may require the provision of examples of behaviors that raise concerns that could result in an FFDE (Fischler et al. 2011). A review of the reasons for referrals of officers who underwent FFDEs in the New York City Metropolitan Area (Guller and Gallegos 2010) found that 34% were referred as a result of an accusation of domestic violence, 15.7% for aggressive or bizarre job behavior, 14.2% for stress, and 5.3% for alcohol abuse. Other less frequent reasons

for referral included abuse of sick time, depression, suicidal ideation, extended administrative leave, posttraumatic stress disorder, bipolar disorder, anxiety, drug abuse, extreme family stressors, off-duty conduct, or health-related issues (Guller and Gallegos 2010).

The threshold for referral of law enforcement officers is lower than that for other types of jobs because of the potential danger to public safety. When considering an officer's fitness for duty, evaluators may need to apply a higher standard; persons who might be fit to continue or resume other employment would not necessarily be found fit for a law enforcement position because of the officer's need to carry a firearm. Public safety concerns have led courts to uphold the right of a department to order an FFDE (see, e.g., *Brownfield v. City of Yakima* 2010; *Conte v. Harcher* 1977; *Yin v. State of California* 1997).

FFDEs can also help agencies satisfy the Occupational Safety and Health Act of 1970 (OSHA) requirement that employers provide a workplace free of recognized hazards likely to cause death or serious harm (Fischler et al. 2011). At the same time, the department's response to problematic behavior or complaints should respect the civil rights of the individual officer and be consistent with agency policies governing FFDE, employee contracts, and state and federal law and regulations such as the Americans With Disabilities Act (1990) and the Family and Medical Leave Act (1993). Law enforcement FFDE examiners should be familiar with the statutory and case law applicable to their jurisdictions.

The IACP has recommended that examiners performing FFDEs be licensed psychologists or psychiatrists with requisite education, training, and experience and be "competent in the evaluation of law enforcement personnel" (IACP

2013, p. 2). The referring agency should provide enough information to help the examiner conduct a thorough evaluation. Such information should include documentation of the objective evidence that forms the basis for mandating the FFDE (Glancy et al. 2015; IACP 2013). Additional records that may inform the FFDE are listed in Table 30–1.

In addition to a review of records, interviews with coworkers may help distinguish if the problem is indicative of a long-standing pattern of disruptive behavior or represents a recent change, perhaps in response to a specific stressor. Consideration of current relationships with coworkers and supervisors is important, especially given the need to work closely with colleagues and the tight social network among police (Pinals and Price 2013). The effect of the officer's working environment also should be considered.

After obtaining informed consent, the examiner should perform a detailed psychiatric interview to assess for a psychiatric disorder or substance use disorder and should offer an opinion about prognosis and likely response to treatment. Clinical interviews may need supplemental psychological or neuropsychological testing (Anfang and Wall 2006; IACP 2013). Evaluators should focus on impairment that may be related to mental illness or to alcohol or substance use disorder. Mental health clinicians cannot assess whether deficits in performance were the result of non–mental health medical issues or a lack of training or experience.

A recommendation regarding fitness for duty should take into account that officers must be able to carry firearms as an essential job function. The report will need to address whether or not continuing to carry service-issued firearms is contraindicated because of a psychiatric illness, personality disorder, alcohol or substance use disorder, or side effects of treatment. The effects of any mental condition on judgment, reaction time, memory, and fine motor skills should be carefully assessed.

Although controversy exists regarding whether officers have a higher risk of suicide than the general population, officers unquestionably use firearms as a means of committing suicide in the vast majority of cases (Stuart 2008). Many officers referred for FFDEs already have been placed on "light" or limited, often administrative, duties. This job status usually includes restrictions on carrying weapons. However, under high-risk circumstances and prior to undergoing an FFDE, if officers are still carrying service-issued firearms, weapon removal and referral for emergency psychiatric assessment is recommended. A return-to-work evaluation can be considered once risk of danger to self or others is mitigated (Mohandie and Hatcher 1999).

The evaluator should be aware of the agency's policy and any relevant laws governing the extent of personal information revealed in the report (Anfang and Wall 2006; Glancy et al. 2015; IACP 2013). Depending on departmental policy, the report provided to the department will become part of the confidential personnel record, although confidentiality cannot truly be guaranteed. Thus, the report should contain only the information necessary to document the presence or absence of job-related personality traits, characteristics, disorders, propensities, or conditions that would interfere with the performance of essential job functions. The amount of feedback given to supervisors should be limited to issues related to referral questions (IACP 2013).

The psychiatric evaluator's primary functions are to provide comprehensive evaluation and to express opinions on

---

TABLE 30–1. Records useful for a law enforcement fitness-for-duty evaluation

Job description

Performance evaluations

Commendations

Citizens' letters of appreciation or complaint

Disciplinary history

Internal affairs investigations

Use of force incidents

Remediation efforts and their results

Involvement in critical incidents

Earlier periods of disability and related information, such as causes, treatment, etc.

Medical and psychiatric treatment records

Source. Adapted from Anfang et al., in press; International Association of Chiefs of Police 2013.

fitness. The evaluator can designate the officer as one of the following:

- Fit for unrestricted duty
- Fit for light duty pending effects of treatment
- Fit for duty with mandatory treatment
- Temporarily unfit for duty but could improve with treatment
- Permanently unfit for duty with little likelihood of remediation

Evaluators also may suggest a return-to-work agreement or set of mandated conditions for returning to work.

Most departments consider having an officer assigned to light duty preferable to having the officer out on medical leave (Pinals and Price 2013). However, departments are not required to create light-duty positions as a form of reasonable accommodation, and the development of a light-duty policy is a function of managerial discretion. Unless prohibited by departmental policy, law, or contractual agreements, evaluators should document the extent of impairment and provide an estimate of the time needed until the evaluee can be returned to full duty (IACP 2013; Miller 2007). Evaluators may be asked to opine about causation or

any work restrictions or to suggest reasonable accommodations consistent with the Americans With Disabilities Act.

The content of the report should be responsive to the referral questions while at the same time respecting relevant law, informed consent, officer's authorization, the employer's labor agreements, as well as policies and procedures relevant to the evaluation and report. It is important to realize that information derived from the evaluation could be discoverable if the officer files a grievance or legal challenge. Evaluators should note caveats to the evaluation such as the voluntariness of participation and any pending legal matters (IACP 2013).

Conclusion

The intersection of mental health and law enforcement is a growing area of interest for many psychiatrists. Expanding collaborations between mental health service providers and law enforcement, working with police-based jail diversion programs, providing mental health training for police, performing reviews of officer-assisted suicides, and completing police FFDEs are aspects of the work often undertaken in this arena.

Key Concepts

- Community models of systematized responses to mental health crises include 1) police-based, specialized mental health response; 2) mental health–based, specialized mental health response; and 3) police-based, specialized police response.

- Mental health training aimed toward reducing stigma, maximizing deescalation skills, and improving communication skills is an important addition to other types of police education and can improve overall knowledge.

- "Suicide by cop" refers to an incident in which suicidal individuals intentionally engage in life-threatening and dangerous behavior specifically to provoke officers to kill them.

- Suicide by cop may be driven by a desire to accomplish the goal of being killed and/or creating an opportunity for self-expression.

- Fitness-for-duty evaluations in law enforcement are unique and require awareness of boundaries of informed consent and sensitivity to police as public safety officials who carry weapons.

References

Americans With Disabilities Act of 1990, Pub. L. No. 101-336, 104 Stat. 328 (1990)

Anfang SA, Wall BW: Psychiatric fitness-for-duty evaluations. Psychiatr Clin North Am 29(3):675–693, 2006 16904505

Anfang SA, Gold LH, Meyer DJ: Guideline for the forensic assessment of disability. J Am Acad Psychiatry Law (in press)

Borum R: Improving high risk encounters between people with mental illness and the police. J Am Acad Psychiatry Law 28(3):332–337, 2000 11055532

Brownfield v City of Yakima, 612 F3d 1140, 2010

City and County of San Francisco v Sheehan, 575 U.S., 135 S. Ct. 1765, 2015

Clark R, O'Hara A: 2012 Police suicides: the NSOPS study. 2012. Available at: http://www.policesuicidestudy.com/id16.html. Accessed January 13, 2017.

Compton MT, Esterberg ML, McGee R, et al: Brief reports: crisis intervention team training: changes in knowledge, attitudes, and stigma related to schizophrenia. Psychiatr Serv 57(8):1199–1202, 2006 16870973

Conte v Harcher, 365 N.E.2d 567 (Ill. App 1977)

Cory DM, Borum R: Forensic assessment for high risk occupations, in Forensic Psychology, 2nd Edition, Vol 11. Edited by Otto RK, Weiner IB. Hoboken, NJ, Wiley, 2013, pp 263–293

Cotton D: The attitudes of Canadian police officers toward the mentally ill. Int J Law Psychiatry 27(2):135–146, 2004 15063638

Deane MW, Steadman HJ, Borum R, et al: Emerging partnerships between mental health and law enforcement. Psychiatr Serv 50(1):99–101, 1999 9890588

Dewey L, Allwood M, Fava J, et al: Suicide by cop: clinical risks and subtypes. Arch Suicide Res 17(4):448–461, 2013 24224677

Dupont R, Cochran S: Police response to mental health emergencies—barriers to change. J Am Acad Psychiatry Law 28(3):338–344, 2000 11055533

Edinger J, Boulter S: Police use of TASERs in the restraint and transport of persons with a mental illness. J Law Med 18(3):589–593, 2011 21528742

Family and Medical Leave Act, Pub. Law No. 103-3, 107 Stat. 6, 1993

Fischler GL, McElroy IIK, Miller L, et al: The role of psychological fitness for duty evaluations in law enforcement. Police Chief 78:72–78, 2011

Fisher WH, Roy-Bujnowski KM, Grudzinskas AJ Jr, et al: Patterns and prevalence of arrest in a statewide cohort of mental health care consumers. Psychiatr Serv 57(11): 1623–1628, 2006 17085611

Fyfe JJ: Policing the emotionally disturbed. J Am Acad Psychiatry Law 28(3):345–347, 2000 11055534

Glancy GD, Ash P, Bath EP, et al: AAPL Practice Guideline for the Forensic Assessment. J Am Acad Psychiatry Law 43 (2, suppl):S3–S53, 2015 26054704

Graham v Connor, 490 U.S. 386, 109 S.Ct. 1865 (1989)

Green TM: Police as frontline mental health workers: the decision to arrest or refer to mental health agencies. Int J Law Psychiatry 20(4):469–486, 1997 9436056

Guller M, Gallegos G: Police and public safety officer fitness-for-duty evaluations in the New York Metropolitan area: referral types and outcomes: 2009 and 2010. 2010. Available at: https://www.google.com/url?sa=t&rct=j&q=&esrc=s&source=web&cd=1&ved=0ahUKEwiH6ZvczdbUAhUk3YMKHW8-B08QFggmMAA&url=http%3A%2F%2Fwww.thei-acp.org%2Fportals%2F0%2Fdocuments%2Fpdfs%2FFFDE_in_NYC_Guller_%26_Gallegos.pdf&usg=AFQjCNGY4qZwR1dwGyJA1h97C4hMmSHEQA. Accessed May 24, 2016.

Homant RJ, Kennedy DB: Suicide by police: a proposed typology of law enforcement officer-assisted suicide. Policing 23:339–355, 2000

Hutson HR, Anglin D, Yarbrough J, et al: Suicide by cop. Ann Emerg Med 32(6):665–669, 1998 9832661

International Association of Chiefs of Police: Psychological Services Section: Psychological Fitness for Duty Evaluation Guidelines. Philadelphia, PA, International Association of Chiefs of Police, 2013

International Association of Chiefs of Police: Psychological Services Section: Pre-employment Psychological Evaluation Guidelines. Orlando, FL, International Association of Chiefs of Police, 2014a

International Association of Chiefs of Police: Report of National Symposium on Law Enforcement Officer Suicide and Mental Health: Breaking the Silence on Law Enforcement Suicides. Washington, DC,

Office of Community Oriented Policing Services, 2014b

Kesic D, Thomas SD, Ogloff JR: Mental illness among police fatalities in Victoria 1982–2007: case linkage study. Aust NZ J Psychiatry 44(5):463–468, 2010 20397789

Kesic D, Thomas SD, Ogloff JR: Estimated rates of mental disorders in, and situational characteristics of, incidents of nonfatal use of force by police. Soc Psychiatry Psychiatr Epidemiol 48(2):225–232, 2013 22744175

Kirst M, Francombe Pridham K, Narrandes R, et al: Examining implementation of mobile, police-mental health crisis intervention teams in a large urban center. J Ment Health 24(6):369–374, 2015 26383041

Lindsay M, Lester D: Suicide by Cop. Amityville, NY, Baywood, 2004

Livingston JD: Contact between police and people with mental disorders: a review of rates. Psychiatr Serv 67(8):850–857, 2016 27079990

McKenzie IK: Forcing police to open fire: a cross-cultural/international examination of police-involved, victim-provoked shootings. Journal of Police Crisis 6:5–25, 2006

Miller L: Officer-involved shooting: reaction patterns, response protocols, and psychological intervention strategies. Int J Emerg Ment Health 8(4):239–254, 2006 17131770

Miller L: The psychological fitness-for-duty evaluation. FBI Law Enforcement Bulletin 76:10–22, 2007

Mohandie K, Hatcher C: Suicide and violence risk in law enforcement: practical guidelines for risk assessment, prevention, and intervention. Behav Sci Law 17(3):357–376, 1999 10481134

Mohandie K, Meloy JR: Clinical and forensic indicators of "suicide by cop." J Forensic Sci 45(2):384–389, 2000 10782957

Mohandie K, Meloy JR, Collins PI: Suicide by cop among officer-involved shooting cases. J Forensic Sci 54(2):456–462, 2009 19220654

Munetz MR, Griffin PA: Use of the Sequential Intercept Model as an approach to decriminalization of people with serious mental illness. Psychiatr Serv 57(4):544–549, 2006 16603751

National Alliance on Mental Illness: What is CIT? 2017. Available at: https://www.nami.org/Get-Involved/Law-Enforcement-and-Mental-Health/What-Is-CIT. Accessed January 13, 2017.

Neitzel AR, Gill JR: Death certification of "suicide by cop." J Forensic Sci 56(6):1657–1660, 2011 21827474

O'Brien AJ, McKenna BG, Thom K, et al: Use of tasers on people with mental illness A New Zealand database study. Int J Law Psychiatry 34(1):39–43, 2011 21126765

Occupational Safety and Health Act, Pub. L. No. 91-596, 84 Stat. 1590, 1970

Pinals DA: Forensic services, public mental health policy, and financing: charting the course ahead. J Am Acad Psychiatry Law 42(1):7–19, 2014 24618515

Pinals D, Price M: Fitness for duty evaluations in law enforcement, in Clinical Guide to Mental Disability Evaluations. Edited by Gold LH, Vanderpool DL. New York, Springer Science and Business Media, 2013, pp 369–392

Price M: Commentary: the challenge of training police officers. J Am Acad Psychiatry Law 33(1):50–54, 2005 15809239

Price M, Pinals DA: Law enforcement and mental health professionals: a collaborative approach to training. Law Enforcement Executive Forum 6:61–73, 2006

Reilly A: In Mass., more mental illness training for police. WGNH News, 2014. Available at: http://news.wgbh.org/post/mass-more-mental-illness-training-police. Accessed January 13, 2017.

Reuland M, Schwarzfeld M, Draper L: Law Enforcement Responses to People With Mental Illness: A Guide to Research-Informed Policy and Practice. Council of State Governments Justice Center. 2009. Available at: http://www.nccpsafety.org/assets/files/library/LE_Responses_to_Mental_Illnesses_-_Policy_and_Practice.pdf. Accessed January 13, 2017.

Silverstone PH, Krameddine YI, DeMarco D, et al: A novel approach to training police officers to interact with individuals who may have a psychiatric disorder. J Am Acad Psychiatry Law 41(3):344–355, 2013 24051586

Stuart H: Suicidality among police. Curr Opin Psychiatry 21(5):505–509, 2008 18650696

Teller JL, Munetz MR, Gil KM, et al: Crisis intervention team training for police officers responding to mental disturbance calls. Psychiatr Serv 57(2):232–237, 2006 16452701

U.S. Department of Justice, Federal Bureau of Investigation, Criminal Justice Information Services Division: 2012 Law enforcement officers killed and assaulted. 2012. Available at: https://ucr.fbi.gov/leoka/2012. Accessed January 13, 2017.

Vermette HS, Pinals DA, Appelbaum PS: Mental health training for law enforcement professionals. J Am Acad Psychiatry Law 33(1):42–46, 2005 15809237

Violanti J, Paton D: Police trauma: psychological aftermath of civilian combat. Policing 23:268–272, 2000

Watson AC, Corrigan PW, Ottati V: Police responses to persons with mental illness: does the label matter? J Am Acad Psychiatry Law 32(4):378–385, 2004 15704622

Wilson EF, Davis JH, Bloom JD, et al: Homicide or suicide: the killing of suicidal persons by law enforcement officers. J Forensic Sci 43(1):46–52, 1998 9456524

Wolfgang ME: Suicide by means of victim-precipitated homicide. J Clin Exp Psychopathol Q Rev Psychiatry Neurol 20: 335–349, 1959 13845724

Yin v State of California, 95F.3d 864 9th Circuit (1996), cert. denied, 117 S.Ct. 955 (1997)

Military Forensic Psychiatry

Kaustubh G. Joshi, M.D.

Military forensic psychiatry is an amalgamation of three unique fields: the military, law, and psychiatry. Military and civilian legal systems share some similarities but also differ in significant ways. Common evaluations and procedures exist in both settings; however, military forensic psychiatry also encompasses evaluations and procedures not found in the civilian sector, such as courts-martial and command-directed mental health evaluations. This chapter is not intended to serve as a complete guide to military forensic psychiatry, but rather provides an overview of this distinctive field.

Military Criminal Law Authority

Military criminal law has hierarchical sources of rights. In *United States v. Marrie* (1995), the court reiterated that the sources of those rights are the U.S. Constitution, the Uniform Code of Military Justice (http://www.ucmj.us) and other federal statutes, executive orders containing the Military Rules of Evidence, Department of Defense (DoD) directives, service-specific directives, and federal common law. The principle source is the U.S. Constitution and the secondary source is the Uniform Code of Military Justice; the highest source takes precedence unless a lower source creates rules that provide greater protections for the individual than the Constitution requires (Joshi et al. 2014).

Courts-Martial

Courts-martial, which are governed by the Uniform Code of Military Justice, are the military's version of criminal trial courts. The *Manual for Courts-Martial United States*, 2012 Edition (U.S. Department of Defense 2012), is the official guide to conducting courts-martial. All the rules pertaining to courts-martial (i.e.,

Rules of Courts-Martial [RCMs]) are found in this manual. The three different types of courts-martial are general, special, and summary. General courts-martial are equivalent to felony trials, special courts-martial are similar to misdemeanor trials, and summary courts-martial are analogous to a justice of the peace court (Gilligan 1997).

The military does not have permanently established trial courts for prosecuting service members. Courts-martial are established or convened as needed by commanders who possess the authority to do so (Joshi et al. 2014). The commander is referred to as the convening authority (CA), who convenes a court-martial by issuing an order, or "referral," according to RCM 601(a), that an accused service member will be tried by a specific court-martial. The military justice system refers to the defendant as the accused, hence the use of the word *accused* throughout this section. The military judge and counsel are appointed in accordance with service-specific regulations. The CA "details" (i.e., appoints) qualified service members to serve as potential members of a "panel" (military equivalent of a jury) (Montalbano 2014). Unlike civilian juries, panel members decide both the verdict and the sentence.

RCM 921 governs the guilt phase and RCM 1006 governs the sentencing phase of a court-martial. Courts-martial panel members are usually of different ranks, and persons of higher rank are not permitted to use their rank to influence another panel member. According to Title 10 U.S. Code §816 and §825a, a general court-martial must have at least five panel members; in death penalty cases there must be at least 12 panel members. A special court-martial must have at least three panel members, whereas a summary court-martial does not have panel members. CAs may detail as many panel members to a court-martial as they choose as long as the minimum number is met.

All of the panel members must be commissioned officers if the accused is a commissioned officer. If the accused is a warrant officer, then commissioned officers and warrant officers may be on the panel. If the accused is an enlisted member, then the panel may comprise commissioned officers, warrant officers, and, if the accused requests it, enlisted members. If an enlisted accused requests to be tried by a panel that includes enlisted members, then at least one-third of the panel members must be enlisted. All panel members of the court-martial are required to be senior or equal in rank to the accused.

A secret ballot is conducted for each charge. A two-thirds vote of the court-martial panel members is required for a defendant to be found *guilty* in non–death penalty cases. If the vote is less than the two-thirds, then a *not guilty* verdict must be returned. Because of this rule, military trials cannot result in hung juries. Death penalty cases require a unanimous vote for guilt and sentencing.

Any panel member may propose a certain sentence derived from sentencing guidelines. Voting is done by a secret written ballot on each sentence proposal. A three-fourths vote is required for life imprisonment (with or without parole) or confinement for more than 10 years; a two-thirds vote is required for lesser sentences. In computing the number of votes required to convict or adopt a sentence, any fraction is rounded up to the next whole number. After the sentence is announced, the court-martial is adjourned and posttrial review processes begin (Joshi et al. 2014).

Sanity Boards

A *sanity board* is an evaluation of competency to stand trial, criminal responsibility, or both. It is also referred to as a "706 inquiry," derived from RCM 706 (Montalbano 2014). The threshold for ordering this evaluation is low if there is a concern about the accused's mental state. This evaluation can be ordered by the CA prior to or after referral for a court-martial. Attorneys on either side of the case, the judge, or the accused can also request a 706 inquiry. This request is submitted in writing to either the CA or the judge. A 706 inquiry is a compelled evaluation, and failure to cooperate can result in the exclusion of defense expert evidence under Military Rules of Evidence 302(d) (U.S. Department of Defense 2012).

RCM 706(c)(1) defines the composition of a sanity board as "one or more persons." This rule states that "each member of the board shall be either a physician [psychiatrist or nonpsychiatrist] or a clinical psychologist" and "normally, at least one member of the board shall be a psychiatrist or a clinical psychologist." The sanity board member(s) are officially appointed by the CA or the judge. Once appointed, the prosecution (also known as trial counsel or government counsel) serves as the point of contact in ensuring that the evaluators receive relevant documents. The prosecution also makes travel arrangements and arranges for the accused to be present for the evaluation (Montalbano 2014).

A forensically trained psychiatrist or psychologist is not required for a sanity board. In *United States v. Best* (2005), the Court of Appeals for the Armed Forces opined that a prior treatment relationship with the accused did not constitute a conflict of interest that would invalidate the results of the sanity board. Thus, having previously diagnosed or treated the accused does not automatically preclude participation of a clinician. However, clinicians can decline to participate in the sanity board if they believe their participation would violate their professional ethics (Montalbano 2014) (see Chapter 3, "Ethics in Forensic Psychiatry").

The evaluator(s) must "make separate and distinct findings as to each of the following questions" [taken directly from RCM 706(c)(2)], commonly referred to as "the four questions" of the sanity board:

A. At the time of the alleged criminal conduct, did the accused have a severe mental disease or defect?[1]
B. What is the clinical psychiatric diagnosis?
C. Was the accused, at the time of the alleged criminal conduct and as a result of such severe mental disease or defect, unable to appreciate the nature and quality or wrongfulness of his or her conduct?
D. Is the accused presently suffering from a mental disease or defect rendering the accused unable to understand the nature of the proceedings against the accused or to conduct or cooperate intelligently in the defense?

The evaluator is asked to determine the accused's mental state currently and at the time of the alleged offense, in addition to determining whether the accused has the capacity to stand trial, whether the accused would have been criminally responsible at the time of the alleged of-

---

[1]The term "severe mental disease or defect" does not include an abnormality manifested only by repeated criminal or other antisocial conduct, or minor disorders, such as nonpsychotic behaviors or personality defects.

fense, and whether the diagnosis at the time of the alleged offense was "severe." Although the *Manual for Courts-Martial United States*, 2012 Edition (U.S. Department of Defense 2012), offers partial guidance as to what conditions may be classified as "severe," there is significant room for clinical judgment (Montalbano 2014). The manual does not specify whether "psychiatric diagnosis" refers to the current diagnosis, the diagnosis at the time of the alleged offense, or both (Montalbano 2014).

RCM 909 governs capacity to stand trial, and RCM 916(k) governs lack of criminal responsibility. Addressing competency to stand trial before addressing criminal responsibility is recommended, because ensuring competency provides a safeguard against an incompetent accused disclosing potentially incriminating information. The military standard for capacity to proceed with a court-martial is based on the *Dusky* standard for competency to stand trial (*Dusky v. United States* 1960) (see Chapter 18, "Evaluation of Competencies in the Criminal Justice System"). Military courts have affirmed the application of the *Dusky* standard in a military setting (*United States v. Proctor* 1993). According to RCM 909, the accused is presumed to have the capacity to stand trial and has the burden of proving incompetency to stand trial by a preponderance of evidence.

Historically, the military court system has followed the federal court system's criminal responsibility standard. Congress passed the Comprehensive Crime Control Act of 1984 in response to the public outcry that developed after John Hinckley, Jr., was adjudicated not guilty by reason of insanity for his assassination attempt on President Ronald Reagan. Title IV of this act was the Insanity Defense Reform Act; the burden of proof

shifted from the government to the defense, and insanity became an affirmative defense (Montalbano 2014) (see Chapter 19, "Evaluation of Criminal Responsibility").

The military court system has a two-stage process for determining criminal responsibility, which is delineated in RCM 921(c)(4). The government first has to prove elements of the case beyond a reasonable doubt. If the panel members vote for a finding of guilty, then the panel members proceed with a second vote on criminal responsibility. The panel members are instructed that the accused is presumed to be criminally responsible and the defense must prove by clear and convincing evidence that the accused was not criminally responsible. A simple majority vote is required to find that the accused lacked criminal responsibility. If a majority vote is not secured, then the finding of guilty stands. Mental disease or defect does not otherwise constitute a defense, and thus a defense of diminished capacity (i.e., lacking the mental ability to form specific intent) is not possible.

After conducting the sanity board evaluation, the examiner generates two reports, often referred to as the "short form" (abbreviated report) and the "long form" (full narrative report). The short form contains a statement consisting only of the board's ultimate conclusions as to all questions specified in the order and is submitted to the accused's commanding officer, the investigating officer (if any), all counsel in the case, the CA, and the military judge. In practice, the short form is usually submitted to the defense counsel, government counsel, military judge, and CA; these parties disseminate the short form to other individuals on an as-needed basis.

The long form is typically sent only to defense counsel to safeguard the accused's Fifth Amendment rights against self-incrimination; however, the long form can be sent to the accused's commanding officer on request (which is rare). This rule, RCM 706(c)(3), also allows the long report to be sent to medical personnel under certain circumstances to coordinate treatment. Government counsel gains access to the long form only when the insanity defense is raised.

If the sanity board finds lack of capacity to stand trial, subsequent procedures depend on whether the finding of incompetence occurs before or after referral for a court-martial (Montalbano 2014). RCM 909(c) governs adjudication prior to referral. In summary, the CA can agree with the finding and forward the charges for further proceedings. The accused is usually committed to the custody of the attorney general (Montalbano 2014). However, the CA can also disagree with the finding of incompetency and take any action authorized under RCM 401, including referral of the charges to trial.

RCM 909(d) governs adjudication after referral. In summary, if the military judge agrees that the accused is incompetent to stand trial, the accused is committed to the custody of the attorney general (Montalbano 2014). The attorney general will then send the accused to a federal hospital in the Federal Bureau of Prisons for competency restoration. The Federal Bureau of Prisons will place the accused based on internal considerations, such as space availability (Montalbano 2014). If the judge disagrees with the finding of incompetency, then the trial proceeds.

The initial hospitalization for competency restoration may not exceed 4 months under Title 18 Section 4241(d) of the U.S. Code (2012). If the accused's mental illness has responded to treatment such that the capacity to stand trial has been re-stored, the general court-martial CA regains custody of the accused. In the event that the accused's mental condition has not improved at the end of the 4-month period, RCM 909 allows for an "additional reasonable period" of hospitalization if "there is a substantial probability the accused will attain the capacity to permit the trial to proceed in the foreseeable future."

If the accused does not regain capacity to stand trial and the charges are dismissed, the accused is subject to civil commitment under Title 18 Section 4246. If civil commitment is pursued, this section states that a hearing will be held and "if the court finds by clear and convincing evidence that the person is presently suffering from a mental disease or defect as a result of which his release would create a substantial risk of bodily injury to another person or serious damage to property of another, the court shall commit the person to the custody of the Attorney General."

RCM 1102A governs the disposition of a service member adjudicated not guilty by reason of insanity. The service member is entitled to a hearing "not later than 40 days" following adjudication to determine whether ongoing confinement is justified (Montalbano 2014). The military judge or CA will order a further psychiatric or psychological evaluation of the accused, and the resulting report is transmitted to the military judge for use in the posttrial hearing.

The accused has the burden of proof to demonstrate readiness for release from commitment. The standard of proof for release depends on the nature of the offense. RCM 1102A states the following: "if the offense involves bodily injury to another person or serious damage to the property of another (or substantial risk of such injury or damage), the accused must prove by clear and convincing evidence that his release would not create a substantial risk of bodily injury to another person or serious damage to property of another due to a present mental disease of defect; for other offenses, the accused must prove by preponderance of the evidence." If the accused has not met the standard of proof to be released, he or she is committed to the custody of the attorney general. The attorney general can exert efforts to get a state government to assume responsibility of caring for and monitoring the insanity acquittee, but the attorney general cannot mandate a state government to assume this responsibility (Montalbano 2014).

Command-Directed Mental Health Evaluations

Governed by Department of Defense Instruction (DoDI) 6490.04, *command-directed mental health evaluations* (CDMHEs) are unique in that they have no equivalent civilian counterpart (U.S. Department of Defense 2013). Service members can be ordered to undergo a mental health evaluation by their commanders (who must have the authority to administer judicial punishment). These evaluations are allowable because commanders need to ensure that the service member does not have a mental illness that would preclude him or her from fulfilling duty requirements (e.g., deploying, carrying a weapon, possessing a specific security clearance).

The commander's ability to request these evaluations is not unconditional. Service members are afforded due process protections due to the potential adverse impact on their military service. The commander must consult with a mental health provider to ensure that the reason for requesting a CDMHE is appropriate and not punitive. Once the provider approves the request, commanders must notify service members in writing using authorized forms that they have been commanded to undergo this evaluation. Commanders must also notify the service member of the date and time of the evaluation (Joshi et al. 2014).

A CDMHE is conducted by a psychiatrist, doctoral-level licensed psychologist, licensed clinical social worker possessing a master's or doctoral degree, or psychiatric nurse practitioner (Joshi et al. 2014). The service member is provided an informed consent form to read and sign prior to the evaluation. The provider also verbally discusses the nature and purpose of the evaluation and the limitations of confidentiality. The provider delineates the rights the service member has during the evaluation, including the right to not participate.

If the service member participates in the evaluation, the provider will give results and recommendations to the commander in accordance with local clinic policy (Joshi et al. 2014). The service member is also entitled to the same feedback. If the service member declines to participate, the provider notifies the commander; the commander then consults with legal staff to determine future course of action. Under no circumstances can a commander order a service member into mental health treatment.

Involuntary Psychiatric Hospitalization

Involuntary psychiatric hospitalization to a military treatment facility (MTF) is also governed by DoDI 6490.04, which is the military's version of civil commitment. The military's civil commitment process has two distinct differences from that of civil commitment in the civil sector: 1) involuntary psychiatric hospitalization and subsequent reviews are clinician driven without judicial oversight, and 2) no appellate process is available (Joshi et al. 2014). The psychiatrist can involuntarily hospitalize a service member to a psychiatric unit of an MTF if the service member presents an imminent danger to self or others and/or has a mental illness causing a deterioration of functioning such that hospitalization is the least restrictive form of treatment. A service member cannot be involuntarily hospitalized under DoDI 6490.04 to a civilian facility; however, a service member can be involuntarily hospitalized to a civilian facility under applicable state laws should an MTF not be available (Joshi et al. 2014).

The service member receives written notification of the reasons for involuntary psychiatric hospitalization and about due process rights. DoDI 6490.04 requires that an independent physician conduct a review of continued need for involuntary psychiatric hospitalization within 72 hours of initial hospitalization. A psychiatrist almost always performs this review because nonpsychiatric providers are frequently uncomfortable rendering such an opinion. If the facility has only one psychiatrist, and that psychiatrist is already providing treatment to the service member, a nonpsychiatric provider would render an opinion regarding continued need for involuntary psychiatric hospitalization (Joshi et al. 2014). During the review, the independent reviewer informs the service member of the right to have legal counsel present. The reviewer generates a report that is placed in the service member's chart after each review, and the service member is informed of the results after each review.

If the service member requires continued involuntary hospitalization, another review is conducted within 5 business days after the 72-hour review. Subsequent reviews after the initial 5-day review are conducted every 5 business days until the service member no longer meets criteria for involuntary psychiatric hospitalization. No mechanism is available for the service member to appeal the reviewer's decision. Although the service member can consult with legal staff at any point, no legal process can override the reviewer's decision (Joshi et al. 2014).

Fitness-for-Duty Evaluations

Military members sometimes develop physical or mental illnesses that can interfere with job performance. DoD medical systems make every attempt to provide treatment for military members' condition(s) with the goal of returning individuals to their job assignments without restrictions (Charissis 2014). Title 10 Chapter 61 of the U.S. Code outlines the DoD disability evaluation system (Armed Forces 2012). The DoD provides additional directives and instructions that are implemented through service-specific regulations. The goal of the disability evaluation system is to provide for a physically and mentally fit military capable of deploying at a moment's notice while balancing the interests of the government and individual service members (Charissis 2014).

A service member's duties may be temporarily restricted to allow the service member to undergo treatment. Each service has its own procedures regarding temporary duty restriction. Generally, the service member is returned to unrestricted duty should the medical condition(s) respond to treatment within certain time parameters and if the medical treatment does not significantly interfere with the service member's duty performance.

If a service member is unable to resume unrestricted job performance after the allotted time or if it becomes apparent to the treating provider that the service member will not return to duty even after exhausting the temporary restriction time frame, the treating provider can refer the service member to the Integrated Disability Evaluation System (IDES). The IDES provides near-simultaneous processing of the service member through the DoD and the Department of Veterans Affairs (VA) systems. The DoD retains the responsibility for determining fitness for duty, and the VA retains the responsibility for determining a percentage rating for unfitting conditions (Charissis 2014). The IDES referral is a one-page form (VA Form 21-0819) documenting the conditions that interfere with duty performance (Charissis 2014).

Having a mental illness does not automatically render a service member unfit for duty. Each of the service-specific instructions outlines conditions that are appropriate for IDES referral, the conditions under which they are potentially "unfitting," and the processes for adjudication of fitness for duty (U.S. Air Force 2013; U.S. Department of the Army 2011; U.S. Department of the Navy 2002). Generally, a condition is potentially unfitting if it meets all of these criteria (Charissis 2014):

- It significantly interferes with the individual's military service (e.g., job duties, ability to deploy, ability to possess a specific security clearance).
- It compromises the health or well-being of the service member or other individuals if the service member were to remain in the service.

- It adversely affects the best interests of the U.S. government if the individual were to remain in the military.

The service-specific instructions list potentially unfitting conditions: psychotic disorders, mood disorders, anxiety disorders, somatoform disorders, dissociative disorders, organic mental conditions (e.g., neurocognitive disorder), and eating disorders. The symptoms of one or more of these diagnoses must interfere with the individual's performance of duties and require ongoing treatment for the service member to be determined unfit for duty (Charissis 2014).

Each service branch instruction also discusses psychiatric conditions that do not constitute a physical disability. Instead of being rendered physically unable to perform their duties, service members with these conditions would be considered administratively unsuitable (Charissis 2014). Such conditions include (but are not limited to) personality disorders, paraphilias and other sexual disorders, substance-related disorders, intellectual disability, disorders of childhood development, learning disorders, adjustment disorders, and attention-deficit/hyperactivity disorder.

Once an IDES referral has been made, the treating provider prepares a narrative to document the service member's medical condition(s), treatment course, response to treatment, prognosis, and onset of condition(s) (prior to service or not), as well as to indicate whether the condition has been permanently aggravated by military service (Charissis 2014). This narrative is called the *medical evaluation board (MEB) report*. The service member's commander also submits a statement describing the impact of the condition(s) on job duties and ability to deploy, as well as whether adverse personnel action is being considered against the service member.

These documents and other additional documents are collected for the *physical evaluation board* (PEB), which informally adjudicates the case. Prior to PEB adjudication, the service member also undergoes compensation and pension examinations at the VA, which assigns disability ratings to the service member's unfitting conditions. The treatment provider who wrote the MEB should comment on the discrepancies (if any) between the compensation and pension examination and the MEB report and attempt to reconcile the differences for the PEB members (Charissis 2014). The service member can also submit a statement for the PEB members to consider regarding the condition(s) and impairment in functioning from the service member's point of view; the statement can also contain a rebuttal to the MEB report.

After all the necessary documents are compiled (including civilian treatment records), the case file is sent to the PEB members to informally adjudicate the case (often referred to as the "informal PEB"). The informal PEB is composed of three service members: two line officers and one medical officer. The informal PEB makes the following determinations (Charissis 2014):

- A determination of fitness for each condition
- For each unfitting condition, a determination of whether the condition existed prior to military service
- For each unfitting condition, an opinion on combat relatedness
- A finding on whether each unfitting condition is consideZred to be permanent

Several factors are considered when making a determination of fitness: whether the condition impairs the service member's ability to perform key aspects of his or her duties; whether retention of the service member poses a danger to the service member or to other service members; and whether the accommodation of the service member on active duty poses an unreasonable burden to his or her command (Charissis 2014).

If the service member is found fit for all conditions, the findings are sent to the service member and he or she is not referred to the VA for disability rating. If the service member has been found unfit for any condition, the finding is sent to the VA for assignment of a rating scheme, returned to the PEB for finalization, and sent to the service member (Charissis 2014). If the service member accepts the findings or does not respond within a specified time, the case is finalized and the service member cannot appeal the informal PEB's decisions. If the service member appeals the informal PEB's decisions, the case is referred to the formal PEB.

A formal PEB is a *de novo* hearing intended to make findings regarding a service member's fitness for continued service and eligibility for disability benefits (Charissis 2014). The service member is assigned military counsel to prepare the case, and the service member may choose to hire a civilian attorney at his or her own expense. Counsel advises the service member of the case's essential legal considerations and assists with argument presentation at the formal PEB (Charissis 2014).

The formal PEB consists of two line officers and one medical officer (all senior military officers). The medical officer, who may have a particular medical specialty, has the experience to adjudicate cases across the medical spectrum (Charissis 2014). The formal PEB is not adversarial. The service member has the right to appear personally at the formal PEB (or by telephone if the service member cannot be physically present) and to present additional material to the formal PEB. The service member can provide sworn testimony and witnesses. PEB members can question the service member and witnesses testifying in the formal board. Once counsel has presented the case, counsel can make closing statements and the service member can make additional statements (Charissis 2014).

After the hearing ends, the board members make a decision based on a vote of the board members. The service member receives a written rationale outlining the reasons for the decision. If the decision was not unanimous, the rationale for the decision is accompanied by a minority rationale (Charissis 2014). An informal PEB or formal PEB can render several decisions: return to duty with or without limitations, medical separation, permanent medical retirement, or temporary medical retirement (also known as temporary duty retirement list, or TDRL). Service members placed on TDRL status require periodic reevaluation every 18 months to determine the status of their condition(s), and the case is then sent back to the PEB for a review (Charissis 2014). The service member can appeal the decision of the formal PEB; the appeals process varies by service.

Conclusion

The military is a unique culture with its own laws and procedures. Mental health practitioners working within the military system should be aware of the similarities with and differences from the civilian system. Military forensic psychiatry relies on a vast array of regulations with which practitioners must familiarize themselves prior to working in this sector.

Key Concepts

- Courts-martial are the military criminal courts. These differ significantly from civilian courts, including in their lack of a requirement for a unanimous verdict for all offenses.

- Capacity to stand trial and criminal responsibility evaluations are conducted through a process known as a sanity board, which utilize standards outlined in *Dusky* and the federal criminal responsibility statute.

- Involuntary psychiatric hospitalization in a military treatment facility is clinician driven and lacks judicial oversight.

- Commanders may order service members to undergo a mental health evaluation but may not order them into mental health treatment.

- Fitness-for-duty evaluations involve a complicated process, and each branch of the service has unique regulations pertaining to determining fitness and suitability for duty.

References

Armed Forces: Title 10 U.S. Code Chapter 61 §1201–1222. Washington, DC, U.S. Government Printing Office, 2012

Charissis M: Updates on disability proceedings, in Forensic and Ethical Issues in Military Behavioral Health. Edited by Ritchie CE. Washington, DC, Office of the Surgeon General: Borden Institute, 2014, pp 114–122

Comprehensive Crime Control Act of 1984. Available at: https://www.congress.gov/bill/98th-congress/senate-bill/1762. Accessed January 14, 2017.

Dusky v United States, 362 U.S. 402, 80 S.Ct. 788 (1960)

Gilligan FA: Military law, in Principles and Practice of Military Forensic Psychiatry. Edited by Lande RG, Armitage DT. Springfield, IL, Charles C Thomas, 1997, pp 28–56

Joshi KG, Benedek DM, Johnson DE: The military forensic psychiatry training program, in Forensic and Ethical Issues in Military Behavioral Health. Edited by Ritchie CE. Washington, DC, Office of the Surgeon General: Borden Institute, 2014, pp 92–95

Montalbano P: Sanity board evaluations, in Forensic and Ethical Issues in Military Behavioral Health. Edited by Ritchie CE. Washington, DC, Office of the Surgeon General: Borden Institute, 2014, pp 39–73

United States v Best, 61 M.J. 375 (2005) (Court of Appeals Armed Forces)

United States v Marrie, 43 M.J. 35, 37 (1995) (Court of Appeals Armed Forces)

United States v Proctor, 37 M.J. 330 (1993) (Court of Military Appeals)

U.S. Air Force: Aerospace Medicine: Medical Examinations and Standards. Air Force Instruction 48–123. Washington, DC, U.S. Air Force, 2013

U.S. Code, Title 18 U.S. Code Chapter 313 § 4241, § 4246. 2012. Available at: http://uscode.house.gov/view.xhtml?path=/prelim@title18/part3/chapter313&edition=prelim. Accessed January 14, 2017.

U.S. Department of the Army: Medical Services: Standards of Medical Fitness. Army Regulation 40–501. Washington, DC, Department of the Army, 2011

U.S. Department of Defense: Manual for Courts-Martial United States, 2012 Edition. Washington, DC, Department of Defense, 2012

U.S. Department of Defense: U.S. Department of Defense Instruction 6490.04: Mental Health Evaluations of Members of the Military Services. Washington, DC, Department of Defense, 2013

U.S. Department of the Navy: Department of Navy (DON) Disability Evaluation Manual: SECNAV Instruction 1850.4E. Washington, DC, U.S. Department of the Navy, 2002

CHAPTER 32

The Internet and Telepsychiatry

Patricia R. Recupero, J.D., M.D.

Since the last edition of this textbook was published in 2010, the body of published research on the intersection of mental health and information and communications technology (ICT) has expanded significantly. Although most of the recent studies have focused on clinical applications of ICT, the forensic use of ICT has also grown in the past several years. Furthermore, the adoption of ICT among the general public has continued its steady rise, reaching further into all segments of society. The Internet and related technologies are increasingly relevant to both clinical and forensic practice. This chapter describes several ways in which the Internet and other ICT (such as telepsychiatry) may impact the practice of forensic psychiatry.

The Information Revolution

Evidence gathered from the Internet or from personal computers, mobile phones, and data storage logs plays an increasingly important role in investigations and legal proceedings. In the past, forensic psychiatrists would have interviewed family members or others for collateral information; today, collateral information often includes some evidence gathered from the Internet or electronic communications. Judges and attorneys use social networking profiles and other Internet activity as character evidence for consideration in criminal sentencing, child custody disputes, and other cases. Law enforcement agencies use technology such as Global Positioning System (GPS) monitoring to help enforce restraining orders and to monitor offenders at higher risk for recidivism (Nellis 2010).

The so-called information revolution has also increased the risk of identity theft and hacking. As the amount of information accessible via the Internet continues to grow, forensic psychiatrists can expect to see an increase in cases of bribery, extortion, stalking, or harassment wherein personal information is used as a bargaining chip or a weapon to intimidate victims.

Social Networking

Commentators have noted the Internet's value for enhancing social communication and connecting people who suffer from isolation or alienation in their offline lives. However, the formation of identity groups and communities online may also lead to an increase in social capital and empowerment among people with harmful beliefs or criminal activity. The Internet's versatility for social networking has been exploited by extremist groups (e.g., terrorist organizations and cults), hate groups (e.g., neo-Nazi communities), street gangs (Patton et al. 2016), and individuals with deviant sexual desires, such as pedophilia (Temporini 2012). Internet-based social networking also plays a role in the formation of suicide pacts (Recupero et al. 2008) and the spread of proanorexia communities (Oksanen et al. 2016). As forensic psychiatrists encounter more cases in which the Internet plays a prominent role, understanding how people use ICT and its significance in legal proceedings will be crucial to assisting the courts.

Internet's Impact on Forensic Psychiatry: Civil and Criminal Cases

The Internet may play a significant role in a variety of forensic evaluations, and forensic psychiatrists should be familiar with the wide variety of ways the Internet may be used for criminal activity. Additionally, forensic evaluators should know how online information can be useful in formulating forensic opinions.

Problematic Internet Use

In 1995, psychiatrist Ivan K. Goldberg humorously proposed a new disorder called "Internet addictive disorder" to satirize the diagnostic criteria in the *Diagnostic and Statistical Manual of Mental Disorders*, 4th Edition (DSM-IV; American Psychiatric Association 1994) (Wallis 1997). To his surprise, he received an outpouring of interest from colleagues who had encountered problematic Internet use (PIU) in the course of their clinical practice. Although Goldberg had cautioned that use of the term *addiction* might not be appropriate in describing the problem, many clinicians disagreed. The controversy continues to this day, with some researchers referring to the behavior as "Internet addiction" and others using different terms. The inclusion of Internet gaming disorder as a "condition for further study" in DSM-5 (American Psychiatric Association 2013, pp. 795–798) underscores the need for further research on PIU and its growing importance in psychiatry.

Typically, PIU includes excessive or otherwise troublesome use of chat rooms, online pornography, cybersex, online gaming or gambling, and social networking sites. Problematic use of mobile phones (particularly smartphones and texting) is also common, although distinctions between "the Internet" and "mobile phones" are rapidly becoming outdated as ICT evolves. PIU research has become more specialized and offers many resources for forensic psychiatrists to tailor evidence-based treatment recommendations in individual cases (Franklin and Swan 2015; Kim et al. 2012). Recupero (2008) offers suggestions for the forensic evaluation of individuals with PIU, including the types of cases in which PIU may arise and recommended questions to help guide psychiatric interviews and case formulation.

Cyberharassment, Cyberbullying, and Cyberstalking

The term *cyberharassment* can refer to several different types of harassing behavior that may occur in electronic communications, including general cyberharassment, cyberbullying, and cyberstalking. These behaviors frequently overlap, but state laws provide more specific definitions. Generally, *cyberbullying* refers to electronic harassment of children and adolescents, whereas *cyberharassment* tends to apply more frequently to similar behavior among adults. A related behavior is "trolling," which refers to deliberately annoying, upsetting, or provoking negative emotional reactions through social media. *Cyberstalking* is "the repeated use of the internet or digital electronic communication devices to harass or threaten a specific individual or group of individuals" (Short et al. 2014, p. 133).

The widely reported suicides of cyberharassment victims have catalyzed the passage of anti-cyberbullying laws in several jurisdictions (Barnett 2009). Some states allow criminal prosecution for cyberbullying, but victims and their families may also sue for damages through civil proceedings (e.g., torts). Similarly, a number of states have passed criminal cyberstalking statutes, and others have revised existing stalking laws to include some types of cyberstalking behaviors (Shimizu 2013).

The use of camera phones, palm-sized digital camcorders, and video recording applications on tablet computers and smartphones, together with the disinhibiting social nature of Internet communication, has increased the reach of electronic shaming and public humiliation. Persons who commit social faux pas or whose behaviors elicit fear or judgment from others (e.g., the ranting of a person in an acute phase of mania or psychosis) may be subjected to widespread harassment or shaming by strangers when a covertly filmed video of them is uploaded to the Web and shared via social media. Similarly, the impact on a victim when sexually explicit images are publicly broadcast or distributed without permission can be devastating. These behaviors frequently occur in the context of cyberharassment and may even elicit increased harassment of sexual assault survivors. If the victim is a minor, the images may constitute child pornography.

The Internet contains a large amount of personal information that can be accessed and exploited to intimidate, control, humiliate, or obsessively follow a victim. Some stalkers make use of the Internet's easy access to information, such as a victim's address, phone number, e-mail address, workplace, and friends' and relatives' contact information (e.g., via friend lists on social networking sites). Perpetrators may send the victim threatening or harassing messages through e-mail, texting, or other messaging capabilities, such as by posting defamatory comments or upsetting images on a person's social networking profile. Cyberstalkers and cyberharassers often employ another tactic that would be more challenging to carry out without ICT: the impersonation of the victim or another party in order to inflict some kind of harm. In one case, a man impersonated his victim by posting personal ads in her name, claiming that she had rape fantasies, and placing her home address online (Glancy et al. 2007).

Another common tactic in cyberharassment campaigns is the practice of "doxing," whereby highly personal information and documents are broadcast publicly without the target's permission, usually by anonymous publication on the

Web (Hinduja 2015). Doxing targets frequently find that the harassing behaviors are not confined to cyberspace, and they may receive threatening phone calls, undergo vandalism or destruction of their personal property, receive anonymous e-mailed death threats, or even experience face-to-face confrontations with strangers who obtained home and work addresses online. Targets of some severe and virulent cyberharassment campaigns have been forced to flee their homes due to credible threats of violence, rape, and homicide.

Sex Crimes

In the twenty-first century, the Internet plays a central role in the commission of many sex crimes. The perception of anonymity in cyberspace may embolden Internet users to seek out sexual material they would not be comfortable viewing in the real world or that would be difficult to obtain offline, such as some of the more bizarre paraphilias (McGrath and Casey 2002) as well as violent pornography. Pedophiles trade images and videos through message boards and peer-to-peer file-sharing networks and may even share tips on identifying and grooming potential victims for child molestation or child pornography (Temporini 2012).

ICT also figures prominently into new types of troubling behavior for which existing criminal laws and procedures may not be well adapted. In "revenge porn," for example, a person (e.g., a former romantic partner) who has access to explicit photographs of a victim posts the photos online at a pornographic Web site without the victim's consent. Revenge-porn cases can result in significant emotional harm to the victim, but they are often difficult to prosecute (Henry and Powell 2016). "Sexting" (the practice of taking and sharing sexually explicit images via mobile phones) is problematic when the participants are not over the age of consent. In these cases, images constitute child pornography, and schools and law enforcement departments often struggle to protect youth from exploitation without unduly punishing or pathologizing a practice that has become a common behavior among many adolescents.

Other Criminal Cases

In murder trials, the prosecution may introduce digital evidence that the defendant had been using search engines or other electronic resources to learn about or acquire poisons or other weapons. The Internet allows would-be criminals access to weapons, particularly as increased scrutiny and restrictions are applied to firearm purchases from licensed sellers. Persons unable to purchase firearms legally through licensed dealers can download templates for creating gun components on 3D printers or purchase unregulated firearm components (and instructions for assembly) through Internet channels (Jensen-Haxel 2012). Additionally, social networking appears to be playing a role in the arrangement of contract homicides (Wiederhold 2013), prostitution (Jonsson et al. 2014), and the illegal sale of drugs (Klein and Kandel 2011).

Threat Assessments

Cases of mass homicide have created an increased demand for violence risk assessments. Data generated by ICT, such as transcripts of text conversations, can be helpful to the forensic psychiatrist in conducting a threat assessment. For example, the perpetrators' Internet activity prior to the Columbine High School shootings in 1999 revealed evidence of violent fantasies and suspicious planning (Block 2007). Referrals for threat assessments may also be prompted by content that a person posts online.

Elonis v. United States (2015) is illustrative of the types of cases that forensic psychiatrists may encounter. Anthony Elonis (under the pseudonym Tone Dougie) posted threatening comments and media on Facebook, hinting at violent and homicidal intentions toward his estranged wife, a female coworker, and an FBI agent who had contacted him because of his troubling Internet activity. Elonis's attorney argued that the threatening content was a therapeutic entertainment for him and that his posts were merely the creative outlet of an aspiring rap artist. The U.S. Supreme Court ruled in Elonis's favor. Nevertheless, when considered in light of recent mass shootings and the role of threatening behavior in intimate partner violence, Internet activity hinting at violent plans may provoke genuine fear and concern among others.

When online threats or expressions of suicidal or homicidal ideation are brought to the attention of school officials or authorities, forensic psychiatrists may be asked to offer their opinions regarding the seriousness of the threat. These types of cases may arise, for example, if a student's social networking profile or blog contains disturbing images or writings, such as statements suggestive of suicide plans or photographs of the student posing with weapons. When performing these evaluations, the clinician should obtain as much electronic data as possible and reference these collateral sources in support of his or her opinions and recommendations. For example, texting a friend sarcastic jokes about violent fantasies toward a teacher who has given an adolescent after-school detention may be harmless and commonplace, but concern might be warranted if those communications are accompanied by a 100-page manifesto on the student's laptop describing detailed plans for acquiring a weapon, disposing of the body, and evading detection.

Torts

Problematic Internet behaviors often cause significant emotional harm to victims, who may sue for damages for intentional or negligent infliction of emotional distress or defamation claims. In litigation, assistance from forensic psychiatrists may be necessary to help the court evaluate emotional damages. In cases alleging serious injury (e.g., insurance claims, personal injury lawsuits), attorneys often introduce evidence gleaned from parties' social networking activity to corroborate or refute a claimant's allegations (Gladysz 2012).

In some cases, a physician's use of ICT may be relevant to establish negligence in malpractice proceedings. When a student in California died by suicide, for example, an investigation revealed that a doctor in Colorado had prescribed antidepressants for the young man over the Internet without having conducted a face-to-face examination (Neimark 2009). A patient who enters the name of a medication into a search engine to learn more about the treatment may find, among the top results, links to law firms soliciting clients for torts against the pharmaceutical company that manufactures the drug. Medical information on the Internet may also affect the role of the forensic expert in consultations or in the courtroom. This may be especially problematic for defendant physicians in malpractice litigation, as studies suggest that even individuals with little to no medical training can find accurate diagnoses for medical symptoms through Internet search engines (Siempos et al. 2008).

Disability and Fitness for Duty

ICT can be especially relevant in independent medical evaluations and evaluations for disability and fitness for duty.

A careful review of digital collateral information can help to shed light on the veracity or reliability of an evaluee's self-report. Reviewing text messages, e-mail communications, and social media activity (e.g., status updates or "tweets") for dates selected at random can provide detailed information about an evaluee's daily routines and social and occupational functioning. Internet searches of an evaluee's name may yield unexpected results relevant to a psychiatric assessment (see, e.g., Neimark et al. 2006). In some cases, a professional's Internet activity may prompt a referral for a fitness-for-duty evaluation (e.g., graphic solicitation of sex with accompanying explicit "selfies" on dating Web sites; "unprofessional" or paranoid ranting on social networking sites about one's colleagues, competitors, or clients; or vlogging [video blogging] while noticeably intoxicated).

The disinhibiting nature of computer-mediated communication can also increase the risk of boundary violations and other unprofessional conduct among physicians, therapists, teachers, attorneys, and other professionals (Gabbard et al. 2011; Terry 2012). When professionals or other workers are subjected to adverse employment actions because of information posted online, they may sue for wrongful termination or other claims. For example, a customer service representative placed on involuntary medical leave might bring suit under the Americans With Disabilities Act of 1990 if the discipline were prompted by a tweet about his or her bipolar disorder.

Family Law

Forensic psychiatrists may encounter divorce or child custody cases in which Internet-based behavior or evidence plays a central role. Cybersex and "online affairs" contribute to a significant number of divorce cases today (Varnado 2013), and attorneys often introduce evidence downloaded from social networking sites and other forms of ICT (Gladysz 2012). Individuals with severe problematic Internet use may neglect interpersonal and occupational responsibilities, and this can have implications for custody determinations. When serving as an expert witness or a consultant in family law cases, a psychiatrist should review any available Internet-based documents that may be relevant to the proceedings; attorneys can help to provide access to such data.

Internet's Impact on Psychiatry

Forensic specialists should understand how the Internet is affecting the practice of psychiatry in general. As ICT makes more medical information available to the public, relationships between patients and physicians are changing. For doctors, Internet-facilitated growth in patient autonomy has been a double-edged sword. On the one hand, empowered patients can help their doctors provide the best treatment possible for their ailments. On the other hand, as Alexander Pope noted in his "Essay on Criticism," "a little learning is a dangerous thing" (Pope 1713).

The Web holds an abundance of inaccurate medical information, and Internet pharmacies often sell dangerous drugs without providing the warnings or monitoring that would normally apply in a traditional doctor-patient relationship. Antipsychiatry groups, such as the Church of Scientology and members of the psychiatric "survivor" movement, have prominent Web sites that discourage patients from seeking treatment for psychiatric illness (e.g., The Antipsychiatry

TABLE 32–1. **Risks and protective factors for Internet use by persons with mental illness**

Risk	Protective
Substance use disorders	
Online pharmacies selling controlled substances without a valid prescription	Support groups branching out online
Web sites providing information on how to synthesize drugs and how to abuse different psychoactive substances	Online treatment for addictions; anonymity may make seeking help easier
Peer pressure on the Internet (e.g., baiting for overdoses in chat rooms, adolescents' promotion of drug abuse on social network site profiles)	Information on medical Web sites about how to get treatment for addictions
Depression	
Pro- and how-to suicide material online (Recupero et al. 2008)	Depression and suicide/self-harm support groups
Baiting in Internet chat rooms	Use of Internet to seek support from friends and family
Relationship to problematic Internet use	Informative Web sites (e.g., APA, NIMH)
Bipolar disorder/mania	
Sexual risk taking (e.g., locating sex partners through Internet)	Safe outlets for symptoms of hypersexuality (e.g., cybersex)
Impulse dysregulation (e.g., one-click ordering, bidding on auction sites)	Possible to chat with people in different time zones without calling friends at unreasonable hours of the night
Schizophrenia/psychosis	
Delusions (e.g., thought insertion by computer, conspiracy theory Web sites, persecutory delusions re: cookies, personal information databases online, ideas of reference related to targeted advertising)	Support groups with peers who can help patients to recognize symptoms and to learn and practice techniques for adapting
Perceptual disturbances and confusion about reality in virtual reality/Internet applications	Informational resources for families and friends
Automatic written record of fantasies and delusions	Potential to expand research opportunities to advance treatments (e.g., through patient social networking)
Anxiety	
"Cyberchondria," "medical Googling" by patients	Use of technology (e.g., virtual reality exposure therapy) in treating phobias

Source. APA=American Psychiatric Association; NIMH=National Institute of Mental Health.

Coalition [http://www.antipsychiatry.org], Citizens Commission on Human Rights [http://www.cchr.org/#/home]). Although a thorough discussion of the relationship between Internet use and various psychiatric disorders cannot be presented in a single chapter, some relevant points are listed in Table 32–1, which illustrates sample risk and protective factors by different diagnostic categories. Psychiatrists may find this type of information helpful during case formulation.

Of particular interest to forensic psychiatrists, the Internet figures importantly into factitious illness and malingering. Patients can download and use medical information and media from the Internet to feign injury or illness. Layperson-produced information about Morgellons disease online has been linked to delusional parasitosis (Robles et al. 2011). The public can access Web sites that coach would-be malingerers on behavior and symptoms associated with a greater likelihood of receiving disability benefits; information at these sites includes desired responses to neuropsychological testing and tactics for detecting malingering (Kleinman and Martell 2015). Clinicians have reported several cases of Munchausen by Internet (Cunningham and Feldman 2011) and Munchausen by proxy by Internet (Brown et al. 2014).

Furthermore, the information revolution has increased public access to information that may have been limited to medical and mental health professionals in the past. For example, video-sharing services such as YouTube allow access to free educational videos, designed for nurses- and therapists-in-training, that portray real or simulated patients exhibiting behavioral symptoms of many psychiatric disorders. Evaluees may arrive at appointments armed with knowledge of diagnostic criteria and may behave in such a way as to convey the characteristics of a particular illness. Evaluees may even be aware of techniques designed to identify malingering.

Apps and mHealth

During forensic interviews, psychiatrists may find it helpful and informative to ask evaluees about which software applications (apps) they use. The proliferation and popularity of apps designed for smartphones and tablet computers have dramatically increased in recent years (see Turvey and Roberts 2015). Health-related apps are among the most popular, and a number of software developers offer apps targeted toward behavioral health consumers.

Forensic psychiatrists today have at their disposal a nearly infinite variety of technological tools to help support their professional activities. The functions of these tools often overlap, and distinctions between different technological applications are growing blurred. Numerous apps have been designed specifically for clinicians and other health care professionals (e.g., educational tools for continuing medical education). When using health-related apps, the source of the software may be a concern, particularly when software is available for free download.

Some free apps marketed to mental health professionals are designed and distributed by pharmaceutical companies. Free apps often involve the use of advertisements or data collection (e.g., by installing cookies on the user's device) to recover research and development costs. Furthermore, just as some Web sites and other discussion forums online promote eating disorders or other problematic behaviors, apps can also be used for potentially harmful purposes. Psychiatrists who wish to learn more about several popular mental health apps available at the time of this writing will find the Turvey and Roberts (2015) review helpful.

Telepsychiatry

A growing body of research supports the effectiveness of electronic service delivery models in psychiatry and mental health, including telepsychiatry. Although telepsychiatry is hardly a new phenomenon in the mental health field, its use has expanded rapidly in recent years, largely due to gains in the pace of technological progress and decreasing costs associated with high-quality technology. Traditionally, *telepsychiatry* refers to "[t]he provision of psychiatric treatment via live interactive videoconferencing" (Shore 2013, p. 256), but the model may also be asynchronous or may involve only diagnostic use rather than treatment (e.g., conducting forensic psychiatric evaluations via videoconferencing technology). A strong research base has shown that telepsychiatry is generally safe and effective for clinical use (Bashshur et al. 2016), and the research supporting its forensic use is growing (Antonacci et al. 2008; Khalifa et al. 2008; Lexcen et al. 2006; Manguno-Mire et al. 2007).

Special caution is warranted when determining which software and hardware to use for videoconferencing in telepsychiatry. Not all popular software programs are compliant with the Health Insurance Portability and Accountability Act of 1996 (HIPAA), and physicians have been disciplined for using popular videoconferencing programs to treat patients. Practitioners have developed standards for minimally acceptable technological specifications, such as bandwidth, and practical issues, such as room configurations (Shore 2013). Special considerations may be appropriate when considering the use of videoconferencing technology for forensic evaluations. Forensic specialists who are considering adding videoconferencing-based services to their practices should familiarize themselves with clinical practice guidelines and similar resources regarding their use (Myers et al. 2008; Turvey et al. 2013; Yellowlees et al. 2010).

Electronic Communication

The use of e-mail, text messaging ("texting"), secure messaging through patient portals, and instant messaging technol-

ogy with evaluees or patients appears to be growing more commonplace. Some forms of electronic messaging have become automated, such as e-mail or text alerts when a patient's electronic medical record has been updated or changed as well as electronic reminders about appointments or medications. Because the use of ICT by psychiatrists carries significant ethical, clinical, and legal considerations, any psychiatrist who is considering using electronic communications or developing practice Web sites in clinical or forensic practice should become familiar with the current legal and ethical guidelines from governing bodies regarding the use of ICT (e.g., American Medical Association 2011; Federation of State Medical Boards 2012).

Social Media

Social networking sites (e.g., Facebook, LinkedIn, Twitter, PatientsLikeMe), video-sharing sites (e.g., YouTube), and virtual worlds (e.g., Second Life) have gained important roles in the transmission of health information and education. Many health organizations have begun advertising or public health information campaigns on sites like YouTube, and some practitioners use applications like Second Life to deliver treatments such as group therapy and exposure therapy for anxiety. Social media can also provide forensic psychiatrists with valuable tools for education and information gathering. Forensic evaluees may post content through social networking tools about suicidal ideation, homicidal ideation, or substance abuse that they might not volunteer to the treating clinician or forensic specialist.

As can occur with other electronic communications between psychiatrists and patients or evaluees, significant boundary violations can easily develop, for example, if the psychiatrist sends or accepts friend requests from evaluees, patients, attorneys, or judges on social networking sites or allows public comments on his or her blog or profile. The accessibility of personal data through social networking site profiles and Internet searches is of particular concern for psychiatrists who work with potentially dangerous evaluees. In many cases, the doctor's home address and other personal information can be easily located through a variety of Internet-based tools.

Patients or others who post reviews of physicians on online rating sites such as Yelp and HealthGrades can raise further concerns. Bound by strict laws for the confidentiality of health information, physicians often have little recourse when evaluees, patients, or others post negative reviews online. Blogging or posting content about one's forensic practice on social media must be done extremely carefully to avoid ethical indiscretions. Furthermore, medical professionals may be held to higher standards for professionalism and personal conduct in their Internet activity than are members of the general public (Greysen et al. 2013). Professional organizations that have published ethical guidelines on the use of social media and ICT include the American College of Physicians and Federation of State Medical Boards (Farnan et al. 2013; Federation of State Medical Boards 2012) and the American Medical Association (2011).

Legal and Ethical Risk Management

Because the Internet introduces numerous additional legal risks while potentially increasing existing risks, psychiatrists are advised to seek the advice of legal or risk management professionals in order to minimize their exposure to li-

ability, as well as to ensure they are in compliance with the applicable laws and rules. Malpractice insurance carriers frequently provide informational resources such as newsletters and updates on recent developments in mental health law. Psychiatrists who have a significant Internet presence should be certain to report this to their insurance carrier.

As highly publicized incidents of medical data theft and hacking become more frequent, data-breach insurance is also available for professionals concerned about the potentially devastating financial impact of a health data breach. Clinicians should ensure that their practice's privacy notice conforms to HIPAA. Consultation with an attorney may be advisable if the psychiatrist intends to rely heavily on ICT in clinical or forensic practice (e.g., having an interactive practice Web site, exchanging texts or e-mails with patients or evaluees, conducting forensic interviews or treatment via telepsychiatry, or using virtual worlds or smartphone apps for evaluation or adjunctive treatment). Attorneys can advise psychiatrists regarding their malpractice exposure as well as licensure and jurisdiction issues that may arise if the doctor and evaluee are in different states.

Because nearly all uses of ICT in psychiatry carry some risk to the privacy of sensitive personal health information, evaluees' informed consent should be obtained for the use of these technologies. Evaluees should be informed, for example, if the technology being used will store potentially sensitive and confidential personal information (Turvey and Roberts 2015). Furthermore, some states have laws specifically crafted to regulate the practice of telemedicine, some of which require written consent (Shore 2013). Psychiatrists who use ICT professionally should be certain to familiarize themselves with any applicable federal and state laws that may come into play, including licensure requirements.

Conclusion

The Internet has become one of the defining features of society in the twenty-first century. The pace of technological change is rapid, and the integration of technology into people's lives has far-reaching implications for the practice of general and forensic psychiatry. The connection between ICT and forensic psychiatry is an area of growing importance in the specialty, and the role of electronic media is likely to continue changing and growing as psychiatry evolves as a profession. In the future it will be increasingly important for forensic psychiatrists to pay careful and close attention to the changes in Internet-related technology and culture and to apply sound risk management strategies when introducing new technology into their professional work.

Key Concepts

- Electronic data from information and communications technology are becoming increasingly relevant to the practice of forensic psychiatry.

- Forensic psychiatrists should request and review any relevant electronic data as part of the usual analysis of collateral information.

- Specialized resources and publications are available to assist forensic psychiatrists in evaluating cases involving problematic Internet use.

- Forensic psychiatrists should be familiar with common tactics employed by perpetrators of cyberharassment, cyberstalking, and cyberbullying, as well as the effects on victims.

- Problematic Internet use behaviors and their potential impact change over time as new technologies become available.

- A significant amount of criminal activity today involves the use of Internet and information and communications technology.

- Forensic psychiatrists should be familiar with Internet resources that may affect an evaluee's presentation, particularly with respect to malingering and factitious illness.

References

American Medical Association: Code of medical ethics, opinion 9.124—professionalism in the use of social media. June 2011. Available at: http://www.ama-assn.org/ama/pub/physician-resources/medical-ethics/codemedical-ethics/opinion9124.page. Accessed January 15, 2017.

American Psychiatric Association: Diagnostic and Statistical Manual of Mental Disorders, 4th Edition. Washington, DC, American Psychiatric Association, 1994

American Psychiatric Association: Diagnostic and Statistical Manual of Mental Disorders, 5th Edition. Arlington, VA, American Psychiatric Publishing, 2013

Americans With Disabilities Act. Pub. L. No. 101-336, 1990

Antonacci DJ, Bloch RM, Saeed SA, et al: Empirical evidence on the use and effectiveness of telepsychiatry via videoconferencing: implications for forensic and correctional psychiatry. Behav Sci Law 26(3):253–269, 2008 18548519

Barnett C: Cyberbullying: a new frontier and a new standard: a survey of and proposed changes to state cyberbullying statutes. Quinnipiac L Rev 27:579–624, 2009

Bashshur RL, Shannon GW, Bashshur N, et al: The empirical evidence for telemedicine interventions in mental disorders. Telemed J E Health 22(2):87–113, 2016 26624248

Block JJ: Lessons from Columbine: virtual and real rage. Am J Forensic Psychiatry 28:5–34, 2007

Brown AN, Gonzalez GR, Wiester RT, et al: Care taker blogs in caregiver fabricated illness in a child: a window on the caretaker's thinking? Child Abuse Negl 38(3):488–497, 2014 24393290

Cunningham JM, Feldman MD: Munchausen by Internet: current perspectives and three new cases. Psychosomatics 52(2):185–189, 2011 21397112

Elonis v United States, Slip Op. No. 13-983, 575 U.S. ___, 135 S.Ct. 2001 (June 1, 2015)

Farnan JM, Snyder Sulmasy L, Worster BK, et al; American College of Physicians Ethics, Professionalism and Human Rights Committee; American College of Physicians Council of Associates; Federation of State Medical Boards Special Committee on Ethics and Professionalism*: Online medical professionalism: patient and public relationships: policy statement from the American College of Physicians and the Federation of State Medical Boards. Ann Intern Med 158(8):620–627, 2013 23579867

Federation of State Medical Boards: Model Policy Guidelines for the Appropriate Use of Social Media and Social Networking in Medical Practice. Euless, TX, Federation of State Medical Boards of the United States, 2012

Franklin LD, Swan SA: Psychodynamic treatment of excessive virtual reality environment use. Clin Case Stud 14:482–493, 2015

Gabbard GO, Kassaw KA, Perez-Garcia G: Professional boundaries in the era of the Internet. Acad Psychiatry 35(3):168–174, 2011 21602438

Gladysz LM: Status update: when social media enters the courtroom. I/S: A Journal of Law and Policy for the Information Society 7:688–717, 2012

Glancy GD, Newman AW, Potash MN, et al: Cyberstalking, in Stalking: Psychiatric Perspectives and Practical Approaches. Edited by Pinals DA. New York, Oxford University Press, 2007, pp 212–226

Greysen SR, Johnson D, Kind T, et al: Online professionalism investigations by state medical boards: first, do no harm. Ann Intern Med 158(2):124–130, 2013 23318312

Health Insurance Portability and Accountability Act. Pub. L. No. 104-191, 1996

Henry N, Powell A: Sexual violence in the digital age: the scope and limits of criminal law. Social and Legal Studies 25(4):397–418, 2016

Hinduja S: Doxing and cyberbullying. Cyberbullying Research Center, September 16, 2015. Available at: http://cyberbullying.org/doxing-and-cyberbullying/. Accessed January 15, 2017.

Jensen-Haxel P: 3D printers, obsolete firearm supply controls, and the right to build self-defense weapons under Heller. Gold Gate Univ Law Rev 42:447–496, 2012

Jonsson LS, Svedin CG, Hyden M: "Without the Internet, I never would have sold sex": young women selling sex online. Cyberpsychology 2014. Available at: http://cyberpsychology.eu/view.php?cisloclanku=2014021703. Accessed January 15, 2017.

Khalifa N, Saleem Y, Stankard P: Use of telepsychiatry within forensic practice: literature review on the use of videolink. J Forensic Psychiatry Psychol 19:2–13, 2008

Kim SM, Han DH, Lee YS, et al: Combined cognitive behavioral therapy and bupropion for the treatment of problematic on-line game play in adolescents with major depressive disorder. Comp Hum Behav 28(5):1954–1959, 2012

Klein CA, Kandel S: www.mydrugdealer.com: Ethics and legal implications of Internet-based access to substances of abuse. J Am Acad Psychiatry Law 39(3):407–411, 2011, 21908759

Kleinman SB, Martell D: Failings of trauma-specific and related psychological tests in detecting post-traumatic stress disorder in forensic settings. J Forensic Sci 60(1):76–83, 2015 25425278

Lexcen FJ, Hawk GL, Herrick S, et al: Use of video conferencing for psychiatric and forensic evaluations. Psychiatr Serv 57(5):713–715, 2006 16675769

Manguno-Mire GM, Thompson JW Jr, Shore JH, et al: The use of telemedicine to evaluate competency to stand trial: a preliminary randomized controlled study. J Am Acad Psychiatry Law 35(4):481–489, 2007 18086740

McGrath MG, Casey E: Forensic psychiatry and the Internet: practical perspectives on sexual predators and obsessional harassers in cyberspace. J Am Acad Psychiatry Law 30(1):81–94, 2002 11931372

Myers K, Cain S; Work Group on Quality Issues; American Academy of Child and Adolescent Psychiatry Staff: Practice parameter for telepsychiatry with children and adolescents. J Am Acad Child Adolesc Psychiatry 47(12):1468–1483, 2008 19034191

Neimark G: Boundary violation. J Am Acad Psychiatry Law 37(1):95–97, 2009 19297640

Neimark G, Hurford MO, DiGiacomo J: The Internet as collateral informant (letter). Am J Psychiatry 163(10):1842, 2006 17012705

Nellis M: Eternal Vigilance Inc.: the satellite tracking of offenders in "real time." J Technol Hum Serv 28:23–43, 2010

Oksanen A, Garcia D, Räsänen P: Proanorexia communities on social media. Pediatrics 137(1):e20153372, 2016 26676052

Patton DU, Lane J, Leonard P, et al: Gang violence on the digital street: case study of a South Side Chicago gang member's Twitter communication. New Media and Society 2016 [Epub ahead of print]

Pope A: An Essay on Criticism, 2nd Edition. London, W Lewis, 1713. Available at: http://www.eighteenthcenturypoetry.org/works/o3675-w0010.shtml. Accessed January 15, 2017.

Recupero PR: Forensic evaluation of problematic Internet use. J Am Acad Psychiatry Law 36(4):505–514, 2008 19092069

Recupero PR, Harms SE, Noble JM: Googling suicide: surfing for suicide information on the Internet. J Clin Psychiatry 69(6):878–888, 2008 18494533

Robles DT, Olson JM, Combs H, et al: Morgellons disease and delusions of parasitosis. Am J Clin Dermatol 12(1):1–6, 2011 21110523

Shimizu A: Domestic violence in the digital age: towards the creation of a comprehensive cyberstalking statute. Berkeley J Gender Law Justice 28:116–137, 2013

Shore JH: Telepsychiatry: videoconferencing in the delivery of psychiatric care. Am J Psychiatry 170(3):256–262, 2013 23450286

Short E, Linford S, Wheatcroft JM, et al: The impact of cyberstalking: the lived experience—a thematic analysis. Stud Health Technol Inform 199:133–137, 2014 24875706

Siempos II, Spanos A, Issaris EA, et al: Nonphysicians may reach correct diagnoses by using Google: a pilot study. Swiss Med Wkly 138(49–50):741–745, 2008 19130327

Temporini H: Child pornography and the Internet. Psychiatr Clin North Am 35(4):821–835, 2012 23107565

Terry NP: Fear of Facebook: private ordering of social media risks incurred by healthcare providers. Neb Law Rev 90:703–751, 2012

Turvey CL, Roberts LJ: Recent developments in the use of online resources and mobile technologies to support mental health care. Int Rev Psychiatry 27(6):547–557, 2015 26523397

Turvey C, Coleman M, Dennison O, et al: ATA practice guidelines for video-based online mental health services. Telemed J E Health 19(9):722–730, 2013 23909884

Varnado SS: Avatars, scarlet "A"s, and adultery in the technological age. Ariz Law Rev 55:371–416, 2013

Wallis D: Just click no. The New Yorker Magazine, January 13, 1997, p 28

Wiederhold BK: Are "Facebook murders" a growing trend? Cyberpsychol Behav Soc Netw 16(1):1–2, 2013 23320869

Yellowlees P, Shore J, Roberts L: Practice guidelines for videoconferencing-based telemental health—October 2009. Telemed J E Health 16(10):1074–1089, 2010 2118699

CHAPTER 33

Research in Forensic Psychiatry

Robert L. Trestman, Ph.D., M.D.
Arielle R. Baskin-Sommers, Ph.D.

Landmark Case

***Kaimowitz v. Michigan Dept. of Mental Health,* 1 MDLR 147 (1973)**

Justice-involved individuals exhibit a wide range of behavioral problems and psychopathologies. They represent heterogeneous groups that end up in the judicial or correctional system for varying reasons. Given this heterogeneity, the need to improve the ability to identify factors that predict the causes and likelihood of antisocial behavior associated with psychiatric illness and the treatments administered to those who are justice-involved or incarcerated is real and pressing.

The disproportionate number of evaluees, parolees, and inmates with psychiatric problems provides a rich opportunity to understand the etiology and pathogenesis of mental illness and associated behaviors that may result in criminal convictions and incarceration. Forensic psychiatrists also have the opportunity to develop approaches to mitigate the maladaptive behaviors that have such profound social and personal impact and can result in arrest and incarceration. However, conducting forensic psychiatric research requires consideration of unique issues related to ethics and feasibility.

History of Forensic Psychiatry Research

Although research within the discipline of forensic psychiatry covers a broad spectrum of topics, the evolution of fo-

489

rensic psychiatric scholarship can be conceptualized in terms of three domains: causation, prediction, and intervention. Below are summaries of the application of forensic psychiatry to these domains.

Causation

Antisocial behavior (including impulsive, aggressive, predatory, and/or violent actions) generates physical, emotional, and economic burdens. For example, during 2014, incidents of violent and nonviolent crime in the United States approached 31,000 per day, and the financial impact on society was estimated as over 3 trillion dollars (U.S. Department of Justice 2015). The pervasiveness of these behaviors highlights the importance of identifying those specific causal factors that are etiologically related to the onset and maintenance of antisocial behavior.

The first attempts to describe the factors that contribute to the development of antisocial tendencies focused on the physical makeup of offenders. Empirical studies portrayed criminal behavior as a function of a single factor or trait, such as body type or defective intelligence (Goring 1913). Multigenerational family studies (Dugdale 1877; Goddard 1912) purported that some traits could be identified as socially inferior and that those traits were heritable. This type of research was used to support the pseudoscience of eugenics and related practices, such as the "scientific" breeding of human beings and sterilization of individuals with inferior or dangerous heritable traits.

Current research focuses on genetic studies, which have the potential to parse the heterogeneity of antisocial behavior based on differential levels of risk in the context of other causal factors. Evidence clearly indicates that specific genotypes confer risk for antisocial behavior and aggression as well as psychiatric condi-

tions related to increased risk of behaviors that may result in criminal justice involvement or incarceration (e.g., substance use disorders, borderline personality disorder, bipolar disorder) (Baker et al. 2006; Viding and Frith 2006). However, equally clear evidence demonstrates that the interaction between genetic and environmental mechanisms is of major importance in explaining individual differences in antisocial behavior (Simons et al. 2011).

Genetic and environmental factors increasingly are understood to shape the way in which biological systems develop and function, and thus affect multiple complex psychological processes important in controlling and regulating behavior (Barnes and Jacobs 2013; Caspi et al. 2002; Kim-Cohen et al. 2006). Nevertheless, important gaps in knowledge remain, and a future challenge for forensic psychiatry lies in determining the specific genetic and environmental influences that generate neurophysiological changes that result in the more proximal cognitive, affective, and behavioral risk factors for violence (Glenn and Raine 2014).

Prediction and Forensic Risk Assessment

In the 1970s, the prediction of an individual's potential dangerousness became a focus of attention in forensic psychiatry. At that time, predictions were largely based on clinical judgments. However, research on the accuracy of these predictions (referred to as first-generation risk predictions) demonstrated that clinicians were not much better than chance in predicting future violence (Monahan 1981).

These findings led to the development of actuarial or historical/static schemes to assess for risk for violence (see Chapter 28, "Violence Risk Assessment"). This "second-generation" approach to risk assessment moved away from categorical predictions of "dangerousness" and toward a proportional estimate of violence risk (Monahan 1988). Instruments such as the Psychopathy Checklist—Revised (Hare 2003) and Violence Risk Appraisal Guide (Quinsey et al. 1998) used algorithms to identify individual risk trajectories (Hart et al. 2007; Singh et al. 2014). Unfortunately, these algorithms often demonstrated poor precision and high error rates.

A third generation of risk research focused on "risk management" (see Chapter 28). Structured professional judgment tools for risk assessment, such as the Historical Clinical Risk Management—20 (HCR-20; Webster et al. 1997), use a structured clinical assessment to evaluate an individual's risk and protective factors (Hart and Logan 2011). Unfortunately, the utility of these tools in clinical settings is limited by several practical issues, including concerns regarding validity and the availability of appropriate resources to administer the instruments.

More recently, the risk-need-responsivity approach has been implemented as an integrated risk assessment and classification model (Bonta and Andrews 2007, 2010). This model, originally developed for use with justice-involved individuals, is based on a social learning model of deviance and integrates multiple domains to classify and predict future behaviors. Some disagreement exists regarding the application of the risk-need-responsivity approach as a prediction tool (Taxman et al. 2006). However, the multiple-domain framework used to characterize a person's past and future behavior provides a more integrative assessment than any single measure.

Unfortunately, a lack of precision remains in the development of prediction

tools, the use of those tools as evidence in forensic cases, and the standards that limit how those tools may be applied (Singh et al. 2015). As a result, evidence that includes their use may not be admitted in court proceedings, because such evidence may not meet the criteria for admissibility of scientific evidence (see Chapter 1, "The Expert Witness"). Consistent application of the *Daubert* criteria to scientific evidence was expected to result in a dramatic increase in forensic research–based testimony, but this has not proven true (Dahir et al. 2005; Shapiro et al. 2015). Nevertheless, the use of multiple levels of information across measures has the potential to improve the accuracy of prediction and the utility of these assessments in both clinical and forensic practice.

Intervention

For decades the U.S. judicial and correctional systems have struggled with an identity crisis centered on whether the purpose of incarceration is to punish or rehabilitate offenders. A strong shift toward a rehabilitative model began in the early twentieth century. In the early 1970s, sociopolitical unrest in America prompted a backlash against rehabilitation as a priority (Martinson 1974), and evidence was presented suggesting that rehabilitation did not work. Recent research demonstrates that many correctional treatment programs, particularly those that employ cognitive-behavioral therapies, are in fact effective in reducing impulsive aggression, antisocial behavior, and recidivism (Henwood et al. 2015; Kersten et al. 2016; Rotter and Carr 2013; Zajac 2015).

Progress has been made in developing psychopharmacological agents that have increased treatment effectiveness by targeting specific risk factors, including impulsivity, attention deficits, and underlying psychiatric disorders associated with increased risk of violence (Comai et al. 2012). A growing body of empirical evidence supports the efficacy of the use of antipsychotics for disruptive behavior disorders (Gorman et al. 2015; Henwood et al. 2015; Ipser and Stein 2007) and psychotic disorders, as well as the use of stimulants for conduct disorder and attention-deficit/hyperactivity disorder (Lichtenstein et al. 2012). Promising results have also demonstrated the efficacy of mood stabilizers (Pappadopulos et al. 2006).

In adults with impulsive aggression, treatment with selective serotonin reuptake inhibitors has been found to increase glucose metabolism in the orbitofrontal cortex, suggesting a potential method for improving functioning in brain regions that have been identified as deficient in antisocial populations (Glenn and Raine 2014). Although some research efforts persist in the field of pharmacology of impulsive aggression, notably targeting the serotonergic system, no pharmacological intervention that specifically targets impulsive aggression currently exists (Olivier and van Oorschot 2005). Nevertheless, the broader area of psychopharmacology research regarding medications that may decrease the incidence of offensive behavior is of critical importance and is being vigorously pursued (Umukoro et al. 2013).

Given the heterogeneity of offenders in the United States, developing a unified intervention strategy for all offenders is implausible. However, personalized approaches that target specific components of and motivations for antisocial behavior are emerging as potential interventions for crime prevention. The next steps in research on effective interventions in forensic psychiatry must take a multidimensional approach that considers the individual's environment, predispositions, and biological factors to determine mechanisms of behavior change.

Evolving Ethical Standards

A variety of codes and reports have helped shape the foundation for the ethical conduct of forensic psychiatric research and the ethical principles that guide clinical research with human subjects. The modern history of human subject protections began with the Nuremberg Trials, which exposed the atrocities of Nazi human experimentation during World War II and prompted the creation of the Nuremberg Code in 1949. The three basic elements of the Nuremberg Code—1) voluntary and informed consent, 2) a favorable risk-to-benefit analysis, and 3) the right to withdraw from research without repercussion—became the foundation for subsequent ethics codes and federal research regulations. Despite playing an integral role in the creation of the Nuremberg Code, U.S. federal regulation of research at that time was minimal.

The U.S. government's role in regulating research on human subjects changed following several highly publicized controversies. For example, in 1972, the public learned about the Tuskegee experiment, a 40-year research study in which the U.S. government withheld adequate treatment from a group of poor African American men with syphilis. The publicity about abuses of the rights of vulnerable people spurred reform in human subject regulations and the governing bodies that oversaw those regulations.

In the aftermath of these profound breaches of research ethics, the Policies for the Protection of Human Subjects were adopted in 1974 as official government regulations (Cislo and Trestman

2013). The U.S. National Commission for the Protection of Human Subjects of Biomedical and Behavioral Research was formed the same year and in 1978 published "The Belmont Report: Ethical Principles and Guidelines for the Protection of Human Subjects of Research" (National Commission for the Protection of Human Subjects of Biomedical and Behavioral Research 1978).

The recommendations proposed in the Belmont Report formed the basis of the Common Rule, the current U.S. federal regulations for protection of human subjects in research, codified in 1991 in the Code of Federal Regulations (45 CFR 46, 2005) (U.S. Department of Health and Human Services 1991). The Common Rule outlines requirements for human subject research and for research institutions to assure compliance, such as the requirements for institutional review boards (IRBs). Since the Common Rule was first codified, protections have been added for three populations deemed especially vulnerable to ethical lapses in research practices: pregnant women and fetuses (1975), prisoners (1978), and children (1991). A vulnerable population is one that has diminished autonomy.

Although federal regulation of permitted and proscribed research behavior is necessary to protect human rights, the Common Rule has not been without unintended consequences and controversy. For example, the Institute of Medicine considers prisoners an understudied population in many critical areas (Gostin et al. 2007). However, due to the complexities and ethical prohibitions regarding human research, especially in a federally defined vulnerable population, progress implementing research with this population has been slow.

One of the most significant aspects of the Common Rule is the mandate that all research proposals involving human subjects be reviewed by an IRB. Effective IRBs are critical components of all successful modern research organizations. Each institution's IRB has the responsibility for protecting human subjects of research, training investigators, and reviewing research proposals. Each IRB must develop policies, procedures, and membership consistent with the guidelines delineated in the Common Rule. A large element of research proposal review is affirming that the informed consent process and the informed consent form meet all regulatory standards. Data safety, adverse event monitoring, and periodic review are also components of IRB functioning (Enfield and Truwit 2008).

Whether a study requires IRB approval depends on whether it involves ongoing practice or actual research. In the Belmont Report, the National Commission defines *practice* as "interventions that are designed solely to enhance the well-being of an individual patient or client and that have a reasonable expectation of success" (Belmont Report, Section A). In contrast, the commission defines *research* as "an activity designed to test a hypothesis, permit conclusions to be drawn, and thereby to develop or contribute to generalizable knowledge" (Belmont Report, Section A). Projects that fit the commission's definition of practice are not considered human subject research and do not require IRB approval.

Three ethical principles inform the work of an institution's IRB: 1) respect for persons, 2) beneficence, and 3) justice. The principle of *respect for persons* incorporates two components related to individual autonomy: each individual has the right to self-determination, and "vulnerable" persons with diminished autonomy are entitled to additional protection to prevent exploitation. Four ethical research requirements follow directly from the principle of respect for persons:

1. Participants must voluntarily consent to participate in research.
2. The consent must be informed.
3. Privacy and confidentiality must be protected.
4. The participant has the right to withdraw from research participation without penalty or repercussions.

Informed consent is perhaps the most widely recognized ethical safeguard in clinical care and research. Informed consent consists of three key elements: voluntariness, disclosure, and capacity (Dyer and Bloch 1987). The landmark case of *Kaimowitz v. Michigan Dept. of Mental Health* (1973) highlighted the importance of these elements. The *Kaimowitz* decision emphasized that informed consent has to be based on the disclosure of appropriate information to a competent subject who is in a position to make a voluntary choice. The principal issue before the *Kaimowitz* court was whether an involuntarily detained psychiatric patient could render valid consent to psychosurgery. The court reasoned that because of a patient's "mental condition, the deprivation stemming from involuntary confinement, and the effects of the phenomenon of 'institutionalization,'" the patient's ability to render informed consent is seriously undermined. The court concluded that the coercive environment of the mental institution precludes mental patients from reasoning as equals with their doctors and that this "inherent inequality" renders it impossible for the patient to give a truly voluntary informed consent. The *Kaimowitz* court also concluded that because the effects of psychosurgery are so uncertain, "knowledgeable consent to psychosurgery [is] literally impossible."

Beneficence, the second ethical principle for IRBs, requires that researchers strive to maximize benefit and minimize harm to subjects. In other words, the risks of the research must be justified by the potential benefits to the individual, society, or both.

Finally, the principle of *justice* addresses equal distribution of both benefits and burdens of research and underlies the additional regulatory protections for vulnerable populations. Participant selection must be fair on an individual level, and researchers may not show favoritism when selecting research subjects. Selection must also be fair at the group level, and federal regulations protect certain vulnerable populations—that is, pregnant women, prisoners, and children—from being used as convenient samples. Other vulnerable populations not formally protected by the Common Rule, such as minorities, the poor, and institutionalized individuals, may also be at risk of improper selection for research studies.

Current Directions in Research Domains

Causation

The pervasiveness of antisocial behavior highlights the importance of identifying specific factors etiologically related to the onset and maintenance of such behaviors. Substantial progress in understanding these etiological factors has been made in a variety of disciplines, including the natural, social, and behavioral sciences. Increasingly, research in these fields documents the influence of neural, genetic, and environmental factors on broad classes of antisocial behavior. Across these studies, factors such as dysfunction in the anterior cingulate cortex, exposure to violence, community disadvantage, repeated engagement in the same behavior, and demographic factors such as age and sex appear to be important predictors. Other factors also differentiate subtypes of antisocial behaviors and disorders; these factors include specific genotypes, activation in the amygdala, familial interactions, peer relationships, trait impulsivity, and substance abuse (Baskin-Sommers 2016).

Nonetheless, research examining etiological factors across neuroanatomical, neurophysiological, developmental, social, and epigenetic domains is needed. Designing research to identify specific etiological factors at multiple levels of analysis could facilitate the identification of variables that need to be controlled for or addressed in risk prediction and the development of interventions that are increasingly more efficacious.

Prediction

Understanding or predicting human behavior is extraordinarily difficult, and forensic examination in civil or criminal settings continues to be an area of expanding research. One challenge to understanding or predicting crime is the complexity and heterogeneity of criminal behaviors and the people who engage in them. To date, behavioral factors have been the focus of prediction models. However, using biological markers as predictors holds great potential. For example, Aharoni et al. (2013) found that error-related brain activity, thought to be related to anterior cingulate cortex activity, elicited during performance of an inhibitory task predicted subsequent rearrests among adult offenders, beyond other risk factors (e.g., age, psychopathy score, substance use). Further examination of paradigms such as this may lead to pragmatic and useful tools for predicting the risk of future behavior.

Despite some evidence that standard behavioral factors are reliable predictors of behavior and that using biological

markers has some potential for predicting criminal behavior, increasing evidence indicates that chronic antisocial behavior is due not to one dysfunction but more likely to an interaction among multiple deficits and domains. Thus, for prediction methods to be more valuable, they must take into account the complexity of such behavior and the many factors that influence the onset and maintenance of this behavior.

For example, studies in individuals with schizophrenia (Kubicki et al. 2011) and Alzheimer's disease (Wolz et al. 2011) found that combining brain measures from different units of analysis into a single (weighted) value predicted disorder-specific symptoms more reliably than any of the individual measures. Therefore, prediction models should begin to take into account the influence of multiple factors that span biological and behavioral levels of analysis. Identifying convergence and unique relationships among predictors across levels of analysis, from biological to behavioral, will allow evaluation of the validity of each predictor and assess whether combining information across units of analysis strengthens the predictive power of determining violent or aggressive behavior.

The use of model-based assays to characterize subgroups of individuals by differences in multiple factors and mechanisms provides an opportunity to pursue formal differential diagnoses and profiles. Several relatively inexpensive tools are already available to measure brain activity (e.g., electrophysiology) or well-validated behavioral tasks that tap underlying brain function (e.g., measures of inhibitory control). These measures, combined with traditional risk factors, such as psychopathology (e.g., psychopathy), age, and environment might, for example, be implemented as part of routine risk assessment for parole.

Additionally, once the field of forensic psychiatry identifies specific measures that are representative of key predictive factors, statistical models can be developed (and run in standard programs) to provide a discrete risk propensity for a specific individual (Monahan et al. 2000; Stephan and Mathys 2014). These statistical programs have the potential to accept fields of data that would seem no different to the user than the typical risk assessment programs currently in use. No predictive assessment tool or model is going to be perfect, and the likelihood that a single measure will provide enough sensitivity and specificity for reliably predicting future behavior is slim. Therefore, the future of forensic prediction lies in assessing and modeling multiple factors and their interactions.

Intervention

Psychotherapeutic efforts to reduce the risk of aggressive, violent, or predatory behaviors that might lead to justice involvement are increasing. Early evidence from several psychotherapeutic interventions and benign brain manipulations (e.g., cognitive remediation) indicate some progress toward the goal of reducing or eliminating offensive behaviors. Extensive work with children, adolescents, and their parents (Sukhodolsky et al. 2016) as well as with adults in both community (Ross et al. 2013) and correctional (Kersten et al. 2016) settings suggests that inroads are being made toward the goal of reducing or eliminating such offensive behaviors.

Although the evidence for the use of psychotherapeutic interventions is strong, these therapeutic programs often fail to target specific cognitive-affective deficiencies associated with subtypes of antisocial behavior. Interest in understanding the mechanisms of behavior change

and developing effective treatments that capitalize on this understanding has been increasing during the past decade. Cognitive remediation, a particularly promising and innovative treatment strategy, attempts to train individuals in the specific cognitive skills identified as deficient in various forms of psychopathology. *Cognitive remediation* is specifically designed to target cognitive-affective dysfunctions for offense subtypes; its application has resulted in differential improvement on trained tasks and also has demonstrated generalization to non-trained tasks (Baskin-Sommers et al. 2015). Similarly, evidence suggests that training directed at specific deficits, such as empathy, through targeted interventions results in durable behavior change (Dadds et al. 2012).

Research to determine the specific moderating and mediating factors of these various interventions is still needed (Cornet et al. 2015). No single treatment alone is likely to have a profound effect on an individual's offending behavior, particularly given the heterogeneity of behaviors such as impulsive or predatory aggression and their causes. However, existing research has provided hope that combining psychosocial treatments with targeted biological interventions will lead to improved efficacy of treatment and to the decrease of behaviors that, when related to mental illness, can result in arrest and incarceration.

Conclusion

Research in forensic psychiatry has been shaped by many factors over the past decades. Court decisions and legislative regulations place demands on the nature, quality, and scope of research that may be conducted. Psychometric research, behavioral studies, psychopharmacology, and neuroscience are all elements of this rapidly evolving domain. Although the body of forensic psychiatric research is growing, it remains limited by the relatively small number of researchers dedicated to an enormous field. The future will certainly bring continued and rapid growth to the field and the understanding of causation, prediction, and intervention in human behavior.

Key Concepts

- The complexity and heterogeneity of antisocial behaviors and the people who engage in them present a challenge to understanding or predicting the behaviors or recidivism rates.

- The *Kaimowitz* decision emphasized that to be legally and morally valid, informed consent must be based on the disclosure of appropriate information to a competent subject who is in a position to make voluntary choice.

- The Belmont Report includes three ethical principles that inform the work of any institutional review board: 1) respect for persons, 2) beneficence, and 3) justice.

- The Common Rule is a federal policy regarding human subject protection that outlines requirements for assuring compliance by research institutions; for researchers' obtaining and documenting informed consent; and for institutional review board membership, function, operations, review of research, and record keeping.

- Research that can improve understanding of antisocial behaviors, assessing of future risk, and designing of interventions to decrease risk of engaging in antisocial behaviors must take into account the influence of multiple factors that span biological and behavioral levels of analysis.

References

Aharoni E, Vincent GM, Harenski CL, et al: Neuroprediction of future rearrest. Proc Natl Acad Sci USA 110(15):6223–6228, 2013 23536303

Baker LA, Bezdjian S, Raine A: Behavioral genetics: the science of antisocial behavior. Law Contemp Probl 69(1–2):7–46, 2006 18176636

Barnes JC, Jacobs BA: Genetic risk for violent behavior and environmental exposure to disadvantage and violent crime: the case for gene-environment interaction. J Interpers Violence 28(1):92–120, 2013 22829212

Baskin-Sommers A: Dissecting antisocial behavior: the impact of neural, genetic and environmental factors. Clin Psychol Sci 4(3):501–510, 2016

Baskin-Sommers AR, Curtin JJ, Newman JP: Altering the cognitive-affective dysfunctions of psychopathic and externalizing offender subtypes with cognitive remediation. Clin Psychol Sci 3(1):45–57, 2015 25977843

Bonta J, Andrews D: Risk-need-responsivity model for offender assessment and rehabilitation. Rehabilitation 6:1–22, 2007

Bonta J, Andrews D: Viewing offender assessment and rehabilitation through the lens of the risk-need-responsivity model, in Offender Supervision: New Directions in Theory, Research, and Practice. Edited by McNeil F, Raynor P, Trotter C. New York, Willan, 2010, pp 19–40

Caspi A, McClay J, Moffitt TE, et al: Role of genotype in the cycle of violence in maltreated children. Science 297(5582):851–854, 2002 12161658

Cislo AM, Trestman R: Challenges and solutions for conducting research in correctional settings: the U.S. experience. Int J Law Psychiatry 36(3–4):304–310, 2013 23683885

Code of Federal Regulations: 2005, 45 CFR 46. Available at: http://www.hhs.gov/ohrp/humansubjects/guidance/45cfr46.htm. Accessed January 27, 2016.

Comai S, Tau M, Gobbi G: The psychopharmacology of aggressive behavior: a translational approach: part 1: neurobiology. J Clin Psychopharmacol 32(1):83–94, 2012 22198449

Cornet LJ, de Kogel CH, Nijman HL, et al: Neurobiological changes after intervention in individuals with anti-social behaviour: a literature review. Crim Behav Ment Health 25(1):10–27, 2015 24888269

Dadds MR, Cauchi AJ, Wimalaweera S, et al: Outcomes, moderators, and mediators of empathic-emotion recognition training for complex conduct problems in childhood. Psychiatry Res 199(3):201–207, 2012 22703720

Dahir VB, Richardson JT, Ginsburg GP, et al: Judicial application of Daubert to psychological syndrome and profile evidence: a research note. Psychol Public Policy Law 11:62, 2005

Dugdale RL: "The Jukes": A Study in Crime, Pauperism, Diseases, and Heredity; Also, Further Studies of Criminals. New York, GP Putnam's Sons, 1877

Dyer AR, Bloch S: Informed consent and the psychiatric patient. J Med Ethics 13(1):12–16, 1987 3572986

Enfield KB, Truwit JD: The purpose, composition, and function of an institutional review board: balancing priorities. Respir Care 53(10):1330–1336, 2008 18811996

Glenn AL, Raine A: Neurocriminology: implications for the punishment, prediction and prevention of criminal behaviour. Nat Rev Neurosci 15(1):54–63, 2014 24326688

Goddard HH: The Kallikak Family: A Study in the Heredity of Feeble Mindedness. New York, MacMillan, 1912

Goring C: The English Convict: A Statistical Study. London, HMSO, 1913

Gorman DA, Gardner DM, Murphy AL, et al: Canadian guidelines on pharmacotherapy for disruptive and aggressive behaviour in children and adolescents with attention-deficit hyperactivity disorder, oppositional defiant disorder, or conduct disorder. Can J Psychiatry 60(2):62–76, 2015 25886657

Gostin LO, Vanchieri C, Pope A (eds): Ethical Considerations for Research Involving Prisoners. Institute of Medicine (U.S.) Committee on Ethical Considerations for Revisions to DHHS Regulations for Protection of Prisoners Involved in Research. Washington, DC, National Academies Press, 2007. Available at: https://www.ncbi.nlm.nih.gov/books/NBK19882/. Accessed January 15, 2017.

Hare RD: Manual for the Revised Psychopathy Checklist, 2nd Edition. Toronto, ON, Canada, Multi-Health Systems, 2003

Hart SD, Logan C: Formulation of violence risk using evidence-based assessments: the structured professional judgment approach, in Forensic Case Formulation. Edited by Sturmey P, McMurran M. Chichester, UK, Wiley Blackwell, 2011, pp 83–106

Hart SD, Michie C, Cooke DJ: Precision of actuarial risk assessment instruments: evaluating the 'margins of error' of group v. individual predictions of violence. Br J Psychiatry Suppl 49:s60–s65, 2007 17470944

Henwood KS, Chou S, Browne KD: A systematic review and meta-analysis on the effectiveness of CBT informed anger management. Aggress Violent Behav 25:280–292, 2015

Ipser J, Stein DJ: Systematic review of pharmacotherapy of disruptive behavior disorders in children and adolescents. Psychopharmacology (Berl) 191(1):127–140, 2007 16983542

Kaimowitz v Michigan Dept. of Mental Health, 1 MDLR 147 (1973)

Kersten L, Cislo AM, Lynch M, et al: Evaluating START NOW: a skills-based psychotherapy for inmates of correctional systems. Psychiatr Serv 67(1):37–42, 2016 26278230

Kim-Cohen J, Caspi A, Taylor A, et al: MAOA, maltreatment, and gene-environment interaction predicting children's mental health: new evidence and a meta-analysis. Mol Psychiatry 11(10):903–913, 2006 16801953

Kubicki M, Alvarado JL, Westin C-F, et al: Stochastic tractography study of inferior frontal gyrus anatomical connectivity in schizophrenia. Neuroimage 55(4):1657–1664, 2011 21256966

Lichtenstein P, Halldner L, Zetterqvist J, et al: Medication for attention deficit-hyperactivity disorder and criminality. N Engl J Med 367(21):2006–2014, 2012 23171097

Martinson R: What works? Questions and answers about prison reform. Public Interest 10:22–54, 1974

Monahan J: Predicting Violent Behavior: An Assessment of Clinical Techniques. Beverly Hills, CA, Sage, 1981

Monahan J: Risk assessment of violence among the mentally disordered: generating useful knowledge. Int J Law Psychiatry 11(3):249–257, 1988 3061944

Monahan J, Steadman HJ, Appelbaum PS, et al: Developing a clinically useful actuarial tool for assessing violence risk. Br J Psychiatry 176:312–319, 2000 10827877

National Commission for the Protection of Human Subjects of Biomedical and Behavioral Research: The Belmont Report: Ethical principles and guidelines for the protection of human subjects of research. Bethesda, MD, ERIC Clearinghouse, 1978. Available at: http://www.hhs.gov/ohrp/regulations-and-policy/belmont-report/. Accessed January 15, 2017.

Olivier B, van Oorschot R: 5-HT1B receptors and aggression: a review. Eur J Pharmacol 526(1–3):207–217, 2005 16310769

Pappadopulos E, Woolston S, Chait A, et al: Pharmacotherapy of aggression in children and adolescents: efficacy and effect size. J Can Acad Child Adolesc Psychiatry 15(1):27–39, 2006 18392193

Quinsey VL, Harris GT, Rice ME, et al: Violent Offenders: Appraising and Managing Risk. Washington, DC, American Psychological Association, 1998

Ross J, Quayle E, Newman E, et al: The impact of psychological therapies on violent behaviour in clinical and forensic settings: a systematic review. Aggress Violent Behav 18:761–773, 2013

Rotter M, Carr WA: Reducing criminal recidivism for justice-involved persons with mental illness: risk/needs/responsivity and cognitive-behavioral interventions. SAMHSA, GAINS Center for Behavioral Health and Justice Transformation, October 2013. Available at: https://www.prainc.com/wp-content/uploads/2016/02/ReduceCrimRecidRNR.pdf. Accessed January 16, 2017.

Shapiro DL, Mixon L, Jackson M, et al: Psychological expert witness testimony and judicial decision making trends. Int J Law Psychiatry 42–43:149–153, 2015 26341310

Simons RL, Lei MK, Beach SR, et al: Social environmental variation, plasticity genes, and aggression: evidence for the differential susceptibility hypothesis. Am Sociol Rev 76(6):833–912, 2011 22199399

Singh JP, Fazel S, Gueorguieva R, et al: Rates of violence in patients classified as high risk by structured risk assessment instruments. Br J Psychiatry 204(3):180–187, 2014 24590974

Singh JP, Yang S, Mulvey EP; RAGEE Group: Reporting guidance for violence risk assessment predictive validity studies: the RAGEE Statement. Law Hum Behav 39(1):15–22, 2015 25133921

Stephan KE, Mathys C: Computational approaches to psychiatry. Curr Opin Neurobiol 25:85–92, 2014 24709605

Sukhodolsky DG, Smith SD, McCauley SA, et al: Behavioral interventions for anger, irritability, and aggression in children and adolescents. J Child Adolesc Psychopharmacol 26(1):58–64, 2016 26745682

Taxman FS, Thanner M, Weisburd D: Risk, need, and responsivity (RNR): it all depends. Crime Delinq 52(1):28–51, 2006 18542715

Umukoro S, Aladeokin AC, Eduviere AT: Aggressive behavior: a comprehensive review of its neurochemical mechanisms and management. Aggress Violent Behav 18:195–203, 2013

U.S. Department of Health and Human Services: Federal policy for the protection of human subjects ("common rule"). 1991. Available at: http://www.hhs.gov/ohrp/humansubjects/commonrule/. Accessed January 15, 2017.

U.S. Department of Justice, Federal Bureau of Investigation, Criminal Justice Information Services Division: Crime in the United States, 2014. 2015. Available at: https://www.fbi.gov/about-us/cjis/ucr/crime-in-the-u.s/2014/crime-in-the-u.s.-2014. Accessed January 16, 2017.

Viding E, Frith U: Genes for susceptibility to violence lurk in the brain. Proc Natl Acad Sci USA 103(16):6085–6086, 2006 16606856

Webster CD, Douglas KS, Eaves D, Hart SD: Assessing risk of violence to others, in Impulsivity: Theory, Assessment, Treat-ment. Edited by Webster CD, Jackson MA. New York: Guilford Press, 1997, pp 251–277

Wolz R, Julkunen V, Koikkalainen J, et al; Alzheimer's Disease Neuroimaging Initiative: Multi-method analysis of MRI images in early diagnostics of Alzheimer's disease. PLoS One 6(10):e25446, 2011 22022397

Zajac G: Implementation and outcomes in cognitive-behavioral therapy among female prisoners. Criminol Public Policy 14:295–299, 2015

Landmark Case Index

Subject Index

*Page numbers printed in **boldface** type indicate tables or figures.*